Anesthesia and Analgesia for Veterinary Technicians and Nurses

PROCEDURES

Anesthesia and Analgesia for Veterinary Technicians and Nurses

Sixth Edition

John A. Thomas, DVM

Professor Emeritus
Veterinary Technology
Cuyahoga Community College
Cleveland, Ohio

Phillip Lerche, BVSc, PhD, Dipl ACVA

Professor-Clinical
Department of Veterinary Clinical Sciences
College of Veterinary Medicine
The Ohio State University
Columbus, Ohio

ELSEVIER

Elsevier
3251 Riverport Lane
St. Louis, Missouri 63043

ANESTHESIA AND ANALGESIA FOR VETERINARY TECHNICIANS
AND NURSES, SIXTH EDITION

ISBN: 978-0-323-76011-9

Notice

Practitioners and researchers must always rely on their own experience and knowledge in evaluating
and using any information, methods, compounds or experiments described herein. Because of rapid
advances in the medical sciences, in particular, independent verification of diagnoses and drug dosages
should be made. To the fullest extent of the law, no responsibility is assumed by Elsevier, authors, editors
or contributors for any injury and/or damage to persons or property as a matter of products liability,
negligence or otherwise, or from any use or operation of any methods, products, instructions, or ideas
contained in the material herein.

Previous editions copyrighted 2017, 2011, 2003, 2000 and 1994.

Content Strategist: Melissa Rawe
Content Development Specialist: Deborah Poulson
Publishing Services Manager: Deepthi Unni
Project Manager: Thoufiq Mohammed
Design Direction: Amy Buxton

Printed in Canada

Last digit is the print number: 9 8 7 6 5 4 3 2 1

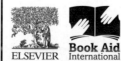

Working together
to grow libraries in
developing countries

www.elsevier.com • www.bookaid.org

Dedication

To my family and friends for their continued support and understanding during the countless hours spent working on this book.

To Phillip, whose professional knowledge and abilities, as well as his instincts as a writer, have made this book possible.

J.T.

To all the veterinary technicians I have worked with in my 25 years at The Ohio State University—it would not have been possible to do what we do for our patients without you. It has been my honor to help you, teach you, work with you, and learn from you.

To John, for his perseverance and infinite patience. His attention to detail and experience of veterinary technician training have been invaluable in bringing this sixth edition to fruition.

P.L.

CONTRIBUTOR

Paul Flecknell, MA, VetMB, PhD, DLAS, DECVA, DECLAM, (Hon) DACLAM, (Hon) FRCVS
Professor of Laboratory Animal Science
Comparative Biology Centre
Newcastle University
Newcastle, Tyne and Wear, UK

REVIEWER

Jim Budde, PharmD, RPh, DICVP
Sun Prairie, Wisconsin

For many decades, the text *Veterinary Anesthesia and Analgesia,* originally under the authorship of Diane McKelvey and K. Wayne Hollingshead, and later John A. Thomas and Phillip Lerche, has been a trusted choice of veterinary technician educators. Now in its sixth edition, this resource for students of veterinary anesthesia and analgesia, with its emphasis on accessibility, consistency, and practical application, has been updated to reflect recent changes in this complex and ever-changing discipline.

Instructors who have used this text in the past will find familiarity in the organization, layout, and general approach; however, recent developments in the field must be reflected in the tone and content of the book over time. Therefore, the authors have worked diligently in writing the sixth edition to update content, include new information about the practice of anesthesia, and remove outdated material. As in past editions, care has been taken to ensure a high degree of uniformity among chapters so that topics discussed in multiple locations are carefully checked for consistency. Additionally, selected charts, tables, boxes, and procedures have been reformatted for clarity and ease of use.

ORGANIZATION

Chapter 1 prepares the reader for the study of veterinary anesthesia and analgesia by covering the following concepts:
- a brief history of veterinary anesthesia
- the role of professional organizations in advancement of the discipline
- how clinical practice guidelines are used to maximize quality of services
- basic terms and definitions
- the role of veterinary technicians or nurses in anesthetic procedures

Chapters 2 through 8 cover the following fundamental principles of veterinary anesthesia and analgesia:
- Chapter 2—Preparation
- Chapter 3—Anesthetic Agents and Adjuncts
- Chapter 4—Anesthetic Equipment
- Chapter 5—Workplace Safety
- Chapter 6—Anesthetic Monitoring
- Chapter 7—Special Techniques (which include local anesthesia, assisted and controlled ventilation, and use of neuromuscular blocking agents)
- Chapter 8—Analgesia

The next four chapters cover application of these fundamentals to specific species or species groups:
- Chapter 9—Canine and Feline Anesthesia
- Chapter 10—Equine Anesthesia
- Chapter 11—Anesthesia of Ruminants, Camelids, and Swine
- Chapter 12—Rodent and Rabbit Anesthesia

The final chapter, Chapter 13—Anesthetic Problems and Emergencies, describes advanced concepts, including:
- reasons that anesthetic problems and emergencies arise
- management of patients that have increased anesthetic risk
- recognition of and responses to common problems and emergencies
- how to perform cardiopulmonary resuscitation (CPR) in veterinary patients

NEW TO THIS EDITION

The content of the sixth edition has been substantially updated to reflect clinical practice guidelines published in recent years, including: (1) 2022 AAHA Pain Management Guidelines for Dogs and Cats; (2) 2020 AAHA Anesthesia and Monitoring Guidelines for Dogs and Cats; and (3) 2018 AAFP Feline Anesthesia Guidelines.

Since publication of the previous edition, there have been many changes in available technology and drugs as well as techniques. For instance, numerous new medicines have become available; touch screen technology is ever more common on veterinary equipment, including multiparameter monitors and even some anesthesia machines; and consensus regarding the need for preanesthetic fasting has changed. The sixth edition includes discussions of these new developments and many more. What follows is a list of significant changes to the sixth edition:
- New content, including (1) discussion of anesthetic safety checklists; (2) calculation, preparation, and administration of constant rate infusions (CRI) to maintain general anesthesia, provide analgesia, and treat complications such as hypotension; (3) discussion of the adverse effects of dead space and strategies to minimize its impact; and (4) monitoring of neuromuscular blockade.
- Expanded coverage of topics, including (1) regulatory considerations for controlled drugs; (2) compressed gas supply; (3) cleaning and disinfecting equipment; (4) management of hypothermia; and (5) behavioral signs of pain.
- Updated information regarding preanesthetic fasting, impact of the ABCB1-1delta (MDR1) gene mutation, and management of high-risk patients.
- Discussion of recently introduced drugs, including medetomidine and vatinoxan hydrochlorides (Zenalpha), liposome-encapsulated bupivacaine (Nocita), transdermal buprenorphine (Zorbium), and frunevetmab (Solensia), as well as drugs not addressed in previous editions such as anxiolytics (e.g., gabapentin and trazodone) and maropitant.
- Discussion of equipment new to this edition, including endotracheal tube (ETT) cuff pressure manometers, adjustable pressure-limiting (APL) occlusion valves, safety pressure relief valves, high pressure alarms, heat and moisture exchangers, electronic anesthetic machines, anesthetic gas analyzers, oxygen analyzers, and multiparameter monitors.
- Revision of quick reference tables for topics that include determination of intravenous (IV) fluid infusion rates, oxygen flow rates, and interpretation of abnormal capnograms; and new tables comparing the injectable anesthetics

propofol and alfaxalone, and the inhalation anesthetics isoflurane and sevoflurane.

- Revised and expanded discussion of topics relating to workplace safety, including minimization of risks associated with exposure to waste anesthetic gases.
- The addition of 49 photographs, 8 drawings, 15 boxes, 6 tables, 2 anesthetic protocols, and 1 procedure.

KEY FEATURES

Rather than being a small animal anesthesia text with large animals addressed separately, this practical resource is intended to be a true multispecies text in which each of the common domestic species (dogs, cats, horses, cattle, camelids, and swine) is discussed throughout. Readers will find the following features in this edition that were present in the previous edition:

- Learning objectives at the beginning of each chapter
- Key terms and a chapter outline at the beginning of each chapter
- Key points at the end of each chapter
- Suggested readings
- Review questions and answers
- Technician notes that emphasize important points and practical tips gleaned from the narrative
- Reference tables and boxes designed to facilitate rapid access to key information such as fluid administration rates; properties of anesthetic drugs; oxygen flow rates; anesthetic protocols; normal and abnormal monitoring parameters; and calculation, preparation, and administration of constant rate infusions
- Step-by-step descriptions of common procedures used during each phase of an anesthetic event, including patient preparation, IV catheter placement, anesthetic induction techniques, endotracheal intubation, anesthetic maintenance techniques, and anesthetic recovery
- A complete glossary with definitions of all key terms
- Revised appendices with supplemental and reference information

EVOLVE RESOURCES

In addition to these features, readers will also have access to the following online resources through Evolve, Elsevier's online portal for instructors and students.

Instructor Resources

- Image collection from the text that can be included in classroom presentations
- PowerPoint lecture outlines with nearly 1000 slides
- NEW! Test bank with more than 1000 questions that include detailed rationales

Student Resources

- Image collection from the text, which can be used for review and study

This established and respected text provides veterinary technician educators, students, and anesthetists with the tools necessary to maximize learning in the classroom and beyond. It is our earnest hope that readers will find this book to be an accessible, useful, and highly valued resource, and will realize as much personal and professional growth from reading it as we have realized in writing it.

ACKNOWLEDGMENTS

The authors would like to thank the following individuals for their contributions to the production of this volume:

Steven Ahern, AA, AAB, and William Fogarty, MEd, for their help in producing many of the photographs in Chapters 2, 3, 4, 5, 6, and 9; and Marie Dagata, graphics specialist, for her help in producing many of the ECG tracings in Chapter 6, including Figs. 6.16 through 6.21, 6.25, 6.26, 6.29, and 6.31.

The Cuyahoga Community College Veterinary Technology Program students for their help through the years with acquisition of many photographs in Chapters 2, 3, 4, 6, and 9. Special thanks to Albert Lewandowski, DVM, who graciously assisted with acquisition of the photographs relating to drugs used in the restraint and capture of wildlife in Chapter 5; and to Linda Kuenzer, RVT, Audrey Kukwa, RVT, Monica Bode, RVT, Carrie Harviel, RVT, BS, Katie Mooney, RVT, Jorden Buddner, RVT, Lauren Kurgan, RVT, and Stephanie Maskovyak, RVT, who graciously volunteered to assist with the acquisition of numerous photographs in Chapters 2, 3, 4, 5, 6, and 9.

Payton Beaver, RVT, Heather Cruea, RVT, VTS (Anesthesia), Aliya Davis, RVT, Tiffany Davis, RVT, Crystal Cole, RVT, Christina Duffey, RVT, Amanda English, RVT, Danni Ensell, RVT, Devin Hainley, RVT, Theresa Hand, RVT, Elise Henning, RVT, Suzanne Huck, RVT, Gladys Karpa, RVT, Aaron Manning, RVT, Amanda Cardenas, RVT, Devin Heilman, RVT, Carl O'Brien, RVT, VTS (Anesthesia), Liz Santschi, DVM, Michael Rings, DVM, MS, Turi Aarnes, DVM, MS, Lisa Sams, DVM, MS, Rebecca Krimins, DVM, Kati O'Donovan, DVM, Kaitie Ban, DVM and Bryce Dooley, DVM, MS, for their help with photographs in several chapters.

As always, Diane McKelvey and K. Wayne Hollingshead, authors of the first three editions of this text, for setting a high standard for veterinary technician educators and for laying the foundation on which subsequent editions rest. Contributing author Paul Flecknell for sharing his knowledge, expertise, and experience.

To the editorial and production staff at Elsevier, including Tina Kaemmerer, Senior Content Development Specialist; Deborah Poulson, Content Development Specialist; Melissa Rawe, Content Strategist; Thoufiq Mohammed, Project Manager; and Deepthi Unni, Publishing Services Manager, for their guidance and support during the many months spent (including in the midst of a pandemic) planning, writing, and producing this text.

John A. Thomas
Phillip Lerche

CONTENTS

Introduction to Anesthesia

LEARNING OBJECTIVES

When you have completed this chapter, you will be able to:

- List two North American professional organizations that offer specialization in anesthesia and analgesia to credentialed individuals and summarize the aims of each.
- Explain the role of clinical practice guidelines in increasing the quality of anesthesia services.
- Define anesthesia, and differentiate topical, local, regional, general, and surgical anesthesia.
- Differentiate sedation, tranquilization, anxiolysis, hypnosis, and narcosis.

- Explain the concept of balanced anesthesia and the advantages of this approach.
- List common indications for anesthesia.
- Describe fundamental challenges and risks associated with anesthesia.
- List the qualities and abilities of a successful veterinary anesthetist.

KEY TERMS

The Academy of Veterinary
  Technicians in Anesthesia
  and Analgesia (AVTAA)
American College of Veterinary
  Anesthesia and Analgesia (ACVAA)
Analgesia
Anesthesia

Anxiolysis
Balanced anesthesia
Epidural anesthesia
General anesthesia
Hypnosis
Local anesthesia
Narcosis

Noxious
Regional anesthesia
Sedation
Surgical anesthesia
Therapeutic index
Topical anesthesia
Tranquilization

A BRIEF HISTORY OF ANESTHESIA

The discovery of inhalant anesthetics during the 19th century marks a major milestone in the history of medicine. It made possible the evolution of surgery from a practice associated with fear, unbearable pain, and high mortality, to one associated with hope, relief, and healing for millions upon millions of patients. In retrospect, it seems impossible that there was a time only a handful of generations ago that humankind did not have the benefit of this branch of medicine that we now cannot imagine a world without.

The early history of medicine includes accounts of the use of plant extracts such as the belladonna alkaloids (from the deadly nightshade plant) and opiates (from the opium poppy) to control pain and produce sleep as early as the 15th century BCE, and these natural compounds remained the only available agents for nearly 3000 years. Between the 1500s and the 1700s, accounts of experimentation with inhaled chemical agents, including diethyl ether, chloroform, and nitrous oxide began to appear, but it was not until the mid-1800s that anesthetic techniques were refined to the point that the practical and widespread use of these agents was possible.

October 16, 1846, is an especially significant date in the history of anesthesia because it was on this day that Boston dentist William T. G. Morton gave the first successful demonstration of the anesthetic properties of diethyl ether at Massachusetts General Hospital (Fig. 1.1). To the amazement of the physicians and medical students in attendance, the patient, who was undergoing removal of a tumor, on receiving the ether, entered a state of insensibility during which the tumor was successfully removed and the surgical pain was alleviated. During the next several months, additional experiments conducted by Morton and others confirmed the value of ether as an effective pain-relieving agent.

Dr. Morton's demonstration attracted the attention of the prominent physician Oliver Wendell Holmes Sr., who, in a letter dated November 21, 1846, suggested adoption of the word *anesthesia* to describe the state of insensibility to pain produced by diethyl ether. Then he accurately and with foresight predicted

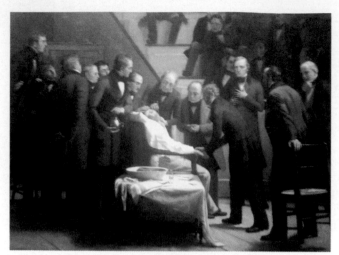

FIG. 1.1 *Ether Day,* or *The First Operation Under Ether* (Robert C. Hinckley, 1882–1893). (From https://commons.wikimedia.org/wiki/File:Ether_Day,_or_The_First_Operation_with_Ether_by_Robert_C._Hinckley.jpg)

that the terms *anesthesia* and *anesthetic* would "be repeated by the tongues of every civilized race of mankind."

Over the next few years, the practice of anesthesia spread widely throughout North America and Europe. However, the veterinary community did not embrace the use of anesthetics as rapidly. Although reports began to appear in the veterinary literature regarding the use of inhalation anesthetics such as ether and chloroform soon after Morton's demonstration, physical restraint remained the preferred method for immobilizing veterinary patients for many years, and anesthesia did not become common practice until well into the 20th century.

In the 1930s, the development of injectable barbiturate anesthetics gave veterinarians an alternative to the inhalant agents, and they became a mainstay of anesthetic practice for many decades. The invention of anesthesia machines and the introduction of many other agents, including the inhalants halothane and methoxyflurane in the 1950s; injectable tranquilizers, including the phenothiazine acepromazine and the alpha$_2$-agonist xylazine in the 1960s; the dissociative ketamine in the 1970s; the inhalant isoflurane and the injectable anesthetic propofol in the 1980s; the inhalant sevoflurane in the 1990s; and many other important agents in the succeeding years, gradually widened the range of effective techniques available to practitioners. During this period, as a result of these and many other developments, the practice of anesthesia evolved into an indispensable and ever-present part of the life of every veterinary professional.

PROFESSIONAL ORGANIZATIONS DEDICATED TO THE PRACTICE OF VETERINARY ANESTHESIA AND ANALGESIA

Over the past 50 years or so, many dedicated individuals have worked to advance the practice of veterinary anesthesia and analgesia by founding professional organizations, establishing certification for specialists, and educating veterinary practitioners regarding best practices in the field. (See Box 1.1 for a partial listing of professional organizations dedicated to the

practice of veterinary anesthesia and analgesia, including web addresses.)

The Academy of Veterinary Technicians in Anesthesia and Analgesia (AVTAA), recognized in 1999 by the National Association of Veterinary Technicians in America–Committee on Veterinary Technician Specialties (NAVTA-CVTS), offers specialization to credentialed veterinary technicians and nurses with an interest in veterinary anesthesia and analgesia through completion of an arduous set of requirements that demonstrates competency in the advanced practice of anesthesia and analgesia. The professional title "VTS (Anesthesia/Analgesia)" after one's name signifies certification as a specialist. A complete list of the specific objectives of the AVTAA may be found in its mission statement (Box 1.2). More information about the AVTAA can be found at http://www.avtaa-vts.org.

In a similar manner, the American College of Veterinary Anesthesia and Analgesia (ACVAA), recognized by the American Veterinary Medical Association (AVMA) in 1975, offers specialization to credentialed veterinarians. The aims of the ACVAA are articulated in its mission statement (see Box 1.3 for the mission statement of the ACVAA). Information about the ACVAA can be found at http://www.acvaa.org.

The **North American Veterinary Anesthesia Society** (NAVAS) is a nonprofit founded in 2019 through a partnership between the ACVAA and AVTAA. Its mission is to make evidence-based guidelines regarding the safe administration of anesthesia and analgesia available to all interested professionals and caregivers. Through a paid subscription, all NAVAS members have access to a library of documents and videos, information about continuing education opportunities, and online discussion forums. More information about the NAVAS can be found at https://www.mynavas.org/.

The remaining organizations listed in Box 1.1 each have unique and specific aims that are posted on their respective website.

CLINICAL PRACTICE GUIDELINES

During the past decade or so, several professional organizations, including the American Animal Hospital Association (AAHA), the American Association of Feline Practitioners (AAFP), and the ACVAA, have published clinical practice guidelines designed to educate practitioners regarding advances in the field of anesthesia and analgesia. (See Box 1.4 for a list of

publications that will be referred to throughout this text.) Whenever possible, the guidelines contained in these documents are evidence based (based on published research), whereas others represent consensus of experts in the field of veterinary anesthesia and analgesia. In either case, these clinical guidelines provide the practitioner (veterinarians, veterinary technicians, and nurses alike) with best practices intended to increase the quality of services provided to the public and consequently decrease the risk that is inherent in the practice of anesthesia. The most recent of these, the 2020 AAHA Anesthesia and Monitoring Guidelines for Dogs and Cats, includes an online resource center that is available at https://aaha.org/anesthesia.

TERMINOLOGY OF ANESTHESIA

The term anesthesia (derived from the Greek word *anaisthesia*, which means "without feeling" or "insensibility") may be defined as "a loss of sensation." By providing a loss of sensation or more specifically, the loss of sensitivity to pain, the development and use of anesthetics solved one of the primary problems associated with the practice of medicine. Now, anesthesia is used daily in most veterinary practices to provide anxiolysis, sedation, tranquilization, immobility, muscle relaxation, unconsciousness, and pain control for a diverse range of indications, including surgery, dentistry, grooming, diagnostic imaging, wound care, and capture and transport of wild animals, just to name a few. The literal definition of the term *anesthesia* accurately describes one of its fundamental effects; however, when viewed from the perspective of current practice, the word falls far short of capturing the many facets of this complex discipline.

> **TECHNICIAN NOTE** Anesthesia is used daily in most veterinary practices to provide anxiolysis, sedation, tranquilization, immobility, muscle relaxation, unconsciousness, and pain control for a diverse range of indications.

Most people associate the word *anesthesia* with general anesthesia, which is only one extreme in a continuum of levels of central nervous system (CNS) depression that can be induced by administration of anesthetic agents (Fig. 1.2). General anesthesia may be defined as a reversible state of unconsciousness, immobility, muscle relaxation, and loss of sensation throughout the entire body produced by administration of one or more anesthetic agents. While under general anesthesia, a patient cannot be aroused, even with painful stimulation. For this reason, general anesthesia is commonly used to prepare patients for surgery or other acutely painful procedures. Surgical anesthesia is a specific stage of general anesthesia in which there is a sufficient degree of analgesia (a loss of sensitivity to pain) and muscle relaxation to allow surgery to be performed without patient pain or movement.

Other states within the continuum of CNS depression include *sedation, tranquilization,* and *anxiolysis.* Sedation refers to drug-induced CNS depression and drowsiness that vary in intensity from light to deep. A sedated patient generally is

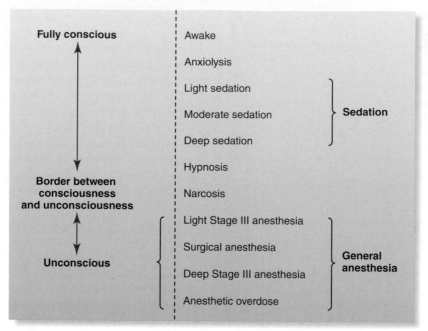

Notes:
- *In addition to CNS depression, most anesthetics cause a variety of other effects such as analgesia and muscle relaxation.*
- *Although most anesthetics cause CNS depression as noted above, some agents such as dissociatives may also stimulate the CNS (see Chapter 3 for a discussion of these agents).*
- *Transient excitement may also occur during some stages of anesthesia (see Chapter 6 for a discussion of the stages and planes of general anesthesia).*

FIG. 1.2 The continuum of levels of central nervous system (CNS) depression induced by anesthetic agents.

minimally aware or unaware of its surroundings but can be aroused by noxious stimulation. Sedation is often used in clinic to prepare patients for diagnostic imaging, grooming, wound treatment, and other minor procedures. Tranquilization is a drug-induced state of calm in which the patient is reluctant to move and is aware of but unconcerned about its surroundings. Although the terms *tranquilization* and *sedation* are not exactly the same in meaning, they are often used interchangeably. Anxiolysis, the reduction of anxiety, is, for practical purposes, synonymous with light tranquilization. However, this term is most frequently used in reference to administration of anxiety-reducing drugs at home prior to a sedative or anesthesia procedure performed in clinic.

The terms *hypnosis* and *narcosis* are also used to describe anesthetic-induced states. Hypnosis is a drug-induced sleeplike state that impairs the ability of the patient to respond appropriately to stimuli. This meaning of this term is somewhat imprecise because it is used to describe various degrees of CNS depression. In this text, hypnosis will be used to mean a sleep-like state from which the patient can be aroused with sufficient stimulation. The term narcosis refers to a drug-induced sleep from which the patient is not easily aroused and that is most often associated with the administration of narcotics.

The effect of anesthetic agents may be selectively directed to affect specific areas or regions of the body. Smaller areas can be targeted by use of local or topical anesthesia. Local anesthesia refers to loss of sensation in a small area of the body produced

by administration of a local anesthetic agent in proximity to the area of interest. Infiltration of local anesthetic into the tissues surrounding a small tumor to facilitate removal is an example of local anesthesia. Topical anesthesia is the loss of sensation of a localized area produced by administration of a local anesthetic directly to a body surface or to a surgical or traumatic wound. Use of ophthalmic local anesthetic drops in the eye before an ophthalmic examination and application of local anesthetic to an open declaw incision for the purpose of pain control are examples of topical anesthesia.

Larger areas can be targeted by use of regional anesthesia, which refers to a loss of sensation in a limited area of the body produced by administration of a local anesthetic or other agent in proximity to sensory nerves. Regional anesthesia can be produced with a variety of techniques, including nerve blocks and epidural anesthesia. For example, a brachial plexus block can be used to anesthetize the forelimb distal to and including the elbow; a maxillary nerve block can be used to anesthetize the upper dental arcade; and epidural anesthesia can be used to provide pain control of the hindquarters and pelvic region.

When anesthetics are administered, it is common practice to administer multiple drugs concurrently in smaller quantities than would be required if each were given alone. This technique, termed balanced anesthesia, maximizes the benefits of each drug, minimizes adverse effects, and gives the anesthetist the ability to produce anesthesia with the degree of CNS depression, muscle relaxation, analgesia, and immobilization appropriate for the patient and the procedure. Premedication with acepromazine and butorphanol, anesthetic induction with a combination of ketamine and midazolam, maintenance with isoflurane, and administration of morphine and lidocaine infusions for analgesia is one example of balanced anesthesia.

> **TECHNICIAN NOTE** Balanced anesthesia maximizes benefits, minimizes adverse effects, and gives the anesthetist the ability to produce anesthesia with the degree of central nervous system depression, muscle relaxation, analgesia, and immobilization appropriate for the patient and the procedure.

THE VETERINARY TECHNICIAN'S ROLE IN THE PRACTICE OF ANESTHESIA

Preparation, operation, and maintenance of anesthetic equipment; administration of anesthetic agents; endotracheal intubation; and patient monitoring under the supervision of a licensed veterinarian are considered part of the credentialed veterinary technician's or veterinary nurse's scope of practice and are a required part of any accredited veterinary technology or veterinary nursing program's curriculum. Competency in each of these areas of responsibility requires an advanced knowledge and skill level that can be achieved only with a substantial commitment of time and effort on the part of the student. Before embarking on a study of anesthesia, the student must be aware of the following fundamental challenges and inherent risks they will face when acting as anesthetist.

- Most anesthetic agents have a very narrow therapeutic index, so the consequences of a calculation or administration error may be serious. Therefore care and attention to detail are critical when dosages are calculated and rates of administration are adjusted.
- Most anesthetic agents cause significant changes in cardiovascular and pulmonary function (e.g., decreased cardiac output, respiratory rate, tidal volume, and blood pressure), which can be dangerous or lethal if not carefully assessed and managed. These changes often occur quickly and without much warning. Consequently, vital signs and indicators of anesthetic depth must be closely monitored.
- The anesthetist must accurately interpret a wide spectrum of visual, tactile, and auditory information from the patient,

anesthetic equipment, and monitoring devices. To do this successfully, they must be able to assess multiple pieces of information rapidly and distinguish those that require action from those that do not.

- The anesthetist must have a comprehensive understanding of the significance of physical parameters (e.g., heart rate, respiratory rate, and reflex responses) and machine-generated data (e.g., blood pressure and oxygen saturation readings). The anesthetist must also be able to use their knowledge to make rapid and decisive judgments regarding patient management and to carry out corrective actions quickly and effectively.
- The potential for patient harm during administration of anesthetics is relatively high when compared with many other procedures. When serious anesthetic accidents occur, they are often devastating not only for the patient, but also for the client and the anesthetist. In addition, after an accident, clients may choose to pursue legal action or file a complaint with the state veterinary medical board if they feel negligence was involved. These factors underscore the importance of maintaining a high standard to maximize the likelihood of a favorable outcome. This high standard includes not only sound practices but also maintenance of detailed and accurate medical records, which are the cornerstone of a solid legal defense should a complaint arise. (See Chapter 6 for more information about anesthetic records.)

In view of each of these risks and challenges, the anesthetist must approach any anesthetic procedure with a genuine willingness to take personal responsibility for the well-being of the patient. Acceptance of this responsibility by the anesthetist is dependent on development of competence and confidence. Ultimately, competence and confidence are acquired only with much study, practice, persistence, an attitude of caring, and a dedication to excellence. Only then can the accomplished anesthetist use their skills and knowledge to protect and improve the life of each and every patient in a way that is infinitely gratifying and unique to this complex and challenging discipline.

> **TECHNICIAN NOTE** The anesthetist must approach each and every anesthetic procedure with a genuine willingness to take personal responsibility for the well-being of the patient.

KEY POINTS

1. General anesthesia is a reversible state of unconsciousness, immobility, muscle relaxation, and generalized loss of sensation, produced by administration of anesthetic agents. It is only one extreme in a continuum of levels of central nervous system (CNS) depression produced by anesthetic agents, which also include anxiolysis, sedation, hypnosis, and narcosis.
2. Many techniques, including sedation, tranquilization, and topical, local, regional, and general anesthesia, are used to produce specific effects appropriate to each patient.
3. Balanced anesthesia (the administration of multiple drugs to the same patient during one anesthetic event) is commonplace in the practice of anesthesia and produces many benefits not possible with administration of a single anesthetic.
4. Anesthesia involves a number of unique risks and dangers, of which the anesthetist must be conscious and aware.
5. The successful practice of anesthesia requires a high level of knowledge, competency, commitment, and acceptance of responsibility on the part of the anesthetist.

REVIEW QUESTIONS

1. A drug-induced state of calm in which the patient is reluctant to move and is aware of but unconcerned about its surroundings.
   a. Sedation
   b. Hypnosis
   c. Narcosis
   d. Tranquilization

2. The term *regional anesthesia* refers to:
   a. Loss of sensation in a limited area of the body produced by administration of a local anesthetic or other agent in proximity to sensory nerves
   b. Loss of sensation in a small area of the body produced by administration of a local anesthetic agent in proximity to the area of interest
   c. Loss of sensation of a localized area produced by administration of a local anesthetic directly to a body surface or to a surgical or traumatic wound
   d. A drug-induced sleeplike state that impairs the ability of the patient to respond appropriately to stimuli

3. A sleeplike state from which the patient can be aroused with sufficient stimulation.
   a. Narcosis
   b. Sedation
   c. Hypnosis
   d. Tranquilization

4. The term *balanced anesthesia* refers to:
   a. The administration of two or more agents in equal volume
   b. Administration of multiple drugs concurrently in smaller quantities than would be required if each were given alone
   c. General anesthesia in which the patient's physiologic status remains stable
   d. The administration of a local and general anesthetic concurrently

5. Evidence-based or consensus recommendations designed to educate practitioners regarding best practices intended to increase the quality of services and decrease risk are referred to as:
   a. Professional papers
   b. Clinical practice guidelines
   c. Best practices for practitioners
   d. Practice standards for veterinary professionals

6. The North American Veterinary Anesthesia Society is an organization recently formed through a partnership between the
   a. AVTAA and VAASG
   b. AVA and ACVAA
   c. ECVAA and AVA
   d. AVTAA and ACVAA

7. Many anesthetic drugs have a narrow therapeutic index. This means that these drugs
   a. Have a low probability of causing death
   b. Must be given in precise amounts
   c. Are only safe in very small doses
   d. Produce relatively less CNS depression

8. Which of the following professional organizations offers credentialing to veterinary technicians and nurses in the practice of anesthesia and analgesia?
   a. NAVAS
   b. AVTAA
   c. VAASG
   d. ACVAA
   e. NAVTA

For the following questions, more than one answer may be correct.

9. With sufficient stimulation, a patient can be aroused from:
   a. Sedation
   b. Narcosis
   c. General anesthesia
   d. Hypnosis

10. Which of the following statements about anesthesia is/are false?
    a. Anesthetic agents have wide therapeutic indices.
    b. There is always a risk to patient safety when anesthetics are administered.
    c. Most anesthetics cause significant changes in cardiopulmonary function.
    d. Administration of anesthetics is routine and thus requires no specialized skills.

SELECTED READINGS

Albin MS, Sim P: Oliver Wendell Holmes, M.C., 1809–1894, poet, physician and anesthesia advocate, *ASA Newsl* 68(10):18–23, 2004.

Jones RS: A history of veterinary anaesthesia, *Anales de Veterinaria de Murcia* 18:7–15, 2002.

Muir W, Hubbell JAE: History of equine anesthesia. In Muir W, Hubbell JAE, editors: *Equine anesthesia: monitoring and emergency therapy*, ed 2, St. Louis, 2009, Mosby Year-Book, pp 1–9.

Muir WW, Hubbell JA, Bednarski RM, Lerche P: *Handbook of veterinary anesthesia*, ed 5, St. Louis, 2012, Elsevier.

Smithcors JF: The early use of anaesthesia in veterinary practice, *Br Vet J* 113:284–291, 1957.

Smithcors JF: *The veterinarian in America 1625–1975*, Santa Barbara, 1975, American Veterinary Publications.

Stevenson DE: The evolution of veterinary anesthesia, *Br Vet J* 119:477–483, 1963.

Tranquilli WJ, Grimm KA: Introduction: use, definitions, history, concepts, classification, and considerations for anesthesia and analgesia. In Grimm KA, Lamont LA, Tranquilli WJ, editors: *Lumb & Jones' veterinary anesthesia and analgesia*, ed 5, Ames, Iowa, 2015, Wiley Blackwell, pp 3–6.

Preparation

LEARNING OBJECTIVES

When you have completed this chapter, you will be able to:
- List the three main elements of preparation for an anesthetic procedure and explain why each is necessary for a successful outcome.
- Explain how a well-designed anesthetic safety checklist can be used to decrease anesthetic complications.
- Explain the importance of effective communication and the role of the veterinary technician or nurse in communication.
- List the reasons for preoperative patient evaluation.
- List the parts of a minimum patient database.
- Take a complete history and identify findings that affect anesthetic event planning.

- Identify ways in which patient signalment influences the anesthetic procedure and patient management.
- Discuss the rationale for obtaining the owner's consent for anesthesia.
- Perform a preanesthetic physical assessment.
- Relate the patient signalment, body weight, and patient condition to the selection and use of anesthetic agents and adjuncts.
- Assign a patient to one of the five physical status classifications as specified by the American Society of Anesthesiologists.
- Describe the components of preanesthetic preparation, including diagnostic testing, choice of protocol, withholding of food, and correction of preexisting problems.

Continued

LEARNING OBJECTIVES—cont'd

- List the reasons why placement of an intravenous (IV) catheter is advisable for all anesthetized patients.
- Describe the types of IV fluids that are used during anesthesia and why each might be chosen.
- List recommended IV fluid infusion rates for patient support during general anesthesia and surgery, and rates for treatment of hypotension, blood loss, and shock.
- Calculate IV fluid infusion rates.

KEY TERMS

Anesthetic Safety Checklists	Extra-label drug use	Obtunded
Anisocoria	Gastric dilatation–volvulus	Oncotic pressure
Attending veterinarian	Homeostasis	Osmolarity
Auscultation	Hypercarbia	Osmotic pressure
Body condition score	Hypotension	Petechiae
Borborygmus	Hypothermia	Physical status classification
Cachexia	Hypoxemia	Purpura
Cardiac output	Hypoxia	Regurgitation
Colloids	Ileus	Reproductive status
Comatose	Infusion rate	Signalment
Consent form	Inotropy	Sloughing
Constant rate infusion	Intact	Solutes
Crystalloids	Lethargic	Stridor
Cyanosis	Level of consciousness	Stuporous
Dead space	Macrodrip	Syncope
Debilitated	Microdrip	Thrombocytopenia
Drip rate	Minimum patient database	Vasodilation
Dyspnea	Miosis	Vesicants
Ecchymoses	Moribund	

PREPARING FOR AN ANESTHETIC PROCEDURE

Careful preparation is the cornerstone of any successful anesthetic procedure. Just as the preparation before painting a room often takes considerably more time than applying the paint, preparation prior to anesthesia is often more time consuming than an anesthetic event itself. There are three main elements of preparation:

1. a general review of the procedure to determine the equipment, supply, anesthetic agent, and personnel needs,
2. preparation of the patient, equipment, associated supplies, and agents that will be administered, and
3. communication with the anesthesia care team prior to commencing the procedure.

Attending to each of the many details of preparation, even for a relatively simple anesthetic procedure, can test the memory of even the most seasoned and experienced anesthetist. Forgetting just one of these details can result in serious or even catastrophic consequences. For instance, forgetting to check the oxygen supply can result in major organ damage, which may lead to an anesthetic fatality. One strategy that has recently gained attention for ensuring that all aspects of preparation are attended to and that the risk of preventable errors is minimized is the use of anesthetic safety checklists. The consistent use of checklists is recommended in the 2020 American Animal Hospital Association (AAHA) Anesthesia and Monitoring Guidelines for Dogs and Cats.

ANESTHETIC SAFETY CHECKLISTS

The use of safety checklists by the aviation industry to increase safety of air travel is well documented as far back as 1935. The use of checklists in healthcare settings to reduce complications and deaths is a much more recent trend. When used properly, checklists are documented to improve outcomes and decrease complications of all types including anesthetic deaths.

Health care checklists may be used in several ways. They may be used to ensure that all equipment is gathered prior to beginning a procedure, that critical steps are not missed when a complex task is performed, or that important points are not omitted when communicating with clients or other team members involved in a procedure.

> **TECHNICIAN NOTE** When used properly, checklists have been shown to improve outcomes and decrease complications of all types, including anesthetic deaths. The consistent use of checklists is recommended in the 2020 AAHA Anesthesia and Monitoring Guidelines for Dogs and Cats.

BOX 2.1 Requirements of an Effective Anesthesia Safety Checklist

- The checklist must be accepted as the right solution for a clearly recognized and articulated problem
- End users and other stakeholders must feel ownership in development of the checklist.
- The checklist should be tailored specifically to the organization in which it is used.
- The checklist must not be overly long or complex; instead, it must be easy to use.
- The end user must be familiar with and have a comprehensive understanding of the checklist.
- The end user must be given flexibility to use clinical judgement when using the checklist.
- The language used in the checklist must be unambiguous and clearly understood by all users.

Modified from Thomassen Ø, Espeland A, Søfteland E, et al: Implementation of checklists in health care; learning from high-reliability organisations, *Scand J Trauma Resusc Emerg Med* 19:53, 2011. http://www.sjtrem.com/content/19/1/53. Accessed February 2022.

BOX 2.2 Summary of Association of Veterinary Anaesthetists Anaesthetic Safety Checklists

The Pre-Induction Checklist
- Patient name, owner consent, and procedure confirmed
- Intravenous (IV) catheter (cannula) placed and patent
- Airway equipment available and functioning
- Endotracheal tube cuffs checked
- Anesthetic machine checked today
- Adequate oxygen supply for proposed procedure
- Breathing system connected, leak-free, and adjustable pressure-limiting valve open
- Person assigned to monitor patient
- Risks identified and communicated
- Emergency interventions available

The Pre-Procedure Checklist
- Patient name and procedure confirmed
- Depth of anesthesia appropriate
- Safety concerns communicated

The Recovery Checklist
- Safety concerns communicated regarding each of the following:
  - Airway
  - Breathing
  - Circulation (fluid balance)
  - Body temperature
  - Pain
- Assessment and intervention plan confirmed
- Analgesia plan confirmed
- Person assigned to monitor patient

Adapted from The Association of Veterinary Anaesthetists (AVA) Anaesthetic Safety Checklist Implementation Manual at https://ava.eu.com/resources/checklists/.

Many years of experience using checklists in a variety of fields, including health care settings, reveal that the use of checklists does not in and of itself reduce risk and increase safety. There are principles that must be followed when developing, implementing, and using a checklist to maximize its effectiveness. A recent study based on interviews of employees of organizations that routinely use checklists (Thomassen et al., 2011) sheds light on issues that must be considered. For instance, the checklist must be recognized as a solution to a clearly recognized and articulated problem (such as failure to check the oxygen supply, perform a leak test, or set the adjustable pressure-limiting valve in the open position when preparing a machine for use). The end users (that is, the anesthesia team) must be given ownership by being intimately involved in the entire process of development and implementation. The checklist must be easy to use and not be overly complex or difficult to understand. (See Box 2.1 for a list of these and other issues that must be considered when developing a checklist.)

The Association of Veterinary Anaesthetists (AVA) has developed an Anaesthetic Safety Checklist Implementation Manual (a.k.a. AVA Checklist—Booklet), which is available at https://ava.eu.com/resources/checklists/. This resource includes three predesigned checklists, intended for use at three specific stages of a general anesthetic procedure (i.e., before anesthetic induction, before commencement of the surgery or procedure, and before recovery). The manual also includes background regarding conception and development, rationale for each item in the three lists, and detailed instructions regarding their use. A summary of the content of the AVA checklists may be found in Box 2.2.

PATIENT PREPARATION

Patient preparation is usually the most involved and labor intensive part of preparing for an anesthetic event. Although monotonous, this important aspect of anesthesia requires careful attention to several diverse tasks. First, the anesthetist must assist the attending veterinarian in developing a minimum patient database—a compilation of pertinent information gleaned from the patient history, physical examination (PE), and diagnostic tests—which the attending veterinarian will use to determine the patient's physical status and anesthetic risk and to select an appropriate anesthetic protocol. Next, the anesthetist must ensure that the patient has been appropriately fasted. They must also provide preanesthetic care for the patient, including medication administration, intravenous (IV) catheterization, fluid administration, stabilization, and any other care ordered by the attending veterinarian. They must confirm that the necessary equipment and supplies are available and in good working order (further described in Chapter 4). Finally, the anesthetist must administer preanesthetic medications ordered by the veterinarian and monitor the patient until the time of induction. Box 2.3 lists "to-do" items during the preanesthetic period. Like the pieces of a puzzle, each step is necessary for a successful outcome. (See Case Presentation 2.1 for an example of the importance of careful patient preparation.)

COMMUNICATION—A KEY TO SUCCESS

A key element of successful patient preparation is effective communication. Veterinarians depend on accurate information

BOX 2.3   Patient Preparation "To-Do" List

Patient History
- Confirm the procedure to be performed
- Gather historical information
- Confirm compliance with fasting instructions
- Confirm vaccines and other preventive care are current
- Inquire about drug allergies or reactions
- Note pertinent medical problems and communicate these to the attending veterinarian

Client Communication
- Present the standard consent form and obtain the client's signature
- Present a fee estimate and obtain the client's signature
- Complete any financial transactions (deposits, payments, insurance)
- Answer the client's questions
- Inform the client of the nature of the procedure, the expected outcome, and the expected time of completion
- Communicate the date and time of discharge if known
- Determine an emergency communication protocol, including client phone number, availability, and schedule

Physical Examination
- Double-check the patient's identity
- Weigh the patient
- Confirm the patient's sex and reproductive status

- Determine the patient's hydration status
- Determine the vital signs
- Perform a physical assessment, focusing on the cardiovascular and pulmonary systems
- Determine the patient's pain score and physical status class
- Communicate to the attending veterinarian any pertinent physical abnormalities
- Note any concurrent conditions that may be best treated while patient is under anesthesia

Direct Patient Preparation
- If patient is hospitalized, make arrangements for preanesthetic fasting
- Perform diagnostic tests, convey results to the attending veterinarian, and highlight abnormal data
- Give medications ordered by the attending veterinarian
- Place IV catheter and administer fluids if indicated
- Administer preanesthetic medications
- Make any necessary preparations for postoperative care

Equipment Preparation
- Gather all necessary equipment
- Prepare the anesthetic machine
- Check that all equipment is in good working order

CASE PRESENTATION 2.1

Maggie, an 8-year-old spayed female Shepherd mix, was presented for removal of a subcutaneous mass located over the chest wall. This patient had originally presented about 1 month earlier for a routine wellness check. At that time, a complete minimum patient database was prepared. The patient was determined to be in good health with the exception of the mass and age-related changes. Routine preoperative blood work and chest radiographs were normal. The attending veterinarian recommended removal and biopsy of the mass to determine whether any additional treatment was necessary. A fee estimate was prepared, the client's questions were answered, and the procedure was explained, including the expected outcome. The doctor expected the surgery to be routine but could not give a long-term prognosis until results of the biopsy were known.

On the day of surgery, the patient was admitted to the hospital and appropriate fasting was confirmed. A consent form was signed, and arrangements were made to communicate the outcome of the surgery with the client later in the day.

The patient was premedicated, induced with an injectable anesthetic, and maintained with gas. The mass was successfully removed and a biopsy was taken. Intravenous fluids were administered at the standard rate, and the patient's heart rate and oxygen saturation were monitored throughout the procedure. After surgery, the patient was transported to the recovery area,

where she was closely monitored. As it was late in the day, the surgeon left the patient in the care of the doctor on duty.

The patient did not begin to recover as rapidly as expected, considering the anesthetic protocol used, but instead remained unconscious for about 45 min. The anesthetist alerted the veterinarian, who assessed the patient for a possible cause of prolonged recovery. Although vital signs were stable, the heart rate was increased (144 beats per minute [bpm]), the heart sounds were muffled, the femoral pulse was weaker than expected, and the pulse varied in intensity with the phase of respiration. At this point, the veterinarian on duty suspected cardiac disease and referred the patient to an intensive care team. Workup revealed pericardial effusion with a mass on the right atrium. The prolonged recovery was felt to be a result of poor heart function and poor tissue perfusion related to the pericardial disease. In view of the preoperative workup, it was probable that the pericardial effusion was not present that the time of the initial workup 1 month previously but had developed between that time and the day of surgery and was present at the time of anesthetic induction.

1. *If you were the client, how might you react to this situation?*
2. *What essential element or elements of patient preparation listed in Box 2.3 were overlooked in this case that, if performed, might have uncovered this problem before anesthetic induction?*

---

at all stages of the procedure to make effective patient care decisions. Clients need clear instructions and answers to questions before the procedure, as well as progress reports and home care instructions after the procedure. In addition, the technician or nurse often acts as a liaison between the doctor and client, conveying necessary information between these two parties.

The bond between most clients and their pets is very strong. Surveys of pet owners over the past several decades consistently show that a vast majority of dog and cat owners consider their pets to be members of the family. Consequently, most clients are very protective of and concerned about the

well-being of their animals, and they are very attuned to real or perceived risks to their safety. The risks inherent in the practice of anesthesia often produce or heighten feelings of anxiety.

These feelings can be minimized, however, when the relationship between health care providers and the client is strong. A strong relationship is based not only on confidence in the competency of the veterinarian and staff but also on assurance that they truly care about the welfare of the patient. The saying, "Clients don't care how much you know until they know how much you care," has become an oft-repeated adage in the veterinary community. Although not originally used in reference to the veterinary profession, anyone with even a little practice experience can tell you that this statement accurately reflects the way most clients feel.

Exceptional communication is probably the best way to convey the caring that clients desire and expect. They feel more confident and less anxious about the procedure when informed. When unanticipated complications occur, clients are thus more able to come to terms with the outcome. A few extra minutes spent answering questions and explaining the risks and benefits before a procedure is well worth the time in terms of increased client satisfaction and lessening the sadness, anger, and disappointment that occur when events do not go as hoped and that, if not adequately addressed, can result in ill will, the loss of a client, or even legal action.

In fact, there is no better predictor of success than the technician's or nurse's communication skills, and for this important reason, communication will remain a centerpiece of this text. (See Case Presentation 2.2 for an example of the importance of good communication.)

THE MINIMUM PATIENT DATABASE

Technicians or nurses soon become accustomed to a wide variety in size, age, temperament, conformation, and condition among the patients they see. Veterinary patients can range in size from 20 g to over 1000 kg, and may be neonatal, pediatric, mature, or geriatric. They may be docile, spirited, fearful, agitated, or aggressive. They may be emaciated, lean, obese, brachycephalic, deep-chested, or pregnant. Some are healthy, and others have varying degrees of illness ranging from mild to critical. Some are brought in for minor procedures; others will undergo complicated and lengthy operations. Given this diversity, it is unrealistic to assume that the same anesthetic techniques will work for all patients. Furthermore, it is dangerous to expect all patients to react to a given anesthetic agent in exactly the same way.

The veterinarian and technician or nurse must therefore gather as much information as possible to uncover any factors that might lead to anesthetic complications. The information, collectively referred to as a *minimum patient database,* is used to make patient care decisions. If the information obtained about a given animal reveals a potential problem, the veterinarian may choose to alter, postpone, or even cancel the anesthetic procedure.

The minimum patient database consists of the following:
1. Patient history, including the patient signalment
2. Complete PE findings
3. Results of a preanesthetic diagnostic workup

Many veterinary clinics routinely recommend that animals scheduled for elective surgery be brought into the clinic for an appointment before the day of surgery so that this information can be gathered. During the visit, the veterinarian may also administer necessary vaccinations, give information about preanesthetic fasting of the animal, obtain signed consent forms, and present a fee estimate. If such an appointment is scheduled several days before the planned procedure, unforeseen problems can be discovered and addressed well in advance of surgery.

TECHNICIAN NOTE An appointment should be scheduled several days before the planned procedure to acquire the minimum patient database so that unforeseen problems can be discovered and addressed well in advance of surgery.

CASE PRESENTATION 2.2

Pixie, a 9-year-old, spayed female Yorkshire Terrier, presented for a comprehensive oral health assessment and treatment (COHAT) (aka: dental cleaning). A minimum patient database was acquired, and the patient was prepared in a routine manner. The client was educated regarding the condition of the oral cavity; the nature of the procedure, including the probable need for extractions; and follow-up care. The consent form was signed, and a phone number at which the client could be reached during the procedure was obtained.

The COHAT was performed and during the process of assessing the oral cavity, the patient was determined to have grade IV periodontal disease, 10 teeth with advanced mobility, and several more with end-stage, irreversible damage to the periodontal tissues. A total of 17 teeth were extracted with minimal effort. The client was not called because the possibility of extractions had been discussed at the preoperative interview.

It was routine in this clinic to have the veterinary technician meet with the owner at discharge to review what had been done and to provide instructions for home care. During the exit interview, the owner became agitated and very angry and demanded to see the doctor immediately. He expressed anger over the large number of extractions and grave concerns that the patient would be unable to eat normally. He refused to listen to any explanation of the importance of removal of these teeth or the dangers associated with leaving them in. The owner left the clinic in a state of extreme agitation, vowing never to come back. Although the doctor followed up by phone 1 week later to check on the patient's progress, the client's anger had not abated.

1. *What could the staff have done differently in this situation to maximize the likelihood of a positive outcome?*

Before embarking on a study of anesthesia, the student should be familiar with the process required to obtain a patient history as well as the procedures required to perform a complete PE and diagnostic workup. Consequently, the sections that follow will focus specifically on how the anesthetist can best obtain information needed to make effective and safe anesthetic management decisions. Emphasis will be placed on specific historical questions to ask, physical findings to focus on, and diagnostic test results that are most pertinent to anesthetic procedures, as well as the ways in which common abnormal findings from each of these sources of information affect outcomes.

Patient History

A patient history is comprised of information about the patient's health, acquired primarily by asking the client questions. A thorough patient history is an essential part of a minimum patient database and, in fact, is often considerably more important for making effective patient care decisions than the results of diagnostic testing.

Obtaining a thorough patient history requires skill and care and, like all arts, it must be continually practiced and refined. The technician or nurse must know the most important questions to ask as well as the most effective way to frame those questions. Otherwise, the patient history will be incomplete or misleading.

> **TECHNICIAN NOTE** When taking a patient history, emphasize open-ended questions. Avoid leading questions or those that can be answered "yes" or "no."

A common error is to ask a question that can be answered "yes" or "no." For instance, the question, "Does your dog drink a normal amount of water?" will yield a "yes" or "no" answer that reflects that owner's assumption regarding what is normal, as opposed to facts that can be accurately evaluated. In contrast, the question, "About how much water does your dog drink per day?" prompts the owner to quantify the amount of water consumed but not to judge whether they believe the amount to be normal. If the client replies, "About 1 quart (or liter)," the attending veterinarian will then be able to determine whether or not this volume is excessive, despite the owner's opinion regarding its significance.

Another common error is to ask leading questions. In the previous example, the question "Your dog doesn't drink much water, does she?" might bias the owner toward a particular response such as "No, I guess not," resulting in misleading information.

In a busy practice, it is often difficult to set aside adequate time to obtain a good history. Under these circumstances, the technician or nurse may be tempted to take shortcuts or omit questions altogether—an inadvisable practice that will lead to unpleasant surprises. For instance, an owner may not realize that coughing and exercise intolerance may be associated with a heart problem. If an adequate history is not taken, the preexisting heart disease may not be detected, and the technician or nurse may become aware of the problem only when the anesthetized animal is in danger.

When inquiring about signs of illness, the technician or nurse should not only note information the client freely offers but always strive to get as much detail as possible. For instance, if a client indicates that the patient is vomiting, the attending veterinarian will want to know other details in order to interpret its significance. No matter what the sign (e.g., vomiting, coughing, diarrhea, polyuria, seizures, or weakness), it is always helpful to know the following four points,[a] which give the veterinarian specific information necessary to arrive at a diagnosis:

1. The duration (how long has it been going on?)
2. The volume or severity (how much or how severe?)
3. The frequency (how often?)
4. The character or appearance (what does it look like?)

> **TECHNICIAN NOTE** When gathering historical information about signs of illness (e.g., vomiting or coughing), always ask about the following:
> 1. The duration (how long has it been going on?)
> 2. The volume or severity (how much or how severe?)
> 3. The frequency (how often?)
> 4. The character or appearance (what does it look like?)

Confirmation of the Scheduled Procedure

Because miscommunications occur and clerical errors may be made on medical charts, in appointment books, and on surgery

---

[a]Note that although not all of these points may apply to every sign, they apply to most.

schedules, the technician or nurse must verbally confirm the procedure to be performed. Periodically, stories appear in the news about devastating consequences of a miscommunication in the human medical field such as amputation of the wrong limb or administration of chemotherapy to the wrong patient. Similar errors may occur in veterinary patients and frequently result in ill will, patient harm, or legal proceedings.

Attention to this simple but important element of effective communication will prevent these and other embarrassing, dangerous, or potentially devastating errors such as a missed diagnosis from failing to submit a biopsy sample, anesthetizing the wrong patient, neglecting to perform a necessary procedure, or performing a procedure the patient does not need. When confirming the procedure, check the following specifics:

- When performing surgery on a limb, confirm the affected limb (left or right; fore- or hind).
- When a tumor is being removed, be sure that the exact location of the tumor is known. Skin tumors can be obscured by the hair coat and if small, can be extremely difficult to locate unless pointed out by the client. Once the tumor has been located, mark the location by clipping the hair or using a surgical marker.
- If removing tumors or other mass lesions, confirm the owner's wishes regarding histopathology (biopsy) or cytology.
- Determine whether the client wishes the veterinarian to use their judgment regarding decisions that must be made during the procedure (such as the number of teeth that need to be extracted during a **comprehensive oral health assessment and treatment** (COHAT) (aka: dental cleaning) or whether the client would like a telephone call before proceeding.

After confirming this information with the client, be sure it is accurately transferred to the medical record and communicated to the attending veterinarian.

> **TECHNICIAN NOTE** Always confirm the nature of the scheduled procedure when the patient is admitted, including the exact location of tumors or lesions, the affected limb (for procedures involving a limb), and the owner's wishes regarding testing (such as histopathology).

Obtaining a Patient History

When a complete patient history is being obtained, the following specific questions should be answered. (*See* Box 2.4 *for a list of these questions.*)

What is the species, breed, age, sex, and reproductive status of the patient? The species, breed, age, sex, and reproductive status are collectively known as the signalment. The signalment is important in planning the anesthetic procedure, as each data point influences the anesthetic plan, drug doses, and many other actions related to patient management as noted in the following sections.

Species. Each species has unique responses to anesthetic agents and adjuncts as well as unique needs associated with anesthesia. Following are examples of notable species differences that must be considered:

- Horses and cats are more sensitive to opioids than dogs and ruminants. Therefore some of these agents must be used with caution, at lower doses, or not at all in these species.

BOX 2.4 **Questions to Answer When Obtaining a Patient History**

1. What is the species, breed, age, sex, and reproductive status of the patient?
2. Is the patient receiving or has it recently received treatment with any drugs, nutraceuticals, or pesticides? If so, what are they (including name, strength, dose, and frequency of administration)?
3. Is there any history of allergies or drug reactions?
4. Is the patient up to date on routine preventive care?
5. Has the patient ever had or does it currently have any medical problems and, if so, what was the medical or surgical treatment?
6. Does the patient have any signs of illness?
   a. Anorexia
   b. Vomiting or diarrhea
   c. Coughing or sneezing
   d. Polyuria
   e. Polydipsia
   f. Tenesmus
   g. Dysuria
   h. Change in behavior
   i. Exercise intolerance
   j. Weakness
   k. Fainting or seizures
   l. Bleeding
7. Is the patient in pain?

- Each species has unique dosing requirements (e.g., cats require a lower dose of lidocaine but are more resistant to the effects of phenothiazine tranquilizers than dogs).
- Horses tend to have rougher recoveries from inhalant anesthetics than other species.
- The use of anticholinergics should be avoided in ruminants as it can make their saliva thick and ropy, which can lead to airway occlusion. Ruminants may also regurgitate at any point during anesthesia, and the anesthetist should take steps to prevent aspiration.
- Ruminants are more sensitive to xylazine, requiring about one-tenth the dose horses need.
- Cats can tolerate administration of dissociative agents alone, whereas dogs may experience seizurelike activity unless the dissociative agent is combined with another agent.
- Large animals are prone to respiratory depression and dependent lung atelectasis (collapse of a portion of one or both lungs) and thus often require ventilatory support.
- Large animals experience pressure necrosis of tissues lying over pressure points such as the shoulder and hip and thus require measures to pad dependent areas when in lateral recumbency.
- Horses may fracture limbs during anesthetic recovery and thus require special attention during the recovery period.
- Cats, small dogs, and small animal pediatric patients are prone to hypoxemia and hypercarbia caused by increased mechanical dead space.
- Cats and ruminants are prone to airway blockage because of development of excess airway secretions.
- Ruminants are prone to bloat.
- Exotic animals such as birds and reptiles must be managed very differently than common domestic species. The

technician or nurse should consult appropriate references and the veterinarian before administering anesthetics to these animals.

Breed. Differences in anatomy and physiology among the various breeds also may affect an animal's response to anesthetic agents and procedures.

- Boxers and giant breeds of dogs are more sensitive to acepromazine than other breeds, whereas Terriers are resistant.
- Brachycephalic animals are more difficult to intubate and must be watched closely to ensure a patent airway before, during, and after any anesthetic procedure. Also, members of these breeds often require the use of smaller endotracheal tubes than most other breeds.
- Dogs and cats with an ABCB1-1delta (also known as MDR1 or Multidrug Resistance 1) gene mutation may have an exaggerated response to the drugs acepromazine and butorphanol. Although any dog or cat may be affected, herding breeds, including Collies and Australian Shepherds, have an increased incidence of this mutation (see Box 2.5 for more about ABCB1-1delta mutation). Animals with this mutation may require dosage reductions of the drugs mentioned or the use of alternative agents.
- Sighthounds such as Greyhounds and Salukis are sensitive to some anesthetics because of their slow metabolism and their relative lack of body fat compared with other breeds. For instance, these breeds may have prolonged recovery if maintained on propofol for longer than 30 minutes. They are also more sensitive to barbiturates (e.g., thiopental sodium). Consequently, these drugs must be used cautiously or, in some cases, not at all in these patients.
- Greyhounds may become hyperkalemic when undergoing general anesthesia.
- Many exotic or rare-breed animals are perceived to be sensitive to anesthetics by their owners, although many of these idiosyncrasies are not proven.

BOX 2.5 **Facts About Dogs and Cats With ABCB1-1delta (MDR1) Gene Mutation**

- The ABCB1-1delta gene (a.k.a. the Multidrug Resistance 1 [MDR1] gene) is responsible for production of P-glycoprotein, a protein that pumps many drugs out of cells.
- Animals with this mutation have one or two copies of the mutated gene. This makes them more sensitive to certain drugs (including some antiparasitic and chemotherapeutic drugs, as well as the sedative drug acepromazine and the opioid butorphanol).
- Animals with two copies of the mutated gene may have a serious or even fatal sensitivity in some circumstances. Those with one copy are more sensitive to these drugs than normal patients.
- Herding breeds (including Collies and Australian Shepherds) have a relatively high incidence of this mutation, although any breed of dog or cat may have it.
- An ABCB1-1delta gene mutation may cause profound and prolonged sedation from doses of the tranquilizer/sedative drug acepromazine and the opioid butorphanol, normally used in animals without the mutation.
- These patients typically require a reduction of approximately 25%–50% when calculating the dose of these drugs.
- The ABCB1-1delta gene mutation can be detected with a genetic test performed using a blood sample or a cheek swab.

- Draft horses are typically sensitive to sedatives in the same way that giant breed dogs are. They are also more likely to experience complications during recovery because of their large body mass compared with average-sized horses.
- Some breeds have one or more genetic predispositions for underlying conditions that may affect the anesthetic plan. For instance, Cavalier King Charles Spaniels have a genetic predisposition for cardiac disease, and individuals of certain small breeds such as Yorkshire Terriers are predisposed to the development of collapsing trachea.

Age. The age of the patient can be an important consideration when deciding what drugs to use. Neonates (up to 2 weeks of age) or pediatric patients (2 to 8 weeks of age) are much less capable of metabolizing injectable drugs than are adult animals because the necessary liver metabolic pathways are not fully developed. Geriatric patients (those that are >75% of the normal life span for that species and breed) may be unable to tolerate normal doses of some drugs because of poor hepatic or renal function. The result, in either case, may be a slow recovery from anesthesia, particularly if doses of injectable drugs are not adjusted accordingly. In addition, young patients are more difficult to intubate and to catheterize, are more subject to dosing errors, are more prone to hypothermia and hypoxia, and have a weaker respiratory drive. As patients age, they become less able to tolerate the demands that anesthesia places on their major organ systems. These factors put neonatal, pediatric, and geriatric patients at higher risk for complications.

> **TECHNICIAN NOTE** Patients that are very large, very small, very young (<8 weeks old), or very old (>75% of the normal lifespan) respond to anesthetic procedures differently than other animals and have special needs of which the anesthetist must be aware.

Sex and reproductive status. Always confirm the patient's sex by PE. Owners may not be aware of their pet's sex or may misidentify it. If not corrected, misidentification of the patient's sex can lead to an undesirable outcome. For instance, attempting to spay a male cat (because the patient's sex was misidentified by the client and not confirmed by the technician or nurse) is unnecessary for the patient and very embarrassing and difficult to explain to the client.

Reproductive status refers to whether or not the patient has been spayed or castrated and, if the patient is intact, whether or not the patient is being used for breeding. For intact female patients, the database also includes the current estrous cycle status and pregnancy status. These points are of particular importance in terms of the anesthetic plan as well as patient management, as indicated in the following examples.

- When an intact female animal is in heat, the uterus is enlarged and has a more extensive blood supply. These patients also may bleed excessively because of the effects of estrogen on the clotting cascade. For an ovariohysterectomy, these factors increase the length, difficulty, risk, and often the cost of the surgery.

- During pregnancy, the gravid uterus and its blood supply gradually enlarge, reaching a size many times larger than a nongravid uterus. As is the case with estrus, these changes substantially increase the length, difficulty, and risk of an ovariohysterectomy. The prospect of spaying a pregnant animal also creates an ethical dilemma that must be discussed with the client before proceeding.
- Acepromazine is considered to be contraindicated in stallions by many clinicians because it may cause penile prolapse, which can lead to permanent injury and loss of breeding soundness.
- Xylazine has been shown to cause uterine contractions during the third trimester of pregnancy in sheep and cattle.

Is the patient receiving or has it recently received treatment with any drugs, nutraceuticals, or pesticides? Many medications, including anticonvulsants, behavior-modifying drugs, drugs that affect the autonomic nervous system, and antibiotics, may influence the effect of anesthetics.

- Sympathomimetics such as epinephrine increase the incidence of cardiac arrhythmias when given with dissociatives, xylazine, and barbiturates.
- Tricyclic antidepressants such as amitriptyline and clomipramine may predispose patients to cardiac arrhythmias and excessive responses to anticholinergics and central nervous system (CNS) depressants.
- The antibiotic chloramphenicol may prolong the action of propofol and ketamine and may decrease the biotransformation of barbiturate anesthetics, leading to significantly prolonged recovery.
- When given within 14 days of one another, some monoamine oxidase (MAO) inhibitors such as amitraz and selegiline may increase the effects of morphine and other opioids.
- Some antihistamines can increase CNS and respiratory depression when given with opioids and other anesthetic agents that depress these body systems.

Is there any history of allergies or drug reactions? Past adverse reactions to drugs must be documented in the medical record and conveyed to the attending veterinarian. Severe allergic reactions such as anaphylaxis preclude the use of the offending drug in the future. A past history of prolonged recovery, personality changes, organ dysfunction, or other postanesthetic adverse reactions may influence a decision to use these agents and must be brought to the veterinarian's attention. For example, some cats will have prolonged recoveries from ketamine and other dissociatives that can last several days. Some dogs can experience behavioral changes after sedation with acepromazine that can result in aggression and biting. It may be best to choose another agent in the future for a patient experiencing these and other adverse reactions.

Is the patient up to date on routine preventive care? Check the date and type of vaccines administered and the results of fecal analysis and routine testing for contagious diseases such as heartworm disease in dogs and cats and feline leukemia and feline immunodeficiency viruses in cats. The last date of tetanus antitoxoid administration to an equine patient should be known. Many veterinary clinics require current vaccinations before hospitalization to prevent the spread of contagious diseases.

Has the patient ever had or does it currently have any medical problems and, if so, what was the medical or surgical treatment? Information about current and past medical problems is obtained from the patient's medical record or verbally from the client. Animals with preexisting disease, especially those involving the heart, lungs, liver, or kidneys, may be at increased risk for anesthetic complications. One important reason these organs are of concern is that they may be adversely affected by various anesthetic and analgesic agents and, in some cases, adverse effects may be severe (e.g., hypotension caused by isoflurane and other inhalant anesthetics, and respiratory depression caused by the IV anesthetic propofol). Another reason is that normal function of these organs is necessary for effective transport, metabolism, and elimination of these drugs. Therefore, significant liver or kidney disease may result in increased potency of a drug or prolonged duration of action, leading to slow recovery.

Does the patient have any signs of illness? Asking whether the patient has any of the signs listed in the following paragraphs helps the attending veterinarian make a diagnosis, determine risk, and guide patient management decisions. These common signs of disease often indicate a variety of problems, which must be explored and acted on through PE, diagnostic testing, patient treatment and stabilization, or even postponement of the procedure. Remember to determine the details regarding duration, volume or severity, frequency, and appearance or character.

Anorexia, vomiting, diarrhea, coughing, sneezing, polyuria, polydipsia, tenesmus, or dysuria. These signs may indicate one of many disorders which may need to be stabilized before anesthesia. Parvovirus in dogs, upper respiratory infections in cats, inflammatory bowel disease, urinary blockage, endocrine disease, and organ dysfunction are examples of problems associated with these signs. Animals with infectious diseases may also introduce pathogens into the hospital, posing a risk to other patients unless they are placed in an isolation ward.

Change in behavior. Changes in behavior (such as loss of interest in favorite activities, hiding, irritability, or uncharacteristic aggression) may be a sign of CNS disease, pain, systemic illness, and many other conditions, and must be explored to determine a cause.

Exercise intolerance. Exercise intolerance (e.g., sleepiness or depression, uncharacteristic reluctance or refusal to run or play, becoming tired more quickly than usual, lying down a lot, or heavy breathing after exercise) may indicate a variety of problems including heart disease, respiratory disease, anemia, and musculoskeletal pain.

Weakness. Weakness is a nonspecific sign caused by many disorders including heart failure, neuromuscular diseases, anemia, dehydration, and electrolyte abnormalities, and always warrants investigation to determine a cause.

Fainting or seizures. Both fainting episodes and seizures vary widely in appearance and sometimes may be difficult to tell apart. In many cases, these disorders can be differentiated by careful observation, but other cases require careful analysis of information derived from the patient history, PE, and diagnostic tests. Despite any similarities in appearance, these disorders have completely different causes. Fainting (also called syncope) often indicates hypoxemia, low blood pressure, or cardiac disease, whereas seizures are often associated with CNS disease, toxin ingestion, or metabolic disorders such as hypoglycemia.

Bleeding. Any unexplained bleeding including bruising, blood in the urine or stool, or prolonged bleeding after venipuncture or surgery may be a sign of a coagulation disorder which, if unidentified, will increase a patient's risk for intraoperative and postoperative hemorrhage.

Is the patient in pain? This question should be routinely asked as part of the discussion of the patient's presenting complaint. If so, ask the client about the nature of the pain and for an estimate of its severity on a scale of 0–10, with 0 representing no pain and 10 representing the worst possible pain. This information is then used when performing a routine PE to help locate problems that must be addressed.

Other Considerations

Before the procedure, it is advisable to give the owner a written estimate of the expected charges. It is also customary to obtain a signed consent form authorizing anesthesia and surgery. It is illegal in most jurisdictions to undertake surgery or anesthesia on an animal without the owner's written or oral consent and in any case, it is unadvisable. Such consent must be informed, meaning that the owner is warned beforehand of risks associated with the procedure. Standard consent forms (available from practice management consultants and from state and provincial veterinary associations) often state that anesthesia and surgery are never without risk (Fig. 2.1).

> **TECHNICIAN NOTE** Before any anesthetic procedure, *always* give the owner a written estimate of the expected charges and obtain a signed consent form authorizing anesthesia and surgery.

Many consent forms also include a statement giving the veterinarian permission to perform cardiopulmonary resuscitation (CPR) if the patient's condition requires it. Owners should be asked to provide a telephone number at which they may be reached during the day in case an emergency or unforeseen complication should arise. Consent forms may also state that some anesthetic drugs may be used that have not received approval from the Food and Drug Administration for this purpose. This is termed extra-label drug use and is common in veterinary anesthesia.

It is ironic that although cell phones are ubiquitous, clients are often difficult to reach because they rely on voice mail and do not always feel compelled to answer their phones promptly. An inability to contact a client presents a problem, particularly with procedures such as exploratory surgery in which the diagnosis is not known. In these situations, decisions that require the client's input (such as whether to biopsy or remove a tumor or whether to proceed with a difficult, high-risk, or expensive procedure) must sometimes be made quickly. Therefore it is imperative that the client knows to be available by phone or text

affix medical records sticker here

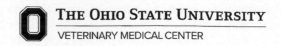
THE OHIO STATE UNIVERSITY
VETERINARY MEDICAL CENTER

General Consent Form

Agreement

The following agreement is made between The Ohio State University Veterinary Medical Center (VMC) and the owner of the animal being presented for care (Owner) or the presenting agent of the owner (Agent).

- **The VMC agrees to provide diagnostic, therapeutic or preventive care to the animal being presented.**
- **As Owner/Agent of this animal, I give permission to the Veterinary Medical Center faculty, staff and students to perform diagnostic, therapeutic or preventive procedures as deemed advisable by the attending clinician after consultation with me.**
- **The Owner/Agent agrees to pay all charges associated with this visit at the time of the animal's release.**
- **It is understood that information from the animal's medical record, fluid and/or tissue samples taken during medical care, and images may be used for teaching or clinical investigation purposes.**
- **It is understood that other veterinarians who care for this animal will have access to the medical record.**
- **I authorize the VMC to provide a copy of my animal's medical record to my insurance company upon their request:** ☐ Yes   ☐ No   ☐ N/A

  Name of Insurance Company:_____

- **The VMC does not participate in third party billing. If my animal does have an insurance policy, I agree to pay all charges associated with this visit at the time of the animal's discharge.**
- **I understand that the VMC treatment team includes a licensed social worker whose role is to provide support to VMC clients and case consultation to the veterinary team when requested. I further understand that these services are free of charge and I have a right to refuse services.**

In the event of an emergency:

☐ **I CONSENT to Cardiopulmonary Resuscitation (CPR)**

☐ **I DECLINE Cardiopulmonary Resuscitation (CPR)**

☐ **Not Applicable**

This signed authorization will become part of the medical record and will remain in effect until revoked by the client.

I certify that I have read and fully understand this authorization. I hereby release The Ohio State University, its faculty, staff and students from any and all claims, except claims for negligence, arising out of or connected with the medical care of the above described animal.

I am the Owner of the animal being presented for care and am over 18 years of age.

Owner Signature:_____   Printed Name:_____   Date:_____

I am the Agent of the owner of the animal being presented for care and am over 18 years of age.

Agent Signature:_____   Printed Name:_____   Date:_____

VMC Witness Signature:_____   Printed Name:_____   Date:_____

Updated 2018-10

FIG. 2.1 Standard consent form for treatment and/or authorization for admission to the hospital. (Courtesy The Ohio State University Veterinary Medical Center.)

at the time of surgery so that they can be contacted immediately should the need arise.

Obviously, a great deal of information must be exchanged before anesthesia is initiated. Although it may be appropriate for a trained receptionist to assist in gathering this information, particularly when a young, healthy animal is scheduled for an elective operation such as castration or ovariohysterectomy, the veterinarian, technician, or nurse should handle more complex cases. The hospital employee who admits a patient and speaks to the owner must not just obtain this information but must also relay that information to the anesthetist by means of a written record or oral report.

In some cases, it may be difficult to obtain the history in person. Some clinics prefer to have the owner fill out a prepared history form, particularly if the clinic has a high volume of patients. In any practice, difficulties may arise when an animal's owner is in a hurry and reluctant to stop and answer questions. However, it is usually possible to obtain a telephone number and call for more information at a prearranged time. Occasionally, the person bringing the animal into the clinic is not the owner and is unfamiliar with the pet. In this case, every effort should be made to contact the owner by telephone to obtain the required information.

Physical Examination and Physical Assessment

A PE is a complete evaluation of a patient's physical condition using the assessor's hands, eyes, ears, and nose. Although the basic technique used to perform a PE is the same whether the examination is performed by a veterinarian, veterinary technician, or nurse, there is a qualitative difference in the way the results of the examination are used by these parties. A veterinarian uses the physical findings to arrive at a diagnosis and plan treatment. In contrast, a veterinary technician or nurse uses physical findings to provide effective patient care, respond to patient needs, and alert the veterinarian to changes in patient condition that influence patient management. The coordinated application of these two very different but complementary approaches enables the veterinary team to provide high-quality care at a level that would not otherwise be possible.

In order to differentiate this contrast in purpose, in this text, the term PE will be used to indicate evaluation by a veterinarian for the purpose of diagnosis and treatment planning, and the term *physical assessment* (PA) will be used to indicate evaluation by a technician or nurse for the purpose of maximizing quality of care and influencing patient management through communication with the attending veterinarian. No value judgment is implied in either term because both PEs and assessments as defined herein are interdependent techniques—equally necessary and of equal importance in the delivery of high-quality patient care. With this in mind, a discussion of this vital part of the minimum patient database follows.

A complete PE should be conducted on every animal scheduled for anesthesia. Although a veterinarian usually does this before scheduling a procedure, the technician or nurse should, in addition, always perform a brief PA immediately before the procedure. Following are common examples of findings revealed during PE or PA that will influence patient anesthetic management.
- *Dehydration* increases the risk of anesthetic complications, including **hypotension**, poor tissue perfusion, and kidney damage.
- *Anemia* decreases the oxygen-carrying capacity of the blood and predisposes the patient to hypoxemia.
- *Bruising lesions* on the skin or mucous membranes, in the absence of trauma, often indicate a clotting disorder, which will increase the risk of potentially life-threatening intraoperative and postoperative bleeding.
- *Respiratory or cardiovascular system abnormalities* increase the risk of anesthetic complications and death.
- *Abnormalities of abdominal organs* such as an enlarged liver or abnormally small kidneys may be associated with abnormal organ function and a reduced ability to metabolize or excrete anesthetic agents.
- *General conditions that require veterinary attention* such as ear mite or flea infestations, otitis externa, dental disease, overgrown nails, and anal sac impaction are conditions that are often most easily treated during the anesthetic procedure. Owners are often not aware these conditions are present and, once informed, will frequently authorize treatment.
- *Physical abnormalities that may influence the procedure.* One example of this is an abdominally retained testicle in a patient presented for castration. This condition increases the complexity and cost of surgery, so the owner must be informed before the veterinarian proceeds.

In most jurisdictions, veterinary technicians or nurses must perform a PA under the supervision of a licensed veterinarian. The veterinary medical licensing board practice act should be consulted to determine the laws regulating technician or nurse duties in your state or province.

TECHNICIAN NOTE The technician or nurse should *always* perform a brief PA immediately before the procedure, to uncover hidden problems that may increase risk or alter patient management.

There are many different ways to approach a PE or PA. Any technique is valid as long as the patient is examined entirely and in a systematic manner (e.g., from head to tail or by organ system). Include each element listed in the following sections, with emphasis on the nervous, cardiovascular, and pulmonary systems, as these systems are generally most affected by anesthetic agents and most directly influence outcome. When possible, it is helpful to have the owner present during the PE or PA to give pertinent history about any physical abnormalities that are found. Any unusual findings must be brought to the attention of the veterinarian because ultimately it is the veterinarian's responsibility to make a diagnosis, formulate an appropriate treatment plan, and advise the owner and hospital staff accordingly.

Patient Identification

In practice, inattention to seemingly simple considerations, such as proper patient identification (ID), may result in undesirable outcomes because they are easily overlooked. Examination of the news will occasionally reveal stories of accidents at human hospitals related to patient ID such as a surgery performed on the wrong patient. Needless to say, serious errors such as these can and do occur in veterinary medicine.

In a busy animal hospital, patients may easily be confused if not positively identified with cage tags and patient ID collars, as well as documentation of external characteristics such as species, breed, size, hair coat length, color, and other visual identifying characteristics. This is because most individuals within a particular breed look very similar. Patients may be placed in the wrong cage, or one may simply be mistaken for another. Therefore, careful attention must always be given to patient ID.

Tags on the front of each cage should identify the patient so that those passing the cage can quickly identify the patient before opening the cage. ID collars confirm patient ID in case a patient is inadvertently placed in the wrong cage.

Before performing any procedure, make a positive patient ID by matching the cage tag, the ID collar, and the patient's external characteristics with the information contained in the medical record. In other words, do whatever needs to be done to make sure the animal in your hands is the correct one!

> **TECHNICIAN NOTE** Identification collars must be placed on *all* patients on admission to the hospital. Before anesthetizing a patient, do whatever you need to do to make sure the animal in your hands is the correct one!

Body Weight

Anesthetic agents as a rule have very narrow therapeutic indexes. Therefore, accurate dosing is critical to a successful outcome. With the exception of inhalant anesthetics, most drug dosages and IV fluid administration rates are calculated according to body weight. All animals should therefore be accurately weighed immediately before any anesthetic procedure. Animals under 5 kg should be weighed on a pediatric scale, and those under 1 kg should be weighed on a gram scale. It is not appropriate to estimate a body weight for purposes of anesthetic administration unless working with a large animal that cannot be weighed because of temperament or lack of a large-animal scale. In this case, techniques will be used to estimate weight based on experience, or in the case of horses, by measurement of girth and length, but must also take into account the patient's body condition score. The basic formula for determining the body weight in horses is as follows:

$$\text{Body weight (kg)} = \frac{\text{Heart girth (cm)}^2 \times \text{Length (cm)}}{11{,}880}$$

where heart girth equals the circumference of the chest behind the point of the elbow, and length equals the distance from the point of the shoulder to the point of the pelvis (tuber ischii).

The current weight should be compared with previous weights (found in the patient's medical record) to determine whether weight gain or loss has occurred. Changes in weight may reflect changes in the patient's food intake, hydration, activity level, or overall state of health.

> **TECHNICIAN NOTE** All animals should be accurately weighed *immediately* before any anesthetic procedure. Animals under 5 kg should be weighed on a pediatric scale, and those under 1 kg should be weighed on a gram scale.

Body Condition Score

A body condition score is a numeric assessment of the patient's weight compared with the ideal body weight. Some professionals use a five-level system, and others use a nine-level system. In the nine-level system, the number 5 represents ideal body weight (*note that some professionals consider 4 or 5 to be normal*). Lower numbers and higher numbers represent a body weight less than or greater than the ideal weight, respectively, with a score of 1 representing extreme cachexia and 9 representing overt obesity (Fig. 2.2). Although it has fewer gradations, the five-level system is similar to the nine-level system, except that a score of 3 represents normal weight and 5 represents overt obesity.

The body condition score is important because changes in body weight influence patient management. Excessive thinness may indicate the presence of an underlying disorder such as hyperthyroidism or chronic parasitism, which may increase patient risk. Animals with little body fat are more prone to hypothermia than patients of normal body weight.

Obesity also poses difficulties for the anesthetist. Obese animals may have compromised cardiovascular function and decreased functional lung volume. In addition, venipuncture and auscultation are more difficult in obese patients. When patients are significantly overweight, anesthetics should be dosed according to lean body weight (excluding body fat) instead of the total body weight. This is because body fat increases the total body weight but not the volume or weight of the nervous tissue on which anesthetics exert their effect. Administration of a dose calculated using total body weight results in an anesthetic overdose. Therefore the anesthetist must use the body condition score along with the actual patient weight to estimate lean body weight.

Assessment of Hydration

Hydration status is assessed using physical parameters that enable the anesthetist to estimate the percentage of dehydration. Table 2.1 outlines these parameters, including skin turgor, position of the eye in the orbit, mucous membrane moisture level, heart rate, pulse strength, and level of consciousness. As these parameters are affected by body fat content, age, and other factors, assessment of hydration is a somewhat subjective procedure at best and is naturally subject to many inaccuracies. For instance, young and obese patients appear more hydrated than they really are, whereas old and cachectic patients appear less hydrated. Panting may dry mucous membranes, causing the patient to appear less hydrated. Therefore, these physical parameters can be expected to give the anesthetist only a general idea of hydration and must be used with other clinical data such as careful serial monitoring of body weight. This is an excellent indicator of hydration, with a sudden loss of 1 kg corresponding to 1 L of fluid loss.

Some clinical chemistry and hematology tests such as the plasma protein (PP) concentration and hematocrit also reflect hydration status and will be discussed in the following section on diagnostic testing.

In any case, if the animal appears significantly dehydrated, this should be corrected before anesthesia, because dehydration will impair tissue perfusion and predispose the patient to hypotension. Fluid administration is further discussed on p. 33.

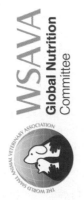

WSAVA
Global Nutrition
Committee

Body Condition
Score

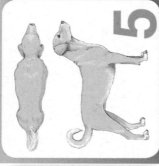
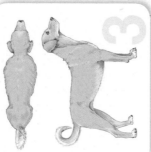
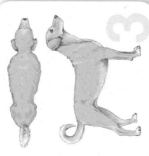
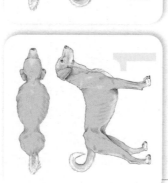

UNDER IDEAL

1. Ribs, lumbar vertebrae, pelvic bones and all bony prominences evident from a distance. No discernible body fat. Obvious loss of muscle mass.

2. Ribs, lumbar vertebrae and pelvic bones easily visible. No palpable fat. Some evidence of other bony prominences. Minimal loss of muscle mass.

3. Ribs easily palpated and may be visible with no palpable fat. Tops of lumbar vertebrae visible. Pelvic bones becoming prominent. Obvious waist and abdominal tuck.

IDEAL

4. Ribs easily palpable, with minimal fat covering. Waist easily noted, viewed from above. Abdominal tuck evident.

5. Ribs palpable without excess fat covering. Waist observed behind ribs when viewed from above. Abdomen tucked up when viewed from side.

OVER IDEAL

6. Ribs palpable with slight excess fat covering. Waist is discernible viewed from above but is not prominent. Abdominal tuck apparent.

7. Ribs palpable with difficulty; heavy fat cover. Noticeable fat deposits over lumbar area and base of tail. Waist absent or barely visible. Abdominal tuck may be present.

8. Ribs not palpable under very heavy fat cover, or palpable only with significant pressure. Heavy fat deposits over lumbar area and base of tail. Waist absent. No abdominal tuck. Obvious abdominal distention may be present.

9. Massive fat deposits over thorax, spine and base of tail. Waist and abdominal tuck absent. Fat deposits on neck and limbs. Obvious abdominal distention.

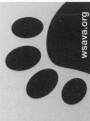
wsava.org

German A, et al. Comparison of a bioimpedance monitor with dual-energy x-ray absorptiometry for noninvasive estimation of percentage body fat in dogs. *AJVR* 2010;71:393-398.
Jeusette I, et al. Effect of breed on body composition and comparison between various methods to estimate body composition in dogs. *Res Vet Sci* 2010;88:227-232.
Kealy RD, et al. Effects of diet restriction on life span and age-related changes in dogs. *JAVMA* 2002;220:1315-1320
Laflamme DP. Development and validation of a body condition score system for dogs. *Canine Pract* 1997;22:10-15.

FIG. 2.2 Nine-level body condition scoring for dogs and cats. **(A)** Body condition scoring system for dogs.

Continued

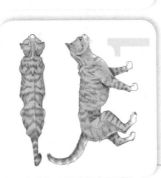
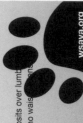
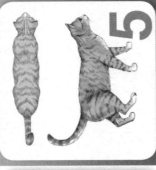
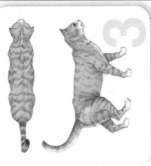
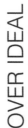
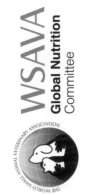

WSAVA
Global Nutrition Committee

Updated on August 13, 2020

Body Condition Score

9   7   5   3   1

UNDER IDEAL

1. Ribs very easily seen on short-haired cats. No fat pads present. Severe abdominal tuck. Lumbar vertebrae and pelvic bones easily seen and felt.

2. Ribs easily seen on short-haired cats. Lumbar vertebrae obvious. Pronounced abdominal tuck. No fat pads present.

3. Ribs easily felt with minimal fat covering. Lumbar vertebrae obvious. Obvious waist behind ribs. Minimal abdominal fat pads.

4. Ribs felt with minimal fat covering. Noticeable waist behind ribs. Slight abdominal tuck. Minimal abdominal fat pads.

IDEAL

5. Well-proportioned. Ribs felt with slight fat covering. Waist seen behind ribs, but not pronounced. Abdominal fat pad minimal.

OVER IDEAL

6. Ribs felt with slight excess fat covering. Waist and abdominal fat pad present but not obvious. Abdominal tuck absent.*

7. Ribs not easily felt through moderate fat covering. Waist not easily seen. Slight rounding of abdomen may be present. Moderate abdominal fat pad.

8. Ribs not felt due to excess fat covering. Waist absent. Obvious rounding of abdomen with prominent abdominal fat pad. Fat deposits present over lower back area.

9. Ribs not felt under heavy fat cover. Heavy fat deposits over lumbar area, face and limbs. Distention of abdomen with no waist. Extensive abdominal fat deposits.

A body condition score of 6/9 may be acceptable in some cats, especially older cats.

wsava.org

Bjornvad CR, et al. Evaluation of a nine-point body condition scoring system in physically inactive pet cats. AJVR 2011;72:433-437.
Laflamme DP. Development and validation of a body condition score system for cats: A clinical tool. Feline Pract 1997;25:13-18.
Teng KT et al., Strong associations of 9-point body condition scoring with survival and lifespan in cats. J Feline Med Surg. 2018;20(12);1110-1118. DOI: 10.1177/1098612X17752198

©2020. All rights reserved.

FIG. 2.2, cont'd (B) Body condition scoring system for cats. (From WSAVA Global Nutrition Committee. https://wsava.org/wp-content/uploads/2020/01/Body-Condition-Score-Dog.pdf and https://wsava.org/wp-content/uploads/2020/08/Body-Condition-Score-cat-updated-August-2020.pdf.)

TABLE 2.1 Physical Signs Associated With Dehydration

Percentage Dehydration	Physical Exam Findings[a]
<5%	Not detectable
~5% (Mild)	Minimal loss of skin turgor Semidry mucous membranes Eyes: normal
~8% (Moderate)	Moderate loss of skin turgor Dry mucous membranes Weak, rapid pulses Enophthalmos (depressed globes within orbits)
>10%	Considerable loss of skin turgor Extremely dry mucous membranes Tachycardia and weak/thready pulses Hypotension Severe enophthalmos Altered level of consciousness

[a]Not all animals will exhibit all signs.

Adapted from Davis H, Jensen T, Johnson A, et al: 2013 AAHA/AAFP fluid therapy guidelines for dogs and cats, *J Am Anim Hosp Assoc* 49(3):149–159, 2013.

TECHNICIAN NOTE Serial monitoring of body weight is an excellent indicator of hydration, with a sudden loss of 1 kg corresponding to 1 L of fluid loss.

TABLE 2.2 Assessment of Level of Consciousness

Signs	LOC (Traditional)	AVPU Scale
Fully conscious, alert, engaged and interested in the environment.	Bright, alert, responsive (B/A/R)	A *(Alert)*
Fully conscious and alert but not engaged due to fear, pain, illness, or any other cause. Subdued or quiet.	Quiet, alert, responsive (Q/A/R)	A *(Alert)*
Mildly depressed. Is aware of surroundings. Can be aroused with minimal difficulty (verbal or tactile stimulus).	Lethargic	A *(Alert)*
Very depressed. Uninterested in surroundings. Responds to but cannot be fully aroused by a verbal or tactile stimulus.	Obtunded	V *(Responds to a verbal stimulus)*
A sleeplike state. Nonresponsive to a verbal stimulus. Can be aroused only by a painful stimulus.	Stuporous	P *(Responds only to a painful stimulus)*
Sleeplike state. Cannot be aroused by any means.	Comatose	U *(Unresponsive)*

AVPU, Alert, verbal, pain, unresponsive; *LOC*, level of consciousness.

Level of Consciousness

Level of consciousness (LOC) refers to the patient's responsiveness to stimuli or how easily it can be aroused and is used to assess brain function. A decreased LOC indicates abnormal brain function and is caused by a variety of factors including hypoxia, drugs, dehydration, and neurologic disease.

The consciousness of healthy patients is often described as alert and responsive or alert and oriented. Patients can further be classified as "bright" if noticeably engaged and interested in the environment, or "quiet" or "subdued" if this is not the case. Therefore "B/A/R" is an abbreviation that may be used to describe patients that are bright, alert, and responsive, and "Q/A/R" may be used for patients that are quiet, alert, and responsive.

Patients with a mildly decreased LOC that can be aroused with minimal difficulty are said to be lethargic. The word *lethargy* is a noun describing this state. Patients that are more depressed and that cannot be fully aroused are referred to as obtunded (noun form: *obtundity*). A stuporous patient (noun form: *stupor*) is in a sleeplike state and can be aroused only with a painful stimulus. A comatose patient (noun form: *coma*) cannot be aroused and is unresponsive to all stimuli, including pain.

A system commonly used in human patients is referred to as the *AVPU scale*. Each letter represents one of four levels of consciousness: *A* for alert (which includes the classifications B/A/R, Q/A/R, and lethargic); *V* for a patient who responds to a verbal stimulus (equivalent to obtunded); *P* for a patient who responds to only a painful stimulus (equivalent to stuporous); and *U* for an unresponsive patient (equivalent to comatose). Although this system is not currently in common use in veterinary medicine, it can easily be applied to veterinary patients. Table 2.2 summarizes the methods used to assess LOC.

Pain Score

Assessment of the patient's level of pain should be included as a routine part of the patient assessment. The pain score will help guide the selection of preanesthetic and anesthetic agents. Refer to Chapter 8 for a discussion of methods used to determine the pain score.

Body Temperature

Body temperature is best determined using a rectal thermometer. Table 2.3 shows normal body temperatures in nonanesthetized animals. A high body temperature most commonly indicates an inflammatory condition, which must be identified and may require pretreatment with antibiotics, antiinflammatories, or other medication. A significantly low body temperature may be associated with one of a number of serious systemic disorders.

General Condition

The patient's general condition refers to findings that are revealed by visually examining the patient at a distance, including gait, temperament, and activity level.

Gait. Gait refers to the manner in which the patient moves. A patient with a normal gait places approximately equal weight

TABLE 2.3   Normal Vital Signs in Nonanesthetized Patients

Species	Body Temperature	Heart Rate	Heart Rhythms[a]				Respiratory Rate and Character
			NSR	SA	First degree AV Block	Second degree AV Block	
Dog	100–102.5°F (37.8–39.2°C)	60–180[b]	✓	✓			10–30 (panting is normal)
Cat	100–102.5°F (37.8–39.2°C)	120–240	✓				15–30
Horse	99–100.5°F (37.2–38°C)	30–45	✓	✓	✓ When at rest	✓ When at rest	8–20
Cow	100–102.5°F (37.8–39.2°C)	60–80	✓	✓			8–20
Sheep/goat	102–104°F (38.9–40°C)	60–90	✓	✓			16–24
All species							Normal effort and V_T

[a]Normal rhythms in each species are indicated by a checkmark.
[b]Owing to the extreme variability in size, large dogs tend to have lower rates, whereas small dogs and puppies have higher rates.
AV, Atrioventricular; *NSR,* normal sinus rhythm; *SA,* sinus arrhythmia; V_T, tidal volume.

on all limbs as it walks. A lame patient places unequal weight on the limbs, limps, or carries a limb, and may have sensitive or painful areas. Any of these signs may indicate a musculoskeletal disorder that may require treatment during the procedure or, in some cases, may indicate a nervous or systemic disorder that would increase anesthetic risk.

Temperament and activity level. The animal's temperament and activity level will affect the selection of anesthetic agents. For instance, an animal that is anxious or excited may override the effects of a phenothiazine tranquilizer. In this case, combining a phenothiazine tranquilizer with an opioid or giving a more potent agent such as an alpha2-agonist may be preferable. An ill patient may be excessively sedated with a standard dose of acepromazine, and the veterinarian may choose to reduce the dose of acepromazine, give a milder agent, or omit sedation entirely. Special handling techniques such as anesthetic chamber induction, or the use of intramuscular (IM) alpha2-agonists or Telazol (tiletamine–zolazepam) may be necessary to restrain feral or extremely aggressive patients without endangering hospital staff.

Exercise intolerance or weakness can indicate a variety of disorders that may affect anesthetic outcome, including anemia, heart disease, or electrolyte disturbances. When observed from a distance, a weak patient will be reluctant to rise, may not stand for long, or may appear unsteady on its feet. An exercise-intolerant patient will tire quickly, may refuse to run or play, or may breathe heavily after exercise. These patients may require alternative anesthetic protocols or treatment before the anesthetic procedure.

Examination of Exterior Surfaces

Examination of exterior surfaces consists of examination of the hair coat, the skin, lymph nodes, mammary glands, and body openings.

Coat condition. The hair coat should be shiny, full, and smooth. A rough hair coat, alopecia, or external parasites should be noted and reported. Although external infestations with ear mites, lice, fleas, ticks, or other parasites may not directly affect the anesthetic management, affected animals may require treatment during or after the anesthetic procedure.

Skin. Part the hair and examine the skin over the entire body, including the ventral surfaces. Run your hands over the entire body surface, because many masses may be hidden in the fur or on a part of the body difficult to see, such as the axilla or groin. Redness, inflammation, masses, or wounds should be noted and reported. Ecchymoses, purpura, or petechiae on the skin or mucous membranes, in the absence of trauma, indicate a clotting disorder, which will increase the risk of potentially life-threatening intraoperative and postoperative bleeding.

Lymph nodes and mammary glands. Examine the superficial lymph nodes and mammary glands for masses or swellings. This is best done with a combination of visual examination and palpation. Lymph nodes, if normal, should be very small or nonpalpable in small-animal patients. Enlarged lymph nodes in any patient may indicate the presence of infection, inflammation, or neoplasia.

Body openings. Examine all body openings for odors and discharges. Intact female patients should be examined for signs of estrus or milk production. Common causes of putrid (foul-smelling) odors include dental disease, external ear infections, abscesses, urogenital infections, diarrhea, and skin infections. Patients with severe kidney failure may have azotemic (urine-like) breath, and patients with ketonemia from complicated diabetes mellitus may have a characteristic odor to the breath. Some of the conditions that cause odors or discharges, such as kidney failure and diabetes, may necessitate treatment before anesthesia. Some, such as pyometra, may necessitate a change in the anesthetic protocol, and many others, including dental disease, abscesses, and ear infections, may require treatment while the patient is anesthetized.

Examination of the eyes, ears, nose, and oral cavity. The eyes, ears, nose, and oral cavity are often referred to as the "eyes, ears, nose, and throat," or EENT. Normal patients should not have discharges, inflammation, or swelling involving the oral cavity, ears, or nose. The eyes should be central, the corneas should be clear, and eye discharge or redness should not be present.

Air should move freely and quietly through the nares during breathing. Stridor may indicate an upper airway infection or obstruction. Any disorder that could impede endotracheal intubation, such as the presence of redundant tissue in the oropharynx, tumors, or jaw fractures, should be noted, because it may be necessary to intubate a patient so affected through a tracheotomy incision. The gingivae and mucous membranes should be pink and should not be inflamed, bleed, or show bruising.

Note the amount of dental tartar. A COHAT (aka: dental cleaning) must be performed using chemical restraint, so it is not uncommon to clean the teeth during the same anesthetic event used to perform another surgery or procedure as long as there is no anticipated detrimental effect of performing both procedures together. Combining two procedures minimizes the number of anesthetic events, decreases the number of visits to the clinic, and in most cases, also costs less. Therefore, identifying dental disease before anesthesia increases safety, value, convenience, and client satisfaction.

> **TECHNICIAN NOTE** A COHAT (aka: dental cleaning) is not uncommonly performed during the same anesthetic event used to perform another surgery or procedure. Combining two procedures minimizes the number of anesthetic events, decreases the number of visits to the clinic, and in most cases, also costs less.

Assessment of the pupillary light reflex. To check the pupillary light reflex (PLR), first observe and compare the size of both pupils, which should be of equal diameter. A patient with pupils of unequal sizes is said to have **anisocoria**. The pupil size depends on the amount of ambient light entering the eye, the patient's level of excitement, the patient's health, and the effect of medications. Next, direct a bright light (usually from a penlight or other portable light source) into the right eye with the beam directed toward the medial aspect of the retina, as this region is more sensitive to light. Note the size of the right pupil (direct reflex). Pupil constriction (**miosis**) is normal, whereas failure to constrict in the presence of light is abnormal. While still directing the light into the right eye, observe the pupil size in the left eye (consensual reflex); in a normal patient, the left pupil should constrict the same amount as the right pupil (Fig. 2.3). Finally, repeat the process on the left eye, looking for both a direct and consensual response. Note that the PLR may be diminished in excited animals or after the administration of some anesthetic agents and adjuncts, including anticholinergics and opioids.

Cardiovascular System Examination

Determination of the heart rate and rhythm. The heart rate and rhythm are generally most easily evaluated by **auscultation** of the heart over the left chest wall at the point of maximal intensity. With experience, the heart rate in beats per minute (bpm) can be accurately determined in small animals by counting the number of beats in 10 seconds and multiplying the number by 6 or by counting the number of beats in 15 seconds and multiplying the number by 4. Large-animal patients have slower heart rates; therefore counting for a period of 30 seconds and multiplying by 2 is more accurate. The heart may be difficult to assess, however, in obese patients, panting dogs, and purring cats, so the anesthetist must be familiar with techniques to deal with these situations. In obese patients (especially cats),

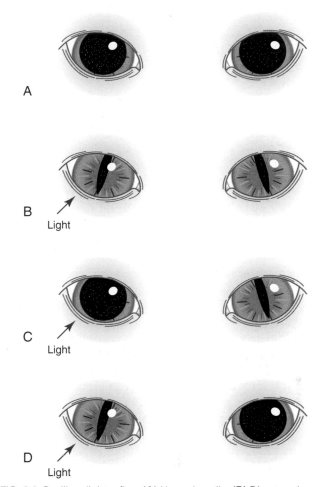

FIG. 2.3 Pupillary light reflex. **(A)** Normal pupils. **(B)** Direct and consensual light reflex (normal). **(C)** Consensual but no direct light reflex (abnormal). **(D)** Direct but no consensual light reflex (abnormal).

the audible intensity of the heartbeat is often decreased. Sometimes, palpation for the apical pulse is helpful to locate the optimal area for placement of the diaphragm of the stethoscope. When the apical pulse is not palpable, the anesthetist must carefully search in the region of the left axilla for a spot where the heart is most audible. This requires systematic, small, measured changes in the position of the stethoscope head until the optimal area is located. A decreased heart sound intensity in a nonobese patient may indicate pericardial or pleural effusion. Suspicion of either of these conditions should be communicated to the attending veterinarian.

> **TECHNICIAN NOTE** The heart rate in beats/minute (bpm) can be accurately determined in small animals by counting the number of beats in 10 seconds and multiplying the number by 6 (or the number of beats in 15 seconds and multiplying the number by 4). In large animals, count the number of beats in 30 seconds and multiply by 2.

When panting prevents the determination of a dog's heart rate, the muzzle can be gently held closed for a brief time to stop the panting, although this will cause some patients to struggle. For these patients, blow gently into the nose or distract the patient. One of these actions may stop the panting long enough to determine the rate. Do not attempt these techniques with aggressive patients if you are concerned for your safety.

Purring in cats can sometimes be stopped by distracting the patient or by turning on the tap in a sink and allowing the patient to see a gentle stream of running water from a distance. If this does not work, gradually bring the patient closer to the stream or increase the flow until the purring stops. Use caution, because some cats are more fearful of water than others and may scratch or bite if brought too close to the water. Placing an alcohol-soaked cotton ball near the cat's nose is another technique that may be effective.

Normal heart rates (see Table 2.3) are generally inversely proportional to body size (faster in smaller species and breeds and slower in larger species and breeds). In all species, pediatric patients tend to have higher rates than adults. Exercise or the stress of handling may cause the heart rate to increase. The heart rate should be measured when the patient is calm, not after stressful events such as inserting a rectal thermometer or collecting a blood sample.

Normal heart rhythms vary according to the species (see Table 2.3). Normal dogs may have either a normal sinus rhythm (NSR) or a sinus arrhythmia (SA). Cats and most other exotic mammals such as rabbits, ferrets, and rodents should always have an NSR, as an SA is not normal in these species. Horses and ruminants usually have an NSR or SA. Horses may also exhibit first- or second-degree atrioventricular (AV) block when at rest but will have an NSR after exercise. The sound of these rhythms is summarized below in the following paragraphs.

Normal sinus rhythm. NSR is a completely regular rhythm with no irregularities or pauses between beats, although the rate may change in response to excitement level.

Sinus arrhythmia. SA is a rhythm in which the heart rate cyclically increases during inspiration and decreases during expiration. This rhythm may be pronounced in young, healthy dogs, and can sound to the inexperienced anesthetist as if there are skipped or premature beats. Abnormal rhythms can be differentiated from SA by observing the respirations while listening to the heart. Abnormal rhythms are not associated with the breathing.

First-degree atrioventricular heart block. First-degree AV heart block is caused by a conduction delay through the AV node and is recognized by a prolonged PR interval on an electrocardiogram (ECG) tracing. This rhythm causes no noticeable change in the heart sounds and therefore can be detected only by electrocardiography.

Second-degree atrioventricular heart block. Second-degree AV heart block is caused by a periodic block of electrical conduction through the AV node and is recognized by missing QRS complexes on the ECG tracing. On auscultation, periodic pauses representing skipped beats are audible. Note that it is not normal for more than one beat to be skipped in a row.

Any abnormal rhythms must be reported to the attending veterinarian, because they may be exacerbated or become life-threatening during anesthesia. (More detail regarding these rhythms may be found in Chapter 6.)

> **TECHNICIAN NOTE** SA is a rhythm in which the heart rate cyclically increases during inspiration and decreases during expiration. This rhythm may be pronounced in young, healthy dogs, and can sound to the inexperienced anesthetist as if there are skipped or premature beats. Abnormal rhythms can be differentiated from SA by observing the respirations while listening to the heart.

Examination for murmurs. During auscultation, also check for heart murmurs. Listen over each valve and place the stethoscope diaphragm into the cranial-most aspect of the left axilla because some murmurs, including those associated with patent ductus arteriosus, are often audible only in this location. Murmurs are caused by turbulence associated with abnormal flow of blood and may indicate a variety of conditions such as a leaking valve, a stenotic valve or vessel, or an abnormal communication between heart chambers, any of which may increase anesthetic risk.

Palpation of the pulse and comparison with the heart rate. In the conscious dog and cat, the pulse is most easily palpated at the femoral artery, on the medial side of the rear leg. The patient should be standing quietly, and the femoral artery should be located by cupping the hand around the medial aspect of the thigh with the pad of the first or second finger in the groin just over the femur (see Chapter 6, Fig. 6.35B). Other sites that may be palpable on medium to large dogs include the metatarsal and metacarpal arteries. In large animals, the pulse may be palpated at the facial artery, digital artery, ventral tail, or auricular artery.

A strong, regular pulse should closely follow each audible heartbeat. If there are more heartbeats than pulses, a pulse deficit exists, which may indicate the presence of cardiovascular disease.

Palpation of the pulse also may give a crude estimate of blood pressure. A weak or nonpalpable pulse suggests hypotension, whereas an exaggerated pulse suggests hypertension. Realize that this is not always reliable because many other factors, including body conformation, drugs, patient temperament, and excitement, may affect either the strength of the pulse or the ability of the anesthetist to feel it.

Assessment of mucous membrane color and capillary refill time. The standard site for assessment is the gingiva at the base of a tooth. Normal mucous membrane color is pink, although the color varies somewhat from patient to patient. Capillary refill time is assessed by applying digital pressure on the gingiva until blanching occurs, releasing the pressure, and then observing the amount of time it takes for the return of normal color (see Chapter 6, Fig. 6.34). Normal refill time is less than 2 seconds in all common domestic species. Pale mucous membranes or prolonged capillary refill times are indicative of decreased perfusion from shock, vasoconstriction, hypotension, or a variety of other conditions. Pale mucous membranes can also be associated with anemia. Cyanotic mucous membranes indicate reduced oxygen saturation, which is a medical emergency. Any of these conditions will increase anesthetic risk and must be treated before the procedure. If the gingivae are pigmented, mucous membrane color and capillary refill time may be observed at other sites, such as the conjunctiva of the lower eyelid, the entrance to the vulva, or the tip of the prepuce.

> **TECHNICIAN NOTE** Pale mucous membranes or prolonged capillary refill time are indicative of decreased perfusion from shock, vasoconstriction, hypotension, or a variety of other issues. Pale mucous membranes can also be associated with anemia. Cyanotic mucous membranes indicate reduced oxygen saturation, which is a medical emergency.

Respiratory System Examination

Determination of respiratory rate and character. The respiratory rate in breaths per minute and the respiratory character are best evaluated by visually observing chest excursions. In most cases, the respiratory rate can be accurately determined in small and large animals by counting the breaths in 30 seconds and multiplying the result by 2. Auscultation is not a particularly useful tool for assessing respiration. As with the heart rate, the respiratory rate is generally inversely proportional to body size and age and will be affected by exercise or stress. Normal dogs may pant during examination. In this situation, as long as the respiratory effort is normal, the rate may be entered in the medical record as "pant" instead of attempting to count the rate. (See Table 2.3 for normal respiratory rates in nonanesthetized animals.)

Respiratory character refers to other aspects of respiration, including effort, relative length of inhalation and exhalation, and regularity. Patients with a normal respiratory cycle should inhale, immediately exhale, and then briefly rest before the next inhalation. Exhalation should be about twice as long as inhalation. Normal respiration should be even, smooth, and minimally visible when the patient is at rest.

Dyspneic patients may exhibit mouth breathing, flared nostrils, excessive panting, exaggerated chest or abdominal movements on inspiration, wheezing, and reluctance to lie down. In extreme cases, a dyspneic animal may exhibit cyanosis. Dyspnea and cyanosis are both medical emergencies and should be brought to the veterinarian's attention immediately. Avoid stressing dyspneic or cyanotic patients, as they are very intolerant of handling and can die during even mild restraint for PE.

> **TECHNICIAN NOTE** Dyspnea and cyanosis are both medical emergencies and should be brought to the veterinarian's attention immediately. Avoid stressing dyspneic or cyanotic patients, as they are very intolerant of handling and can die during examination.

Auscultation of the lungs. Assess the lungs by auscultating each of the four quadrants of the thorax (the right and left anteroventral lung fields and the right and left dorsal lung fields). In normal, calm patients, the lung sounds should be very quiet.

The presence of discontinuous lung sounds (crackles, rales, or rhonchi) or continuous sounds (wheezes) may indicate either pulmonary conditions (including pneumonia, bronchial disease, or asthma) or heart failure.

Abdominal Palpation and Auscultation

The normal abdomen should be soft to the touch and not painful. In small animals, most normal organs are difficult to feel except for a full urinary bladder, full colon, and, in cats, the kidneys. Any firm or painful structure or any organ that feels larger than normal should be reported. Abdominal distention may indicate ascites, pregnancy, organ enlargement, or the presence of tumors. In large animals, abdominal auscultation is used to detect normal borborygmus (gut sounds). Borborygmus should be present in all four abdominal quadrants in horses. In ruminants, normal contraction of the rumen is audible in the left paralumbar fossa.

Preanesthetic Diagnostic Workup

After the history and PE are completed, the veterinarian will decide which diagnostic tests (if any) are recommended for a given patient. The technician or nurse will then obtain appropriate samples (blood, urine, feces, or other samples) and will either perform the tests or forward the samples to a diagnostic laboratory for testing.

There are no universal guidelines for preanesthetic diagnostic tests, but each facility has standard policies. Some tests may be routinely recommended for every animal scheduled for anesthesia; different test groupings may be recommended for different patient groups such as geriatric patients, patients undergoing elective surgeries, and sick patients; or recommended tests may be based on the physical status class. The veterinarian may customize tests on the basis of the patient's age, history, and the results of the PE. Financial and other considerations may affect the number and type of tests the client chooses to approve. If the client declines one or more tests, a waiver should be signed indicating that the client understands the risk of proceeding without the information that would be provided by the declined tests. Table 2.4 lists a sample of preanesthetic diagnostic testing recommendations based on the American Society of Anesthesiologists (ASA) Physical Status Classification. See page 29 for a discussion of this system.

Common preanesthetic diagnostic tests and procedures include the complete blood count (CBC), blood chemistries, parasite screens, complete urinalysis, serologic tests, coagulation screen, ECG, and thoracic radiographs. Other tests may be ordered, based on other conditions or illnesses that may be present. All test results must be recorded in the medical record and reviewed by the attending veterinarian before the commencement of the procedure.

Complete Blood Count

The CBC is a comprehensive evaluation of blood cell numbers and morphology that includes packed cell volume (PCV), PP, hemoglobin, total red blood cell (RBC), white blood cell (WBC), platelet, and absolute leukocyte counts. Normal values for these parameters are given in Table 2.5.

TABLE 2.4 Sample Preanesthetic Diagnostic Test Recommendations based on ASA Physical Status Classification

Species	ASA Physical Status Classification	Age	Recommended Tests
Dogs[a]/cats[b]	PS1 and PS2	<5 years	PCV and PP, and possibly urine specific gravity
	PS1 and PS2	>5 years	CBC/chemistry profile and possibly complete UA
	PS3-PS5	Any age	As ordered by the attending veterinarian
Ruminants	PS1 and PS2	Any age	PCV and PP
	PS3-PS5	Any age	As ordered by the attending veterinarian
Horses	PS1 and PS2	Any age	CBC and PP
	PS3-PS5	Any age	As ordered by the attending veterinarian

[a]Heartworm testing is recommended for all dogs. Some clinics may extend this requirement to feline patients as well.
[b]All cats should be screened for feline leukemia virus (FeLV) and feline immunodeficiency virus (FIV) before anesthesia.
ASA, American Society of Anesthesiologists; *CBC*, complete blood count; *PCV*, packed cell volume; *PP*, plasma protein; *UA*, urinalysis.

TABLE 2.5 Normal Hematologic Values

	Dog	Cat	Horse	Cow
Plasma protein (g/dL)	5.7–7.2	5.6–7.4	6.5–7.8	7–9
PCV (%)	36–54	25–46	27–44	23–35
Hb (g/dL)	11.9–18.4	8.0–14.9	9.7–15.6	8.3–12.3
RBC (10^{12}/L)	4.9–8.2	5.3–10.2	5.1–10.0	5–7.5
Total leukocytes ($\times 10^9$/L)	4.1–15.2	4.0–14.5	4.7–10.6	3.0–13.5
Neutrophil—segmented ($\times 10^9$/L)	3–10.4	3–9.2	2.4–6.4	0.7–5.1
Neutrophil—band ($\times 10^9$/L)	0–0.1	0–0.1	0–0.1	0–0.1
Lymphocytes ($\times 10^9$/L)	1–4.6	0.9–3.9	1–4.9	1.1–8.2
Monocytes ($\times 10^9$/L)	0–1.2	0–0.5	0–0.5	0–0.6
Eosinophils ($\times 10^9$/L)	0–1.3	0–1.2	0–0.3	0–1.5
Basophils ($\times 10^9$/L)	0	0–0.2	0–0.1	0–0.1
Platelets ($\times 10^9$/L)	106–424	150–600	125–310	192–746

Modified from Muir WW, Hubbell JA, Bednarski RM, Lerche P: *Handbook of veterinary anesthesia*, ed 5, St. Louis, 2013, Elsevier.
Hb, Hemoglobin; *PCV*, packed cell volume; *RBC*, red blood cells.

The PCV is a measurement of the percentage of the total blood volume that is made up of whole RBCs. The total RBC count (erythrocyte count) is a direct measurement of the total number of RBCs in a fixed volume of blood. Both tests are indicators of the oxygen-carrying capacity of the blood.

An elevated PCV or RBC count is most often caused by dehydration and is of concern to the anesthetist because of the associated decrease in blood volume, which may adversely affect cardiac output, blood pressure, and tissue perfusion.

In contrast, a decreased PCV or RBC count indicates anemia caused by decreased production, loss, or destruction of RBCs. Anemia results in a decreased capacity to supply oxygen to the tissues. Because the effects of anesthesia often increase the risk of tissue hypoxia, anemia must not be ignored. When a significant anemia is present, the veterinarian may recommend that anesthesia be postponed until it is corrected. A PCV of less than 25% in a dog or less than 20% in a cat, horse, or cow should be reported immediately.

The PP is a measurement of blood protein including albumin, globulins, and fibrinogen. As with an elevated PCV, hyperproteinemia may be associated with dehydration and the same potential adverse consequences mentioned previously.

Hypoproteinemia usually results from decreased protein production by the liver or increased loss from the gastrointestinal tract or kidneys, or from blood loss. Many anesthetics circulate in the blood partially bound to PPs and partially free. Only the portion of the drug that is free and unbound can exert an effect. In patients with hypoproteinemia, the unbound portion proportionately increases, increasing drug potency. Hypoproteinemic patients also have difficulty maintaining adequate blood volume and may develop tissue edema because of the decreased oncotic pressure in the vascular system. For these reasons, a PP less than 4.0 g/dL in a patient of any species should be reported immediately.

The total WBC and absolute leukocyte counts (calculated from the total WBC and the differential WBC counts) measure the total number of leukocytes and the number of each type of leukocyte (neutrophils, lymphocytes, monocytes, eosinophils, and basophils). Changes in these counts may be associated with infection, parasitism, leukemias, and many other conditions that may be exacerbated by anesthesia and surgery or may increase anesthetic risk. The blood smear evaluation reveals changes in blood cell morphology, inclusions, parasites, and other conditions that may influence preanesthetic patient management. Interpretation of these tests is complex and beyond the scope of this chapter.

The platelet count is necessary to evaluate the mechanical component of blood coagulation. Patients with **thrombocytopenia** are at higher risk for abnormal intraoperative and postoperative bleeding, and their condition must be stabilized before surgery. Any decrease in platelet numbers should be reported to the attending veterinarian immediately.

TECHNICIAN NOTE The following findings should be reported to the attending veterinarian immediately:
- A PCV <25% in a dog or <20% in a cat, horse, or cow
- A PP <4.0 g/dL in any species
- Any decrease in the platelet count
- Any coagulation test result outside the normal range

Urinalysis

The complete urinalysis provides information about both the urinary and nonurinary systems. Kidney function is of particular interest to the anesthetist, as it plays an important role in regulating electrolyte and water balance, blood pressure, and elimination of many anesthetics. If there is protein in the urine or if the urine specific gravity is less than 1.030 in a canine sample, 1.035 in a feline sample, or 1.025 in a large-animal sample, the veterinarian should be notified because further tests may be needed to assess kidney function accurately.

Abnormalities in the macroscopic examination findings (color, clarity, and odor), biochemical analysis, and microscopic examination findings also may reveal evidence of diabetes mellitus, liver or kidney disease, or other systemic disorders that may affect patient anesthetic management. Abnormalities in any of these parts of the urinalysis should be reported and investigated.

Blood Chemistry Tests

A wide variety of blood chemistry tests is available to assess circulating enzymes, electrolytes, proteins, metabolites, and metabolic products. These tests give information about organ health and function, help the veterinarian formulate the anesthetic plan, screen for conditions that increase patient risk or influence perianesthetic patient management, and allow preparation for potential complications. Chemistry tests are often grouped in preanesthetic profiles that may assess one body organ such as the kidney, the liver, or the pancreas, or may provide a comprehensive evaluation of all organ systems. Chemistry tests commonly assayed may be found in Table 2.6.

As with any other diagnostic testing, some chemistry tests are typically used routinely to assess any patient regardless of historical findings or physical exam findings, whereas others are used only for patients with specific risk factors. For instance, in the case of cats, the AAFP Feline Anesthesia Guidelines recommend retroviral testing in all patients up to 2 years of age, test selection based on clinical judgement of the attending veterinarian in patients between 3 and 6 years of age, general chemistry screening (along with CBC and urinalysis) in all patients 7 years of age or older, and a T4 in all patients over 10 years of age. Each of the tests already mentioned (retroviral testing, general chemistry screening, and T4), as well as other tests, such as NT-proBNP screening for asymptomatic heart disease, may be indicated on some animals of any age based on signalment, history, and physical exam findings.[b] In any case, the interpretation of chemistry tests is complex, so any abnormalities should be reported to the veterinarian.

Blood Coagulation Screens

Blood coagulation screens evaluate the chemical, and sometimes mechanical, components of blood coagulation. This is particularly important before nonelective surgeries because various disorders may adversely affect blood coagulation and put surgery patients at high risk for intraoperative and postoperative hemorrhage. A coagulation panel, including prothrombin time (PT) and activated partial thromboplastin time (APTT), should be performed on any patient that may have a preexisting coagulation disorder (such as those with end-stage liver disease) or animals of breeds known to be

TABLE 2.6 Chemistry Assays Commonly Used to Evaluate General Health

Kidney health	BUN; Creatinine; SDMA; Potassium and other electrolytes; Blood gases
Liver health	ALT (Ca, Fe), AST, SDH (LA), GLDH (Ru), AP, GGT Bilirubin; bile acids
Pancreas health	Amylase, lipase, TLI (Ca, Fe), PLI (Ca, Fe), triglycerides
Endocrine system health	Glucose, cholesterol, triglycerides, Thyroid (T4), cortisol levels Electrolytes (e.g., sodium, potassium and chloride) Minerals (calcium, phosphorus, and magnesium)
Skeletal and cardiac muscle health	CPK (CK), NT-proBNP (primarily Fe)
Energy metabolism	Glucose, triglycerides, fructosamine, lactic acid (primarily Eq)
Protein metabolism	Total protein, albumin, globulin, A:G ratio
Pulmonary function and metabolic processes	Blood gases (PaO, PaCO$_2$, HCO$_3$ [bicarbonate], and pH)—(primarily for Eq patients)
Inflammation	Fibrinogen and SAA (Eq)
Infectious disease	Heartworm (Ca, Fe) FeLV, FIV (Fe)

[a]Note interpretation of chemistry assays is complex as most are influenced by multiple organ systems and conditions. Therefore some of these assays may be used to assess multiple organ systems, physiologic processes, or conditions.
A:G, Albumin:globulin; ALT, alanine aminotransferase; AP, Alkaline phosphatase; AST, aspartate aminotransferase; BUN, blood urea nitrogen; NT-proBNP, N-terminal pro hormone B-type natriuretic peptide; Ca, canine; CPK or CK, creatine phosphokinase; Eq, equine; Fe, feline; FeLV, feline leukemia virus; FIV, feline immunodeficiency virus; GGT, gamma glutamyltranspeptidase; GLDH, glutamate dehydrogenase; PaCO$_2$, arterial partial pressure of carbon dioxide; PaO$_2$, arterial partial pressure of oxygen; PLI, pancreatic lipase immunoreactivity; Ru, ruminants; SAA, serum amyloid A; SDH, sorbitol dehydrogenase; SDMA, symmetric dimethylarginine; TLI, trypsinlike immunoreactivity.

commonly affected by hereditary coagulation disorders, such as Doberman Pinschers, Rottweilers, and Scottish Terriers. Coagulation panels may be performed at reference laboratories or in house. Any abnormal coagulation test result should be reported to the attending veterinarian immediately. The buccal mucosal bleeding time is an in-house screening test that can be used in any patient, including those with normal platelet counts and coagulation panels, if there is evidence of abnormal primary hemostasis (abnormal formation of a platelet plug) (Procedure 2.1).

> **TECHNICIAN NOTE** The buccal mucosal bleeding time is an in-house screening test that can be used in any patient, including those with normal platelet counts and coagulation panels, if there is evidence of abnormal primary hemostasis (abnormal formation of a platelet plug).

Electrocardiogram

The ECG records the electrical activity of the heart, allowing the veterinarian to assess heart rhythm. Although not routine,

[b]Robertson SA, Gogolski SM, Pascoe P, et al: AAFP feline anesthesia guidelines. *J Feline Med Surg* 20:602–634, 2018.

PROCEDURE 2.1 Buccal Mucosal Bleeding Time

The **buccal mucosal bleeding time** is an in-house coagulation screen that gives an estimation of platelet function. It can be easily performed on any anesthetized animal but may also be performed on conscious patients.

This test primarily evaluates platelet function, but results may be abnormal in patients with other problems such as thrombocytopenia and von Willebrand disease. In contrast, results may be normal in patients with other coagulation disorders.

Equipment
- Spring-loaded lancet that makes two side-by-side cuts of a standard length and depth, such as the Simplate II (6 mm long and 1 mm deep), Surgicutt Adult (5 mm long and 1 cm deep), or Surgicutt Junior (2.5 mm long × 0.5 mm deep).
- Stopwatch
- Filter paper
- Roll gauze

Procedure
1. Place the patient in lateral recumbency.
2. Fold the lip back and tie with gauze so the mucosa of the lip cranial to the tie is slightly engorged (Fig. 1).

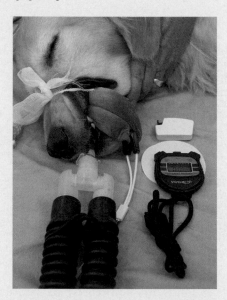

3. Activate the lancet on the lip cranial to the tie, but away from major blood vessels.
4. Start the stopwatch (Fig. 2).

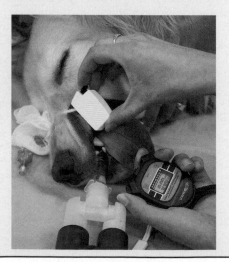

5. Wick blood from the area with the filter paper (without touching the incisions) at 5-s intervals until blood no longer appears from the incisions (Fig. 3).

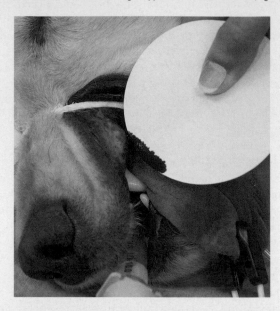

6. Stop the stopwatch when the bleeding stops.
7. Release the gauze.
8. Report the time from when the incision was made to blood clotting (Fig. 4).

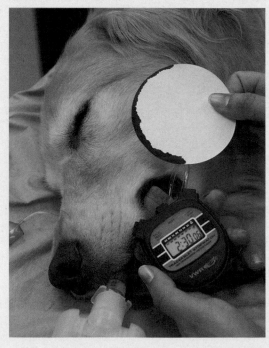

9. If clotting takes longer than 15 min, stop the test, release the gauze, apply pressure to the cuts, and report as ">15 min."

Note. Normal values: Dog, <4 min (Simplate II and Surgicutt Adult); Cat, <2 min (Surgicutt Junior).

an ECG is recommended for those patients with known or suspected heart disease, chest trauma, gastric dilatation–volvulus, splenic disease, electrolyte disturbances, or those that are on medications that affect heart rhythm. The ECG also can be used to screen for cardiac disease in geriatric or other high-risk patients. Because most anesthetic agents alter heart rate, cardiac output, and oxygen consumption to some degree, patients with heart disease are at much greater risk for anesthetic complications. (ECGs are further discussed in Chapter 6.)

Radiography

Although not routine, thoracic radiography is warranted in animals that show signs of cardiac or pulmonary disease. Thoracic and abdominal radiographs are indicated for animals with major trauma (such as those that have been hit by a car) to rule out conditions that could increase anesthetic risk or require modification of the protocol such as diaphragmatic hernia, pneumothorax, pleural effusion, pulmonary contusions, bladder rupture, or intraabdominal bleeding.

Miscellaneous Tests

Depending on patient need, existing illness, the geographic location of the practice, and other factors, other diagnostic tests may be routinely performed before anesthesia. For example, most veterinary practices in areas where heartworm disease is endemic require a heartworm test for all dogs and, in some cases, cats before any anesthetic procedure.

DETERMINATION OF THE PHYSICAL STATUS CLASSIFICATION

Before selecting the anesthetic protocol, the attending veterinarian should evaluate the minimum patient database and assign a physical status classification. The most widely accepted classification system is the one adopted by the ASA, which is summarized in Table 2.7. This system is used to assess the patient's overall health preoperatively by placing the patient into one of five grades ranging from a normal, healthy patient (class PS1) to one that is moribund and not expected to survive without the surgery (class PS5). A sixth class (PS6) signifies a brain-dead organ donor and so is not commonly applied to veterinary patients. Patients undergoing emergency anesthesia may also be assigned an additional letter E regardless of class (e.g., PS2E or PS5E). Clinically, this system is most often used to guide the selection of an appropriate anesthetic protocol based on the patient's physical status.

The physical status classification system is commonly understood as a way to gauge anesthetic risk. It is not always an accurate predictor of overall risk level, however, because it does not take into account a number of important factors that affect outcome such as the patient's age, the risk inherent in the procedure being performed, and quality of postoperative care. Instead, it should be viewed as a basis for anesthetic event planning, for communication between colleagues, and for recordkeeping. In general, class PS1 and class PS2 patients can be anesthetized with standard anesthetic protocols. Class PS3 to PS5 patients often require special, individually tailored protocols, and should be stabilized before surgery if possible.

Physical status classification is somewhat subjective and may change over time. Two anesthetists might disagree, for example, on whether a patient with moderate anemia should be assigned to class PS2 or class PS3. A patient in shock might be downgraded to a lower risk classification after receiving appropriate IV fluid therapy. Nevertheless, this system gives the anesthetist some basis for making patient management decisions that are appropriate for the patient. The physical status class should be recorded in the animal's medical record and in the anesthetic logbook.

> **TECHNICIAN NOTE** In general, class PS1 and class PS2 patients can be anesthetized with standard anesthetic protocols. Class PS3 to PS5 patients often require special protocols and should be stabilized before surgery if possible.

TABLE 2.7	American Society of Anesthesiologists Physical Status Classifications		
Classification	**Risk**	**Criteria**	**Representative Conditions**
PS1	Minimal	Normal, healthy patient	Patients undergoing elective procedures (ovariohysterectomy, castration, or declaw)
PS2	Low	Patient with mild systemic disease	Obese patient Mild dehydration Low-grade heart murmur
PS3	Moderate	Patient with severe systemic disease	Anemia Moderate dehydration Compensated major organ disease
PS4	High	Patient with severe systemic disease that is a constant threat to life	Ruptured bladder Internal hemorrhage Pneumothorax Pyometra
PS5	Extreme	Moribund patient that is not expected to survive without the operation	Severe head trauma Pulmonary embolus Gastric dilatation–volvulus End-stage major organ failure

Modified from Bassert JM, Beal AD, Samples OM: *McCurnin's clinical textbook for veterinary technicians*, ed 10, St Louis, 2022, Elsevier.

SELECTION OF THE ANESTHETIC PROTOCOL

As mentioned in the previous sections, the technician or nurse acting as an anesthetist should not hesitate to discuss abnormal findings from the minimum database with the veterinarian because such information may lead to changes in the planned anesthetic protocol. The presence of severe disease does not necessarily require that the procedure be postponed or canceled, although this may be the wisest course in some situations. It does often require the selection of agents with which the anesthetist may be less familiar but that are less likely to produce adverse effects. For example, the attending veterinarian may choose to use etomidate instead of propofol in a geriatric dog with heart failure because etomidate is much less likely to affect cardiovascular function adversely.

If the patient is very ill, the veterinarian may decide that the animal's condition must be stabilized before an anesthetic is administered. Patients that are severely dehydrated, profoundly anemic, or have a serious systemic disease or electrolyte imbalance are poor anesthetic risks. Every attempt should be made to correct these conditions before anesthesia, if time allows. If the planned procedure is not immediately necessary to save the patient's life, it is possible that anesthesia may safely be postponed.

Factors That Influence Selection

In all jurisdictions in the United States and Canada, the veterinarian is the only health care provider legally allowed to choose (i.e., prescribe) anesthetic drugs for animals. In most hospitals, however, the veterinarian establishes one or two standard anesthetic protocols for patients of physical status class P1 and P2, with which the technician or nurse will quickly become familiar. However, each patient must be evaluated individually based on the minimum patient database, and changes must be made to the standard protocol when necessary. Although a technician or nurse with a strong knowledge base can help the veterinarian make an appropriate choice by communicating observations and suggestions regarding the patient, ultimately, the attending veterinarian bears responsibility for the patient and must make the final decision regarding the anesthetic protocol.

When choosing the anesthetic protocol, the following factors must be considered.

Facilities and Equipment

Some anesthetic protocols require the use of specialized equipment. For example, isoflurane and sevoflurane require the use of a precision vaporizer and an oxygen supply. In some circumstances, such as equine field anesthesia, the use of a machine is impractical or impossible.

Familiarity With the Agent

Although for most patients any one of several anesthetic protocols is likely to result in a successful outcome, practitioners frequently choose the protocol with which they are most familiar. It is seldom advisable to anesthetize a high-risk patient with a new combination of drugs that the anesthetist may have heard or read about but has never tried before.

Nature of the Procedure

Procedures vary in their duration and complexity. They also require different degrees of analgesia, immobilization, muscle relaxation, and CNS depression. For example, local anesthesia may be suitable for short procedures such as a skin biopsy in which the patient requires only anesthesia of the biopsy site and physical restraint but no CNS depression. However, general anesthesia is required for thoracic or abdominal surgery, which necessitates unconsciousness, immobility, generalized visceral and somatic analgesia, and muscle relaxation.

Circumstances Specific to the Procedure

Anesthetics that may be appropriate for animals undergoing a routine operation (such as ovariohysterectomy or orchiectomy) may not be appropriate for a nonelective surgical procedure. For example, a cesarean section will require a protocol that minimizes respiratory depression in the neonates. In contrast, excellent muscle relaxation may be important for a fracture repair.

Cost

In a situation in which two agents are comparable in terms of patient safety, it is reasonable to choose the less-expensive option. In other situations, such as the presence of cardiac disease, it may be important to choose a cardiac-sparing drug such as etomidate even though it is considerably more expensive than a ketamine–midazolam mixture or propofol.

Degree of Urgency

Critically injured animals may require rapid induction of anesthesia to initiate emergency therapy. For example, a patient that is in danger of shock because of ongoing uncontrolled hemorrhage cannot wait 15 to 20 minutes for a premedication given subcutaneously or IM to take effect. Selection of agents that allow preservation of adequate blood pressure and rapid induction is desirable in this case.

PREINDUCTION PATIENT CARE

During the preinduction period, the technician or nurse should ensure that the patient has been fasted and receives appropriate nursing care, fluid therapy, medication administration, and any other care ordered by the veterinarian. All treatments should be recorded in the medical record. A checklist of procedures may be helpful, particularly if more than one person is responsible for preanesthetic care.

Withholding Food Before Anesthesia

Animals that are anesthetized without prior fasting are prone to a variety of mild to serious complications that result from reflux of stomach contents into the distal esophagus, aspiration of stomach contents into the pulmonary tree, and bloating in ruminants (see Chapter 11).

Esophageal reflux commonly occurs during the anesthetic period as a result of decreased lower esophageal sphincter tone and flow of stomach acid into the esophagus that occurs when a patient is in a prone position. Esophageal reflux may cause irritation, inflammation, or, in extreme cases, severe tissue

TABLE 2.8 Fasting Recommendations for Dogs and Cats

Patient Status	Food Withholding Time (Hours)	Water Withholding Time (Hours)	Notes
Healthy adult	4–6	None	Consider small amount of treats in hospital to facilitate gentle handing/decrease patient stress.
Adult <2 kg in body weight	≤1–2	None	May offer pate-consistency wet food during preop period. Schedule procedure as first case of the day.
Neonatal and pediatric patients (<8 weeks old)	≤1–2 *(note that some authors recommend none)*	None	May offer pate-consistency wet food during preop period. Schedule procedure as first case of the day.
Diabetic adult	2–4	None	Give 50% of normal amount of pate-consistency wet food and $1/2$ normal insulin dose 2–4 h prior to induction. Schedule procedure as first case of the day.
Patient with a history of or at risk for regurgitation	6–12	6–12	Consider 10%–25% of normal amount of pate-consistency wet food 4–6 h prior to induction
Emergent cases	As soon as possible	As soon as possible	Stabilize prior to induction

Other recommendations include (1) administration of ongoing oral medications (such as anxiolytics and analgesics) with 1–2 TBSP of wet food or coating pills in an edible pastelike material; and (2) a small amount of treats after arrival at the hospital to facilitate low stress handling in healthy patients based on the attending veterinarian's clinical judgement.
Modified from Grubb T, Sager J, Gaynor JS, et al: 2020 AAHA anesthesia and monitoring guidelines for dogs and cats, *J Am Anim Hosp Assoc* 56(2):59–82, 2020.

damage of the distal esophagus, resulting in stricture, and is recognized as a common cause of postoperative nausea, dysphagia, vomiting, and anorexia.

Vomiting is an active expulsion of stomach contents, preceded by retching, that occurs only in conscious patients. In contrast, regurgitation is a passive process that may occur in an unconscious or conscious patient, is not preceded by retching, and results in the flow of stomach contents into the esophagus and mouth. Pulmonary aspiration occurs if the patient vomits or regurgitates during a time when the swallowing reflex is decreased or absent. Pulmonary aspiration is always serious and may lead to pneumonia that is difficult to treat, permanent disability, and in some cases, even immediate respiratory arrest and death.

To prevent vomiting and minimize reflux during the anesthetic period, food should be withheld from most patients except for neonatal, pediatric, and some exotic patients. Traditionally, food withholding for 8 to 12 hours and water withholding of 2 to 4 hours in adult dogs and cats has been recommended. In recent years, however, many clinicians have begun to reconsider traditional fasting recommendations based on clinical experience and research that has suggested that the incidence of gastric reflux, regurgitation, and vomiting are significantly influenced by a variety of factors in addition to the duration of the fasting period. Other factors include the type and volume of food eaten before the fast and the patient's anxiety level. For instance, anxiety, a large meal size, and consuming food with low moisture content (i.e., dry food) may slow gastric emptying and increase the risk. In addition, excessive withholding can negatively impact hydration as well as secretion of digestive juices into the stomach. Based on these findings, many clinicians now recommend shorter fasting for many patients. A summary of current recommendations in the 2020 AAHA Anesthesia and Monitoring Guidelines for Dogs and Cats may be found in Table 2.8. Current fasting recommendations for large animals may be found in Table 2.9.

TABLE 2.9 Fasting Recommendations for Large Animals

Species	Food Withholding Time (Hours)	Water Withholding Time (Hours)
Horses	8–12	0–2
Adult cattle	24–48	8–12
Small ruminants	12–18	8–12
Neonatal and pediatric patients (<8 weeks old)	None	None

If a patient is known to have eaten within the recommended fasting period and the surgery cannot be postponed, the veterinarian may choose to administer a preanesthetic with antiemetic properties (such as acepromazine), an agent that is likely to induce vomiting (such as xylazine or dexmedetomidine in small animals) in order to empty the stomach, or proceed with heightened monitoring for regurgitation or vomiting. Other drug choices that may be used to minimize the negative consequences of vomiting, reflux, and regurgitation include antiemetics (such as maropitant), promotility drugs (such as cisapride), and antacids (such as omeprazole).

TECHNICIAN NOTE Pulmonary aspiration is always serious and may lead to pneumonia that is difficult to treat, permanent disability, and in some cases, even immediate respiratory arrest and death of the patient. Unless told otherwise by the attending veterinarian, food should be withheld from all patients prior to sedation or general anesthesia except for neonatal, pediatric, and some exotic patients.

Regardless of which recommendations are followed, there is always some risk of reflux, regurgitation, or vomiting during the anesthetic or recovery period. Consequently, the technician or nurse must watch carefully for and be prepared to respond, and must ensure that fluids are administered as prescribed because fasted patients are at higher risk for dehydration, especially if ill.

Fasted patients sometimes vomit foam, bile, or mucus. At other times, food may be vomited if a disorder exists that prevents the stomach from emptying, such as a foreign body, ileus, or a stricture. If regurgitation occurs in the anesthetized patient, there is some protection against aspiration if a lubricated and cuffed endotracheal tube is in place. This is the reason that the endotracheal tube must be left in place during recovery until the animal regains the swallowing reflex. (Methods for preventing and managing regurgitation and vomiting during anesthesia are discussed further in Chapter 13.)

Animals undergoing gastrointestinal procedures such as enterotomy, colonoscopy, or intestinal biopsy may require longer withholding times, enemas, or cathartics to minimize the amount of ingesta within the gastrointestinal tract at the time of surgery.

The anesthetist should be aware that, although preanesthetic fasting is often recommended as noted previously, delayed return to normal feeding during the postoperative period is detrimental. Many seriously ill animals are anorexic and may refuse to eat. For example, a dog with severe trauma that requires prolonged hospitalization may be too uncomfortable, frightened, or weak to eat, and by the time it is released, it may have gone without eating for several days. This lack of adequate intake impedes the healing process and prolongs recovery. For these reasons, efforts should be made to reestablish caloric intake by hand-feeding palatable foods, feeding by syringe bolus, or using feeding tubes or total parenteral nutrition.

Patient Stabilization

Seriously ill patients may require significant nursing care for stabilization before surgery. For example, a patient with a pneumothorax and femoral fracture will need to have the pneumothorax stabilized before the fracture repair is performed. This care can be labor and time intensive but is a very important part of minimizing patient risk. Veterinary technicians or nurses are usually intimately involved in this process of stabilization. At times (e.g., with a patient with a gastric torsion or uncontrolled internal bleeding), the veterinarian may decide that the risk of delaying surgery outweighs the increased anesthetic risk and will elect to proceed. These patients often pose the greatest test of the anesthetist's skills and knowledge.

INTRAVENOUS CATHETERIZATION AND FLUID THERAPY
Reasons for Intravenous Catheterization

IV catheterization and fluid therapy is an essential part of patient stabilization prior to anesthesia as well as prevention and treatment of common complications of anesthesia and surgery including vasodilatation, hypotension, and hypovolemia. Placement of an IV catheter and fluid administration is therefore recommended as a standard of care to maintain blood volume and support blood pressure for all patients undergoing general anesthesia but is especially important for the following patient groups:

- Patients undergoing any procedure that may result in significant blood loss (such as a cesarean section or removal of a splenic tumor)
- Debilitated or dehydrated patients
- Patients with organ dysfunction or failure
- Patients with electrolyte abnormalities (e.g., hyperkalemia).
- Patients undergoing prolonged anesthesia (more than 1 hour)
- Patients at risk for hypotension or shock. Even mild hypotension is a potential problem in anesthetized animals because it leads to decreased blood flow to the kidneys and other vital organs.

In addition to the reasons just mentioned, IV catheterization and fluid therapy has a number of other important benefits:

1. IV access allows rapid administration of emergency drugs such as epinephrine.
2. An IV catheter can be used for constant rate infusion (CRI) of anesthetics, analgesics, electrolytes, or other drugs such as insulin. CRI is a slow, continuous administration of a drug at a rate sufficient to achieve the desired effect. For example, propofol is administered by CRI to maintain general anesthesia or to control seizures in patients with status epilepticus. Drugs given by CRI are either administered through an IV catheter with a syringe pump or added to an IV fluid bag and given via an administration set and IV catheter (see Chapter 9 for a detailed discussion of CRIs).
3. Vesicants (drugs that damage tissues if injected perivascularly, such as some chemotherapeutic agents) can be administered safely. Some vesicants are so irritating to tissues that injection of even an extremely small amount can cause tissue irritation and sloughing. Perivascular injection is much more likely when a syringe and needle are used.
4. Incompatible drugs can be administered more easily via an IV catheter. For example, diazepam and hydromorphone will precipitate when mixed because hydromorphone is water soluble and diazepam is not. When administering this drug combination intravenously, each drug must be injected separately with saline flush between to prevent mixing. Sequential injections are very cumbersome to administer by venipuncture with a needle and syringe without the risk of inadvertent perivascular injection or without breaking aseptic technique.

Choosing and Placing a Peripheral Intravenous Catheter

Two main types of IV catheters can be used for fluid and drug administration in veterinary patients: peripheral IV catheters and central IV catheters (Fig. 2.4). Central catheters are single- or multiple-lumen catheters are long enough to reach from the point of entry (often the external jugular vein) to the great veins near the heart (often the cranial vena cava). They are intended

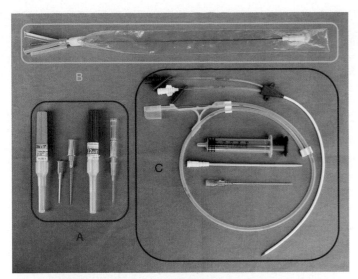

FIG. 2.4 Intravenous catheters. **(A)** Over-the-needle peripheral intravenous (IV) catheters (20- and 22-gauge). **(B)** Through-the-needle peripheral IV catheter. **(C)** Double-lumen central IV catheter.

for long-term use in critical care patients that may be receiving multiple fluids or medications, that require frequent blood draws, or that receive vesicants such as some chemotherapeutic agents. These catheters are not routinely used for general anesthesia or surgery.

In contrast, when administering drugs or fluids to support patients undergoing anesthesia and surgery, peripheral catheters are most frequently used. Peripheral catheters are relatively short catheters that are placed into a peripheral vein (a vein outside of the chest or abdomen) such as the cephalic and accessory cephalic (dogs and cats), lateral saphenous (dogs), medial saphenous (cats), or external jugular (small and large animals). Both over-the-needle and through-the-needle catheters may be used in peripheral veins. Both types of catheters have one lumen through which fluids, drugs, or blood products can be infused, and consequently are classified as single-lumen catheters.

Over-the-needle catheters are more commonly used in general practice for patients receiving anesthesia and, in most cases, serve this purpose well because they are inexpensive, readily available, and relatively easy to place. Procedure 2.2 shows the sequence of events used to place an over-the-needle catheter in a small animal patient. Typically, 16- to 24-gauge, ¾- to 2-inch catheters are used in small animal anesthesia, small ruminants and pigs, and 12- to 16-gauge, 5¼-inch catheters are used in cattle and horses.

Through-the-needle catheters are significantly longer than over-the-needle catheters (typically 8 to 12 inches). They are most often placed in the jugular vein. Unlike over-the-needle catheters, through-the-needle catheters are infrequently used for anesthesia because the additional length of these catheters is not necessary when performing most anesthetic procedures, and they are more complex and time consuming to place, especially if the technician or nurse is not experienced with their use.

> **TECHNICIAN NOTE** When placing and maintaining an IV catheter for use during surgery:
> - Choose a catheter of sufficient length to minimize the risk of dislodgement.
> - Choose a catheter of large diameter.
> - Choose a location that will not interfere with the procedure.
> - Use an administration set with an injection port or place a T-port between the catheter hub and the administration set.
> - After positioning the patient, check that fluids are flowing freely.
> - Avoid excessive catheter and patient movement during transfer.
> - Administer IV drugs slowly.
> - Use saline flush following IV injection of a drug.

When used for anesthetic management, the basic principles of catheter placement and maintenance are no different than when used for any other purpose. However, there are several special considerations that apply specifically to catheter maintenance and fluid administration during anesthesia.

- It is important to choose a catheter of sufficient length and to secure it carefully to prevent it from being dislodged during patient transfer (such as from surgical preparation to the operating room to recovery).
- When possible, choose a large-diameter catheter in case rapid fluid administration is necessary, as would be the case with excessive blood loss or hypotension.
- The catheter must be placed in a location that will not interfere with the procedure. For instance, if an orthopedic procedure is to be performed on the left forelimb, the catheter must be placed in the right forelimb, a hindlimb, or some other site.
- Be sure to use an administration set with an injection port or place a T-port between the catheter hub and the administration set so that IV medications can be administered when necessary. Procedure 2.3 shows the sequence of events used to administer medications through the port of an IV administration set or through a T-port.
- Because surgery patients are placed in various positions most conducive to exposure of the surgery site, limb ties or the limb position itself may impede the flow of fluids. This must be kept in mind when positioning and securing the patient to ensure that fluids are flowing freely.
- Excessive movement of the catheter and patient during patient transfer may result in the introduction of air into the vein (known as an *air embolism*) through the administration line. This must be avoided because a large air embolus is life-threatening.
- Drugs administered via an IV catheter must be given slowly. Most drugs should be given over a period of 15 to 60 seconds, although some, such as sodium bicarbonate and potassium chloride, must be given much more slowly.
- When administering drugs IV, be sure to flush the entire dose of drug into the vein after each bolus. This will prevent dosage errors.

FLUID ADMINISTRATION

All animals have a fundamental physiologic need for a constant source of oxygen delivered to all body tissues in quantities necessary to perform basic metabolic functions. An absence of

PROCEDURE 2.2   Placing an Over-the-Needle Intravenous Catheter in a Small Animal Patient

Equipment (Fig. 1)
- **a,** Catheter (20–24 gauge, ¾ to 1½ inches long for cats; 16–22 gauge, 1–2 inches long for dogs)
- **b,** Two approximately 6-inch-long strips of 1-inch porous adhesive tape; one approximately 6-inch-long and one approximately 3-inch-long strip of ½-inch tape
- **c,** Clipper with #40 blade
- **d,** 1:1 Chlorhexidine surgical scrub/water-soaked cotton balls and alcohol-soaked cotton balls
- **e,** ½-inch plastic strip with antiseptic ointment
- **f,** T-port, cap, or administration set (both the catheter and T-port should be flushed with saline before catheterization)

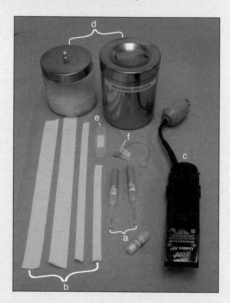

Procedure

1. Clip a generous area over the vein from the medial to lateral aspect of the limb. Prepare the area using standard aseptic technique using chlorhexidine/water-soaked cotton balls alternated with alcohol-soaked cotton balls a total of three times each or until the skin is clean. Place a 6-inch strip of ½-inch tape over the catheter hub. Have an assistant hold off the vein. Locate the vein, apply tension in a ventral direction to tense skin, and position the catheter with the needle fully inserted and with the bevel up (Fig. 2).

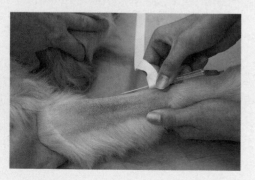

2. Advance the catheter and needle assembly as a unit through the skin and the near wall of the vein. Blood will flash back into the needle hub when the vein is entered. Check that the catheter and needle assembly is directed exactly parallel to the vein, then advance the unit a few more millimeters until the end of the catheter is firmly seated in the vein (Fig. 3).

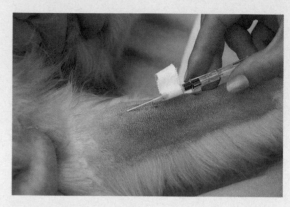

3. Holding the needle stationary, advance the catheter over the end of the needle until inserted to the hub. Remove the needle. Have the assistant apply firm pressure proximal to the skin insertion site to prevent bleeding (Fig. 4).

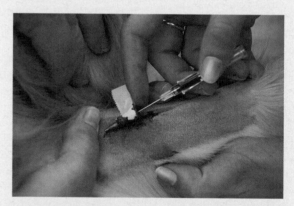

4. Quickly attach a T-port, cap, or administration set line to the catheter hub. Apply the first piece of tape to secure the catheter (Fig. 5).

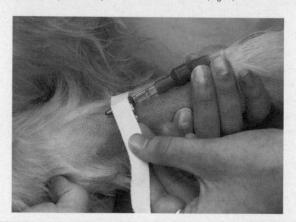

PROCEDURE 2.2—**Placing an Over-the-Needle Intravenous Catheter in a Small Animal Patient—cont'd**

5. Flush the catheter with several milliliters of normal saline through the injection port. Twist the 3-inch-long-strip of ½-inch tape into a "bow-tie" configuration (Fig. 6).

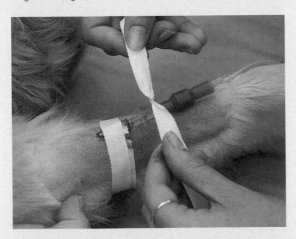

6. Apply the tape under and then around the catheter hub in a crisscross fashion (Fig. 7).

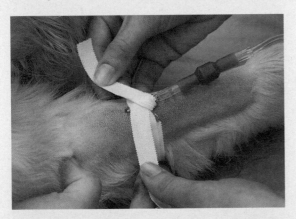

7. Apply a small amount of chlorhexidine ointment to the plastic strip (Fig. 8).

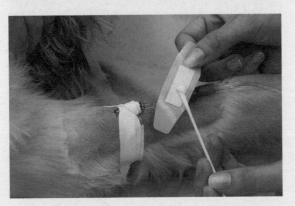

8. Apply the plastic strip over the insertion site (Fig. 9).

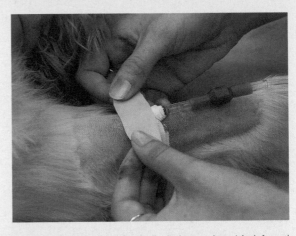

9. Tear a ½-inch V in a 6-inch length of 1-inch tape about 1 inch from the end. Slip it under the catheter, with the torn area directly under the catheter hub (Fig. 10).

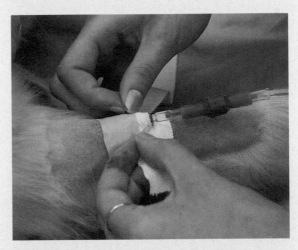

10. Apply the remainder of this length of tape over the plastic strip to secure (Fig. 11).

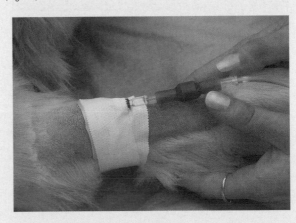

11. Apply the remaining 6-inch-long strip of 1-inch tape around the administration set line or T-port to create a tension loop (see Procedure 2.3, Fig. 1).

PROCEDURE 2.3 Giving an Intravenous Injection Through an Intravenous Administration Set Port or T-Port

Procedure

1. Prepare the medication or induction agent. Cleanse the injection port with alcohol. Intravenous (IV) fluids should be flowing at the standard infusion rate (Fig. 1).

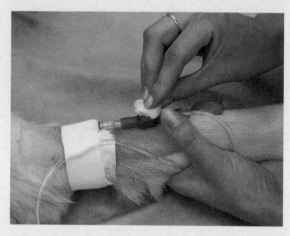

2. Insert the needle into the injection port. Pinch off the administration set line between the injection port and the fluid bag to prevent the backflow of agent into the fluid bag during injection (Fig. 2).

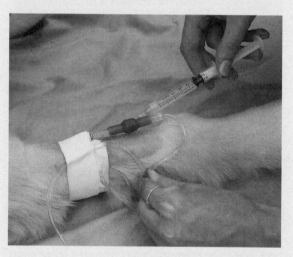

3. Give the medication at an appropriate rate as dictated by the attending veterinarian. For most medications, a slow IV bolus is appropriate. When induc-

ing general anesthesia, inject an appropriate initial volume following the guidelines in Chapters 9, 10, and 11 (Fig. 3).

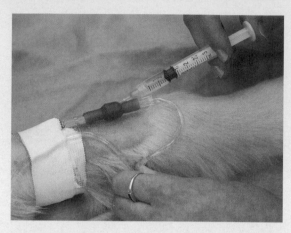

4. After injection, release the administration set line so that the entire dose of medication is flushed into the patient. This is necessary because typically as much as 0.5–2 mL of agent will remain in the fluid line and catheter until flushed through (Fig. 4).

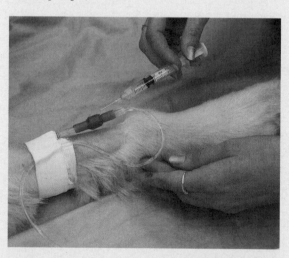

5. When administering an induction agent, administer additional doses to effect by following steps 2, 3, and 4. As soon as the patient is at an adequate anesthetic depth to permit intubation, remove the needle and syringe to prevent accidental overdose.

---

adequate oxygen will rapidly damage any tissues so deprived and will result in cell death in high-demand tissues such as the brain and heart muscle within minutes.

One of the primary functions of the cardiovascular and respiratory systems is to supply this need by extracting oxygen from the air and conveying it directly to every cell in the body. For this reason, agents that adversely affect cardiopulmonary function have the potential for decreasing oxygen delivery. As nearly all anesthetic agents adversely affect these systems, constant attention to cardiopulmonary support is one of the cornerstones of the successful practice of anesthesia.

There are several specific ways in which anesthetic agents affect cardiopulmonary function. Almost all anesthetic agents

decrease the force of heart muscle contraction (referred to as negative inotropy) and cause bradycardia. These factors in turn decrease the flow of blood from the heart (cardiac output). Almost all agents also relax the muscle tone of blood vessels, which in turn causes an increase in the intravascular volume (vasodilation). Together, the decreased cardiac output and vasodilation cause hypotension and decrease the perfusion of tissues with blood.

Administration of IV fluids is one of the primary tools available to the anesthetist to support oxygen delivery. Fluids increase circulating blood volume and cardiac output—two physiologic changes that support blood pressure and tissue perfusion.

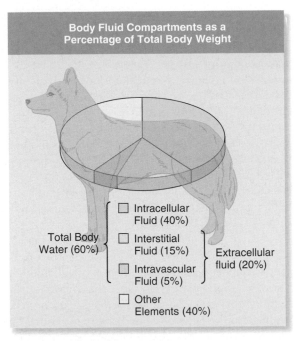

Body Fluid Compartments as a Percentage of Total Body Weight

Total Body Water (60%)

☐ Intracellular Fluid (40%)
☐ Interstitial Fluid (15%)
☐ Intravascular Fluid (5%)
☐ Other Elements (40%)

Extracellular fluid (20%)

FIG. 2.5 Body fluid compartments.

Composition of Body Fluids

Water is the most prevalent substance in the body. In adult animals, about 60% of the body weight is water. Because of the variation associated with age and body fat content, young and lean patients have a somewhat higher percentage, whereas old and obese patients have a somewhat lower percentage. Body water is separated by cell membranes into intracellular (within the cells) and extracellular (outside the cells) fluid compartments. The extracellular fluid (ECF) compartment is subdivided by the vascular endothelium into the interstitial fluid compartment (fluid in the tissues outside the cells) and the intravascular compartment (fluid within the vascular system).

Of the 60% of the body weight that consists of water, about two-thirds (or 40% of the body weight) is intracellular fluid (ICF). Although estimates of ECF vary widely (about 15% to 30% of body weight for small animals), most clinicians use a figure of 20% for the purpose of calculating fluid needs. About three-quarters of the ECF (15% of the body weight) is interstitial fluid (fluid between the cells), and one-quarter (5% of the total body weight) is intravascular fluid (plasma) (Fig. 2.5). When blood cells are added, blood volume is considered to be 8% to 9% of body weight in dogs and large animals and 6% to 7% of body weight in cats. The figures 80 to 90 mL/kg for dogs and large animals and 50 to 60 mL/kg for cats[c] are commonly used for the purpose of calculating blood volume.

Body fluids consist of water and **solutes.** Body fluid solutes are either atoms or molecules dissolved in body water. The solutes most important in fluid therapy are small–molecular-weight, electrically charged particles called *ions*, large–molecular-weight PPs called **colloids,** and small nonionic particles such as glucose and small proteins.

Electrolytes are substances that when dissolved separate into positively charged ions called *cations* (so called because they migrate toward the cathode during electrolysis) and negatively charged ions called *anions* (so called because they migrate toward the anode). Sodium chloride (NaCl or table salt) is an example of an electrolyte; when dissolved, it separates into the cation sodium and the anion chloride. Important cations in body fluids include sodium (Na^+), potassium (K^+), magnesium (Mg^{2+}), and calcium (Ca^{2+}). Important anions include chloride (Cl^-), bicarbonate (HCO_3^-), phosphates (HPO_4^{2-}, $H_2PO_4^-$), and proteins.

Solutes serve diverse purposes. Electrolytes provide osmotic pressure and are essential for many fundamental physiologic processes such as blood clotting, heart function, and neuromuscular function. Proteins participate in a wide variety of processes including drug transport, regulation of blood pressure by providing oncotic pressure, and blood clotting. Glucose provides energy to the cells.

Fluid Homeostasis

Homeostasis refers to a constant state within the body created and maintained by normal physiologic processes. Maintenance of fluid homeostasis is a highly delicate and dynamic process. In health, water and solutes constantly move through cell membranes between fluid compartments as needed to maintain solute concentrations within a narrow and specific range. Many solutes move freely between body compartments by passive diffusion along gradients from areas of high concentration to those of low concentration. Others are confined to or concentrated in a particular space. For instance, owing to its extremely large size, albumin does not travel freely through the normal vascular endothelium but tends to concentrate within the intravascular space. Another example is K^+, which because of active transport through the cell membranes, is concentrated within the cells (98% of K^+ is located within the cells). In contrast, Na^+ is largely excluded from the cells and thus is found in high concentrations in the extracellular space.

Consequently, the concentration of each of the major solutes often differs widely among the fluid compartments. For instance, ICF is very rich in K^+, Mg^{2+}, proteins, HPO_4^{2-}, and $H_2PO_4^-$ when compared with ECF. In contrast, ECF has much higher concentrations of Na^+, Cl^-, and HCO_3^- (Fig. 2.6).

The balance of water and solutes in body fluids is governed by a number of principles, which, if understood, help the anesthetist administer fluids in a way that provides the most benefit to the patient. Some of these principles are as follows:

- At any given time, the number of negatively and positively charged particles in any given fluid compartment must be equal. Thus if the number of positively charged particles in a compartment increases, the number of negatively charged particles must increase by the same amount. This state of electrical balance in any fluid compartment is called *electroneutrality.*
- In health, a solute concentration or **osmolarity** of approximately 300 mOsm/L is maintained in all body fluids. Conditions including dehydration, exercise, heat stroke, and some cases of vomiting and diarrhea that involve primarily water loss will increase the osmolarity, and others such as chronic congestive heart failure, in which large quantities of solutes are lost, will decrease it.

[c]Robertson SA, Gogolski SM, Pascoe P, et al: AAFP feline anesthesia guidelines. *J Feline Med Surg* 20:602–634, 2018.

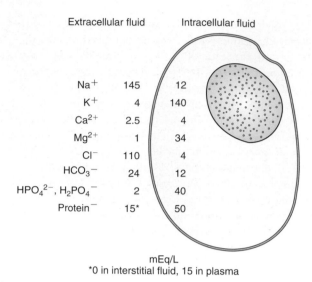

Extracellular fluid   Intracellular fluid

Na$^+$	145	12
K$^+$	4	140
Ca^{2+}	2.5	4
Mg^{2+}	1	34
Cl$^-$	110	4
HCO$_3^-$	24	12
HPO$_4^{2-}$, H$_2$PO$_4^-$	2	40
Protein$^-$	15*	50

mEq/L
*0 in interstitial fluid, 15 in plasma

FIG. 2.6 Comparison of the average electrolyte concentrations in the extracellular and intracellular fluid compartments. (Modified from DiBartola S: *Fluid, electrolyte, and acid-base disorders*, ed 4, St. Louis, MO, 2012, Elsevier.)

- The solutes in each fluid compartment provide osmotic pressure, which draws water into that compartment in proportion to the number of particles present. For example, if the osmolarity in the vascular space increases or decreases, water will follow, increasing or decreasing the blood volume respectively.
- Small particle solutes such as ions diffuse freely through vascular endothelium, taking water with them. Thus they equilibrate relatively quickly between the intravascular and interstitial fluid spaces. The interstitial fluid compartment is about three times the size of the intravascular compartment. Therefore only about one-quarter of fluid administered intravenously remains in the vascular space after equilibration.
- Colloids including albumin do not diffuse freely through vascular endothelium. Their presence in the vascular space provides colloid osmotic pressure (also called oncotic pressure) that tends to draw water into the blood vessels and is thus important for the maintenance of blood volume and pressure.
- The plasma concentration of certain solutes such as potassium and calcium must be kept in a very narrow range in order to maintain normal muscle and heart function. Relatively small deviations in levels of these cations can cause significant clinical signs and can endanger the patient.

> **TECHNICIAN NOTE** The plasma concentration of certain solutes such as potassium and calcium must be kept in a very narrow range in order to maintain normal muscle and heart function. Relatively small deviations in levels of these cations can cause significant clinical signs and can endanger the patient.

Fluid Needs During Anesthesia

During anesthesia, many factors including disease conditions, surgery, and effects of drugs often disrupt fluid homeostasis and require the anesthetist to intervene. Appropriate fluid therapy requires knowledge of the nature of fluid losses associated with disease conditions. Following are some common associations with general anesthesia:

- Fluid losses that occur from dehydration and many general disease conditions initially deplete the ECF space. For this reason, when replacing recent fluid losses in patients with disease, dehydration, or anorexia, fluids should be chosen with solute profiles similar to ECF.
- Perioperative hemorrhage involves fluid loss from the intravascular space, part of the ECF space. Thus, as in the previous example, fluids should be chosen with solute profiles similar to ECF unless hemorrhage is profound.
- Profound perioperative hemorrhage involves significant loss of albumin, blood cells, and other constituents of blood in addition to electrolytes and water. To support patients experiencing severe perioperative hemorrhage, administration of blood products may be necessary to provide RBCs or hemoglobin to support oxygen-carrying capacity and in some cases, clotting factors and platelets to support normal coagulation.
- Patients with perioperative hemorrhage may also benefit from hypertonic saline or colloid solutions, both of which draw water into the vascular space and raise blood pressure.
- Patients with low albumin may require colloids or blood plasma (fluids containing large solutes), which provide osmotically active particles that remain in the vascular space for longer periods and help maintain blood volume and pressure.

Classification of Intravenous Fluids

All IV fluids are solutions consisting of one or more solutes dissolved in water. Most IV fluids contain one or more electrolytes. Dextrose, a naturally occurring form of glucose, is another ingredient present in some fluids. Some fluids also contain the buffers lactate, gluconate, or acetate, which are converted to HCO$_3^-$ by the liver and help regulate pH. Others contain colloids (large-molecular-weight solutes).

There are many IV solutions, each with different solute profiles. These fluids are classified as either crystalloids or colloids, based on the molecular weight of the primary solutes they contain.

Crystalloids and colloids may also be classified, according to the mix and quantity of solutes, as isotonic, hypotonic, or hypertonic; replacement or maintenance; and balanced or unbalanced. Isotonic fluids have an osmolarity near that of blood plasma (300 mOsm/L). Hypotonic and hypertonic fluids have an osmolarity significantly lower or higher than plasma, respectively. Replacement fluids have high concentrations of Na$^+$ and Cl$^-$ (as ECF does) and are designed to replace fluid losses such as those that occur from hypovolemia or dehydration. Maintenance fluids have lower concentrations of Na$^+$ and Cl$^-$ but somewhat more K$^+$ (as total body water does) and are designed to maintain fluid balance over a longer period. Balanced fluids contain a solute profile similar to that of ECF, whereas unbalanced fluids do not.

> **TECHNICIAN NOTE** Replacement fluids have high concentrations of Na$^+$ and Cl$^-$ (as ECF does) and are designed to replace fluid losses. Maintenance fluids have lower concentrations of Na$^+$ and Cl$^-$ but somewhat more K$^+$ and are designed to maintain fluid balance over a longer period.

Crystalloid Solutions

Crystalloid solutions (also referred to as *crystalloids*) contain water and small-molecular-weight solutes such as electrolytes that pass freely through vascular endothelium. In addition to electrolytes, some crystalloids contain dextrose and alkalinizing agents (buffers). Table 2.10 shows the composition of selected commercially available crystalloid fluids. Other constituents are sometimes added to commercially available crystalloids, including 50% dextrose, potassium, and B-complex vitamins. Crystalloids are routinely used in most anesthetized patients, except those that have low blood protein, low RBC mass, or low platelet count. These solutions are generally appropriate, provided the PCV is 20% or greater and the PP is 3.5 g/dL or greater.

Isotonic crystalloid solutions. The most commonly used isotonic crystalloid fluids in veterinary patients are subclassified as polyionic replacement solutions. These balanced solutions contain several ions (most often sodium, potassium, and chloride and in some cases, magnesium and/or calcium) in concentrations that reflect the solute composition of ECF. This subclass of crystalloid solutions is the first choice for fluid therapy of healthy patients undergoing anesthesia and routine surgery as well as correction of hypovolemia and dehydration, as long as the PCV is over 20% and the PP is over 3.5 g/dL. Lactated Ringer's solution (LR), Plasma-Lyte R (PLR), Plasma-Lyte A pH 7.4 (PLA), Normosol-R pH 7.4 (NR), and Iso-Lyte S pH 7.4 (ILS) are examples of some commonly used solutions in this class.

These fluids all have somewhat similar solute profiles, with the following exceptions. Each contains one or two buffers (lactate, gluconate, and/or acetate), but the concentration of buffer differs among these five solutions. PLR, PLA, NR, and ILS contain magnesium, whereas LR does not. LR and PLR contain calcium, whereas PLA, NR, and ILS do not. Because calcium may cause transfused blood to clot, neither LR nor PLR may be administered with blood products.

Normal saline solution (NS) (a.k.a. *physiologic saline, 0.9% saline,* or *sodium chloride 0.9%*) is an isotonic fluid that contains only sodium and chloride ions in water and is therefore an unbalanced replacement solution. Normal saline is recommended as the preferred fluid in some specific circumstances (e.g., patients with hypochloremic metabolic alkalosis, hypercalcemia, and for administering blood transfusions). NS is also used to bathe exposed tissues during surgery, to flush IV catheters, and to flush body cavities. Normal saline is somewhat more acidic (pH of approximately 5.0) than polyionic solutions and does not contain any potassium, and therefore can cause hypokalemia if not supplemented.

> **TECHNICIAN NOTE** Isotonic polyionic replacement crystalloids are the first choice for fluid therapy of healthy patients undergoing routine surgery as well as many sick patients as long as the PCV is over 20% and the PP is over 3.5 g/dL.

Hypertonic crystalloid solutions. Concentrated saline solution (3%, 7%, and 23.4% [diluted to ≤7.5%]) is given with isotonic crystalloids in acute care settings to treat patients with hypovolemic, traumatic, or endotoxic shock. Hypertonic saline rapidly but temporarily draws water into the intravascular space and supports blood pressure but, like other crystalloids, rapidly diffuses into the interstitial space and so must be followed with colloids if the patient needs long-term blood volume expansion.

These solutions are seldom used during the perioperative period but may be used in special circumstances such as profound hemorrhage when blood products are unavailable, or for patients with increased intracranial pressure or low sodium.

Hypotonic crystalloid solutions. Normosol-M in 5% dextrose (NM5) and Plasma-Lyte 56 in 5% dextrose (PL5) are hypotonic fluids that are subclassified as polyionic maintenance solutions. These fluids are designed for sick patients that need maintenance fluid therapy over a longer period of time. They contain less sodium and chloride and more potassium than the corresponding replacement solutions and consequently more closely reflect the solute composition of total body water. These solutions also contain lower concentrations of a buffer than their replacement counterparts and contain dextrose. Although these fluids are technically isotonic (approximately 368 mOsm/L), once infused, the dextrose in these solutions is rapidly metabolized to CO_2 and water and the osmolality drops to 111 mOsm/L/L. Consequently, these fluids are classified as hypotonic.

Five percent dextrose in water (D5W) is a solution that contains dextrose as the only solute. For the reason previously mentioned, D5W is classified as hypotonic (as opposed to isotonic as its osmolality of 253 mOsm/L would suggest). Plain 5% dextrose is used to replace the pure water deficit that accompanies simple dehydration or heat stroke. It is not suitable for patients in shock as a result of blood loss, however, because it does not expand the blood volume, and it should not be used as a sole maintenance fluid because it will dilute the electrolytes contained in total body water.

Other polyionic replacement solutions, (such as LR, PLR, PLA, NR, ILS, half-strength [0.45%] or full-strength [0.9%] saline) containing 2.5% or 5% dextrose are commercially available or may be mixed in house. The osmolality of these fluids varies according to the concentration of electrolytes they contain.

Although solutions containing dextrose are not used for replacement fluid therapy, they are used for specific purposes. Dextrose solutions with or without electrolytes are used to support blood glucose in neonatal, hypoglycemic, or debilitated patients and in patients with diabetes mellitus that are receiving insulin. They may also be used as a part of the therapy for hyperkalemia.

Colloid Solutions

Colloid solutions (also referred to as *colloids*) contain large-molecular-weight solutes that do not freely diffuse across vascular endothelium and therefore stay in the intravascular space. Colloids are used to support the expansion of blood volume and blood pressure. During the perioperative period, colloids are used for patients with PP less than 3.5 g/dL. There are two basic types of colloids.

Synthetic colloid solutions. Synthetic colloid solutions contain the very-large-molecular-weight solutes hetastarch (hydroxyethyl starch), dextran, pentastarch, or gelatin products. Like natural colloids, these solutes tend to remain in the

TABLE 2.10   Solute Composition of Selected Commercially Available Crystalloid Fluids

Fluid	Dextrose (g/L)	Na+ (mEq/L)	Cl− (mEq/L)	K+ (mEq/L)	Ca2+ (mEq/L)	Mg2+ (mEq/L)	Buffer[a] (mEq/L)	Osmolarity (mOsm/L)	pH kcal/L	Fluid Type[b]
0.9% NaCl	0	154	154	0	0	0	0	310	pH 5.0 0 kcal/L	R/U/I
Lactated Ringer's solution	0	130	109	4	4	0	28 (L)	272	pH 6.5 9 kcal/L	R/B/I
Plasma-Lyte R	0	140	103	10	5	3	47 (A) 8 (L)	312	pH 5.5 11 kcal/L	R/B/I
Plasma-Lyte A (pH 7.4) Normosol R (pH 7.4)	0	140	98	5	0	3	27 (A) 23 (G)	294	pH 7.4 18 kcal/L (21 kcal/L-PLA)	R/B/I
Iso-Lyte S (pH 7.4)	0	141	98	5	0	3	29 (A) 23 (G)	295	pH 7.4	R/B/I
Normosol-M w/5% dextrose Plasma-Lyte 56 w/5% dextrose	50	40	40	13	0	3	16 (A)	368 (111 w/o D)	pH 5.5 170 kcal/L	M/I or H[c]
5% dextrose	50	0	0	0	0	0	0	253	pH 3.2–6.5 170 kcal/L	D/I or H[c]
3% NaCl	0	513	513	0	0	0	0	1030	pH 5.0 0 kcal/L	HTS
7% NaCl	0	1198	1198	0	0	0	0	2396	pH 5.0 0 kcal/L	HTS

[a]Buffers used: A, Acetate; G, gluconate; L, lactate.
[b]Fluid types: B, Balanced; D, dextrose solution; H, hypotonic; HTS, hypertonic saline; I, isotonic; M, maintenance; R, replacement; U, unbalanced.
[c]Note that, because of the rapid metabolism of dextrose, these solutions may be classified as hypotonic.
Modified from Plumb D: Plumb's veterinary drug handbook, ed 9, Ames, 2018, Wiley-Blackwell.

intravascular space, expanding the blood volume. Depending on the agent, 30% to 60% of a synthetic colloid remains in the plasma after 24 hours, and a smaller percentage remains in the plasma for as long as days to weeks after administration. Hetastarch is the most commonly used synthetic colloid in veterinary patients. VetStarch (Abbott Animal Health) is a solution of 6% hydroxyethyl starch in 0.9% saline labeled specifically for veterinary use.

Blood products. Blood products such as plasma and whole blood contain albumin and other natural colloids. During the perioperative period, blood products are used for a variety of indications including anemia, hypoproteinemia, coagulation disorders, and thrombocytopenia. Whole blood or packed RBCs are used to support the oxygen-carrying capacity of blood for patients that have profound blood loss. Plasma is primarily used to support the expansion of blood volume or treat hypoproteinemia.

Intravenous fluid selection and administration rates.

Fluid therapy is an inexact science. Although there are generally accepted fluid choices and administration rates for animals that are in shock, ill, experiencing blood loss, or undergoing surgery, each patient must be managed in a unique manner appropriate to its condition. Even though these standard rates are used as a starting point, ultimately, the veterinarian will use their professional judgment to determine the final rate for each patient.

Fluid Therapy During Anesthesia and Surgery

As mentioned in the previous section, isotonic polyionic replacement crystalloids including LR, PLR, PLA, NR, and ILS are the first-choice fluid for healthy patients undergoing routine surgery, as well as many sick patients as long as the PCV is over 20% and the PP is over 3.5 g/dL. Consequently, these fluids are used in the vast majority of anesthetized patients.

Recommended prescribed IV administration rates for crystalloid fluids during general anesthesia and surgery are as follows:
- The 2013 AAHA/AAFP Fluid Therapy Guidelines for Dogs and Cats recommend an initial rate of 5 mL/kg/h in dogs and 3 mL/kg/h in cats followed by a reduced rate if the patient is anesthetized for more than 1 hour, with a total of no more than 10 mL/kg/h for maintenance and any necessary replacement.[d]
- Fluid infusion rates recommended for large animals are typically in the range of 2 to 5 mL/kg/h.

Until relatively recently, for both small and large animals, a rate of 10 mL/kg/h during the first hour followed by 5 mL/kg/h for the remainder of the procedure was commonly used as a standard IV administration rate-a rate substantially higher than current recommendations and one that does not take into account important physiologic considerations such as the relatively high susceptibility of cats to overhydration.

Ultimately, the attending veterinarian must select the best rate for each patient based on its specific needs, the available scientific evidence, and their own experience. For this reason, the technician or nurse may encounter a variety of different

---

BOX 2.6 Recommended Fluid Administration Rates During Anesthesia and Surgery

Rates Typically Recommended for Dogs and Cats[a]
- The total rate (including maintenance and replacement) should be under 10 mL/kg/h.
- Initial rate for dogs: **5 mL/kg/h**
- Initial rate for cats: **3 mL/kg/h**
- Reduce the rate by 25% every hour until the maintenance rate is reached provided the patient remains stable
- The fluid type and rate should be adjusted based on ongoing monitoring and assessment.
- Decrease rates in patients with cardiovascular and renal disease

Rates Typically Recommended for Large Animals
- Initial rate: 2–5 mL/kg/h

[a]Adapted from the 2013 AAHA/AAPF Fluid Therapy Guidelines for Dogs and Cats.

---

standards in the workplace and must become familiar with the standard rates at their place of employment. (See Box 2.6 for a summary of recommended fluid administration rates.)

Regardless of which of these recommendations is followed, each is higher than the volume needed to maintain hydration in a patient that is normal and awake because they are intended to compensate for the **vasodilation**, decreased cardiac output, and increase in insensible fluid loss that can occur during anesthesia. Tables 2.11 and 2.12 consist of calculated infusion rates in mL/h (based on the commonly prescribed rates previously discussed) for dogs and cats, respectively, as well as calculated rates for managing various complications in the remaining columns.

TECHNICIAN NOTE The 2013 AAHA/AAFP Fluid Therapy Guidelines for Dogs and Cats recommend an initial rate of 5 mL/kg/h in dogs and 3 mL/kg/h in cats, followed by a reduced rate if the patient is anesthetized for more than 1 hour, with a total of no more than 10 mL/kg/h for maintenance and any necessary replacement. Fluid infusion rates recommended for large animals are typically in the range of 2–5 mL/kg/h.

Hypotension is a frequent occurrence in anesthetized patients due to blood loss, decreased cardiac output, peripheral vasodilation, or other factors. In otherwise healthy patients, hypotension associated with peripheral vasodilation (not associated with blood loss) may respond to a decrease in anesthetic depth. If not, a bolus of isotonic crystalloid IV fluids can be given rapidly at a rate of 3 to 10 mL/kg (dogs and LAs) or 3 to 5 mL/kg (cats), followed by a repeat bolus if needed. If the response to 1 to 2 boluses is inadequate, colloids should be considered, titrated slowly to effect at a rate of 5 to 10 mL/kg (dogs) and 1 to 5 mL/kg (cats) while monitoring blood pressure every 3 to 5 minutes.[e] As an alternative, in normally hydrated

---

[d]These rates are also recommended in the 2020 AAHA Anesthesia and Monitoring Guidelines for Dogs and Cats as well as the 2018 AAFP Feline Anesthesia Guidelines.

[e]Note that the AAFP 2018 Feline Anesthesia Guidelines recommend a balanced electrolyte fluid bolus of 3 to 10 mL/kg up to a maximum of 15 mL/kg over 5 to 15 minutes to treat hypotension in feline patients. The AAHA 2020 Anesthesia and Monitoring Guidelines for Dogs and Cats recommend a crystalloid bolus of 5 to 20 mL/kg and/or a colloid bolus of 1 to 5 mL/kg for both dogs and cats.

TABLE 2.11   Canine IV Fluid Infusion Rates (mL/unit time) During Anesthesia and Surgery

Indication and Prescribed Rate / Body weight (kg)	Standard Rate During Anesthesia and Surgery[a] (5 ml/kg/h) / Infusion Rate in mL/h	Treatment of Hypotension Associated With Peripheral Vasodilatation (3–10 ml/kg rapidly. Repeat once if needed) / Volume in mL to be Given Rapidly	Treatment of Excessive Blood Loss or Hypotension (20 ml/kg over 15 min. Repeat once if needed) / Volume in mL to be Given Over 15 min	Treatment of Shock With Crystalloids (~20 ml/kg rapidly. Give additional boluses as necessary up to 80–90 ml/kg) / Volume in mL to be Given Rapidly	Treatment of Shock with Colloids (5 ml/kg as a bolus over 15–20 min, repeat up to max. of 4 doses) / Volume in mL to be Given over 15–20 min	Treatment of Shock With Hypertonic Saline (4–5 ml/kg slowly over 5 min followed by isotonic crystalloids) / Volume in mL to be Given Slowly over 5 min
2.0	10	6–20	40	40	10	8–10
2.5	13	7.5–25	50	50	13	10–13
3.0	15	9–30	60	60	15	12–15
3.5	18	10.5–35	70	70	18	14–18
4.0	20	12–40	80	80	20	16–20
4.5	23	13.5–45	90	90	23	18–23
5.0	25	15–50	100	100	25	20–25
6.0	30	18–60	120	120	30	24–30
7.0	35	21–70	140	140	35	28–35
8.0	40	24–80	160	160	40	32–40
9.0	45	27–90	180	180	45	36–45
10.0	50	30–100	200	200	50	40–50
11.0	55	33–110	220	220	55	44–55
12.0	60	36–120	240	240	60	48–60
13.0	65	39–130	260	260	65	52–65
14.0	70	42–140	280	280	70	56–70
15.0	75	45–150	300	300	75	60–75
16.0	80	48–160	320	320	80	64–80
17.0	85	51–170	340	340	85	68–85
18.0	90	54–180	360	360	90	72–90

Weight						
19.0	95	57–190	380	380	95	76–95
20.0	100	60–200	400	400	100	80–100
22.0	110	66–220	440	440	110	88–110
24.0	120	72–240	480	480	120	96–120
26.0	130	78–260	520	520	130	104–130
28.0	140	84–280	560	560	140	112–140
30.0	150	90–300	600	600	150	120–150
32.0	160	96–320	640	640	160	128–160
34.0	170	102–340	680	680	170	136–170
36.0	180	108–360	720	720	180	144–180
38.0	190	114–380	760	760	190	152–190
40.0	200	120–400	800	800	200	160–200
42.0	210	126–420	840	840	210	168–210
44.0	220	132–440	880	880	220	176–220
46.0	230	138–460	920	920	230	184–230
48.0	240	144–480	960	960	240	192–240
50.0	250	150–500	1000	1000	250	200–250
55.0	275	165–550	1100	1100	275	220–275
60.0	300	180–600	1200	1200	300	240–300
65.0	325	195–650	1300	1300	325	260–325
70.0	350	210–700	1400	1400	350	280–350
75.0	375	225–750	1500	1500	375	300–375
80.0	400	240–800	1600	1600	400	320–400
85.0	425	255–850	1700	1700	425	340–425
90.0	450	270–900	1800	1800	450	360–450
95.0	475	285–950	1900	1900	475	380–475
100.0	500	300–1000	2000	2000	500	400–500

USING THIS TABLE

This table lists infusion rates for each of the indications listed in Fig. 2.9. For rates listed as a range, the clinician will select an appropriate rate within the range based on the patient's needs. The infusion rate should be programmed into a fluid pump or syringe pump. Boluses that are to be given rapidly may be given by gravity as rapidly as possible or by using a pressure infusion bag.

[a]Note: Rates are reduced after the 1st hour *(see Box 2.6 for details)*. Recommendation based on the 2013 AAHA/AAPF Fluid Therapy Guidelines for Dogs and Cats.

IV, Intravenous.

TABLE 2.12   Feline IV Fluid Infusion Rates (mL/unit time) During Anesthesia and Surgery

Indication and Prescribed Rate	Standard Rate during Anesthesia and Surgery[a] (3 ml/kg/h)	Treatment of Hypotension Associated with Peripheral Vasodilatation (3–5 ml/kg rapidly. Repeat once if needed.)	Treatment of Excessive Blood Loss or Hypotension (10 ml/kg over 15 min. Repeat once if needed.)	Treatment of Shock with Crystalloids (~12.5 ml/kg rapidly. Give additional boluses as necessary up to 50–55 ml/kg.)	Treatment of Shock with Colloids (2.5–3 ml/kg as a bolus over 15–20 min, repeat up to max. of 4 doses.)	Treatment of Shock with Hypertonic Saline (2–4 ml/kg slowly over 5 min followed by isotonic crystalloids)
Body Weight (kg)	Infusion Rate in mL/h	Volume in mL to be Given Rapidly	Volume in mL to be Given Over 15 min	Volume in mL to be Given Rapidly	Volume in mL to be Given over 15–20 min	Volume in mL to be Given Slowly over 5 min
2.0	6	6–10	20	25	5–6	4–8
2.5	7.5	7.5–12.5	25	31	6–7.5	5–10
3.0	9	9–15	30	37.5	7.5–9	6–12
3.5	10.5	10.5–17.5	35	44	9–10.5	7–14
4.0	12	12–20	40	50	10–12	8–16
4.5	13.5	13.5–22.5	45	56	11–13.5	9–18
5.0	15	15–25	50	62.5	12.5–15	10–20
6.0	18	18–30	60	75	15–18	12–24
7.0	21	21–35	70	87.5	17.5–21	14–28
8.0	24	24–40	80	100	20–24	16–32
9.0	27	27–45	90	112.5	22.5–27	18–36
10.0	30	30–50	100	125	25–30	20–40
11.0	33	33–55	110	137.5	27.5–33	22–44
12.0	36	36–60	120	150	30–36	24–48

USING THIS TABLE

This table lists infusion rates for each of the indications listed in Fig. 2.9 For rates listed as a range, the clinician will select an appropriate rate within the range based on the patient's needs. The infusion rate should be programmed into a fluid pump or syringe pump. Boluses that are to be given rapidly may be given by gravity as rapidly as possible.

[a]Note: Rates are reduced after the 1st hour (see Box 2.6 for details). Recommendation based on the 2013 AAHA/AAPF Fluid Therapy Guidelines for Dogs and Cats.

IV, Intravenous.

patients, a bolus of colloids can be given initially instead of a bolus of crystalloids.

Patients with excessive bleeding or excessive hypotension will need significantly higher rates of administration. Healthy young dogs tolerate an IV infusion rate of up to 40 mL/kg, with half of this given over the first 15 minutes. As mentioned previously, cats are more susceptible to overhydration than dogs, and for this reason, the infusion rate should not exceed 20 mL/kg, with half of this given over the first 15 minutes. Large-animal infusion rates are similar to those used in dogs. Overhydration in these species is unlikely, however, because the infusion rate is somewhat limited by the size of the catheter. Colloid administration should be considered if there is a lack of response to crystalloid boluses and decreased inhalant concentrations are being delivered.

When blood loss occurs, at least 3 mL of crystalloid fluids must be given for every 1 mL of blood lost. This is because the interstitial fluid compartment is about three times the volume of the intravascular compartment and, like all crystalloids, these fluids equilibrate throughout the entire ECF compartment. In contrast, if a colloid or a whole blood transfusion is given, the amount of colloid or blood given should approximately equal the amount of blood lost. A saturated 3 × 3 or 4 × 4 gauze sponge holds an average of about 3 to 6 or 5 to 10 mL of blood, respectively. Although not a completely reliable measure, these guidelines can be used to estimate approximate blood loss during surgery. After an initial infusion, additional volumes of colloid or blood must be based on the results of laboratory testing.

> **TECHNICIAN NOTE** Crystalloid IV infusion rates for healthy young patients with excessive bleeding or excessive hypotension are up to 40 mL/kg (dogs and large animals) or up to 20 mL/kg (cats), with half of this given over the first 15 min. Colloid administration should be considered if there is a lack of response to crystalloid boluses and decreased inhalant concentrations are being delivered.

The crystalloid IV infusion rates for animals in shock are even higher (e.g., 80 to 90 mL/kg for dogs and for large animals, and 50 to 55 mL/kg for cats[f]). In a clinical setting, for patients with blood loss, hypotension, or shock, 25% of the calculated shock dose is commonly administered rapidly, and the patient is reevaluated. Further boluses are given as necessary. If two boluses have not stabilized the patient, administration of a colloid should be considered. Because of the complexity involved in determining administration rates, the technician or nurse should consult with the veterinarian about the optimum rate and should carefully monitor the total volume of fluids being given to the patient during surgery.

> **TECHNICIAN NOTE** Crystalloid IV infusion rates for animals in shock are 80–90 mL/kg for dogs and large animals and 50–55 mL/kg for cats. Many clinicians recommend an initial bolus of 25% of the calculated shock dose, reevaluation of the patient, and additional boluses as necessary. If two boluses have not stabilized the patient, administration of a colloid should be considered.

Hypertonic Saline. Sometimes 3% and 7% hypertonic saline solutions are administered in small volumes to patients with shock and blood loss when blood volume expansion is necessary. The standard rate of administration for 7% hypertonic saline is 4 to 5 mL/kg for dogs and large animals and 2 to 4 mL/kg for cats,[g] given slowly over a 5-minute period, followed by administration of isotonic crystalloids. If hypertonic solutions are given too quickly, serious side effects can occur, including hypotension; bradycardia; rapid, shallow breathing; and bronchoconstriction. Therefore the rate of administration must be monitored carefully.

> **TECHNICIAN NOTE** For blood volume expansion in large and small animals, administer 7% hypertonic saline IV at a rate of 4–5 mL/kg for dogs and large animals and 2–4 mL/kg for cats, given slowly over a 5-min period, followed by administration of isotonic crystalloids.

Colloids. Synthetic colloids are administered IV in moderate volumes (10 to 20 mL/kg/day for dogs and large animals and 5 to 10 mL/kg/day for cats) to animals with shock, hypotension, or blood loss. Because colloids expand blood volume, the infusion rate and total volume of colloids administered must be watched closely to prevent volume overload. These agents can also infrequently cause coagulation disorders, acute kidney injury, and rarely, allergic reactions. If given too rapidly, hetastarch can induce nausea and vomiting. Therefore colloids should be administered to dogs and large animals as a bolus of 5 mL/kg over 15 to 20 minutes and to cats as a bolus of 2.5 to 3 mL/kg over 15 to 20 minutes, with reassessment before giving additional boluses. It is not recommended to exceed a total colloid dose of 20 mL/kg/day for dogs and large animals and 10 to 20 mL/kg/day (typically 10 mL/kg/day) for cats.[h] These solutions may also be administered as a CRI of 1 to 2 mL/kg/h.

In recent years, controversy has arisen regarding the use of synthetic colloids based on studies in human patients that have shown adverse outcomes, especially in patients with conditions that may lead to systemic inflammatory response syndrome (SIRS), such as severe trauma, critical illness, and sepsis. Therefore, although these agents may be used to treat shock, hypotension, and blood loss, especially if there is no response to crystalloids, most experts recommend caution in patients that

[f]Davis H, Jensen T, Johnson A, et al: 2013 AAHA/AAFP fluid therapy guidelines for dogs and cats. *J Am Anim Hosp Assoc* 49(3):149–159, 2013.

[g]Davis H, Jensen T, Johnson A, et al: 2013 AAHA/AAFP fluid therapy guidelines for dogs and cats. *J Am Anim Hosp Assoc* 49(3):149–159, 2013.
[h]Davis H, Jensen T, Johnson A, et al: 2013 AAHA/AAFP fluid therapy guidelines for dogs and cats. *J Am Anim Hosp Assoc* 49(3):149–159, 2013.

are at high risk for adverse effects, particularly those with pre-existing kidney disease, SIRS, sepsis, or coagulation disorders.

> **TECHNICIAN NOTE** Synthetic colloids should be administered to dogs and large animals as a bolus of 5 mL/kg over 15–20 min and to cats as a bolus of 2.5–3 mL/kg over 15–20 min, with re-assessment before giving additional boluses, up to a maximum of 20 mL/kg/day for dogs and large animals and 10–20 mL/kg/day (typically 10 mL/kg/day) for cats.

Adverse Effects of Fluid Administration

If fluid administration is too rapid, the volume may overwhelm the circulation and cause problems such as pulmonary or cerebral edema. This condition is known as *volume overload*. Animals weighing less than 5 kg and those with cardiac or renal disease are at greatest risk. For these patients, a slower infusion rate of crystalloid fluids during anesthesia and surgery may be more appropriate. When monitoring any anesthetized patient that is receiving IV fluids, the anesthetist should be alert for signs of overhydration. These include ocular and nasal discharge, chemosis (edema and swelling of the conjunctiva), subcutaneous edema, increased lung sounds, increased respiratory rate, and dyspnea. When the patient is awake, coughing and restlessness may be seen. Although not commonly done, measurement of central venous pressure (see Chapter 6) allows early detection of overhydration and is recommended for patients receiving more than the recommended volume of fluids.

Another potential adverse effect of excessive fluid administration is dilution of the RBCs and PPs, a condition known as *hemodilution*. Anemic patients, hypoproteinemic patients, and patients that lose a lot of blood from tissue oozing during surgery are at particular risk. In these patients, fluid therapy should therefore be based on careful monitoring of the PCV, PP, and physical parameters.

> **TECHNICIAN NOTE** Signs of overhydration include ocular and nasal discharge, chemosis (edema and swelling of the conjunctiva), subcutaneous edema, increased lung sounds, increased respiratory rate, and dyspnea. When the patient is awake, coughing and restlessness may be seen.

To avoid overhydration, fluids should either be administered using a fluid pump or monitored carefully. In either case, the fluid bag should be labeled with a scale indicating the starting fluid level and anticipated fluid levels by the hour so that the volume of fluid administered can be closely monitored. The use of a burette is advisable for small patients because it allows accurate measurement and administration of small volumes of fluids rather than direct administration from a bag or bottle. See Fig. 2.7 for an illustration of fluid infusion pumps, a scale, and a burette.

Calculating Fluid Administration Rates

When fluids are administered, the prescribed rates (in volume/body weight/unit time) listed in the previous section must be converted into a form that will allow the anesthetist to program an infusion pump or set the roller clamp on an infusion set. Conversion requires the use of mathematic formulas. Any

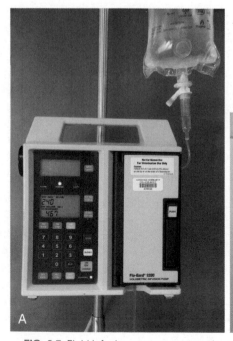
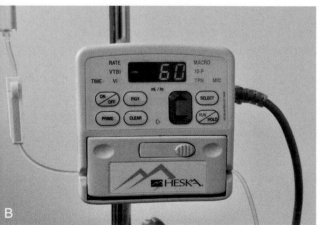

FIG. 2.7 Fluid infusion pumps, tape scale, and burette. **(A)** Flo-Gard Infusion pump. Place the administration set line in the pump as indicated in the owner's manual. Most pumps require an infusion rate in milliliters per hour and a total volume to be infused (VTBI) in milliliters. Note that this pump is programmed to deliver 240 mL/h, and the VTBI is 467 mL. Most pumps will stop and sound an alarm if an occlusion or air bubble is detected in the line. Consequently, infusion pumps must be monitored frequently to ensure proper operation. **(B)** Vet/IV 2.2 Infusion Pump, Heska, Loveland, CO.

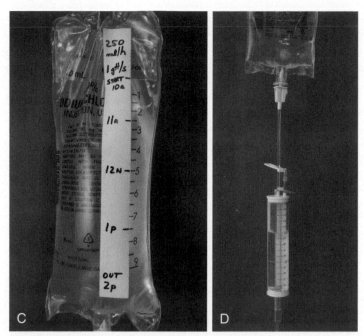

FIG. 2.7, cont'd (C) Tape scale used to monitor the fluid administration rate. The tape should be labeled with the infusion rate (250 mL/h in this case) and the drip rate (1 gtt/s in this case) and should have lines drawn indicating the expected fluid level each hour. This way, any staff member can determine whether the patient has received the proper volume of fluids. Even if using an infusion pump, tape scale helps to ensure that the proper volume of fluids is being delivered. **(D)** Burette. Used to administer small volumes of fluids to small, pediatric, or exotic patients. The burette is filled with the total volume of fluids to be infused by opening the clamp between the burette and the fluid bag. When it is filled to the desired level (in this case 100 mL), the upper clamp is closed. The lower clamp is then opened to allow the fluids to flow into the patient at the desired rate. (A, Courtesy Baxter; https://www.baxter.com. B, Courtesy Heska; https://www.heska.com/.)

discussion of fluid rate calculations can be confusing, however, because the terminology of fluid administration is not standard throughout the literature. So, to avoid confusion, the discussion that follows will begin with a list of terms and definitions related to fluid administration rate calculations (Box 2.7).

The infusion rate (mL/h) is the value used to program an IV infusion pump, and the drip rate (gtt/min or gtt/s) is the value

used to adjust the administration set roller clamp. In order to perform the necessary calculations, the anesthetist must be familiar with the formulas used to determine these rates as well as the delivery rates of available administration sets.

There are two general types of administration sets. Macro-drip sets deliver fluids at a rate of 10 or 15 drops per milliliter and work best to deliver fluids at infusion rates equal to or

---

BOX 2.7 Terms Related to Fluid Administration Rate Calculations

Prescribed Rate
- The fluid administration rate ordered by the attending veterinarian.
- Expressed in **milliliters per unit body weight per unit time.** Most often **mL/kg/h.**

Infusion Rate
- The rate at which fluids should be administered, expressed in **milliliters per unit time.** Most often **mL/h.** (Determined by multiplying the following: **Patient body weight × Prescribed rate.** May also require a conversion factor to change pounds to kilograms.)

Delivery Rate
- The number of drops of fluid that must fall inside the drip chamber of an administration set to deliver 1 mL of fluid expressed in drops per milliliter **(gtt/mL).** (Determined by looking on the packaging of the administration set [see Fig. 2.8].)

Drip Rate
- The rate at which fluids should be administered expressed in **drops per unit time.** Most often **gtt/min.** (Determined by multiplying the following: **Infusion rate × Conversion factor for hours to minutes × Delivery rate.)**
- If necessary to make it easier to set the rate, this figure may be reduced to **drops per 10 or 15 s** (usually calculated using a proportion) or **drops per second** (usually calculated by multiplying the drip rate [drops per minute] by the conversion factor for minutes to seconds).

Infusion Time
- The total time over which the fluids will be administered expressed in **hours.**

Infusion Volume
- The total volume of fluids to be administered expressed in **milliliters** or **liters.** (Determined by multiplying the following three values: **Patient body weight × Prescribed rate × Infusion time.)**

Note: Before fluid infusion rates are calculated, units must be converted so that they are the same (e.g., if working in milliliters per kilogram per hour, then all values involving body weight must be in kilograms).

greater than 100 mL/h. Microdrip sets deliver fluids at a rate of 60 drops per milliliter and work best for infusion rates less than 100 mL/h (Fig. 2.8).

As an alternative, the appropriate set can be chosen on the basis of the patient's body weight. When giving fluids to anesthetized patients, macrodrip sets are appropriate for patients that weigh 20 kg or more when using a prescribed rate based on AAHA/AAFP guidelines, and microdrip sets are appropriate for patients that weigh less than 20 kg. This guideline works well unless delivering fluids at very high rates, as for shock therapy, in which case the guideline based on the infusion rate will work better. If the appropriate set is not used, the anesthetist will find it difficult to adjust the drip rate accurately if the fluids are administered by gravity (without the use of an IV fluid pump).

Calculation of fluid administration rates may be divided into two basic steps. (1) Use the patient's body weight and the prescribed rate to calculate the infusion rate in milliliters per hour. (2) Using the infusion rate, the delivery rate, and conversion factors, calculate the drip rate in drops per minute or some other unit of time. Box 2.8 and Fig. 2.9 summarize the steps required to calculate infusion rates and drip rates during the perioperative period for routine administration during surgery and for treatment of blood loss, hypotension, and shock. Tables 2.11 and 2.12 consist of calculated infusion rates in mL/h (based on the commonly prescribed rates) for dogs and cats, respectively.

TECHNICIAN NOTE When administering IV fluids by gravity (without the use of an IV fluid pump), use a macrodrip set (10 or 15 gtt/mL) for infusion rates ≥100 mL/h. Use a microdrip set (60 gtt/mL) for infusion rates <100 mL/h. When administering fluids at the prescribed rates based on AAHA/AAFP guidelines, a macrodrip set is most appropriate for dogs over 20 kg in body weight, whereas a microdrip set should be used for cats and dogs that weigh <20 kg.

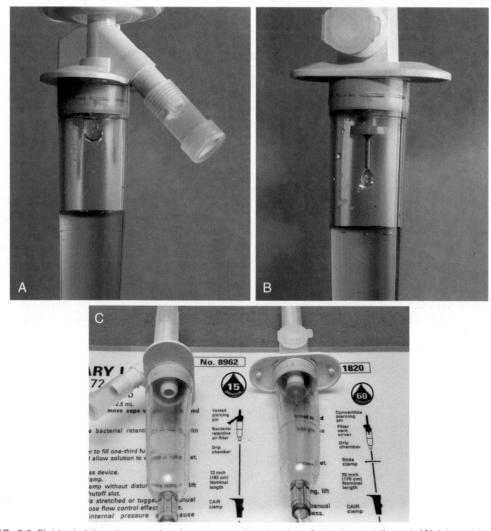

FIG. 2.8 Fluid administration set chambers, comparing the size of the drops delivered. **(A)** Macrodrip set chamber (15 gtt/mL). Used for infusion rates ≥100 mL/h. Compare the size of this drop with **(B)** microdrip set chamber (60 gtt/mL). Used for infusion rates of <100 mL/h. **(C)** Macrodrip (15 gtt/mL) and microdrip (60 gtt/mL) fluid administration sets on the left and right, respectively. Note that the delivery rate in gtt/mL is listed on the package *(see the drop icons circled in red)*.

BOX 2.8 Calculating Fluid Administration Rates

Step 1: Calculate the Infusion Rate
a. Determine the patient's body weight (lb or kg).
b. Determine the prescribed rate (mL/kg/h).
c. Calculate the infusion rate (mL/h).

Example 1
The doctor orders intravenous (IV) fluids for a **55-lb dog** at a rate of **5 mL/kg/h** for a 1-h surgery. What is the infusion rate in mL/h?
Set up the problem this way:

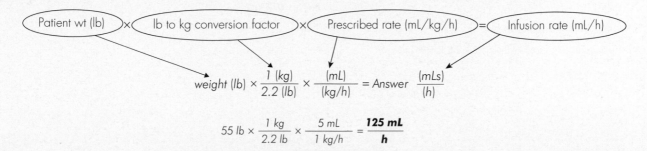

$$ \text{weight (lb)} \times \frac{1 \text{ (kg)}}{2.2 \text{ (lb)}} \times \frac{\text{(mL)}}{\text{(kg/h)}} = \text{Answer} \; \frac{\text{(mLs)}}{\text{(h)}} $$

$$ 55 \text{ lb} \times \frac{1 \text{ kg}}{2.2 \text{ lb}} \times \frac{5 \text{ mL}}{1 \text{ kg/h}} = \mathbf{\frac{125 \text{ mL}}{h}} $$

Example 2
The doctor orders IV fluids for treatment of shock in a **12-lb** cat at a rate of **55 mL/kg. You are to give one-quarter of the calculated dose rapidly.** What is the infusion rate in milliliters?
Set up the problem this way:

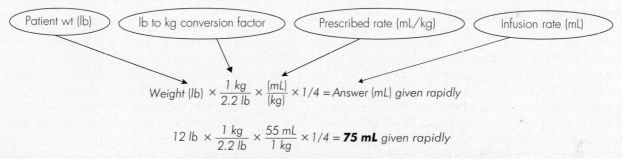

$$ \text{Weight (lb)} \times \frac{1 \text{ kg}}{2.2 \text{ lb}} \times \frac{\text{(mL)}}{\text{(kg)}} \times 1/4 = \text{Answer (mL) given rapidly} $$

$$ 12 \text{ lb} \times \frac{1 \text{ kg}}{2.2 \text{ lb}} \times \frac{55 \text{ mL}}{1 \text{ kg}} \times 1/4 = \mathbf{75 \text{ mL}} \text{ given rapidly} $$

Because this cat is being treated for shock, the calculated dose of fluids will be given rapidly instead of at a constant rate.

Step 2: Calculate the Drip Rate
a. Choose the appropriate administration set and note the delivery rate (in drops per milliliter) by looking at the package.
  • Choose a *microdrip* set if the rate is <100 mL/h (all microdrip sets deliver **60 gtt/mL**).
  • Choose a *macrodrip* set if the rate is ≥100 mL/h (the delivery rate will be **10 or 15 gtt/mL** depending on the set chosen).
b. Calculate the drip rate (gtt/min).

Example 1
The **55-lb dog** in Step 1, Example 1 requires an infusion rate of **125 mL/h**. What administration set should you use and what is the drip rate? Available sets include a 60 gtt/mL microdrip set and a 15 gtt/mL macrodrip set.
Set up the problem this way:

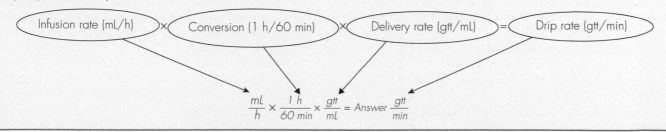

$$ \frac{mL}{h} \times \frac{1 \text{ h}}{60 \text{ min}} \times \frac{gtt}{mL} = \text{Answer} \; \frac{gtt}{min} $$

Continued

BOX 2.8   Calculating Fluid Administration Rates—cont'd

You should choose a macro administration set because the infusion rate is >100 mL/h

$$125 \, \frac{mL}{hr} \times \frac{1 \, hr}{60 \, min} \times \frac{15 \, gtt}{mL} = \frac{\textbf{31 gtt}}{\textbf{min}}$$

Example 1 (Continued)

i. If desired, convert the drip rate to gtt/sec, gtt/10 s, or gtt/15 s.

It is often easier to set the drip rate if you convert it to a smaller unit of time (number of drops in 10 or 15 s or drops/s).

Conversion to drops per second:

$$\frac{31 \, gtt}{min} \times \frac{1 \, min}{60 \, sec} = \frac{\textbf{0.5 gtt}}{\textbf{sec}}$$

Conversion to drops in 10 s: cross-multiply and solve for the unknown.

$$\frac{31 \, gtt}{60 \, sec} = \frac{gtt}{10 \, sec}$$

$$31 \, gtt \times 10 \, sec = gtt \times 60 \, sec$$

$$gtt = \frac{31 \, gtt \times 10 \, sec}{60 \, sec}$$

Answer = **5 gtt in 10 sec** or **1 gtt in 2 sec**

OTHER PREANESTHETIC CARE

In addition to the care summarized on the previous pages, the veterinarian may direct the technician, nurse, or another staff member to provide additional preoperative nursing care including administration of medications.

Antibiotics are often ordered for animals that have infections or that are scheduled for procedures involving a contaminated area (such as gastrointestinal or dental procedures). Administration of pain medication before painful procedures, a practice known as *preemptive analgesia* (discussed further in Chapter 8), is proven to be considerably more effective than waiting until the pain is manifest, and significantly improves patient recovery.

Some patients may require a variety of other medications such as insulin, anticonvulsants, or antiemetic or antiinflammatory drugs. The technician or nurse should actively seek specific instructions from the veterinarian regarding the care required as the well-being of the patient and the outcome of the procedure are significantly influenced by the attention that is given to this final but important facet of patient preparation.

KEY POINTS

1. Effective communication is key to the ability of the veterinary health care team to provide high-quality patient care. The veterinary technician or nurse often acts as a liaison between the attending veterinarian, the client, and other members of the health care team.
2. Effective use of anesthetic safety checklists help to minimize errors and improve outcomes when gathering and preparing equipment, performing complex procedures, and communicating among team members.
3. During the preanesthetic period, the technician or nurse has many duties. They must help the attending veterinarian develop a minimum patient database, ensure that fasting instructions were followed, place an intravenous (IV) catheter, administer fluids, stabilize the patient, prepare equipment, and administer medications.
4. An accurate and complete patient history is at least as important, if not more important, than the results of diagnostic tests in shaping patient management. Acquisition of a patient history requires skill in choosing and framing questions.
5. There are many ways in which patient signalment influences response to anesthesia. The anesthetist must consider these factors when managing patients.
6. Dehydration, anemia, abnormal bleeding, respiratory or cardiovascular system disease, kidney or liver dysfunction, and conditions that require treatment while the patient is under anesthesia are physical findings that may influence anesthetic management.
7. Immediately before any procedure, definitively identify and weigh the patient; assess body condition, hydration, level of consciousness, vital signs, and general condition; and determine a pain score.
8. Before any procedure, always present a consent form and fee estimate and acquire signatures.
9. No single anesthetic protocol is ideal for all patients. Rather, the anesthetic techniques and agents used are tailored to the

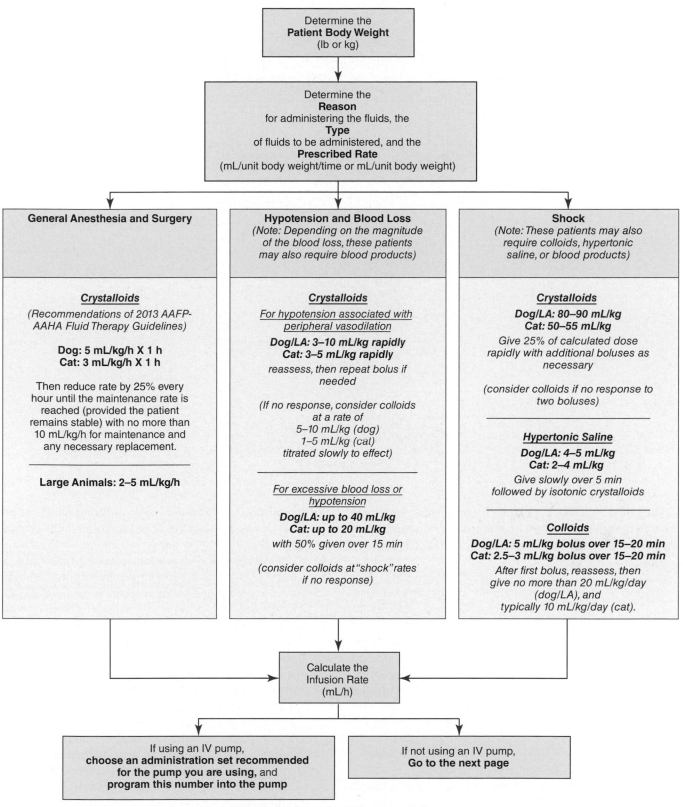

FIG. 2.9 Flow chart for fluid rate calculations.

Continued

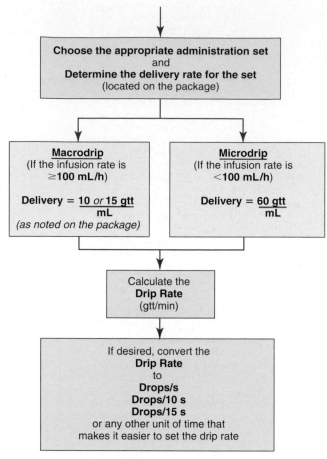

FIG. 2.9, cont'd

needs of the individual patient. Factors such as previous or concurrent illness, nature of the procedure, urgency, and preference of the veterinarian are all considered in selecting a protocol.

10. Diagnostic tests such as the complete blood count (CBC), chemistries, urinalysis, radiography, and electrocardiography may provide valuable information regarding the patient's ability to tolerate anesthesia and anesthetic planning.

11. The physical condition of the patient should be assessed before initiating any procedure. The patient should be assigned to a physical status classification based on physical condition as outlined by the American Society of Anesthesiologists.

12. The patient should be in stable condition, when possible, before being anesthetized. Preexisting problems such as dehydration or shock should be corrected.

13. IV catheter placement gives the anesthetist the ability to administer IV anesthetics safely, provide fluid support, maintain anesthesia via constant rate infusion (CRI), and administer emergency drugs to patients if needed.

14. Knowledge of fluid homeostasis and composition of body fluids enables the anesthetist to administer fluids safely and effectively.

15. Crystalloids may be classified according to the mix and quantity of solutes as isotonic, hypotonic, or hypertonic; replacement or maintenance; and balanced or unbalanced.

16. Isotonic crystalloid solutions are routinely used in most anesthetized patients, except those with a plasma protein level less than 3.5 g/dL, a packed cell volume (PCV) less than 20%, or a low platelet count.

17. Colloids and/or blood products may be used to support expansion of blood volume, blood pressure, oxygen-carrying capacity, and/or blood coagulation in patients with low plasma protein, PCV, and/or platelet count.

18. An initial fluid infusion rate of 5 mL/kg/h in dogs and 3 mL/kg/h in cats, followed by a reduced rate if the patient is anesthetized for more than 1 hour, is recommended by the authors of the 2013 AAHA/AAFP Fluid Therapy Guidelines for Dogs and Cats. Infusion rates of 2 to 5 mL/kg/h are typically used for large animals.

REVIEW QUESTIONS

1. In gathering a patient history, which of the following would be the best way to frame a question about a patient's exercise level?
   a. "Your dog does not exercise much, does he, Mrs. Jones?"
   b. "Does your dog exercise, Mrs. Jones?"
   c. "How many times a week does your pet go for a walk or exercise, Mrs. Jones?"
   d. "You don't give your dog as much exercise as you should, do you, Mrs. Jones?"

2. Which of the following examples of species associations is not correct?
   a. Horses and cats are more sensitive to opioids than dogs and ruminants.
   b. The use of anticholinergics is recommended in ruminants to avoid airway occlusion.
   c. Horses may fracture limbs during anesthetic recovery and thus require special attention during the recovery period.
   d. Large animals are prone to respiratory depression and dependent atelectasis and thus often require ventilatory support.

3. Which of the following statements regarding physical examination findings is incorrect?
   a. Dehydration increases the risk of hypotension.
   b. Anemia predisposes the patient to hypoxemia.
   c. Patients with bruising may be at higher risk for potentially life-threatening intraoperative and postoperative bleeding.
   d. A dog with a body condition score of 8/9 will require more anesthetic per unit body weight than a dog of the same breed with a body condition score of 5/9.

4. You are evaluating a patient's LOC and find the patient in a sleeplike state, nonresponsive to a verbal stimulus but arousable by a painful stimulus. This patient is:
   a. Lethargic
   b. Obtunded
   c. Stuporous
   d. Comatose

5. You are evaluating a patient's hydration. The skin elasticity is mildly slowed, the patient's mucous membranes are tacky, the CRT is 1.5 seconds, but the eyes are in a normal position in the orbit. Your patient is:
   a. Hydrated
   b. Approximately 5% dehydrated
   c. Approximately 8% dehydrated
   d. Greater than 10% dehydrated

6. Which of the following fasting times is least advisable?
   a. Dog: 4 to 6 hours
   b. Horse: 2 to 4 hours
   c. Cow: 24 to 48 hours
   d. Small ruminant: 12 to 18 hours

7. Which of the following is not a crystalloid solution?
   a. Lactated Ringer's solution
   b. Normal saline solution
   c. Hetastarch
   d. 5% Dextrose

8. Using the ASA Physical Status Classification system, a patient that is moderately anemic or moderately dehydrated would be classified as:
   a. Class PS1
   b. Class PS2
   c. Class PS3
   d. Class PS4
   e. Class PS5

9. Which of the following signs of disease in a calm canine patient would be most significant in terms of the potential to increase the risk of anesthesia?
   a. Increased respiratory effort
   b. Lethargy
   c. A body temperature of 103.4°F
   d. A sinus arrhythmia

10. Which of the following species or breeds must be watched especially closely during any anesthetic procedure to ensure a patent airway?
    a. Brachycephalic breeds
    b. Exotic breeds
    c. Cats and horses
    d. Sighthounds

11. Using a prescribed fluid administration rate of 5 mL/kg/h for the first hour of anesthesia and a macrodrip administration set with a delivery rate of 15 gtt/mL, a 53-lb patient would require which of the following infusion and drip rates?
    a. 265 mL/h; 1 gtt/s
    b. 121 mL/h; 1 gtt/s
    c. 121 mL/h; 1 gtt/2 s
    d. 121 mL/h; 1 gtt/4 s

12. Which of the following statements regarding IV catheter placement and use in anesthesia patients is incorrect?
    a. Choose an administration set with an injection port.
    b. Give all IV drugs slowly unless told otherwise.
    c. Always follow IV injections administered through a catheter with a sterile saline flush.
    d. Choose a catheter that is small in diameter to minimize the risk of bleeding.

13. Which of the following general guidelines about body fluids in a normal adult animal is incorrect?
    a. About 40% of the body weight is water.
    b. About two-thirds of the total body water is inside the cells.
    c. Blood plasma makes up about 5% of the total body weight.
    d. Dogs have a larger total blood volume per unit body weight than cats.

14. The fluid type most appropriate to replace moderate losses from dehydration would be:
    a. Colloids
    b. Hypertonic saline
    c. Isotonic crystalloids
    d. 50% dextrose

15. Which of the following figures represents a fluid infusion rate as defined in this chapter?
    a. 10 mL/kg/h
    b. 100 mL/h
    c. 1 gtt/s
    d. 500 mL total

16. The delivery rate of a microdrip administration set is:
    a. 10 gtt/mL only
    b. 10 or 15 gtt/mL
    c. 20 or 60 gtt/mL
    d. 60 gtt/mL only

17. Which of the following statements regarding electrolyte composition of fluids is incorrect?
    a. Extracellular fluid contains more sodium than intracellular fluid.
    b. Intracellular fluid contains more potassium than intravascular fluid.
    c. The osmolarity of intracellular fluid is similar to that of extracellular fluid.
    d. Intravascular fluid has more negatively charged particles than positively charged particles.

18. Regarding fluid infusion rates, which of the following is true?
    a. Standard shock doses of fluids are about the same as doses used during routine surgery.
    b. Surgery patients with blood loss may require colloids instead of crystalloids.
    c. Crystalloids are generally given at lower administration rates than colloids to treat shock.
    d. Hypertonic saline is administered in large volumes to patients in shock.

19. Which of the following is *not* a sign of fluid overload?
    a. Ocular and nasal discharge
    b. Hypotension
    c. Increased lung sounds and respiratory rate
    d. Dyspnea

20. Which of the following heart rhythms is not normal in a resting horse?
    a. NSR
    b. SA
    c. Second-degree AV block
    d. Third-degree AV block

ANSWERS TO CASE PRESENTATIONS

Case Presentation 2.1

Question #1: Clients react in different ways to any set of circumstances, so there are many possible feelings a client may experience depending on their relationship with the animal, their understanding of the problem, their relationship with the doctor, and a variety of other factors. Even so, it would certainly be expected that a client might feel alarmed and upset at this unexpected outcome and perhaps frustrated or angry that the pericardial disease was not detected and discussed before surgery. The client also might feel anxious and unsure what to do after receiving the unexpected news of a serious condition in a pet that was thought to have a relatively minor and treatable problem.

Maggie's owner was very angry and felt that the problem should have been detected before the surgery was performed. He felt that if he had known that the pericardial disease was present, he might not have authorized surgery. Not only had he paid the expense of the workup and surgery, but also was facing the much higher expenses of treating the cardiac problem—expenses that he was not prepared to incur. He also questioned whether or not he was being told the truth.

Question #2: There are two elements of patient preparation that were overlooked. *First, the client was not asked about the patient's condition on the day of surgery.* As happened in this case, a patient's condition will sometimes change between the time of the initial exam and the day that surgery is scheduled, especially when the two are separated for a significant period of time. Knowledge of changes in a patient's condition enables the attending veterinarian to make appropriate changes in the treatment plan before anesthetic induction, thus avoiding a complication such as this. In this particular case, the owner had not noticed any change in condition and

so the problem would not have been revealed but, in many other cases, owners neglect to tell the staff about changes in a patient's condition unless asked.

Second, a PA focusing on the cardiovascular and pulmonary systems was not performed. If a PA had been performed, the abnormal heart rate, heart sounds, and pulses would likely have been detected. Then the client could have been contacted by the attending surgeon before surgery and an informed decision could have been made regarding the best course of action to take with full knowledge of the cardiac disease. Regardless of the outcome, in all likelihood, the client would have been confident that everything possible had been done to help Maggie.

Outcomes of the Case

Owing to the seriousness of the problem and additional costs that would be associated with further workup and treatment, the owner elected to have the patient euthanized. On necropsy, the presence of an inoperable, malignant heart-based mass was confirmed by biopsy.

Case Presentation 2.2

Question #1: This case illustrates how easily seemingly small omissions in communication can lead to misunderstandings, dissatisfaction, anger, and even the loss of a client. The client's perception of the quality of care is most often closely related to whether or not their expectations have been met, so if there is an unexpected outcome, the client may react strongly. In this situation, even though the owner was informed that extractions would be necessary, he assumed perhaps two or three at the most, and he had no previous experience to prepare him for the large number that was needed in this case. Consequently, the gap between his expectation and the outcome was wide.

With experience, veterinary professionals learn to anticipate circumstances that have the potential to lead to misunderstandings and to circumvent unmet expectations with good communication. Options in this case would have been to write an estimated number of extractions on the release form and call the client if the actual number was going to exceed this figure, or call the client in any case when it was clear that the number of extractions was going to be high. If the client had been warned and had not been surprised with this information during the exit interview, it is likely that he would have left happy, satisfied, and confident that everything possible had been done to protect the health of his pet.

SELECTED READINGS

Adamik KN, Yozova ID: Colloids yes or no?—A "Gretchen question" answered, *Front Vet Sci* 8:624049, 2021. https://doi.org/10.3389/fvets.2021.624049.

Auckburally A: Fluid therapy and blood transfusion. In Duke-Novakovski T, DeVries M, Seymour C, editors: *BSAVA manual of canine and feline anaesthesia and analgesia*, ed 3, Glouchester, UK, 2016, British Small Animal Veterinary Association.

Chohan AS, Davidow EB: Clinical pharmacology and administration of fluid, electrolyte, and blood component solutions. In Grimm KA, Lamont, LA, Tranquilli WJ, editors: *Lumb & Jones' veterinary anesthesia and analgesia*, ed 5, Ames, IA, 2015, John Wiley & Sons, Inc., pp 386–413.

Davis H, Jensen T, Johnson A, et al: 2013 AAHA/AAFP fluid therapy guidelines for dogs and cats, *J Am Anim Hosp Assoc* 49(3):149–159, 2013.

DiBartola S, Bateman S: Introduction to fluid therapy. In DiBartola S, editor: *Fluid, electrolyte, and acid-base disorders*, ed 3, St. Louis, MO, 2011, Saunders, pp 325–344.

Donohoe C: *Fluid therapy for veterinary technicians and nurses*, West Sussex, UK, 2012, John Wiley & Sons.

Fielding CL, Magdesian KG: *Equine fluid therapy*, West Sussex, UK, 2015, John Wiley & Sons.

Grubb T, Sager J, Gaynor JS, et al: 2020 AAHA anesthesia and monitoring guidelines for dogs and cats, *J Am Anim Hosp Assoc* 56(2):1–24, 2020.

Hansen BD: Technical aspects of fluid therapy. In DiBartola S, editor: *Fluid, electrolyte, and acid-base disorders*, ed 4, St. Louis, MO, 2011, Saunders, pp 351–385.

King LG, Boag A: *BSAVA manual of canine and feline emergency and critical care*, ed 3, Glouchester, UK, 2016, British Small Animal Veterinary Association.

Lake T, Green N: *Essential calculations for veterinary nurses and technicians*, ed 3, St. Louis, MO, 2017, Elsevier, pp 89–96.

Liss D, Norkus CL: Fluid therapy, electrolyte abnormalities, and acid-base disorders. In Norkus CL, editor: *Veterinary technician's manual for small animal emergency and critical care*, ed 2, West Sussex, UK, 2019, John Wiley & Sons., pp 385–416.

Macintire D, Drobatz K, Haskins S, Saxon W: *Manual of small animal emergency and critical care medicine*, ed 2, Ames, IA, 2012, Blackwell.

Mathews KA: Monitoring fluid therapy and complications of fluid therapy. In DiBartola S, editor: *Fluid, electrolyte, and acid–base disorders*, ed 4, St. Louis, MO, 2011, Saunders, pp 386–404.

Muir WW, de Morais SA, Seeler DC: Acid–base balance and fluid therapy. In Grimm KA, Tranquilli WJ, Lamont LA, editors: *Essentials of small animal anesthesia and analgesia*, ed 2, Ames, IA, 2011, Blackwell, pp 240–273.

Muir WW, Hubbell JA, Bednarski RM, Lerche P: *Handbook of veterinary anesthesia*, ed 5, St. Louis, 2012, Elsevier.

Pascoe PJ: Perioperative management of fluid therapy. In DiBartola S, editor: *Fluid, electrolyte, and acid–base disorders*, ed 4, St. Louis, 2011, Saunders, pp 405–435.

Plumb DC: Plumb's Veterinary Drugs. https://plumbs.com/solutions/plumbs-veterinary-drugs/.

Posner LP: Pre-anaesthetic assessment and preparation. In Duke-Novakovski T, DeVries M, Seymour C, editor: *BSAVA manual of canine and feline anaesthesia and analgesia*, ed 3, Glouchester, UK, 2016, British Small Animal Veterinary Association, pp 6–12.

Robertson SA, Gogolski SM, Pascoe P, et al. AAFP feline anesthesia guidelines, *J Feline Med Surg* 20:602–634, 2018.

The Association of Veterinary Anaesthetists. *Guidelines for safer anaesthesia*. 2018. https://ava.eu.com/wp-content/uploads/2018/01/AVA-Safer-Anaesthesia-Guidlines-Booklet-VET-Web.pdf. Accessed August, 2021.

Thomassen Ø, Espeland A, Søfteland E, et al: Implementation of checklists in health care; learning from high-reliability organisations, *Scand J Trauma Resusc Emerg Med* 19:53, 2011. http://www.sjtrem.com/content/19/1/53. Accessed February, 2022.

Tranquilli WJ, Grimm KA: Introduction: use, definitions, history, concepts, classification, and considerations for anesthesia and analgesia. In Grimm KA, Lamont LA, Tranquilli WJ, editors: *Lumb & Jones' veterinary anesthesia and analgesia*, ed 5, Ames, IA, 2015, John Wiley & Sons, Inc., pp 3–10.

Trent KB: Venous access. In Norkus CL, editor: *Veterinary technician's manual for small animal emergency and critical care*, ed 2, West Sussex, UK, 2019, John Wiley & Sons., pp 35–44.

Wellman ML, DiBartola SP, Kohn CW: Applied physiology of body fluids in dogs and cats. In DiBartola S, editor: *Fluid, electrolyte, and acid–base disorders*, ed 4, St. Louis, 2011, Saunders, pp 2–25.

Anesthetic Agents and Adjuncts

OUTLINE

LEARNING OBJECTIVES

When you have completed this chapter, you will be able to:

- Classify anesthetic agents and adjuncts based on route of administration, time of administration, principal effect, or chemistry.
- Differentiate agonists, partial agonists, agonist–antagonists, and antagonists based on their action and effect; list anesthetics and adjuncts that can be reversed.
- Describe the effect of protein binding, lipid solubility, and redistribution on the pharmacokinetics and pharmacodynamics of injectable anesthetics.
- Apply principles of safe administration of anesthetic agents and adjuncts.
- List anesthetic agents and adjuncts commonly used as preanesthetic medications and describe their indications, mode of action, effects, adverse effects, and use.

- List injectable anesthetic drugs in common use and describe their indications, mode of action, effects, adverse effects, and use.
- Define dissociative anesthesia, describe the actions and effects of dissociative anesthetics, and explain ways in which these drugs differ from other injectable anesthetics.
- List the inhalation anesthetic agents in common use and describe their indications, mode of action, effects, adverse effects, and use.
- Define vapor pressure, partition coefficient, minimum alveolar concentration (MAC), and rubber solubility; explain the ways in which these properties affect the action and use of inhalant anesthetic agents.
- Describe the uptake, distribution, and elimination of the commonly used inhalation anesthetic agents.

KEY TERMS

Adjunct	Colic	Nystagmus
Agonist–antagonists	Cortisol	Parasympatholytics
Agonists	Dead space	Partial agonists
Analeptic agent	Desiccated	Pharmacodynamics
Anesthetic agent	Dysphoria	Pharmacokinetics
Antagonists	Enantiomer	Preanesthetic medications
Anticholinergics	Fasciculations	Reversal agents
Anxiolytics	Hypoventilation	Somatic analgesia
Apnea	Macroemulsion	Status epilepticus
Apneustic respiration	Microemulsion	Synergistic (supra-additive)
Ataxia	Mydriasis	Tachycardia
Bagging	Myoclonus	Tidal volume
Behavioral disinhibition	Neuroleptanalgesia	Visceral analgesia
Cataleptoid state	Neuromuscular blockers	Windup

INTRODUCTION TO ANESTHETIC AGENTS AND ADJUNCTS

An anesthetic agent may be defined as any drug used to induce a loss of sensation with or without unconsciousness. The term adjunct is used to describe a drug that is not a true anesthetic but that is used during anesthesia to produce other desired effects such as anxiolysis, sedation, muscle relaxation, analgesia, reversal, neuromuscular blockade, or parasympathetic blockade. Because adjuncts are used as a part of balanced anesthesia, they are traditionally included in the study of anesthetic agents. Anesthetic agents and adjuncts may be classified a number of ways.

First, they may be classified on the basis of the route of administration. Inhalant agents are administered from an anesthetic machine into the lower respiratory tree via an endotracheal tube or mask. Injectable agents are injected intravenously, intramuscularly, subcutaneously, intraperitoneally, intralesionally, or into a number of other locations. Oral agents are given by mouth, and topical agents are applied to a body surface such as the skin or mucous membranes.

Another way these agents may be classified is based on the time period at which they are given during the course of an anesthetic procedure. Drugs given before general anesthesia are referred to as preanesthetic medications. Drugs used to induce general anesthesia are referred to as *induction agents*, and those used to maintain general anesthesia are referred to as *maintenance agents*.

A third way anesthetic agents and adjuncts may be classified is according to their principal effect. Local anesthetics induce a loss of sensation in a localized area of the body. In contrast, general anesthetics induce a loss of sensation over the entire body, accompanied by unconsciousness. Anxiolytics, sedatives, and tranquilizers are agents that cause anxiolysis, sedation, and tranquilization, respectively. Analgesics prevent and control pain. Muscle relaxants decrease muscle tone. Neuromuscular blockers, although infrequently used in general practice, are used to relax or paralyze skeletal muscles during ophthalmic, orthopedic, or other surgeries. Anticholinergic agents are used to decrease effects of parasympathetic nervous system (PNS) stimulation such as bradycardia and excessive salivation.

Finally, reversal agents lessen or abolish the effects of other anesthetic agents and are therefore used to "wake" the patient after sedation or anesthesia.

Many of the agents used in anesthesia cause two or more of these effects, depending on the dose and the circumstances under which they are used. For instance, morphine causes sedation and is an excellent analgesic. The injectable drug dexmedetomidine causes moderate to profound sedation, analgesia, and good muscle relaxation when given alone but can be used in combination with other agents to induce general anesthesia. The intravenous (IV) anesthetic alfaxalone induces general anesthesia at clinically used doses but can also be used as a sedative when given by intramuscular (IM) injection. As a consequence, classification of these agents on the basis of the principal effect is somewhat arbitrary.

The final way anesthetic agents and adjuncts may be classified is based on their chemistry. For the student, this is perhaps the most useful method of classification because the agents within a given class tend to have similar properties and effects. For this reason, the anesthetic agents and adjuncts discussed herein will be presented this way. Tables 3.1 to 3.4 summarize the principal effects and adverse effects of the anesthetic agents and adjuncts.

Clinically Important Properties of Anesthetic Agents

Before embarking on a study of anesthetic agents and adjuncts, a general knowledge of pharmacokinetics (the effect the body has on a drug) and pharmacodynamics (the effects a drug has on the body) is necessary. After administration, most drugs are distributed throughout the body by the blood. Each drug binds to specific receptors in one or more "target tissues." After binding to specific receptors, the drug stimulates the receptor, causing one or more specific effects. In the case of anesthetic agents and adjuncts, the primary target tissue is most often the central nervous system (CNS), and the most common effect is depression and/or stimulation of one or more parts of the CNS.

Many factors influence the amount of anesthetic available to bind to receptors such as the percentage of the drug that is floating free in the blood plasma versus the amount bound

TABLE 3.1   Principal Central Nervous System Effects of Anesthetic Agents and Adjuncts

Agent Class	CNS Activity	Intracranial Pressure	Analgesia	Body Temperature	Other CNS Effects
Anxiolytics (gabapentin and trazodone)	− (anxiolysis/ sedation-both drugs)	− (gabapentin) 0 (trazodone)	+ (gabapentin) 0 (trazodone)	0	Ataxia (both); anticonvulsant activity (gabapentin); possible agitation or excitement, behavioral disinhibition (trazodone)
Anticholinergics	− (atropine) 0 (glycopyrrolate)		0	0	
Acepromazine	− − (Ca, Eq, Bo) − (Fe),		0	Decreased	Excitement; aggression
Benzodiazepines	− (old, ill) + (young, healthy)	0 to −	0	0	Disorientation; aggression; ataxia; anticonvulsant activity
Alpha$_2$-agonists	− − − (especially SA, small Ru, foals)	+ (in SA because of vomiting)	+ + (short duration, somatic and visceral)	Decreased	Aggression; ataxia; cattle lie down; muscle tremors (Eq)
Opioids	− to − − − (Ca) − to + + + (Fe, Eq, Ru)	0 (+ only if hypoventilating)	+ + + (agonists) + + (agonist–antagonists) (somatic and visceral)	Decreased (Ca) Increased (Fe, possibly Eq, Ru)	Disorientation (Ca, if not in pain); excitement, dysphoria (Fe, Eq, Ru)
Propofol	− to − − −	−	0	Decreased	Muscular activity that resembles seizures
Etomidate	− to − − −	0	0 to +		Anticonvulsant activity; decreased O$_2$ consumption
Alfaxalone	− to − − −	−	0	Decreased	
Barbiturates	− to − − − (+ at low doses)	− (0 if normal respiration)	0	Decreased	Excitement during recovery and induction, especially if given too slowly
Dissociatives	Both + and − (dissociative anesthesia)	+	+ + (somatic) 0 to + (visceral)	Decreased	Seizurelike activity; intact reflexes
Guaifenesin	−		0		Ataxia
Halogenated inhalants	− to − − −	+	0	Decreased	Malignant hyperthermia in susceptible patients

Notes on use of this table:
- 0 indicates minimal to no effect.
- − indicates a decrease in the parameter indicated (where − is mild; − − is moderate; − − − is marked).
- + indicates an increase in the parameter indicated (where + is mild; + + is moderate; + + + is marked).
- Effects of drugs depend on many factors, including species, differences among specific agents within a class, dose, and drug interactions. Therefore quantifications of the principal effects (mild, moderate, Marked) are approximations.
- The information regarding opioids includes those of agonists, partial agonists, and agonist–antagonists. When reading this, note that effects of agonists are generally more pronounced than those of agonist–antagonists or partial agonists).

Bo, Bovine; *Ca,* canine; *CNS,* central nervous system; *Eq,* equine; *Fe,* feline; *Ru,* ruminants; *SA,* small animals; −, depression; +, stimulation.

TABLE 3.2 Principal Cardiovascular System Effects of Anesthetic Agents and Adjuncts

Agent Class	Heart Rate	Cardiac Output	Blood Pressure	Cardiac Arrhythmias	Other Cardiovascular Effects
Anxiolytics (gabapentin and trazodone)	0	0	0	0	
Anticholinergics	++/+++	0/+	0/+	++ (atropine) + (glycopyrrolate)	Atropine, low doses: temporary bradycardia
Acepromazine	− or + secondary to hypotension	−	− −/− − −	− (protects against arrhythmias)	Vasodilation; high doses may cause low HR (Ca)
Benzodiazepines	0 (diazepam: − if given rapidly IV)	0	0 (diazepam: − if given rapidly IV)	0	
Alpha₂-agonists	− − −	− −/− − −	− −/− − − − (following an initial period of hypertension)	++ (especially early)	Initial hypertension resulting from vasoconstriction; pale mucous membranes
Opioids	− to − − −	0	0	0	Morphine: hypotension secondary to histamine release
Propofol	−	−	− (transient); − − in some patients	0 (alone) + (with epinephrine)	
Etomidate	0	0	Transient −, then 0	0	
Alfaxalone	0/+	0/−	− (dose dependent)	0/+ (thought to be due to hypoxemia and/or hypercapnia)	
Barbiturates	− or +	− to − − − (dose-dependent)	− to − − − (dose-dependent)	+++ (especially bigeminy)	
Dissociatives	+	+	+	+	Increased O₂ consumption; decreased inotropy
Guaifenesin	Mild + (transient)	0	− (transient)	0	
Halogenated inhalants	Variable	−/− − (dose-dependent)	−/− −	0 (except halothane: ++)	Vasodilation

Notes on use of this table:
- 0 indicates minimal to no effect.
- − indicates a decrease in the parameter indicated (where − is mild; − − is moderate; − − − is marked).
- + indicates an increase in the parameter indicated (where + is mild; ++ is moderate; +++ is marked).
- Effects of drugs depend on many factors, including species, differences among specific agents within a class, dose, and drug interactions. Therefore quantifications of the principal effects (mild, moderate, marked) are approximations.
- The information regarding opioids includes those of agonists, partial agonists, and agonist–antagonists. When reading this, note that effects of agonists are generally more pronounced than those of agonist–antagonists or partial agonists).

Ca, Canine; *HR,* heart rate; *IV,* intravenously; *−*. depression; *+*. stimulation.

to blood proteins and how easily the drug penetrates the brain. After a drug acts on the receptors, it will eventually be metabolized and ultimately eliminated from the body. The speed with which this takes place is, in turn, influenced by a number of variables such as liver and kidney health, movement of the drug between tissues, and route of administration. Understanding of factors that affect these processes is necessary to use these drugs safely.

Agonists, Partial Agonists, Mixed Agonist–Antagonists, and Antagonists

Anesthetic agents and adjuncts differ according to the degree to which they stimulate target tissue receptors. Agonists bind to and stimulate tissue receptors. Most anesthetics and adjuncts are classified as agonists.

Some drug classes such as the alpha₂-adrenergics and opioids include drugs that are classified as antagonists. Antagonists bind to but do not stimulate receptors. These drugs are

given after an agonist of the same class to "wake" the patient from anesthesia or sedation. They are therefore called *reversal agents* because they reverse the effects of the corresponding agonist. Specifically, most antagonists competitively bind to receptors and displace the corresponding agonist, blocking further action.

The opioid class also includes some partial agonists and agonist–antagonists. Partial agonists bind to and partially stimulate receptors. Agonist–antagonists bind to more than one receptor type and simultaneously stimulate at least one and block at least one. Both partial agonists and agonist–antagonists are sometimes used to partially block the effects of pure agonists.

Effects and Adverse Effects of Anesthetic Agents and Adjuncts

When learning about anesthetic agents and adjuncts, the student anesthetist must understand the major effects associated

TABLE 3.3 Principal Respiratory and Gastrointestinal System Effects of Anesthetic Agents and Adjuncts

Agent Class	Respiratory Rate	Tidal Volume	Salivary, Respiratory, GI Secretions	GI Motility	Other Respiratory and GI Effects
Anxiolytics (gabapentin and trazodone)	0	0	0 0		Vomiting and/or diarrhea; changes in appetite (both)
Anticholinergics	0	0	− (atropine); − − (glycopyrrolate) (except for Ru)	− −/− − − Colic (Eq); bloat (Ru)	Bronchodilation; thickening of secretions (Fe, Ru)
Acepromazine	0 (− with other agents)	0 (− with other agents)	0	−	Antiemetic
Benzodiazepines	0 (diazepam: apnea if given rapidly IV)	0	0		Appetite stimulation (Fe, Ru)
Alpha₂-agonists	−/− − (especially Ru)	−/− − (especially Ru)	0	−	++ vomiting (Fe > Ca); gastric distension (Ca); bloat, regurgitation (Bo); bloat, ileus (Eq)
Opioids	− (minimal except at high doses)	− (minimal except at high doses)	+/++ (SA)	Stimulation (+), then ileus (-)	++ vomiting (SA) diarrhea, then constipation
Propofol	− −/− − − (including apnea)	− −/− − −	0		Antiemetic
Etomidate	0 (temporary apnea), then may +	0	0	0	Nausea and vomiting (induction, recovery)
Alfaxalone	− −/− − − (including apnea)	− −/− − −	0		
Barbiturates	− −/− − − (including apnea)	− −/− − −	++/+++	− then +	Sneezing and coughing
Dissociatives	0	0	++/+++		Apneustic respiration at high doses (common in Eq)
Guaifenesin	0	0	0	+	Apneustic respiration at high doses
Halogenated inhalants	− to − − −	− to − − −	0	−	Isoflurane: may vomit; Desflurane: coughing

Notes on use of this table:
- 0 indicates minimal to no effect.
- − indicates a decrease in the parameter indicated (where − is mild; − − is moderate; − − − is marked).
- + indicates an increase in the parameter indicated (where + is mild; ++ is moderate; +++ is marked).
- Effects of drugs depend on many factors, including species, differences among specific agents within a class, dose, and drug interactions. Therefore quantifications of the principal effects (mild, moderate, marked) are approximations.
- The information regarding opioids includes those of agonists, partial agonists, and agonist–antagonists. When reading this, note that effects of agonists are generally more pronounced than those of agonist–antagonists or partial agonists).

Bo, Bovine; *Ca*, canine; *Eq*, equine; *Fe*, feline; *GI*, gastrointestinal; *IV*, intravenously; *Ru*, ruminants; *SA*, small animals; −, depression; +, stimulation.

with each drug in order to use them safely and effectively. The magnitude of many of these effects, whether desirable or undesirable, is related to the dose of the drug given, that is, it is "dose dependent" (e.g., both the CNS depression and the respiratory depression caused by propofol increase in intensity as the dose increases). Some of these effects are desirable (e.g., loss of consciousness, muscle relaxation, and analgesia), whereas others are undesirable (e.g., respiratory depression, hypotension, and ataxia). The undesirable effects are often referred to as "adverse effects," "side effects," or "adverse reactions." In this text, effects and adverse effects are discussed together and can be differentiated in most cases simply by determining whether any given effect is desirable or undesirable.

TECHNICIAN NOTE Many commonly used general anesthetics are not analgesics but indirectly provide pain control during the anesthetic period by producing a state of unconsciousness. Therefore when these agents are used, analgesia must be provided in the perioperative period by the use of true analgesics such as the opioids.

Analgesic Effects of Anesthetics and Adjuncts

When an anesthetic protocol is being chosen for animals that are experiencing pain or that are undergoing a painful procedure, it must be kept in mind that analgesia must be provided

TABLE 3.4 Other Principal Effects of Anesthetic Agents and Adjuncts

Agent Class	Ocular Effects	Muscle Tone	Urogenital System Effects	Crosses Placental Barrier	Other Effects
Anxiolytics (gabapentin and trazodone)	0	0	0	+ (gabapentin)	Possible serotonin syndrome (trazodone)
Anticholinergics	+/++ mydriasis (Fe > Ca)	0		Yes (atropine); minimally (glycopyrrolate)	PLR may be depressed; decreased lacrimal secretions
Acepromazine	Third eyelid prolapse; decreased IOP	0	Penile prolapse (Eq, Bo)	Yes—slowly	Antihistamine effect; decreased PCV
Benzodiazepines	Decreased IOP	− − −		Yes	Muscular fasciculations (Eq); diazepam: IM injection painful
Alpha$_2$-agonists	Increased IOP because of vomiting	− − −	Premature parturition (Bo); increased urine production	Yes	Transient hyperglycemia; reaction to loud noises; sweating, muscle tremors (Eq)
Opioids	Miosis (Ca); mydriasis (Fe, LA); increased IOP (only if hypoventilating)	0	Urine retention; decreased urine production	Yes—slowly	Reactions to loud noises; sweating (Eq); increased motor activity (Eq)
Propofol	Decreased IOP	− −/− − −		Yes	Muscle twitching during induction (Ca)
Etomidate	0/increased IOP	− −		Yes	Excitement and muscle activity during induction, recovery; intravenous injection painful
Alfaxalone	Decreased IOP	− −/− − −		Yes	Excitement during recovery
Barbiturates	Decreased IOP	0/−		Yes	Tissue irritation if not injected IV
Dissociatives	Open, central, dilated; 0/+ nystagmus; increased IOP	0 to +++ (muscle twitching)		Yes	Increased sensitivity to sensory stimuli; behavior changes during recovery
Guaifenesin		− −		Yes	Excitement during induction if used alone; tissue irritation if not injected IV
Halogenated inhalants		−/− − (isoflurane)		Yes	Sevoflurane: excitement, muscle fasciculations during recovery

Notes on use of this table:
- 0 indicates minimal to no effect.
- − indicates a decrease in the parameter indicated (where − is mild; − − is moderate; − − − is marked).
- + indicates an increase in the parameter indicated (where + is mild; ++ is moderate; +++ is marked).
- Effects of drugs depend on many factors, including species, differences among specific agents within a class, dose, and drug interactions. Therefore quantifications of the principal effects (mild, moderate, marked) are approximations.
- The information regarding opioids includes those of agonists, partial agonists, and agonist–antagonists. When reading this, note that effects of agonists are generally more pronounced than those of agonist–antagonists or partial agonists).

Bo, Bovine; *Ca,* canine; *Eq,* equine; *Fe,* feline; *IM,* intramuscular; *IOP,* intraocular pressure; *IV,* intravenously; *LA,* large animals; *PCV,* packed cell volume; *PLR,* pupillary light reflex; *Ru,* ruminants; *SA,* small animals; −, depression; +, stimulation.

before, during, and after the anesthetic event. Many commonly used general anesthetics, including halogenated inhalant agents, propofol, alfaxalone, and etomidate, produce unconsciousness but little to no pain control and so are not true analgesics.

Animals are, however, not aware of pain while unconscious. Consequently, general anesthetics provide lack of awareness of pain by producing a state of unconsciousness. In other words, when the patient is under surgical anesthesia, pain is not consciously perceived, but it recurs with the return of consciousness. This can lead to the perception that patients do not need pain control when these agents are used. It is important to realize that pain that is not consciously perceived by the patient causes undesirable physiologic changes in the body that can lead to postoperative pain that is difficult to control and that can compromise the well-being of the patient.

Therefore the use of general anesthetics must be preceded, accompanied, and followed by administration of true analgesics if pain control is necessary. A number of anesthetic agents and adjuncts are used for this purpose, including opioids, local anesthetics, alpha$_2$-agonists, and dissociatives. These agents produce analgesia regardless of the patient's level of consciousness. In other words, these agents work whether the patient is "asleep" (unconscious) or "awake" (conscious) and consequently provide analgesia during the pre-, intra-, and postoperative periods (see Chapter 8 for more information about the use of these agents as analgesics).

Protein Binding

Anesthetic drugs travel in the bloodstream freely or bound to carrier proteins such as albumin. The amount of this protein binding affects the way the drug acts in patients with decreased plasma protein due to disease because only the free (unbound) molecules are able to cross cell membranes and enter the brain to induce anesthesia, whereas the molecules bound to proteins are not. In hypoproteinemic animals (that is, those with total plasma protein less than 3 g/dL) there is less plasma protein to bind the drug and more in the active, unbound form. Consequently, doses of a highly protein-bound drug that are suitable for healthy animals may have exaggerated effects in these patients and so may need to be reduced. Propofol, which is approximately 95% to 99% protein bound, is an example of such a drug.

Lipid Solubility

The tendency of a drug to dissolve in fats, oils, or lipids is referred to as *lipid solubility* and is related to the ability to penetrate the fatty layer of cell membranes. Many injectable anesthetics (such as propofol) are highly lipid soluble and therefore pass into brain cells quickly, causing a faster onset of action than other drugs with low lipid solubility. Lipid solubility is also related to duration of action. Drugs with high lipid solubility are rapidly removed from the brain by a process known as *tissue redistribution*.

Tissue Redistribution

Tissue redistribution is a phenomenon that occurs because of the way in which some drugs are distributed to various tissues based on blood flow. After IV administration, absorption is most rapid in tissues with very high blood flow, known as the *vessel-rich group* (the CNS, heart, liver, kidney, and endocrine tissues), which make up only about 10% of total body weight but receive about 75% of the total blood flow. Absorption is less rapid in muscle, which makes up about 50% of the body weight but receives only 20% of the blood flow, and slowest in fat, which makes up about 20% of body weight but receives a meager 5% of the blood flow (Fig. 3.1).

Within seconds of IV injection, a redistributed drug is dispersed throughout the body via the bloodstream. Large amounts of the drug rapidly reach the brain because of the excellent blood supply this organ receives.

Once the drug concentration in the blood falls below that in the brain tissue, it begins to leave the brain and reenter the circulation, where it is redistributed to muscle, fat, and other body tissues. When using such a drug, the animal shows signs of recovery (within 5 to 10 minutes in the case of propofol) as the concentration in the brain decreases although the drug is still present in other tissues (see Fig. 3.2 for a graphic representation of the process of redistribution).

Following redistribution, the drug is gradually released from the muscle and fat and is most often eliminated from the body by liver metabolism and excretion of the metabolites in urine.

Route of Administration

Most anesthetic agents and adjuncts are available in injectable form. Some formulations may be given by one route only (such as etomidate injection, which can only be given intravenously), whereas other formulations can be administered by multiple routes (such as the analgesic agent butorphanol, which can be given by IV, IM, or subcutaneous [SC] routes among others). Onset of action, duration of action, and dose vary with each of these routes. Of the three injectable routes mentioned, SC administration of a drug is associated with the slowest onset of action and longest duration. IM administration results in a somewhat faster onset (15 to 20 minutes in many cases) and a somewhat shorter duration than SC administration. Drugs given intravenously generally act within seconds to a few minutes and have a shorter duration than if given either intramuscularly or subcutaneously but should be administered slowly and cautiously because potency and the potential for adverse effects are increased when drugs are given by this route.

For agents also available in oral form (such as the anxiolytics trazodone and gabapentin as well as the opioid morphine), the oral route (PO) is generally associated with an even slower onset of action and longer duration than those of any of the injectable routes (Box 3.1 illustrates how route influences onset of action and duration of action). Doses of a drug also may vary among routes of administration. In general, the IV dose of any injectable drug is typically about one-half of the IM or SC dose, although this varies drug to drug. Consequently, a drug formulary or other resource should be consulted for appropriate doses to use for any given route of administration.

Although some injectable agents (formations labeled for injection) such as ketamine, dexmedetomidine, and buprenorphine can be given by mouth (oral transmucosal or OTM), effects of orally administered injectable drugs are often unpredictable. For this reason, this route of administration is usually reserved for patients too aggressive to be handled or for other situations in which it is difficult or impossible to inject the drug. Specific indications for the OTM route will be noted where applicable in the discussion of each drug.

Using Drugs in Combination

Two or more anesthetic agents and/or adjuncts are often used in combination. Some drugs can be safely mixed in the same syringe, whereas others cannot. Incompatible mixtures can produce a variety of harmful or even fatal adverse effects because of loss of potency, change in chemistry, precipitation of one or more of the drugs, or other untoward interactions. For this reason, the anesthetist must observe some general guidelines when faced with a decision to mix two or more drugs.

With the exception of diazepam (a benzodiazepine tranquilizer), most anesthetic agents and adjuncts are water soluble. In general, two or more water-soluble drugs can be safely mixed, but a water-soluble drug and a non–water-soluble drug cannot. The sole exception to the rule is the combination of the water-soluble drug ketamine with diazepam, which can be safely mixed and administered unless visible precipitation occurs. Regardless of these guidelines, *do not mix two or more drugs unless you have reliable evidence that it is safe to do so.* Usually, this information can be found in professional publications such as anesthesia textbooks, drug formularies, and peer-reviewed journals, as well as from experienced anesthetists.

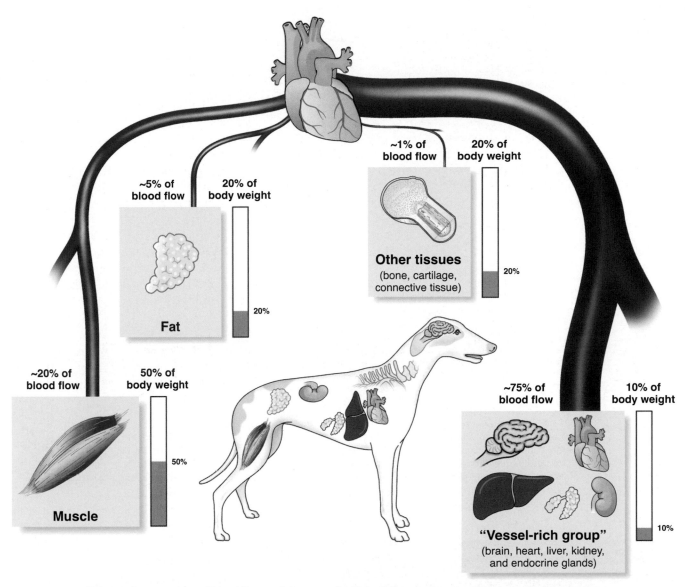

~1% of blood flow   **20% of body weight**

Other tissues
(bone, cartilage, connective tissue)

20%

~5% of blood flow   **20% of body weight**

Fat

20%

~20% of blood flow   **50% of body weight**

Muscle

50%

~75% of blood flow   **10% of body weight**

"Vessel-rich group"
(brain, heart, liver, kidney, and endocrine glands)

10%

FIG. 3.1 A comparison of blood flow and tissue mass. Note that some tissues make up a small proportion of total body weight but receive a relatively large proportion of total blood flow (e.g., approximately 10% of total body weight and approximately 75% of total blood flow in the case of the vessel-rich group), whereas other tissues make up a relatively large proportion of total body weight but receive much less blood flow (e.g., approximately 50% of total body weight and approximately 20% of total blood flow in the case of muscle, and approximately 20% of total body weight and approximately 5% of total blood flow in the case of fat).

> **TECHNICIAN NOTE** With the exception of diazepam, most anesthetic agents and adjuncts are water soluble. In general, two or more water-soluble drugs can be safely mixed, but a water-soluble drug and a non–water-soluble drug cannot. For this reason, when using two or more drugs in the same patient, *do not mix them unless you are sure that it is safe to do so.*

REGULATORY CONSIDERATIONS FOR CONTROLLED SUBSTANCES

Some of the agents covered in this chapter are subject to federal government regulation regarding purchase, handling, and dispensing under the Controlled Substances Act (CSA) in the United States (enforced by the Drug Enforcement Administration [DEA]) and the Controlled Drugs and Substances Act (CDSA) of 1996 in Canada (enforced by the Royal Canadian Mounted Police [RCMP]). Of the agents discussed here, benzodiazepines, dissociatives, alfaxalone, barbiturates, and most opioids fall into this category. Any use of these controlled substances necessitates compliance with strict handling and storage requirements as well as detailed record-keeping requirements owing to the potential for abuse or theft. Specifically, these agents are subject to diversion by people for illicit purposes and, when used in this manner, have the potential to induce psychologic and/or physical dependency. Theft, illegal use, or diversion of a controlled substance is a criminal act that is punishable by imprisonment and/or fines and may adversely affect eligibility for professional licensure.

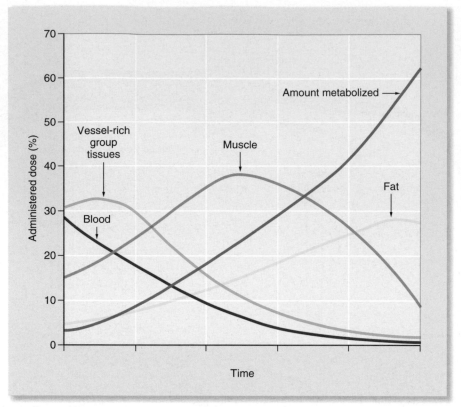

FIG. 3.2 Tissue redistribution of propofol. The height of the line corresponds to the amount of the drug that is in each location at any given time. Note that the drug levels in the vessel-rich organs (central nervous system [CNS], heart, liver, kidney, and endocrine tissue) reach a maximum very rapidly following IV administration, and then decrease gradually as the drug redistributes to the muscle, causing the anesthetic effect to diminish. Over a longer period of time, the drug leaving the muscle redistributes to the fat. During the period of redistribution, the drug is relatively rapidly metabolized and eliminated from the body.

BOX 3.1 How Route of Administration influences Onset of Action and Duration of Action

Route of Administration	Onset of Action	Duration of Action
IV	Fast	Short
IM	↕	↕
SC		
PO	Slow	Long

IM, Intramuscular; *IV,* intravenous; *PO,* per os (orally); *SC,* subcutaneous.

The laws regarding how these agents are classified differ among countries, so veterinary professionals using these drugs must become familiar with the laws where they practice. In the United States, the Controlled Substances Act assigns each drug to one of five drug schedules (I, II, III, IV, or V) according to its potential for abuse. Agents classified as Schedule II substances in the United States cannot be dispensed or drawn into a syringe except under the direct supervision of a licensed veterinarian. Table 3.5 lists the DEA schedules and commonly used anesthetic drugs in each schedule.

Use of controlled drugs takes place within a "closed system" of distribution. This means that anyone who handles these substances, including manufacturers, distributors, and veterinarians, must be registered with the DEA and is assigned a unique number that identifies the registrant. Registrants must maintain an accurate inventory of these drugs; carefully account for the distribution, transfer, and use of these drugs; and ensure that these agents are stored in a secure location. Although not registered with the DEA, veterinary technicians and nurses are often intimately involved with record keeping, ordering, and storage in addition to administering these drugs.

Record Keeping

Maintenance of accurate records enables the DEA to trace any drug from the time of manufacture to its consumption by or administration to the patient. For veterinary practitioners, these records include an inventory of all substances every 2 years and an accounting of the use of each drug on a day-to-day basis in a controlled substance log.

The inventory must include:
- The date the inventory was taken, including whether it was taken at the beginning or end of the day

TABLE 3.5 Drug Enforcement Administration (DEA) Controlled Substances Used in the Practice of Veterinary Anesthesia

Schedule	Description	Examples of Drugs Used for Veterinary Anesthesia and Analgesia
I	No currently accepted medical use	N/A
II	High potential for abuse	Narcotics (opioid agonists) (carfentanil, codeine, etorphine, fentanyl, hydromorphone, meperidine, morphine, oxymorphone, sufentanil, thiafentanil)
		Narcotic antagonist (diprenorphine)
		Barbiturate (pentobarbital)
III	Less potential for abuse than Schedule I or II drugs	Narcotics (the opioid partial agonist buprenorphine)
		Dissociatives (ketamine; tiletamine [in Telazol])
		Barbiturates (thiamylal; thiopental)
IV	Less potential for abuse than Schedule III drugs	Narcotics (opioid agonist–antagonists such as butorphanol and pentazocine)
		Benzodiazepines (diazepam; midazolam; lorazepam; alprazolam)
		Alfaxalone
		Barbiturate (methohexital)
V	Less potential for abuse than Schedule IV drugs	(No commonly used anesthetic drugs are in this schedule)

- The finished form of the drug (e.g., injectable, tablets, oral liquid)
- The amount of each drug on hand (e.g., volume for liquid drugs, number of tablets)
- The drug concentration (e.g., 10 mg/mL, 100-mg tablets)
- The number of containers of each drug (e.g., five 10-mL bottles, two 500-tablet bottles)

It should also include the name, address, and DEA registration number of the registrant and the signature of the person who took the inventory.

The accounting of drug use is generally in the form of a log with the date the drug was administered or dispensed, identification of the patient and client, the amount or quantity administered or dispensed, and the signature of the person who administered or dispensed the drug. See Fig. 3.3 for an example of a controlled substance log. This record is often used to track the quantity on hand by subtracting the amount used or dispensed from the total amount on hand.

The controlled substance inventory and logs must be filled out in indelible ink and kept for a minimum of 2 years. The log should be in the form of a bound booklet with numbered pages as opposed to a binder, which allows pages to be easily removed or added. The log for Schedule III, IV, and V substances must be in a readily retrievable form and must also be kept separate from all other records, including those for Schedule II drugs. All records should be available for inspection at any time.

Ordering Controlled Substances

When ordering controlled drugs from a supplier, the ordering process for schedule II drugs is more stringent than that for schedules III, IV, and V. Schedule II drugs require use of a special order form that is issued only to registered persons (DEA Form 222) or use of the DEA Controlled Substance Ordering System (CSOS).

Form 222 is preprinted with the name and address of the customer (a DEA registrant) and must be filled out in triplicate. After completing the order form, two copies are forwarded to the supplier, one of which is then forwarded to a DEA office, and the third is retained by the purchaser. This system helps to ensure that only authorized individuals are able to order these drugs and allows careful tracking of the drug from the distributor to the individual who is prescribing and dispensing the drug. In contrast, no special order form is necessary for Schedule III and IV agents; however, when filling these orders, the supplier must verify that the purchaser is registered with the DEA, and both parties must keep detailed records of all transactions.

Anywhere Animal Hospital

Drug: **Ketamine**   Container Size: **10 mL**   Strength: **100 mg/mL**   Form: **Injectable**   Controlled Status: **III**

Date administered	Client name	Patient name and ID #	Patient species	Reason	Bottle #	Amount drawn up	Amount given	Amount wasted	Balance	Initials of person who drew up drug	Initials of witness
Starting Balance (from previous page)					#5				10 mL	N/A	JAB
8/17/21	Longo	Rocko #1234	Canine	Induction	#5	1.3 mL	0.9 mL	0.4 mL	8.7 mL	JAB	KMT

FIG. 3.3 Example of a controlled substance log.

Schedule II drugs may also be ordered by using the CSOS system. This electronic ordering system uses a technology known as public key infrastructure (PKI), which verifies the identity of those individuals and computers used in ordering these drugs and encrypts the information so that others cannot read it. To use this system, the customer must apply for and be issued a digital certificate and a private key (a passcode known only to that individual) that is used to exchange information securely. The CSOS system allows suppliers of these drugs to check that the order is legitimate and has not been tampered with and that the order has come from a DEA registrant, whose identity is verified before the order is shipped. The CSOS system can also be used to order Schedule III, IV, and V drugs, although it is not required.

Storage Requirements for Controlled Substances

Schedule II through V controlled substances must be stored in a securely locked, substantially constructed cabinet or safe. If the safe or cabinet can easily be picked up, it must be securely affixed to a substantial object such as a wall or the floor. In the case of mobile units, locked storage containers must be built in or permanently mounted to the vehicle. Refrigerated drugs must be kept in a lockbox affixed to the inside of the refrigerator; ideally, the refrigerator should also be locked. Furthermore, containers of controlled substances must not be left unattended on countertops or in other public areas. After a dose is withdrawn from a bottle containing a controlled substance, the bottle should be immediately returned to locked storage.

Controlled substance storage containers must be placed in a location intended to secure the drugs from unauthorized individuals and to discourage theft. This means that storage areas should be kept out of sight and away from public areas. Because most thefts of controlled substances are by employees, policies must be in place to minimize access. Ideally, the storage will have two uniquely keyed locks so that two keys are required to gain access. Access to the storage should be limited to the registrant and a minimum number of other authorized persons. Keys or combinations to safes or padlocks should be secured in a location that is not near the storage area.

Thiafentanil and etorphine hydrochloride (highly potent opioid agonists used to immobilize wild animals) and diprenorphine (a highly potent opioid antagonist used to reverse the effects of thiafentanil and etorphine in wild animals) must be stored in a safe or a steel cabinet. These substances are highly dangerous to humans and therefore must be used with great caution. (Precautions regarding safe use of these substances are detailed in Chapter 5.)

In the event of unexplained significant loss or suspected or known theft of a controlled substance, the registrant must notify the DEA Diversion Field Office within one business day, and DEA Form 106 must be completed and submitted. Although not specifically required by federal law, local police should also be notified.[a]

---

[a]DEA: *Drugs of abuse—a DEA resource guide/2022 edition.* https://www.dea.gov/sites/default/files/2022-12/2022_DOA_eBook_File_Final.pdf.

BOX 3.2 DEA Prescription Writing Requirements for Controlled Substances

Schedule II Controlled Substances

Prescriptions must be written on a prescription blank and signed by the practitioner.

Prescriptions may only be telephoned into the pharmacy in the event of an emergency.

Prescriptions for these drugs may not be refilled.

Schedule III and IV Controlled Substances

Prescriptions for these drugs may be written or oral.

These prescriptions may be refilled up to five times within 6 months from the date of the prescription.

From DEA: Drugs of abuse: a DEA resource guide, 2022 edition. https://www.dea.gov/sites/default/files/2022-12/2022_DOA_eBook_File_Final.pdf

Prescribing Controlled Substances

When prescribing controlled substances, such as oral analgesics, for home use, practitioners must take precautions to prevent diversion. This includes following DEA requirements regarding the prescription writing, keeping prescription blanks in a secure location, and taking measures to prevent illegal alteration of prescriptions—for instance, by writing out the quantity of a dispensed drug in longhand in addition to as a number (e.g., 60 [sixty] tablets). (See Box 3.2 for DEA prescription writing requirements.)

PREANESTHETIC MEDICATIONS

The following agent classes are usually classified as preanesthetic medications because they are most often administered during the preanesthetic period. These agents are either given alone or, more often, in combination with one another as a part of balanced anesthesia.

- Anxiolytics
- Anticholinergics
- Tranquilizers and sedatives
  - Phenothiazines
  - Benzodiazepines
  - Alpha$_2$-adrenoceptor agonists (alpha$_2$-agonists)
- Opioids
- Antiemetics

Reasons for the Use of Preanesthetic Medications

The principal reasons for giving commonly used preanesthetic medications follow. Table 3.6 summarizes these benefits.

1. To decrease patient stress and anxiety prior to travel to the hospital.
2. To calm or sedate an excited, frightened, or vicious animal. Sedation not only enhances patient comfort and reduces anxiety, but also facilitates safe and stress-free patient handling.
3. To reduce the risk of perioperative nausea, vomiting, and associated complications.
4. To minimize adverse effects of concurrently administered drugs. All anesthetic agents and adjuncts cause undesirable adverse effects in addition to their desired action. For example, ketamine causes excessive salivation in some patients,

TABLE 3.6 Principal Reasons for Giving Preanesthetic Agents

Preanesthetic Agent Class	Provide Anxiolysis, Tranquilization, and/or Sedation	Ease of Induction and Recovery	Reduce Amount of General Anesthetic Required	Reduce Risk of Nausea, Vomiting, and Associated Complications	Minimize Bradycardia and Salivation	Provide Analgesia	Provide Muscle Relaxation
Anxiolytics	+++ (anxiolysis) + (sedation)	0	0	0	0	0	0
Anticholinergics	0	0	0	0	+++	0	0
Acepromazine	++ (tranq. and/or sedation)	++	+	+	0	0	0
Benzodiazepines	+ (tranq.)/0	++	+	0	0	0	++
Alpha$_2$-agonists	+++ (tranq. and/or sedation)	+++	+++	(may cause vomiting)	0	++	++
Opioid agonists; partial agonists; agonist–antagonists	+/++ (sedation)	++ (most prominent with agonists)	++ (most prominent with agonists)	(agonists may cause vomiting; less common with methadone, partial agonists, and mixed agonists/ antagonists)	0	+++ (agonists > partial agonists or agonists/ antagonists)	0
Antiemetic - maropitant	0	+ (recovery)	+ (inhalants)	+++	0	(some evidence of visceral analgesia in dogs)	0

0 = does not have the effect listed.
+, ++, or +++ = produces the effect to a slight, moderate, or great degree, respectively.

and alpha$_2$-agonists may cause profound bradycardia or heart block. Anticholinergics are sometimes given to decrease these exaggerated parasympathetic effects.

5. To reduce the required dose of concurrently administered agents. For example, administration of a sedative during the preanesthetic period will often decrease the amount of general anesthetic required to produce surgical anesthesia.

6. To produce smoother anesthetic inductions and recoveries. During induction and recovery, patients pass through a period of involuntary excitement. While passing through this stage, they can be dangerous to themselves and to personnel, inflicting bites or experiencing bone fractures or other serious injuries in extreme situations.

7. To decrease pain and discomfort before, during, and after surgery. As noted previously, most general anesthetic agents have limited or no analgesic effect, so in many cases, adjuncts must be given to provide the necessary level of pain control.

8. To produce muscle relaxation. Muscle relaxation is particularly important during some procedures, including orthopedic and ocular surgery. Preanesthetic medications such as benzodiazepines and alpha$_2$-agonists are often given concurrently with general anesthetics to produce the desired amount of muscle relaxation.

Preanesthetic medications often have other uses. For example, tranquilizers are used to calm patients for transport, physical examination, radiographic procedures, and wound treatment.

They are helpful in preventing animals from chewing wounds and bandages. Benzodiazepines are administered IV to stop seizures, anxiolytics are used for behavior modification, phenothiazines have antiemetic properties, and many opioids are effective cough suppressants.

The veterinarian will decide which preanesthetic medications to give based on the nature of the procedure, patient need, personal preference, and other factors, as well as the route and time of administration.

With the exception of anxiolytics, preanesthetic medications are usually given via the IV or IM route. As mentioned previously, the onset of action depends on the route used. Because of this, patients given sedatives by the IM or SC route should be left undisturbed until peak action is reached (approximately 15 to 20 minutes in most cases) because excitement or stimulation during the interim can sometimes override the effects of these agents when either of these routes is used.

TECHNICIAN NOTE Patients given sedatives by the IM or SC route should be left undisturbed until peak action is reached because excitement or stimulation during the interim can sometimes override the effects. Drugs given intravenously should be administered slowly and cautiously because potency and the potential for adverse effects are increased when drugs are given by this route.

Anxiolytics

Anxiolytics are a diverse group of agents administered at home prior to travel to the hospital for examination, anesthesia, surgery, or other stressful procedures (e.g., radiography, blood or urine sample collection, ultrasound exam). The use of anxiolytics has gained attention in recent years as one component of a comprehensive approach designed to minimize the negative effects of stress, anxiety, and fear on our patients. *(See Fear Free at https://fearfreepets.com/ for more information about this approach to patient care.)*

In addition to improvement in general well-being, there are numerous benefits of this approach, including improved effectiveness of and response to treatment; decreased likelihood of injury to the patient or personnel; improved relationships among clients, patients, and members of the care team; and ultimately, better outcomes. Consequently, many experts, including the authors of the 2020 AAHA Anesthesia and Monitoring Guidelines and the authors of the 2018 AAFP Feline Anesthesia Guidelines, now recommend use of anxiolytics as one aspect of balanced anesthesia for any patient that experiences any amount of fear, anxiety, or stress.

Two of the most commonly recommended agents used for this purpose are gabapentin and trazodone. Neither of these drugs is a traditional anesthetic, tranquilizer, or sedative, although sedation is one of the effects of both drugs. Both are available in oral formulations and so can be administered at home by the client on the day of and, if needed, the day before the scheduled visit.

Gabapentin

Gabapentin is a drug originally developed as a human anticonvulsant that is now widely used off-label as an anxiolytic and adjunctive analgesic in veterinary patients. It is also used as an anticonvulsant in veterinary patients with seizures not well controlled with other drugs. Gabapentin is not currently FDA approved for use in animals. Although not controlled by the DEA at the time of this writing, gabapentin has been classified as a Schedule V controlled substance by several states including Michigan, Kentucky, West Virginia, Tennessee, and Alabama.

Mode of action and pharmacology. Gabapentin is structurally related to the inhibitory neurotransmitter gamma-aminobutyric acid (GABA) but does not appear to act by binding with GABA receptors or by altering GABA pharmacokinetics. The precise mode of action of gabapentin is unknown, but it appears to inhibit release of excitatory neurotransmitters such as glutamate and norepinephrine by decreasing calcium movement into cells. In dogs and cats, the peak effect of gabapentin occurs approximately 1 to 3 hours after oral administration. It has a relatively short half-life (within the range of 2 to 4 hours) in cats and dogs.

Effects. Gabapentin has three main effects on the nervous system:

- Analgesic properties that are felt to be most effective for chronic pain involving a neuropathic component (pain involving disease of or damage to a nerve).
- In dogs and cats, it reduces anxiety in a similar way to tranquilizers.
- Anticonvulsant properties.

Adverse effects. Because few studies have been done on the use of gabapentin in animals at the time of this writing, there is not a lot of data concerning dosing and adverse effects. However, based on available reports, gabapentin appears to have a very favorable safety profile, and adverse effects that do occur are generally temporary and mild. The most commonly reported adverse effects of gabapentin are sedation and ataxia, which are more pronounced at higher doses. GI effects, such as hypersalivation and vomiting, have also been reported.

> **TECHNICIAN NOTE** Major effects and adverse effects of gabapentin are as follows:
> - Analgesia, especially for neuropathic pain
> - Anxiolysis
> - Anticonvulsant properties
> - Sedation
> - Ataxia
> - GI effects

Use of gabapentin. In cats, gabapentin has become a favorite drug of many clinicians to reduce fear responses to handling, examination, and minor procedures such as sample collection. It is generally recommended at a dose of 50 to 100 mg/cat (the correlates to approximately 10 to 20 mg/kg in the average-sized cat) given orally the morning of the appointment at least 2 to 3 hours before travel. In cats, the powder from the capsule can be added to a small amount of wet food (~1 tablespoon).

Recommendations regarding the dosage of gabapentin vary widely. For instance, published dosages typically range from 10 to 30 mg/kg or even higher in dogs and 5 to 20 mg/kg in cats, depending on the reason it is being prescribed. When used to treat chronic pain or seizures, the recommended dosing frequency is generally between 6 and 12 hours. For these reasons, the dose must be tailored to the needs of each patient.

Gabapentin is available in a variety of formulations including tablets, capsules, and oral solution. The commercially available oral solution (Neurontin) contains xylitol (a commonly used sugar substitute for a variety of products). Xylitol is toxic to dogs and can cause life-threatening hypoglycemia due to release of insulin at high doses or liver toxicity if ingested in very large amounts. Therefore this formulation should not be used in dogs and should be used cautiously in cats, although currently used doses are not known to cause a problem in this species.

Gabapentin is primarily eliminated by the kidneys, so caution should be used when giving it to patients with renal disease.

Trazodone

Trazodone was originally developed as an antidepressant for use in humans. Recently, it has gained popularity as a drug to reduce stress, fear, and anxiety in dogs prior to veterinary visits in a similar way to that previously described for gabapentin in cats. Trazodone may also be used in dogs for a variety of other indications including treatment of anxiety disorders, relief of situational anxiety (such as that precipitated by storms, fireworks, or hospitalization), and facilitation of confinement following orthopedic surgery. It is a noncontrolled drug that, like gabapentin, is not FDA approved for use in animals at the present time.

Mode of action and pharmacology. Trazodone is a drug with properties similar to selective serotonin-reuptake inhibitors (SSRIs) that increases the activity of the neurotransmitter serotonin in the CNS. It does this by inhibiting the system that removes serotonin from the synapse, causing it to last longer. In addition, it antagonizes several nervous system receptors, which in turn inhibit or stimulate release of other neurotransmitters including glutamate, dopamine, and norepinephrine.

Effects on major organ systems. In the CNS, trazodone induces behavioral changes, resulting in sedation and anxiolysis necessary to treat situational anxiety and achieve postoperative calming.

Adverse effects. There is limited research on the use of this drug in veterinary patients, although in one study, approximately 80% of dogs had no adverse effects, and those effects that were seen were predominately mild, with sedation, sleepiness, lethargy, and ataxia being most common. Less commonly reported adverse effects include nervous system effects (agitation, excitement, and behavioral disinhibition), GI system effects (vomiting, diarrhea), and changes in appetite. Based on adverse effects seen in humans, cardiac arrhythmias and hypotension are also possible. Many of these effects would be expected to occur more commonly when higher doses are given.

Serotonin syndrome is a rare but potentially serious adverse effect that can result from simultaneous administration of trazodone and certain other agents including other behavior-modifying drugs (such as monoamine oxidase inhibitors [MAOIs], SSRIs, and tricyclic antidepressants [TCAs]). Therefore under these circumstances, it is important to educate clients to watch for signs of serotonin syndrome, which can be nonspecific and challenging to recognize. These signs include changes in heart rate and rhythm, hypertension, tachypnea, hyperthermia, nervous system effects, and vomiting or diarrhea.

> **TECHNICIAN NOTE** Major effects and adverse effects of trazodone are as follows:
> - Sedation
> - Anxiolysis
> - Drowsiness
> - Ataxia
> - GI effects (vomiting or diarrhea)
> - Changes in appetite
> - Agitation or excitement
> - Behavioral disinhibition
> - Serotonin syndrome (due to interaction with other drugs)

Use of trazodone. Trazodone is used as an anxiolytic by many clinicians to reduce fear responses to veterinary visits for anesthetic procedures, examination, and minor procedures, such as sample collection. The recommended dose for dogs is in the range of 3 to 7.5 mg/kg, given 1 to 2 hours prior to travel to the clinic. Some clinicians also recommend a dose be given the night before. Although not specifically mentioned for use in

cats in either the 2020 AAHA Anesthesia and Monitoring Guidelines or the 2018 AAFP Feline Anesthesia Guidelines, other references suggest use of this drug in cats at a dose of approximately 50 mg/cat PO (which correlates to approximately 10 mg/kg in the average-sized cat) 1 to 2 hours prior to travel.

It is best to try a test dose before the actual day of the visit so that the dose and timing can be adjusted based on the response to the medication. Trazodone may be given with or without food, but if vomiting occurs, it may help to administer it with a small amount of food.

Other Anxiolytics and Combination Protocols

There are several sedatives that may be used as anxiolytics to prevent fear, anxiety, and stress associated with travel and veterinary visits including acepromazine, benzodiazepines, and oral transmucosal dexmedetomidine gel. Detailed discussions of these drugs follow in the section entitled "Sedatives and Tranquilizers."

Anticholinergics

Also known as parasympatholytics, anticholinergics are noncontrolled drugs that are most commonly used to prevent and treat bradycardia and to decrease salivary secretions arising from parasympathetic stimulation. The two anticholinergic agents commonly used in veterinary medicine are atropine and glycopyrrolate. Atropine is a relatively old drug, derived from the deadly nightshade plant, that was used for many years to decrease excessive respiratory secretions and laryngospasm caused by the irritating effects of ether and the excess secretions caused by the barbiturates. Glycopyrrolate is a newer synthetic quaternary ammonium compound. Both drugs may be given by the IV, IM, SC, or intratracheal (IT) route. When these drugs are used as preanesthetics, the IM and IV routes are most commonly employed. The IT and IV routes are used in emergency situations in which rapid action is essential. Atropine is approved for use in several domestic species, and glycopyrrolate is approved for use in dogs and cats.

Mode of Action and Pharmacology

Acetylcholine is the primary neurotransmitter in the PNS responsible for parasympathetic effects (also referred to as *cholinergic effects*). The PNS has two types of receptors for acetylcholine. The nicotinic receptors are located on the postganglionic neurons at the junction with the preganglionic neurons, and the muscarinic receptors are located on the target organs (Fig. 3.4). Anticholinergics competitively block binding of the neurotransmitter acetylcholine at the muscarinic receptors and therefore may be referred to as antimuscarinic agents.

The vagus nerve (tenth cranial nerve) provides parasympathetic innervation to numerous target organs including the heart, lungs, gastrointestinal (GI) tract, some secretory glands, and the iris of the eye. During surgery, the vagus nerve may be stimulated by endotracheal intubation, traction on visceral organs during abdominal surgery (known as the *viscerovagal reflex*), manipulation of the eye during ocular surgery (known as the *oculovagal reflex*), and by some drugs, including the alpha$_2$-agonists, opioids, and common general anesthetics. Increased binding of acetylcholine to the muscarinic receptors

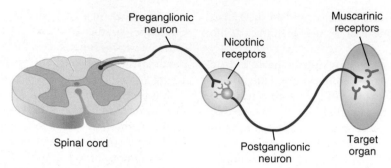

FIG. 3.4 The parasympathetic nervous system. The preganglionic neuron releases acetylcholine at the nicotinic receptors. The postganglionic neuron releases acetylcholine at the muscarinic receptors of the target organ. Anticholinergics affect only the muscarinic receptors.

caused by vagal stimulation results in observable parasympathetic effects at the target organs, such as bradycardia, bronchoconstriction, excess tear and saliva production, excess production of respiratory system secretions, increased GI motility, and miosis. By blocking the muscarinic receptors, anticholinergics help to reverse and prevent these parasympathetic effects (thus the alternative name *parasympatholytics*).

After IM injection, atropine begins to act in about 5 minutes, reaches peak effect in about 10 to 20 minutes, and has a duration of action of 60 to 90 minutes. Glycopyrrolate has a similar onset of action, reaches peak effect in about 30 to 45 minutes, and has a duration of action of 2 to 3 hours, although salivary secretions can be suppressed for up to 7 hours. In order to allow time to reach the peak effect, either agent should be administered intramuscularly at least 20 to 30 minutes before anesthetic induction. When given intravenously, the onset of action of atropine is about 1 minute and peak effect is about 3 to 4 minutes after injection. This makes this drug ideal for treatment of bradycardia in emergency situations such as cardiopulmonary resuscitation (CPR).

Effects and Adverse Effects involving Major Organ Systems

Central Nervous System

- Anticholinergics are not sedatives and therefore have limited CNS effects, although atropine can cause mild sedation in some patients at therapeutic doses. Glycopyrrolate is less likely to cause CNS effects because it does not cross the blood–brain barrier.

Cardiovascular System

- These agents prevent bradycardia, which is often associated with anesthesia and surgery, and which routinely cause the heart rate to increase. However, when given at low doses, atropine may induce a temporary bradycardia. This is because atropine blocks a second type of muscarinic receptor located on presynaptic nerve terminals that normally inhibits acetylcholine release. The atropine-induced blockade of these receptors releases acetylcholine, resulting in bradycardia until the postsynaptic receptors are also blocked.
- Arrhythmias. After IV injection, anticholinergics may induce temporary first- or second-degree atrioventricular (AV) block, followed by sinus tachycardia. Although glycopyrrolate is less arrhythmogenic than atropine, either drug

may also induce other cardiac arrhythmias including ventricular arrhythmias. For these reasons, these drugs should be avoided in animals with preexisting rapid heart rates (more than 140 beats per minute [bpm] in dogs, 180 bpm in cats, 60 bpm in horses, and 100 bpm in ruminants) or heart disease (such as congestive heart failure or hyperthyroid-associated cardiomyopathy in cats).

Respiratory system

- Reduction and thickening of respiratory and salivary secretions. The use of anticholinergics in cats is associated with the production of thick mucus secretions within the airways. Even though these drugs decrease the volume of the secretions, the increased viscosity may predispose the patient to airway blockage. For this reason, some veterinarians do not use anticholinergics in this species. Anticholinergics are not recommended in ruminants at all except to treat intraoperative bradycardia or for CPR. This is because these drugs do not decrease the amount of salivary secretions in these species but instead cause the saliva to become thick and ropy, which places these patients at risk of respiratory obstruction.
- Bronchodilation. Anticholinergics increase the diameter of the bronchioles. This results in increased anatomic dead space, which may put the patient at risk of hypoventilation and hypoxemia (low blood oxygen). The bronchodilatory effect may be useful in patients with previously diagnosed bronchoconstriction (e.g., cats with feline asthma).

Other Effects and Adverse Effects

- Mydriasis. This effect is not commonly seen when dogs are given the usual preanesthetic doses but may be seen in cats. When monitoring patients, the anesthetist must remember that the pupillary light reflex (PLR) may be depressed and therefore unreliable in patients given anticholinergics.
- Reduction of GI tract and salivary secretions. Several anesthetic agents, particularly ketamine and thiobarbiturates, induce copious production of saliva. Administration of an anticholinergic prior to or along with these drugs will lessen this effect and can lead to dry mouth.
- Reduction of lacrimal secretions. Corneal drying is a risk of general anesthesia because the patient's eyes remain open. Corneal drying, if severe or prolonged, will result in keratitis and corneal ulceration. For this reason, the corneas

of animals receiving anticholinergics should be protected from drying by instilling a ¼- to ½-inch strip of ophthalmic lubricating ointment in each eye every 2 to 3 hours.

- Anticholinergics inhibit intestinal peristalsis. This can cause gut stasis and colic in horses and bloat in ruminants even at clinical doses. Therefore use of these agents should be avoided in these species.

TECHNICIAN NOTE Major effects and adverse effects of anticholinergics are as follows:
- Prevention of bradycardia
- Increased heart rate
- Cardiac arrhythmias
- Reduction and thickening of respiratory secretions
- Bronchodilation
- Mydriasis
- Reduction of GI, salivary, and lacrimal secretions
- Inhibition of peristalsis

Use of Anticholinergics

Atropine and glycopyrrolate are still used by veterinary anesthetists, although less so than in the past. Many modern anesthetic agents do not cause excessive secretions, and bradycardia is well tolerated by most patients. Because of the potential for significant adverse effects, particularly tachycardia, thickening of mucus secretions, decreased tear production, and mydriasis, many authorities question the routine use of these agents. However, anticholinergics are beneficial for some patients (e.g., those with severe bradycardia, heart block, or excessive salivary secretions).

Atropine or glycopyrrolate is often included in preanesthetic and sedative protocols such as the "BAG" and "SuperBAG" protocols (see Chapter 9). Either agent can also be used to prevent adverse effects associated with reversal of nondepolarizing neuromuscular blocking agents. (See Chapter 7 for more information about neuromuscular blocking agents.)

Although the agents are similar, there are subtle differences between atropine and glycopyrrolate. Glycopyrrolate is slightly less likely to induce cardiac arrhythmias, suppresses salivation more effectively than atropine, and only minimally crosses the placental barrier in pregnant animals. For these reasons, many practitioners prefer this drug as a preanesthetic. Atropine is still considered to be the better choice as an emergency treatment for bradycardia associated with cardiopulmonary arrest, however, because of its faster onset.

Veterinary-labeled atropine products are available in three strengths: SA strength containing 0.54 mg/mL (sometimes listed on the label as 1/120 grain/mL), 0.6 mg/mL, and LA strength containing 15 mg/mL. After calculating a dose, remember to draw the drug of the correct strength into the syringe or an incorrect amount will be administered to the patient. For example, a volume of 0.5 mL of atropine drawn from a solution with a concentration of 15 mg/mL contains nearly 30 times the amount of drug when compared with a solution with a concentration of 0.54 mg/mL.

TECHNICIAN NOTE: Atropine is available in SA and LA strengths that vary in concentration by a factor of nearly 30. When drawing up the drug, remember to check the concentration on the bottle so that you *do not mix up the two!*

Tranquilizers and Sedatives

As mentioned in the introduction, a sedative and a tranquilizer are not exactly the same thing. A tranquilizer is a drug that reduces anxiety but does not necessarily decrease awareness and wakefulness. A sedative is a drug that causes reduced mental activity and sleepiness. Most veterinarians use the terms *sedative* and *tranquilizer* interchangeably, however. This is because the effects of these drugs often overlap, as most of these drugs produce both effects to some degree. For instance, tranquilizing effects predominate in the drug diazepam, whereas dexmedetomidine has primarily sedative effects.

Three classes of tranquilizer or sedative are commonly used in veterinary medicine: phenothiazines, benzodiazepines, and alpha$_2$-adrenoceptor agonists (alpha$_2$-agonists). In addition to tranquilization and sedation, some also cause other effects including ataxia and prolapse of the nictitating membrane (also called the *third eyelid*) (Fig. 3.5). Phenothiazines protect against cardiac arrhythmias and are antiemetics. In contrast, alpha$_2$-agonists are analgesics and can produce vomiting in some patients. Both alpha$_2$-agonists and benzodiazepines are good muscle relaxants.

There are some general risks associated with the use of these medications of which the technician must be aware. After receiving these drugs, patients should not be left unattended on a table or in a cage with an open door because they can easily fall and be injured. Sedatives relax the tissues in the pharynx, which may cause serious and life-threatening respiratory distress in brachycephalic dogs, especially those that exhibit significant respiratory stridor when awake. There are also risks to personnel and owners. Sedated animals may exhibit unusual behavior such as aggression, or may suddenly become aroused and aggressive, particularly if stimulated suddenly (e.g., by pain).

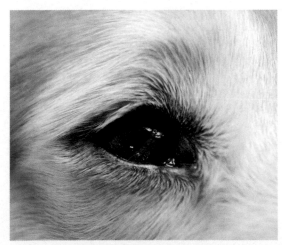

FIG. 3.5 Prolapse of the third eyelid. Note that the cornea is partially covered.

Phenothiazines

Phenothiazines are a group of noncontrolled, water-soluble drugs with somewhat diverse indications. Acepromazine maleate is the only drug in this class that is commonly used as an anesthetic adjunct. Chlorpromazine, a related drug, is occasionally used in veterinary patients as an antiemetic.

Acepromazine maleate (also known as acepromazine or "ace") is used alone or in combination with other drugs as a preanesthetic in a wide variety of large- and small-animal species to provide sedation, to decrease the dose of general anesthetic required, and to ease induction and recovery. It is also used alone or in combination with opioids to provide a mild to moderate level of sedation and tranquilization for minor procedures including wound treatment, grooming, and noninvasive diagnostic tests such as radiography. It is approved for use in dogs, cats, and horses.

When used as a preanesthetic and sedative, acepromazine is usually administered by the IV or IM route. Although it is also available in oral tablet form for tranquilization and sedation of small animals, this route is seldom used in anesthesia. There is currently no available reversal agent.

Mode of action and pharmacology. Acepromazine has a complex mechanism of action that is not fully understood. Major effects include depression of the reticular activating center of the brain and blockage of alpha-adrenergic, dopamine, and histamine receptors. It is metabolized by the liver and crosses the placental barrier slowly. Onset of action is about 15 minutes after IM injection in dogs or IV injection in horses, and peak effect occurs within 30 to 60 minutes. The duration of action is 4 to 8 hours in small animals but may be longer (up to 48 hours) if higher doses are used, or if the drug is given to old, sick, or debilitated patients or patients with liver disease. The duration of action in horses is shorter (1 to 3 hours).

Effects and adverse effects involving major organ systems
Central nervous system
- Calming, sedation, reluctance to move, and decreased interest in the patient's surroundings. Sedation is less pronounced in cats than in dogs and horses and is less pronounced than that seen with alpha$_2$-agonists in all species.
- Acepromazine does not provide pain control but does decrease anxiety in patients in pain that are receiving analgesics concurrently.
- Historically, acepromazine has been avoided in animals with neurologic disease due to concern about induction of seizures; however there is little to no evidence of this. In fact, some research suggests possible anticonvulsant activity.
- Effect on seizure threshold. Although some clinicians avoid using acepromazine in animals predisposed to seizures because of concern that it lowers the seizure threshold, research has failed to back this up. As previously mentioned, there is some evidence that acepromazine may have some anticonvulsant properties.
- Occasionally, acepromazine may induce excitement or aggression rather than sedation. This effect may persist into the postanesthetic period but usually resolves within 48 hours. Owners should be warned that behavioral changes sometimes occur, and care should be used when handling patients returning home within 48 hours of anesthesia.

Cardiovascular system
- Phenothiazines can cause either tachycardia in response to hypotension or bradycardia, especially when given at high doses.
- Antiarrhythmic effect. Some anesthetics, such as barbiturates, have a potential to cause cardiac arrhythmias, which may decrease cardiac output. Phenothiazines protect against ventricular arrhythmias.
- Peripheral vasodilation. This causes hypotension, a reflex increase in heart rate, and increased heat loss leading to hypothermia. Acepromazine also directly decreases cardiac output, although indirectly, through its vasodilatory effect, cardiac output is improved at low doses in normovolemic animals.
- Severe hypotension. Hypotension produced by acepromazine is dose dependent. In animals receiving isoflurane, a significant drop in blood pressure (as much as 20% to 30%) occurs. This contributes to the intraoperative hypotension commonly seen in patients given this combination.

Respiratory system
- At usual clinical doses, acepromazine does not cause significant respiratory depression but worsens depressive effects of other sedative and anesthetic agents.

Other effects and adverse effects
- Antiemetic effect. Even at very low doses, acepromazine helps prevent vomiting during the anesthetic period. It can also be used to prevent vomiting caused by motion sickness.
- Hypothermia. Body temperature decreases due to suppression of thermoregulation and increased loss resulting from vasodilatation. Therefore measures should be taken to maintain body temperature.
- Penile prolapse. In horses and other large animals, acepromazine has been reported to cause prolapse of the penis, which can lead to injury and subsequent permanent paralysis of the retractor penis muscle. For this reason, some veterinarians choose not to use acepromazine in breeding stallions.
- Decreased packed cell volume (PCV). In horses and dogs, the PCV drops within 30 minutes, likely because of increased uptake of red blood cells (RBCs) by the spleen.
- Antihistamine effect. Histamine is a chemical released during an allergic response. Acepromazine prevents the release of histamine and therefore decreases allergic reactions. For this reason, acepromazine should not be used to sedate animals that are to undergo allergy testing.

TECHNICIAN NOTE Major effects and adverse effects of phenothiazines are as follows:
- Calming, sedation, reluctance to move
- Tachycardia or bradycardia
- Antiarrhythmic effects
- Peripheral vasodilation
- Hypotension
- Antiemetic effects
- Hypothermia
- Penile prolapse in horses and other large animals
- Decreased PCV

Use of acepromazine. Patients should be placed in a quiet location free from stimulation between administration and peak effect (approximately 30 to 40 minutes following IM injection) because the sedative effects can be overridden if the patient is stimulated to a sufficient degree.

It has been suggested that the manufacturer's recommended dose for acepromazine is higher than that actually required for preanesthesia and that the dose should be reduced to minimize the danger of adverse effects. The commonly accepted dose range is 0.01 to 0.05 mg/kg in small animals, with a maximum dose of 3 mg in dogs and 1 mg in cats, and 0.03 to 0.05 mg/kg in horses. Higher doses will increase hypotension but not sedation.

The anesthetist should be particularly aware that phenothiazines have increased potency or duration in geriatric animals, neonates, animals with liver or cardiac dysfunction, and generally debilitated patients. Responses to this drug are also species and breed dependent. Doses should be reduced by 25% to 50% in Collies, Australian Shepherds, and other animals suspected of or known to have an MDR1(ABCB1-1delta) mutation *(see Box 2.5 in Chapter 2, for more information about this mutation)*, to minimize the possibility of exaggerated or prolonged sedation. Giant breed dogs, Greyhounds, and Boxers can be very sensitive to this drug and may experience severe bradycardia and hypotension. Terriers and cats are more resistant to its effects. Severe hypotension and bradycardia are treated with IV fluid therapy and anticholinergics.

In horses, care must be taken to ensure that acepromazine is injected into a vein. Inadvertent injection into the carotid artery can cause severe CNS excitement or depression, seizures, and death. The location of the needle can be checked by the following maneuver. After venipuncture, remove the syringe from the needle. Release digital pressure on the vein. If the needle is in the jugular vein, blood flow from the hub will cease. If it is in an artery, blood flow will continue from the hub despite the release in digital pressure.

Although acepromazine has relatively low toxicity, severe overdoses require treatment. Hypotension resulting from overdose is worsened by epinephrine and should instead be treated with phenylephrine or norepinephrine.

> **TECHNICIAN NOTE** The commonly used dose of acepromazine (0.01–0.05 mg/kg in small animals, with a maximum dose of 3 mg in dogs and 1 mg in cats; 0.03–0.05 mg/kg in horses) is significantly lower than the labeled dose. Higher doses will increase hypotension but not sedation.

Benzodiazepines

The benzodiazepines, also referred to as *minor tranquilizers,* are a group of DEA Schedule IV controlled, reversible drugs (with the exception of zolazepam, a component of the combination drug Telazol, which is a Schedule III product) most often used in combination with other agents for their muscle relaxant and anticonvulsant properties. These drugs produce unreliable sedative effects and, in dogs, cats, and horses, may instead produce dysphoria, excitement, and ataxia, especially when administered to young, healthy animals.

Midazolam, zolazepam (a component of Telazol), and diazepam are the most commonly used anesthetic adjuncts in this class. Although not used for anesthesia, lorazepam is used in dogs as an alternative to midazolam and diazepam to treat status epilepticus, and lorazepam, alprazolam, and clonazepam can be used for anxiolysis. Of these agents, only zolazepam is licensed for use in animals in the United States and Canada.

Benzodiazepines are commonly administered by the IM or IV route, although diazepam is irritating and poorly absorbed when administered intramuscularly.

Mode of action and pharmacology. Benzodiazepines depress the CNS. Although the exact mechanism of action is not known, benzodiazepines exert their primary effects by increasing activity of GABA, an inhibitory neurotransmitter in the brain.

The commercially prepared injectable diazepam is mixed with 40% propylene glycol as well as several other ingredients. It is not water soluble and cannot be mixed with water-soluble drugs (except ketamine) and so should not be mixed in a single syringe with these drugs because a precipitate may form. Although not recommended by the manufacturer, diazepam is often combined in the same syringe with ketamine. This combination seldom results in adverse events but should not be used if a visible precipitate forms. In addition, this mixture should not be stored in syringes or other plastic containers because diazepam is very soluble in plastic and over time, is absorbed by syringes, IV bags, and IV tubing. Midazolam and zolazepam are water soluble and so can be used in combination with other water-soluble drugs. Most benzodiazepines have a relatively rapid onset of action (less than or equal to 15 minutes after IM injection for midazolam and zolazepam) and short duration (1 to 4 hours).

> **TECHNICIAN NOTE** Diazepam should not be mixed in a single syringe with water-soluble drugs (except ketamine) because a precipitate may form. Diazepam should not be stored in syringes, IV bags, or other plastic containers because it is absorbed.

Effects and adverse effects involving major organ systems
Central nervous system

- Antianxiety and calming effect. Benzodiazepines, unlike phenothiazines, do not cause significant sedation in healthy young animals unless used in combination with other drugs such as ketamine or opioids. Although their effect as a sole sedative in healthy young animals is inadequate, benzodiazepines are much more effective in geriatric or debilitated animals. Diazepam also enhances the sedation and analgesia of other agents, and its relative safety makes it a popular drug for combination protocols.
- Anticonvulsant activity. To take advantage of this effect, many anesthetists use benzodiazepines in combination with other agents that have the potential to cause seizures, including ketamine and local anesthetics. Benzodiazepines are also preanesthetics of choice for some animals with seizure disorders. Diazepam and lorazepam can be given intravenously

or intrarectally, and midazolam can be given intravenously for treatment of seizures.

- The primary adverse effects of these drugs involve the CNS. Animals, especially those that are young and healthy, receiving these drugs alone may actually become more difficult to control. Dogs may become disoriented and excited, and cats may become dysphoric or aggressive. Horses may have muscle fasciculations, and animals of any large species may become ataxic or recumbent.
- The anesthetist should be aware that benzodiazepines, like phenothiazines, have no analgesic effect and when used alone, are rarely effective in calming animals that are experiencing pain.

Cardiovascular and respiratory systems

- At therapeutic doses, benzodiazepines have few effects on the cardiovascular and respiratory systems and therefore have a high margin of safety. Heart rate, blood pressure, and cardiac output are minimally affected. This property makes them particularly useful for anesthesia of high-risk and geriatric animals.

Other effects and adverse effects

- Skeletal muscle relaxation. Benzodiazepines are excellent skeletal muscle relaxants and often are used to counteract the muscle rigidity seen with agents such as ketamine and etomidate.
- Potentiation of general anesthetics. Premedication with benzodiazepines decreases the requirements for many general anesthetics including the inhalant agents.
- Effect on neonates. Benzodiazepines cross the placenta and may cause CNS depression in neonates delivered by cesarean section (C-section).
- Adverse effects specific to diazepam: Diazepam is painful and poorly absorbed when administered intramuscularly. Diazepam should be given by slow IV injection because if given rapidly, it can cause pain, bradycardia, hypotension, and apnea.

TECHNICIAN NOTE Major effects and adverse effects of benzodiazepines are as follows:
- Antianxiety and calming *only* in old or ill patients
- Anticonvulsant activity
- Disorientation and excitement in young, healthy dogs
- Dysphoria and aggression in cats
- Muscle fasciculations in horses
- Ataxia or recumbency in large animals
- Few cardiopulmonary effects
- Skeletal muscle relaxation
- Pain on IM injection of diazepam

Use of benzodiazepines. Midazolam and diazepam are both commonly used in combination with other agents to induce anesthesia. Although it is not possible to induce anesthesia in a healthy animal through the use of these drugs alone, they are an effective supplement to other agents. In particular, the combination of ketamine and midazolam has gained wide acceptance as a safe and effective IV induction agent in small animals,

horses, and ruminants. When this combination is used in small animals, diazepam may be substituted for midazolam. Midazolam may also be administered concurrently with opioids, propofol, alfaxalone, or etomidate to achieve safe, smooth induction for high-risk patients. If diazepam is given in combination with opioids, propofol, alfaxalone, or etomidate, separate syringes should be used to administer each drug through an IV catheter with saline flush given after each drug.

Midazolam and diazepam are light-sensitive and for this reason are often provided in brown glass vials. If in a clear glass container, these drugs should be stored away from light.

Midazolam has some advantages over diazepam. It is water soluble and therefore can be mixed with other preanesthetic and anesthetic agents. It is less irritating to tissues and is also more reliably absorbed after IM or SC injection. Both midazolam and diazepam produce unreliable sedation in dogs when used alone but are excellent sedatives in swine and some exotics including ferrets, rabbits, and birds.

In small mammals and birds, midazolam is usually used in combination with ketamine and/or opioids for sedation and intubation. It can also be administered before induction of anesthesia with propofol, alfaxalone, or etomidate to increase muscle relaxation and reduce adverse effects.

Zolazepam is available only mixed with tiletamine in the combination product Telazol. This powdered product requires reconstitution with sterile water and is discussed more in the section covering dissociative anesthetics.

The benzodiazepine antagonist flumazenil can be administered IV to reverse the effects of benzodiazepines. This drug is especially useful for animals that are slow to recover from benzodiazepines or when performing cardiopulmonary resuscitation on patients that have received benzodiazepines.

Alpha$_2$-Adrenoceptor Agonists

Alpha$_2$-adrenoceptor agonists (also written as *alpha$_2$-agonists* or *α_2-agonists*) are a group of noncontrolled, reversible agents used alone and in combination with other anesthetics and adjuncts in both large- and small-animal patients for sedation, analgesia, and muscle relaxation. They are commonly given before minor procedures such as radiography, wound treatment, or bandaging and subsequently reversed with an alpha$_2$-adrenoceptor antagonist. This allows the patient to be sequentially sedated and "awakened" so that it can be sent home a short time after completion of the procedure. Xylazine (Rompun, AnaSed), dexmedetomidine (Dexdomitor), detomidine (Dormosedan), and romifidine (Sedivet) are members of this class of drugs. Medetomidine, a predecessor to dexmedetomidine, is one component of the combination drug Zenalpha (see p. 77 for a discusson of this drug). These drugs are most often administered intramuscularly or intravenously. SC injection is less reliable and not recommended. Alpha$_2$-agonists have considerable potential for adverse effects. These are reported most commonly when the drugs are given by the IV route.

Mode of action and pharmacology. Alpha$_2$-agonists act on alpha$_2$-adrenergic receptors (also called *alpha$_2$-adrenoceptors*) of the sympathetic nervous system (SNS) both within the CNS and peripherally, causing a decrease in the release of the neurotransmitter norepinephrine. When these drugs are combined with other tranquilizers or analgesic agents, the result tends to be additive or synergistic (supra-additive) in nature.

The SNS has several different types of receptors (alpha, beta, and dopaminergic). In general, stimulation of the SNS is associated with the "fight-or-flight response." For this reason, the CNS depression induced by alpha$_2$-agonists does not at first glance seem logical. This paradoxical effect occurs, however, because stimulation of the alpha$_2$-receptors does not cause the fight-or-flight response but instead causes sedation, analgesia, bradycardia, hypotension, and hypothermia. These unique effects make these particular SNS stimulants useful sedatives and analgesics.

Alpha$_2$-agonists are metabolized in the liver, and the metabolites are excreted in the urine. Adequate hepatic and renal function are therefore important requirements for any animal receiving these drugs.

The onset and duration of action are similar with all currently available alpha$_2$-agonists. After injection, sedation occurs rapidly (within 5 to 15 minutes of IV injection or 15 to 30 minutes of IM injection) and lasts about 1 to 2 hours in most cases. Complete recovery takes about 2 to 4 hours if the drug is not reversed.

Effects and adverse effects involving major organ systems
Central nervous system
- Alpha$_2$-agonists are potent sedatives. Sedation is dose dependent and can be profound in small animals, small ruminants, and foals. In horses, effects include a lowered head ("knees-to-nose" position), relaxed facial muscles, and a drooping lower lip. When the drugs are combined with other agents, sedation may be sufficient for minor or even major surgical procedures (referred to as "standing sedation").
- Analgesia. Unlike phenothiazines and benzodiazepines, alpha$_2$-agonists provide analgesia. When combined with other analgesics and sedatives, they may provide sufficient analgesia to allow surgical procedures to be performed. Although the sedative effect of alpha$_2$-agonists may last for several hours, the analgesia may be short-lived (approximately 20 minutes for xylazine) and should be supplemented with another agent, typically an opioid, if a prolonged effect is required.
- Temporary behavior changes. Patients that are excited before administration may become agitated and aggressive when touched, and any patient may move or startle in response to loud noises.
- Horses may experience muscle tremors and may kick in response to loud noises.
- Cattle frequently lie down. Excessive doses given intravenously may cause falling from ataxia and sedation.

Cardiovascular system
- Alpha$_2$-agonists have a significant effect on the cardiovascular system. After injection, there is an early dose-dependent vasoconstriction that results in a brief period of hypertension and reflex bradycardia, during which the mucous membranes may look pale. Various cardiac arrhythmias including first- and second-degree AV block may also occur during this time (see Chapter 6 for a discussion of these arrhythmias). These effects are more pronounced when the drug is given intravenously. This phase is followed by a decrease in cardiac output, hypotension, and a further drop in heart rate due to decreased sympathetic tone.
- Dramatic decreases in heart rate (e.g., down to 30 to 50 bpm in dogs), blood pressure, and cardiac output with a resultant decrease in tissue perfusion can occur with these agents, especially when given at high doses. Because of these serious effects, the use of alpha$_2$-agonists should be avoided in animals that are debilitated or that have cardiovascular disease.

Respiratory system
- Alpha$_2$-agonists depress the respiratory system, especially in ruminants. Although the effect is minimal at lower doses, high doses or concurrent administration of other agents can significantly decrease tidal volume and respiratory rate. Brachycephalic dogs and horses with upper respiratory obstruction may become dyspneic. For these reasons, as a general rule, alpha$_2$-agonists should not be administered to animals showing signs of respiratory disease.

Other effects and adverse effects
- Muscle relaxation. These drugs are useful adjuncts to general anesthetics for procedures in which muscle relaxation is necessary.
- Increased effects of other anesthetics. When these agents are given as a preanesthetic or concurrently with general anesthetics, the required doses of the anesthetics are substantially reduced (e.g., up to a 50% reduction of propofol and inhalant agents).
- GI effects. Many cats and some dogs vomit within a few minutes of receiving these agents. Because affected patients may have decreased swallowing reflexes, the airway must be protected to prevent aspiration of stomach contents by placing the head in a dependent position as soon as retching is noted. Dexmedetomidine is less likely to cause vomiting than xylazine. Dogs may develop gaseous distension of the stomach that is visible on radiographs and may need to be relieved. Cattle may salivate, bloat, and regurgitate stomach contents. Rarely, horses may develop gas colic (intestinal bloat).
- Hyperglycemia. Alpha$_2$-agonists reduce the secretion of insulin by the pancreas, causing transient hyperglycemia, which is not harmful to the animal but may confound the interpretation of blood samples collected during this period.
- Hypothermia. Alpha$_2$-agonists decrease thermoregulation and shivering, leading to hypothermia.
- Increased urination. Alpha$_2$-agonists may increase urination because they interfere with the release of antidiuretic hormone and owing to their antiinsulin effect, which causes glucosuria.
- Premature parturition. Xylazine causes increased intrauterine pressure in cattle and has the potential to cause abortion in the last trimester.
- Horses may sweat.
- Accidental intraarterial injection in horses can result in excitement, seizures, and collapse. The maneuver described on page 73 may be used to check needle placement.

Use of alpha$_2$-agonists. Careful monitoring of vital signs is always essential for patients receiving these drugs, all of which should be used with caution. All members of this class can be given in standard doses to young, healthy patients but should be avoided or used with great caution in geriatric, diabetic, pregnant, pediatric, or sick patients.

To reduce the incidence of bradycardia, some veterinarians give atropine or glycopyrrolate as premedication. However, this is not always effective and may in fact increase the workload of the heart and myocardial oxygen consumption. If used, anticholinergics must be administered 10 to 20 minutes before these agents are given or bradycardia may worsen and other arrhythmias may develop. Anticholinergics should also be avoided with alpha$_2$-agonist–ketamine combinations because prolonged tachycardia can occur. If excessive bradycardia occurs, the best treatment is administration of an appropriate reversal agent.

Alpha$_2$-agonists can be absorbed through skin abrasions and mucous membranes, and as little as 0.1 mL of dexmedetomidine can cause hypotension and sedation in humans. Hospital employees handling these agents should ensure that any of the drug spilled on human or animal skin is immediately washed off.

Xylazine. Xylazine has been available since the 1960s and was the first widely used alpha$_2$-agonist in both large- and small-animal species. It is supplied as a 2% solution (20 mg/mL)

for small-animal use and as a 10% solution (100 mg/mL) for equine use. Therefore to avoid a serious overdose, it is very important to look carefully at the label before drawing up a dose.

For many decades, xylazine has been frequently used alone or in various combinations with ketamine, opioids, and other agents in dogs, cats, and other small animals. It has now been largely replaced by dexmedetomidine in these species, although it may be used as an emetic in cats to treat toxicities and drug overdoses. It is still used in large animals as a preanesthetic and sedative, in combination with butorphanol for minor procedures, and in combination with ketamine and guaifenesin (a combination known as "triple drip") to produce total IV anesthesia. Cattle have a much lower tolerance for xylazine, requiring only about one-tenth the dose needed by horses.

Dexmedetomidine. Dexmedetomidine is currently the most commonly used alpha$_2$-agonist in dogs and cats, having greater potency and fewer adverse effects than xylazine. It is supplied as a 0.5 mg/mL solution (Dexdomitor) (Fig. 3.6—left) and as a 0.1 mg/mL solution (Dexdomitor 0.1) (see Fig. 3.6—right) for sedation, analgesia, and preanesthesia in dogs and cats, and is marketed along with a corresponding antagonist, atipamezole (Antisedan) (see Fig. 3.6—center). Dexdomitor 0.1 contains dexmedetomidine at one-fifth the concentration of Dexdomitor and is intended for use in dogs weighing less than 20 lb (9.1 kg) and cats weighing less than 7 lb (3.2 kg) to increase dosing accuracy and convenience in these patients.

Dexdomitor (0.5 mg/mL) and Antisedan are packaged such that equivalent volumes of the two drugs can be used sequentially to sedate and wake a patient for short or minor diagnostic, surgical, or therapeutic procedures. In contrast, the volume of Antisedan needed to reverse the effects of Dexdomitor 0.1 is approximately one-fifth the volume of Dexdomitor 0.1 given. Dexmedetomidine is labeled for IM use in dogs and cats and IV use only in dogs, although it has been used in many other species, including horses, and exotic animals.

The manufacturer recommends that the dose of dexmedetomidine be determined according to body surface area in dogs so that smaller patients receive relatively more and larger patients receive relatively less. Charts based on this dosage scheme are

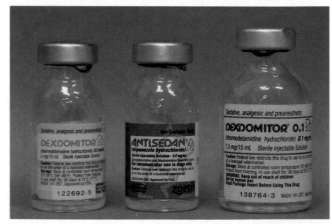

FIG. 3.6 Dexdomitor (0.5 mg/mL) *(left)*, Antisedan (5.0 mg/mL) *(center)*, and Dexdomitor 0.1 (0.1 mg/mL) *(right)*. (Courtesy Zoetis; https://www.zoetis.com.)

supplied with the drug, with progressively increasing doses listed for patients of various body weights for "sedation/analgesia in dogs," "preanesthesia in dogs," and "sedation/analgesia and preanesthesia in cats." Low doses of dexmedetomidine given as a preanesthetic are generally more effective than acepromazine in reducing general anesthetic requirements and do not cause as profound a degree of hypotension when given with isoflurane.

Like xylazine, dexmedetomidine is also used in combination with other agents. For instance, one combination in widespread use is dexmedetomidine (10 μg/kg) and butorphanol (0.2 mg/kg). The two drugs can be mixed in the same syringe and given intramuscularly. Dexmedetomidine can also be mixed with opioids and ketamine to produce CNS depression of varying degrees ranging from mild sedation to general anesthesia, depending on the specific combination and dose (e.g., the popular combinations "kitty magic" and "doggie magic" [dexmedetomidine, butorphanol, and ketamine]).

Animals should be left in a quiet environment for 10 to 15 minutes after injection to allow the drug to take maximum effect. If a short, minimally invasive procedure is planned (such as an ear flush, bandage change, or radiography), the sedation provided by dexmedetomidine–butorphanol and other combinations may be adequate without a general anesthetic. The sedation can be supplemented with a local block if minor surgery such as suturing a laceration or removal of a superficial skin tumor is planned. Although these patients are usually too awake for intubation, some veterinarians choose to provide supplemental oxygen by face mask. Caution should be exercised when dexmedetomidine combinations are used for minor operations because sudden arousal has been reported even in heavily sedated patients.

If the sedated animal is to undergo more extensive surgery, an injectable or inhalant general anesthetic (e.g., propofol or isoflurane) can be given. The dose of general anesthetic required will be significantly less than that required for a nonsedated animal, and caution must be exercised to avoid overdosage.

Pain may be associated with IM injection of dexmedetomidine. Do not give anticholinergics with high doses of dexmedetomidine because paradoxic bradycardia may result.

Oral transmucosal dexmedetomidine gel (Sileo [Zoetis]) is a special formulation of dexmedetomidine labeled for treatment of noise phobias in dogs. The recommended dosage is based on body surface area. The drug is packaged in dosing syringes that allow the owner to determine the proper amount to give by using a table that converts body weight to an appropriate number of dots from 1 to 10 that correspond to the correct setting on the syringe. Some clinicians may also use this product as a general anxiolytic prior to veterinary visits. Although it may be appropriate for this indication, it is important to remember that adverse effects seen with the injectable form of this drug such as profound sedation, changes in cardiovascular function, respiratory depression, and paradoxical aggression may occur and consequently, this must be taken into consideration.

Medetomidine and vatinoxan hydrochloride. Zenalpha® (Dechra Veterinary Products, LLC) is a combination drug containing the alpha2-agonist medetomidine and the alpha2-antagonist vatinoxan hydrochloride that became available in the European Union in 2021 and in the United States in 2022. Medetomidine is an equal mixture of two enantiomers (drugs that are mirror images of one another)—dexmedetomidine (which has sedative and analgesic properties) and levomedetomidine (which is an inactive drug). Therefore, medetomidine is approximately one-half the potency of pure dexmedetomidine. Vatinoxan is an alpha2-adrenoceptor antagonist that acts in the peripheral nervous system to selectively block adverse effects (including the cardiovascular effects) of dexmedetomidine, such as bradycardia, vasoconstriction, and hypertension.

This drug combination, which is labeled for sedation in physical status class I and II dogs, is designed to preserve the analgesic and sedative effects of dexmedetomidine but maintain the heart rate and blood pressure at nearly normal levels. There are other differences between the clinical effects of Zenalpha and dexmedetomidine that are detailed in the product insert. Like dexmedetomidine, the manufacturer's recommended dosage is based on body surface area as opposed to patient weight.

Detomidine. Detomidine, which is available as an injectable and also an equine oral transmucosal gel, is used in horses to produce sedation, analgesia, and muscle relaxation. This drug is similar to xylazine, producing similar beneficial and adverse effects, but has approximately twice the duration of action. It is commonly given with butorphanol to produce standing sedation. It is also used to provide analgesia for colic pain.

Romifidine. Romifidine is similar to other drugs in this class but produces less ataxia than either detomidine or xylazine.

Alpha2-Antagonists

Yohimbine, tolazoline, and atipamezole are alpha2-antagonists that can be used to reverse the effects of alpha2-agonists. Because of the adverse cardiovascular effects and long duration of sedation that can occur after administration of alpha2-agonists, use of an antagonist is often desirable. Yohimbine and tolazoline are used to reverse the effects of xylazine in dogs, cats, ruminants, horses, and exotic species. Atipamezole is used to reverse the effects of dexmedetomidine in dogs, cats, and exotic species.

Mode of action and pharmacology. These agents work by displacing the agonist from the alpha2-receptors. Alpha2-antagonists preferentially bind to the receptors, thus reversing the effect of the corresponding agonist.

Effects and adverse effects. The major effect of alpha2-antagonists is reversal of the sedative and cardiovascular effects of the corresponding agonist. Alpha2-antagonists have few adverse effects at clinical doses but can have significant adverse effects if too much is given. Doses should be based on the amount of the agonist that was given and the length of time since agonist administration, and should be reduced if more than 30 minutes have elapsed. Adverse effects affect the GI, neurologic, and cardiovascular systems, and include excitement, muscle tremors, hypotension, tachycardia, salivation, vomiting, and diarrhea. Because of the potential for tachycardia, these agents should not be given when anticholinergics have also been given.

Patients whose sedation is reversed with these agents may exhibit excitement, apprehension, or aggression. Therefore the anesthetist should be vigilant when monitoring these patients because they may "wake up" very rapidly, causing injury to themselves or personnel.

> **TECHNICIAN NOTE** Alpha$_2$-antagonists have few adverse effects at clinical doses but can have significant adverse effects if too much is given. Doses should be based on the amount of the agonist that was given and the length of time since agonist administration and should be reduced if more than 30 minutes have elapsed. When given intravenously, these agents should be given *slowly!*

Use of alpha$_2$-antagonists. Alpha$_2$-antagonists will reverse all of the clinical effects of alpha$_2$-agonists, both detrimental (bradycardia) and beneficial (analgesia). To maintain analgesia it may be necessary to administer another analgesic agent just before the reversal. The anesthetist must also realize that alpha$_2$-antagonists do not reverse the effects of other drugs given concurrently (e.g., dissociatives, opioids, general anesthetics). Because the duration of action of alpha$_2$-antagonists is generally short, resedation may occur, in which case, an additional dose may be necessary.

The dose of these drugs is expressed as a ratio of the agonist dose to the antagonist dose.[b] In other words, an agonist–antagonist ratio of 10:1 means that if 0.1 mg/kg of the agonist was given, the correct dose for the antagonist is 0.01 mg/kg (one-tenth the agonist dose). An agonist–antagonist ratio of 2:1 means that 0.1 mg/kg of the agonist should be followed by 0.05 mg/kg of the antagonist (one-half the agonist dose). When given intravenously, alpha$_2$-antagonists should be given slowly.

Tolazoline. Tolazoline is a nonspecific alpha-antagonist (it binds to both alpha$_1$ and alpha$_2$ receptors) primarily used to reverse the sedative and cardiovascular effects of xylazine in ruminants. The dose is calculated using a 1:10 agonist–antagonist ratio (0.1 mg/kg of xylazine is reversed with 1 mg/kg of tolazoline).

Yohimbine. Yohimbine is primarily used to reverse the sedative and cardiovascular effects of xylazine in dogs, cats, horses, and exotic species. The calculated dose is based on a 10:1 agonist–antagonist ratio in dogs and horses and a 2:1 ratio in cats.[c] (In a dog, 1 mg/kg of xylazine is reversed with 0.1 mg/kg of yohimbine.)

Atipamezole. Atipamezole (Antisedan) is packaged as a specific antagonist for dexmedetomidine and medetomidine. Atipamezole is labeled for IM injection only and should be given by this route unless IV administration is necessary for emergency resuscitation. The dose of atipamezole is based on an agonist–antagonist ratio of about 1:10. As the formulation of atipamezole is 10 times more concentrated than the concentration of dexmedetomidine in Dexdomitor (atipamezole 5 mg/mL, dexmedetomidine

0.5 mg/mL), equal volumes of these drugs should be administered to dogs. Cats are more sensitive to the effects of atipamezole, so ideally, a little over half of this dose should be used in this species (an agonist–antagonist ratio of about 1:6). When Dexdomitor 0.1 is given to a dog or a cat, the volume of atipamezole required for reversal is only about one-fifth or one-eighth of the volume of Dexdomitor 0.1 given, respectively. Because of marked side effects such as hypersalivation and CNS excitement, atipamezole should not be given intravenously to cats. Reversal of effects typically occurs 5 to 10 minutes after IM injection.

Opioids

Opioids are derivatives of opium, an extract of a species of poppy called *Papaverum somniferum.* Opioids include both naturally derived compounds called *opiates* and synthesized compounds.

This is a versatile class of drugs used for analgesia, sedation, and, when combined with other agents, anesthetic induction. Opioids are classified as agonists, partial agonists, agonist–antagonists, or antagonists, depending on their predominant effects.

Commonly used opioids include the agonists morphine, hydromorphone, methadone, fentanyl, meperidine, and oxymorphone; the partial agonist buprenorphine; the agonist–antagonists butorphanol and nalbuphine; and the antagonist naloxone. Lesserused opioid agonists include alfentanil, remifentanil, and sufentanil, as well as etorphine and thiafentanil, two agonists used for wild animal capture. With the exception of the antagonists and nalbuphine, opioids are controlled drugs and include several that are in class II (including morphine, methadone, hydromorphone, meperidine, fentanyl, and oxymorphone). They may be administered by a wide variety of routes including IV, IM, SC, oral, rectal, and transdermal, as well as subarachnoid and epidural routes (two different types of "spinal injections"). They have a wide safety margin and can be used in both healthy and debilitated patients. Information on the use of opioids as induction agents is found in Chapters 9, 10, and 11, and detailed information on specific opioid agents and their use for analgesia is presented in Chapter 8.

Mode of Action and Pharmacology

Opioids produce similar effects to natural chemicals present in the body called *endogenous opioid peptides,* which include β-endorphins, dynorphins, and enkephalins. Although the mode of action of opioids is not completely understood, it has been the subject of a great deal of research over the past several decades that has yielded much information. Although opioid receptors are found on neurons throughout the body, the analgesic and sedative effects are chiefly the result of their action on receptors located in the brain and spinal cord.

Three major types of opioid receptor have been identified: mu (μ), kappa (κ), and delta (δ), each of which has two or more subtypes. This variety of receptors produces a wide spectrum of effects because each opioid agent differs in its action at each of these sites and therefore in its overall effects on the body.

Opioid agonists exert their effects primarily by binding to and stimulating the mu and kappa receptors and are the best drugs available for moderate and severe pain. Partial agonists

[b]Lemke KA: Anticholinergics and sedatives. In Tranquilli WJ, Thurmon JC, Grimm KA, editors. *Lumb & Jones' veterinary anesthesia and analgesia,* ed 4, Ames, IA, 2007, Blackwell, pp 225.

[c]Lemke KA: Anticholinergics and sedatives. In Tranquilli WJ, Thurmon JC, Grimm KA, editors. *Lumb & Jones' veterinary anesthesia and analgesia,* ed 4, Ames, IA, 2007, Blackwell, pp 226.

only partially stimulate the opioid receptors. Agonist–antagonists do not stimulate the mu receptors but instead, stimulate the kappa receptors. Pure antagonists bind to but do not stimulate mu or kappa receptors. They are therefore called *reversal agents* because they displace agonists from the receptors and block their effects. These antagonists have no clinical effect on their own but are used to reverse the effects of the pure agonists, partial agonists, and mixed agonist–antagonists.

With few exceptions, opioids have a relatively short duration of action (0.5 to 3 hours). Exceptions are buprenorphine, which has a significantly longer duration (6 to 8 hours), and morphine, which has a duration of 6 to 8 hours in horses.

In people, prolonged use of some opioid agents can lead to physical dependence (addiction). Human patients given morphine develop a tolerance for its effects in approximately 2 to 3 weeks. Not all opioids are addictive. Those with minimal or antagonistic activity at mu receptors (e.g., butorphanol) have less potential for causing physical dependence.

Effects and Adverse Effects Involving Major Organ Systems

Central nervous system

- Opioid agents may cause CNS depression or excitement. The exact effect depends on the dose, route, agent used, species, the patient's temperament, and pain status.
- In dogs, the predominant effect is sedation, which tends to be greater with agonists and milder with partial agonists and agonist–antagonists. Most dogs exhibit CNS depression within 60 seconds of IV administration and 15 minutes of IM administration. If high doses of opioid agonists are given (particularly to a sick animal), a sleeplike state called *narcosis* may be produced.
- In contrast, cats, horses, and ruminants exhibit CNS stimulation that is more pronounced with pure agonists. This may include bizarre behavior patterns, for example, excitement, increased motor activity, or dysphoria (a state characterized by anxiety or restlessness), particularly if the drug is given intravenously. For this reason, some opioids (e.g., morphine) must be used at low doses in these species, and IV injection is avoided. Dogs that are not in pain may show a similar reaction (e.g., whining and barking) after opioid administration, particularly if given by rapid IV injection or if a tranquilizing agent is not used concurrently.
- Analgesia. Opioids have long been considered to be the most effective agents for the treatment of pain. The degree of analgesia varies among members of the class: pure agonists such as morphine and hydromorphone are more effective for treatment of severe pain than the partial agonists such as buprenorphine or the mixed agonist–antagonists such as butorphanol. Opioids are particularly useful when included in premedication for patients undergoing surgery for painful conditions (e.g., repair of fractures). Because most commonly used general anesthetics have limited analgesic properties (e.g., isoflurane, sevoflurane, propofol, alfaxalone, and etomidate), the analgesic effect of opioids remains one of the chief indications in veterinary patients.
- Opioids tend to increase intraocular and intracranial pressures because of their tendency to depress ventilation which,

in turn, increases the partial pressure of carbon dioxide in arterial blood ($Paco_2$). Therefore they should be avoided or used cautiously in patients with head trauma and other CNS disorders as an elevation in $Paco_2$ leads to an increase in intracranial pressure.

Cardiovascular system

- Opioids typically cause a vagus-induced bradycardia which may be pronounced, especially if the drugs are given with other agents that slow the heart rate (such as alpha$_2$-agonists). This is a dose-related effect that is less pronounced in animals pretreated with atropine.

Respiratory system

- Although these drugs have the potential to decrease respiratory rate and tidal volume, this effect is often minimal at low dose rates (such as those used for pain control) and in the absence of preexisting CNS depression.
- Some dogs pant after administration of opioid agonists. This is because of a direct effect on the thermoregulatory center of the brain, which mistakenly interprets normal body temperature as being elevated.
- Opioids can cause severe respiratory depression, particularly at higher doses or when given with another drug that is a respiratory depressant, such as dexmedetomidine or isoflurane. The resulting decrease in both respiratory rate and tidal volume can lead to decreased blood oxygen levels (Pao_2) and increased carbon dioxide levels ($Paco_2$). Some opioids such as butorphanol, which does not stimulate the mu receptors, cause minimal respiratory depression.

Other Effects and Adverse Effects

- Changes in body temperature. Dogs become hypothermic and will pant as a result of resetting of the thermoregulatory center in the hypothalamus. Cats become hyperthermic for unknown reasons.
- Opioids can cause several adverse GI effects, including salivation and vomiting in small-animal patients. Initially, many agents also cause an increase in peristaltic movement, resulting in diarrhea, vomiting, and flatulence. Pretreatment with atropine or acepromazine usually moderates this effect. After the initial stimulation of peristalsis, a prolonged period of GI stasis may occur, resulting in constipation. GI stasis, or ileus, is of particular concern in horses because it can predispose them to developing colic. Given the emetic effect of some opioid agents (particularly morphine), these drugs should be avoided in animals in which vomiting would be detrimental (e.g., animals with GI obstruction).
- Increased responsiveness to noise. Some patients will startle in reaction to loud noises, requiring caution to ensure that the patient does not fall off a table or out of an open cage.
- Changes in pupil size. Opioids cause miosis in dogs and mydriasis in cats, ruminants, and horses.
- Sweating in horses.
- Decreased urine production and urine retention.
- Morphine and meperidine may cause facial swelling and hypotension after rapid IV administration because of histamine release.

- Drug interactions. Some opioids, particularly meperidine, may cause a potentially fatal reaction known as *serotonin syndrome* when given to animals receiving MOIs such as selegiline or TCAs such as clomipramine. Although the incidence of this reaction in veterinary patients is unknown, these combinations should be avoided until future studies clarify the risk.

TECHNICIAN NOTE Major effects and adverse effects of opioids are as follows:

- CNS depression or excitement depending on the dose, route, agent used, species, patient's temperament, and pain status
- CNS depression in dogs (except for those not in pain)
- CNS stimulation (excitement, dysphoria, and increased motor activity) in cats and large animals
- Excellent somatic and visceral analgesia
- Dose-dependent bradycardia and respiratory depression that can be pronounced
- Panting in dogs
- Hypothermia in dogs and hyperthermia in cats
- Salivation and vomiting in small animals
- Initial vomiting, diarrhea and flatulence, then ileus and constipation
- Colic and sweating in horses
- Increased responsiveness to noise
- Miosis in dogs and mydriasis in cats and large animals
- Decreased urine production and urine retention

Use of Opioids

Opioid agonists, partial agonists, and agonist–antagonists are used in many ways in veterinary anesthesia. They are a common component of preanesthetic protocols. For high-risk patients, some anesthetists prefer to use an opioid such as morphine or hydromorphone as the sole preanesthetic agent. More commonly, however, opioids are mixed with a tranquilizer (such as acepromazine, midazolam, or dexmedetomidine) and/or an anticholinergic (atropine or glycopyrrolate) and given during the preanesthetic period. Many combinations are used; see Protocols 9.2 and 9.3 in Chapter 9 for common combinations used in small animals.

Ideally, these combinations should be chosen on the basis of individual patient need and drawn up into a syringe immediately before use. Some practices prepare these mixtures in advance and administer a set dose by IM or SC injection according to patient weight. This is more convenient than individual preparation, but there is some risk of inappropriate treatment, particularly if the patient is geriatric or debilitated or has significant organ dysfunction (e.g., liver disease).

Opioids are also used to prevent and treat postoperative pain (see Chapter 8 for a complete discussion of analgesia) and are often used in combination with a tranquilizer to achieve a state of profound sedation and analgesia termed neuroleptanalgesia.

Neuroleptanalgesia

Neuroleptanalgesia is a state of profound sedation and analgesia induced by the simultaneous administration of an opioid and a tranquilizer. Animals given neuroleptanalgesics generally lie quietly in lateral or sternal recumbency (adult horses stand quietly) but can be aroused by sufficient noise or surgical stimulation. Therefore, neuroleptanalgesia is commonly used for procedures that require significant CNS depression and analgesia but not general anesthesia.

Opioids commonly used for neuroleptanalgesia include morphine, methadone, buprenorphine, butorphanol, fentanyl, and hydromorphone. Tranquilizers that may be combined with opioids include acepromazine, midazolam, xylazine, and dexmedetomidine. Virtually any combination of these drugs may be used according to the veterinarian's preference.

Neuroleptanalgesics are commonly used to induce sedation in patients undergoing minor procedures including wound treatment, porcupine quill removal, and diagnostic procedures such as endoscopy or radiography, but they are seldom used to induce anesthesia in cats because of unacceptable side effects (excitement, mania) and are generally not suitable for routine induction of anesthesia in healthy young dogs because the level of sedation is not sufficient to permit intubation in these patients unless supplemented with an inhalation agent such as isoflurane or sevoflurane given by mask. However, neuroleptanalgesics may have a profound effect in high-risk or debilitated dogs (including those with hepatic, renal, and CNS disorders) and are a useful alternative to propofol, alfaxalone, or ketamine induction in these animals. Although this type of induction is slow and may cause some respiratory depression and bradycardia, it is safe for most patients, especially if the patient is subsequently intubated and ventilation is assisted.

The two drugs are often mixed in the same syringe (as long as diazepam is not included), although they may be injected separately. They are given intramuscularly or by slow IV injection and may be administered after pretreatment with anticholinergics although this is not required, provided the heart rate is carefully monitored. If bradycardia is excessive, the anticholinergic can be administered later.

Neuroleptanalgesics provide a wide margin of safety in most patients, but care must be taken to administer them slowly intravenously because if they are injected rapidly, CNS stimulation may occur. The anesthetist must also be prepared to intubate and ventilate the patient if necessary because respiratory depression may be profound.

Several procedures have been described for induction of anesthesia with neuroleptanalgesics, including the following:

- Administration of an anticholinergic and tranquilizer intramuscularly 15 minutes before slow IV injection of the opioid.
- Administration of an anticholinergic intramuscularly, followed 15 minutes later by slow IV administration of the tranquilizer–opioid mixture. If diazepam is selected as the tranquilizing agent, the opioid should be given first, followed 1 to 2 minutes later by diazepam because if diazepam is given before the opioid has taken effect, excitement may be seen. In young dogs, acepromazine offers more reliable sedation than diazepam and can be given at the same time as the opioid.
- Alternating small doses of hydromorphone or fentanyl and midazolam or diazepam by slow IV injection until the animal is adequately anesthetized.

- IM administration of the tranquilizer–opioid mixture. If using diazepam, two syringes are used because these drugs cannot be mixed together.

When the procedure is over, the opioid in neuroleptanalgesic combinations can be reversed with naloxone. However, the tranquilizer component may or may not be reversible depending on whether or not a specific antagonist is available. A detailed discussion of opioid reversal follows.

> **TECHNICIAN NOTE** Neuroleptanalgesics must be administered slowly intravenously because if they are rapidly injected, CNS stimulation may occur. The anesthetist must also be prepared to intubate and ventilate the patient if necessary because respiratory depression may be profound.

Opioid Antagonists

One distinct advantage of using opioids is their reversibility, which allows undesirable effects to be antagonized in situations in which the patient is in danger and allows the anesthetist to "wake" or partially wake the patient after sedation with these agents. The opioid antagonist naloxone hydrochloride is commonly used to reverse the CNS and respiratory depression caused by administration of opioid agonists, partial agonists, or agonist–antagonists. It is administered by IM or slow IV injection and can be used in dogs, cats, horses, and exotic mammals. Although not used in domestic animals, naltrexone is a longer-lasting antagonist that is used in wild animals to reverse the effects of ultrapotent opioids such as etorphine and thiafentanil.

Agonist–antagonists such as butorphanol can also be used to partially reverse the effects of pure agonists. Realize that opioid antagonists are effective in reversing opioid agents only and cannot be used to reverse the effects of phenothiazines, benzodiazepines, or other nonopioid agents.

Mode of action and pharmacology. Although as with many other anesthetics and adjuncts, the exact mechanism of action of naloxone is not known, it is believed to bind competitively to the mu, kappa, and sigma receptors. Naloxone acts within 2 minutes of IV administration and 5 minutes of IM administration; it has a duration of action of 30 to 60 minutes and in some cases, may last longer.

Effects and adverse effects. The primary effect of naloxone is reversal of both the desirable and undesirable effects of an opioid agonist, partial agonist, or agonist–antagonist, which include sedation, dysphoria, panting, respiratory depression, hypotension, bradycardia, GI effects, and analgesia. The action of opioid antagonists is often dramatic, causing the patient to appear nearly unaffected shortly after administration. The respiratory depression caused by buprenorphine may be unresponsive, however, because this agent binds tightly to the mu receptors and is not easily displaced.

Adverse effects are rare at clinical doses, although sudden loss of analgesic effects resulting from routine use may precipitate excitement, anxiety, and SNS stimulation, resulting in tachycardia and cardiac arrhythmias. Total reversal of analgesia can be avoided by using an agonist–antagonist such as butorphanol that has some analgesic effect.

> **TECHNICIAN NOTE** Opioid antagonists should be administered by IM or slow IV injection. They reverse both the desirable and undesirable effects of an agonist, partial agonist, or agonist–antagonist, including sedation and analgesia. The action of opioid antagonists is often dramatic, causing the patient to appear nearly unaffected shortly after administration.

Use of opioid antagonists. Reversal of opioid effects through the use of an antagonist is not necessary for routine anesthesia. However, the technique is extremely useful in emergencies, after an overdose, or to reverse opioid effects after neuroleptanalgesia for nonpainful procedures. Ideally, the dose should be titrated based on the length of time that has passed since the agonist was given. For instance, if a significant length of time has passed since administration of the agonist, the attending veterinarian may choose to administer a lower dose initially and give additional doses if needed based on patient response. Opioid antagonists are also helpful in reviving neonates delivered by C-section if the dam was given opioids. One drop of naloxone placed under the tongue of each puppy or kitten is usually sufficient to reverse the respiratory depression caused by fentanyl, morphine, or other opioid agonists.

In cases where the duration of action of the drug being reversed is longer than the duration of action of naloxone, signs of CNS or respiratory depression recur (a phenomenon referred to as *renarcotization*). In these cases, additional doses may be needed.

Antiemetics
Maropitant

Maropitant is an antiemetic intended for the prevention and treatment of acute vomiting in dogs and cats, and prevention of vomiting associated with motion sickness in dogs. It is also commonly used as a preanesthetic medication and has been shown to improve patient outcomes in several important ways that will be detailed in the following paragraphs. In fact, some experts suggest including maropitant as a part of preanesthetic protocols for patients over 4 months of age undergoing both routine and nonroutine anesthetic procedures.

Mode of Action and Pharmacology. Maropitant is classified as a neurokinin-1 (NK_1) receptor antagonist that suppresses both centrally mediated vomiting (i.e., vomiting due to stimulation of the vomiting center in the brain) and peripherally mediated vomiting (i.e., vomiting due to input from the vestibular system and other peripheral nerves) by inhibiting action of a neurotransmitter called Substance P on the NK_1 receptor. In addition to its antiemetic effect, there is evidence that maropitant reduces visceral pain in dogs associated with stimulation of the NK_1 receptor by substance P. It reaches peak blood levels less than 1 hour after SC administration or 2 hours after oral administration and has a relatively long duration of action in dogs and cats.

Effects and Adverse Effects. The usefulness of maropitant as a preanesthetic drug is based on its ability to decrease the risk of complications related to perioperative vomiting and aspiration as well as a number of other desirable effects. It has been shown to significantly decrease the incidence of vomiting and nausea associated with administration of some commonly used anesthetic and analgesic drugs including the opioid agonists morphine and hydromorphone and the alpha$_2$ adrenergic agonist dexmedetomidine. This reduction of vomiting in turn prevents increases in intracranial and intraocular pressure that are often associated with the act of vomiting. It also has been shown to reduce inhalant anesthetic requirements, improve the quality of anesthetic recoveries (as evidenced by decreased random movements, vocalization, and panting in dogs), and promote faster return to normal eating postoperatively.

> **TECHNICIAN NOTE** Maropitant is an antiemetic, commonly administered by SC injection during the preanesthetic period to reduce nausea and vomiting and improve patient outcomes. The injectable form of the drug should be refrigerated before use as this has been observed to reduce pain associated with subcutaneous injection.

A common adverse effect of maropitant is significant pain and vocalization after SC injection. If given IV, it has also been shown to lower blood pressure in animals under inhalant anesthesia, especially if premedicated with acepromazine. Although maropitant is well tolerated by most patients, other, less common adverse effects include lethargy, anorexia, hypersalivation, and allergic reactions.

Maropitant is contraindicated in patients with GI obstruction and toxin ingestion, and caution should be used when administering it to patients with liver dysfunction as it is metabolized and eliminated primarily by the liver.

Use of Maropitant. When using maropitant as a preanesthetic medication, it may be given orally at home by the owner or by injection in the hospital on the day of the procedure. The injectable solution is typically given subcutaneously at a dose of 1 mg/kg (for both dogs and cats) approximately 45 minutes to 1 hour before giving any agents that are known to induce vomiting (such as opioid agonists and alpha$_2$ agonists). The injectable form of the drug should be refrigerated beforehand as this has been observed to reduce the pain associated with injection. If given IV, the drug should be administered slowly over 1 to 2 minutes (typically at a dose of 1 mg/kg for both dogs and cats). As an alternative, the tablet form (licensed for use in dogs) can be sent home with the client. Typically, it is administered at a dose of 2 mg/kg approximately 2 to 3 hours before leaving for the hospital or the night before the procedure. The tablet form has been used off-label in cats, with a recommended dose of 1–2 mg/kg.

Skin contact with injectable maropitant may result in an allergic reaction and sensitivity in some people, so skin exposed to the drug should be washed with soap and water.

INJECTABLE ANESTHETICS, DISSOCIATIVES, AND ADJUNCTS

Injectable anesthetics are drugs characterized by their ability to produce unconsciousness when given alone. They do not necessarily provide all the effects of general anesthesia (such as analgesia and muscle relaxation), however. Consequently these drugs must be used with other agents to produce the complete spectrum of effects of general anesthesia.

Injectable anesthetic agents include propofol, alfaxalone, etomidate, and barbiturates, each of which is used to induce anesthesia. Through use of repeat boluses, or a constant rate infusion (CRI), propofol and alfaxalone can also be used to maintain general anesthesia. Propofol, alfaxalone, and etomidate are used only in small animals, small ruminants, and neonates of any species, but not in adult large animals because of the high expense of these agents. The ultrashort-acting injectable barbiturate anesthetics are no longer used in general practice in the United States owing to changes in anesthetic practice and limited availability.

Although they do not produce unconsciousness when given alone, dissociative agents are included in this discussion of injectable anesthetics because they are frequently used in combination with tranquilizers, opioids, and other injectable agents to produce general anesthesia.

With few exceptions, these agents are administered by IV injection to effect, instead of giving the entire calculated dose at once. "To effect" means that the drug is given in small boluses until the desired level of anesthesia is reached. More about this technique can be found in Chapter 9.

Propofol

Propofol is a short-acting injectable anesthetic with a wide margin of safety that is given intravenously for induction and short-term maintenance of general anesthesia in small animals, small ruminants, exotic animals, and neonates of any domestic species. The DEA proposed placing propofol in Schedule IV of the Controlled Substances Act in October 2010. It has remained uncontrolled at the federal level at the time of writing, although it is controlled at the state level in some states including Georgia, Alabama, and North Dakota. Even in states where it is not controlled, some clinics and institutions elect to treat propofol as a controlled substance and consequently observe the record-keeping requirements of other controlled drugs. Since its introduction to the veterinary market several decades ago, its popularity has gradually increased and, for some time, it has been the most commonly used short-acting injectable agent in small animals for brief procedures or for anesthetic induction before intubation and maintenance with inhalant agents.

Propofol is also administered as an IV bolus followed by a CRI to treat status epilepticus in dogs and cats that do not respond to midazolam or diazepam and phenobarbital.

Mode of Action and Pharmacology

Propofol has a chemical structure unlike that of other anesthetic or preanesthetic agents. It is minimally water soluble and may be formulated either as a macroemulsion or a microemulsion (Box 3.3). The propofol macroemulsion contains propofol at a concentration of 10 mg/mL as well as egg lecithin, glycerin, and soybean oil. It has a milky appearance but is given by the IV route and consequently is the sole exception to the general rule that milky liquids should never be given intravenously. In contrast, the propofol microemulsion contains no lipids and is clear in appearance.

Although the mode of action is not completely understood, propofol appears to augment action of the inhibitory neurotransmitter GABA in a similar manner to other hypnotics. Propofol has a rapid onset because it is highly fat soluble. Propofol is rapidly taken up by vessel-rich tissues such as the brain, heart, liver, and kidneys but is very quickly redistributed to muscle and fat and is subsequently rapidly metabolized. This accounts for the rapid recovery and minimal residual sedative effects seen even after repeated injections.

Propofol has an onset of action of about 30 to 60 seconds as well as a duration of action of 5 to 10 minutes after a single bolus, with complete recovery in 20 minutes (dogs) and 30 minutes (cats). Because metabolism is rapid, propofol is relatively safe and effective in animals with liver or kidney disease.

Effects and Adverse Effects Involving Major Organ Systems

Central nervous system

- Propofol produces a dose-dependent CNS depression ranging from sedation to general anesthesia. Subanesthetic doses produce sedation and lack of awareness of surroundings. Anesthetic doses produce unconsciousness and muscle relaxation. Propofol is not an analgesic.
- Transient excitement and muscle tremors are seen occasionally during induction, especially if injection is slow or the animal has not been premedicated. Paddling, muscle twitching, nystagmus, and opisthotonus (hyperextended head and front legs) can occur and may resemble seizures. This response usually resolves on its own and can be treated with the muscle relaxants midazolam or diazepam if it is severe or if it persists.

Cardiovascular system

- Propofol is a cardiac depressant, producing bradycardia, decreased cardiac output, decreased vascular resistance, and, as a result, transient hypotension.
- Hypotension is often of short duration in animals with normal cardiovascular function, but in some patients, it may be significant and prolonged, especially if the patient is premedicated.

For this reason, propofol should be given cautiously to animals with preexisting hypotension such as patients in shock or those that have blood loss or dehydration.

Respiratory system

- Propofol is a potent respiratory depressant. High doses or rapid injection may cause significant respiratory depression, including apnea. To lessen the respiratory depression associated with the use of propofol, the anesthetist should give the initial bolus gradually over 1 to 2 minutes, carefully titrate the dose to effect, and monitor respiratory rate and depth carefully during the first few minutes after injection.
- Prolonged apnea, decreased oxygen saturation, or cyanosis. If apnea lasts more than 1 minute or if pulse oximetry shows oxygen saturation to be less than 95%, the patient should be intubated and ventilated. The best approach is prevention of hypoxemia by delivering oxygen to the patient (by facemask) for 3 to 5 minutes (so that the patient's lungs will be filled with oxygen rather than air) before inducing anesthesia with propofol.

Other Effects and Adverse Effects

- Some dogs may exhibit muscle twitching during induction. This reaction should not be interpreted as an indicator of inadequate anesthetic depth.
- Good muscle relaxation.
- Antiemetic effect.
- Decreased intracranial and intraocular pressure. This makes propofol a good choice for animals with head trauma and other CNS disorders that involve increased intracranial pressure as well as ocular disorders that involve increased intraocular pressure as long as hypoventilation is avoided.
- Based on experience in people, propofol is known to cause pain on IV injection but does not produce the tissue damage after perivascular injection seen with some other drugs, including barbiturates.
- When given repeat doses or a prolonged CRI, cats can develop Heinz bodies, lethargy, diarrhea, and anorexia, and can experience slow recoveries.
- Individuals of some breeds, including sighthounds, may have prolonged recovery if maintained with propofol for longer than 30 minutes.

TECHNICIAN NOTE Major effects and adverse effects of propofol are as follows:
- CNS depression ranging from sedation to general anesthesia
- Transient excitement, muscle tremors, and seizurelike activity during induction
- Bradycardia, decreased cardiac output, and hypotension that can be significant and prolonged in some patients
- Respiratory depression including apnea, especially after rapid injection or high doses
- Prolonged apnea, decreased oxygen saturation, and cyanosis
- Muscle relaxation
- Antiemetic effect
- Decreased intracranial and intraocular pressure
- Pain on IV injection

Use of Propofol

Propofol should be given slowly intravenously over a period of 1 to 2 minutes until the desired anesthetic depth is reached (see Case Presentations 3.1 and 3.2). IM injection may cause mild sedation and ataxia but does not induce anesthesia because the drug is metabolized too rapidly.

One effective induction method is to give one-quarter of the calculated dose slowly intravenously every 30 seconds until the desired plane of anesthesia is reached. The dose of propofol needed for a patient and the duration of anesthesia depend on the type of premedication used. Do not give propofol too slowly, however, because this can cause paradoxical excitement, making the patient difficult to handle. Propofol is highly protein bound and therefore should be used with caution in patients with significant hypoproteinemia.

Propofol boluses can be given repeatedly every 3 to 5 minutes or as required to maintain anesthesia in dogs and cats up to 20 minutes. Alternatively, propofol can be delivered by CRI. In this procedure, a low dose of propofol (0.1 to 0.4 mg/kg/min) is continuously administered to the patient with a syringe pump (Fig. 3.7) or through an IV line. This method allows the anesthetist to control the depth of anesthesia precisely at a stable plane for up to several hours. Intubation and oxygen administration are advisable for patients unless the period of anesthesia is anticipated to be very brief.

In dogs, recovery from propofol anesthesia is rapid and smooth, even after multiple injections. Because of the rapid recovery seen with this agent, it is useful for patients that need to be released immediately after surgery. Dogs that have received propofol may appear completely recovered within 20 minutes of the final dose. Cats recover within about 30 minutes after a single injection but may experience longer recoveries after multiple injections because they metabolize propofol more slowly.

Administration of tranquilizers decreases the dose of propofol required by as much as 75% and facilitates IV injection in fractious animals. Some premedications, however, may prolong recovery time.

A mixture consisting of propofol and either ketamine or midazolam is used by some clinicians as an alternative to plain

---

CASE PRESENTATION 3.1   Giving an Injectable IV Anesthetic Too Rapidly

Petunia, a 2-year-old, 5 kg, intact female domestic shorthair (DSH) cat was scheduled to be anesthetized. The patient was premedicated with 0.05 mg of hydromorphone per kilogram of body weight by IM injection. Propofol was prepared for induction at a dose of 5 mg/kg, and 25 mg (2.5 mL) was drawn into a syringe. The anesthetist was familiar with anesthetic induction using a combination of midazolam and ketamine intravenously but not propofol, and was used to administering the entire calculated dose quickly. Based on this experience, after approximately 15 min, the anesthetist commenced anesthetic induction by injecting the entire dose of propofol over about 30 s. The patient immediately became unconscious, hypotensive, and apneic. Heart sounds were nearly inaudible. At this point, the anesthetist became concerned and summoned the attending veterinarian. The patient was quickly assessed and was determined to be in a deep level of anesthesia but stable. The patient was immediately intubated, and manual intermittent positive-pressure ventilation was initiated at a rate of approximately one breath every 15 s. The patient remained stable and gradually, over the next 5 min, began to exhibit spontaneous respiratory movements which,

although weak at first, gradually became stronger and more frequent. The rate of manual ventilation was decreased gradually, and after 15–20 min, spontaneous respirations were adequate to allow the patient to breathe on her own.

This case illustrates the importance of using an appropriate injection rate when inducing patients with short-acting IV anesthetics. If these agents are given too quickly, the patient will experience adverse effects, which in the case of propofol include respiratory and cardiovascular depression, apnea, and hypotension. Depending on how much is given, the level of anesthesia may become dangerously deep. For this reason, this agent must be given to effect and must be given slowly in small boluses while the patient is monitored between boluses for signs of readiness for intubation. When short-acting agents are given, a balance must be struck between injecting the drug slowly enough to minimize apnea and other adverse effects but rapidly enough to bring the patient into a plane of anesthesia sufficient to allow intubation. For these reasons, great care must be given to proper injection technique when these agents are used.

CASE PRESENTATION 3.2   Giving an Injectable IV Anesthetic Too Slowly

Snoopy, a 1.5-year-old, 15 kg male Beagle mix was scheduled to be anesthetized. The patient was premedicated with 0.05 mg of acepromazine per kilogram of body weight by IM injection. Propofol was prepared for induction at a dose of 5 mg/kg, and 75 mg (7.5 mL) was drawn into a syringe. After approximately 15 min, the anesthetist commenced anesthetic induction. She first injected 3 consecutive 1.0 mL boluses (a total volume of 3.0 mL) over 3 min in an attempt to bring the patient into a state of readiness for intubation. During this time, the patient was unconscious but exhibited muscle tremors, weak spontaneous movements, and swallowing motions. Although the anesthetist continued to inject additional boluses of 0.5 to 1 mL every few minutes, the patient continued to remain at an anesthetic depth inadequate to allow intubation.

The attending veterinarian was summoned. She saw no evidence that the drug had been given perivascularly and proceeded to determine why this patient had not reached surgical anesthesia. After assessing the situation, she determined that the patient was in no danger and that the induction agent was simply given too slowly.

She suggested that the anesthetist increase the rate of administration. Within 90 s at the increased rate, the patient was at an adequate depth to be intubated. The anesthetic procedure was completed with no further complications.

This case also illustrates the importance of using an appropriate injection rate when inducing patients with short-acting IV anesthetics but for a different reason than in the previous case. When giving these agents, emphasis is often placed on avoiding rapid injection and overdose, but it is equally important to avoid giving the drug too slowly. If the agent is given too slowly, the patient will remain at an inadequate anesthetic depth. This is very frustrating for the anesthetist and may lead to adverse effects from delayed intubation, epinephrine release, and other issues. Even though these drugs must be given slowly to effect to minimize apnea and other adverse effects, they must be given rapidly enough to produce a depth of anesthesia adequate for intubation within a reasonable period of time. Thus as in the previous case, a balance must be achieved that results in a smooth and safe induction.

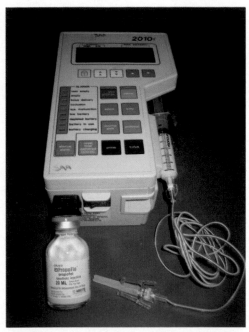

FIG. 3.7 This syringe pump (also known as a *syringe driver*) is set up to administer a constant rate infusion (CRI) of propofol from a 5 mL syringe. The syringe is attached to microbore tubing that has been preloaded with propofol.

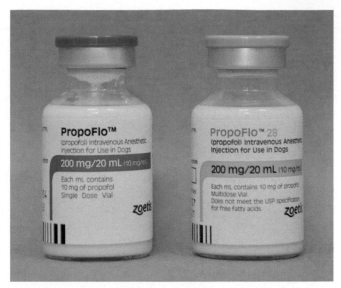

FIG. 3.8 PropoFlo—left side; PropoFlo 28—right side. (Courtesy Zoetis; https://www.zoetis.com.)

propofol to induce general anesthesia. These combinations reduce the dose of each drug needed, which can lessen adverse effects such as propofol-induced hypotension and ketamine-induced muscle rigidity in the case of ketamine and propofol (a mixture often referred to as "ketofol"). Ketofol is prepared by mixing 2 mg/kg of ketamine and 2 mg/kg of propofol in the same syringe. Like propofol, the combination is then administered to effect.

Handling and Storage

Propofol macroemulsion (Fig. 3.8) should be shaken thoroughly before use. Although generally stable, it should not be used if the liquid appears separated, if large droplets or particles are visible, or if discolored.

One significant disadvantage of propofol macroemulsion is the poor storage characteristics of this agent. Because the product contains soybean oil, egg lecithin, and glycerol, it will support bacterial growth unless formulated with a preservative. Unopened, the shelf life is approximately 3 years. Ampules and bottles should be handled in a strictly aseptic manner and, once they have been opened, the manufacturer recommends that unused product be discarded within 6 hours of opening to avoid contamination, although some authorities suggest that unused propofol can be stored for up to 24 hours provided that sterile technique is used for opening, dispensing, and storing the product. Unfortunately, detailed studies on the storage characteristics of propofol have not been published, but the incidence of infection from contaminated drug appears to be low.

PropoFlo 28 (Zoetis) (see Fig. 3.8—right side) is a macroemulsion that contains benzyl alcohol as a preservative, which is labeled for use in dogs only due to the possibility of benzyl

alcohol toxicity in cats. Providing that strict aseptic technique is observed when drawing up this drug, the contents can be stored at room temperature for 28 days after opening. According to the AAFP Feline Anesthesia Guidelines (based on results of studies), propofol containing 2% benzyl alcohol is safe and appropriate for induction of anesthesia in cats but should not be used as an infusion due to the potential for accumulation of benzyl alcohol.

> **TECHNICIAN NOTE** Propofol should be handled in a strictly aseptic manner. The manufacturer recommends that unused propofol macroemulsion that contains no preservative should be discarded within 6 hours of opening to avoid contamination. Unused portions of PropoFlo 28 can be stored at room temperature for up to 28 days after opening.

Alfaxalone

Alfaxalone is a controlled, short-acting injectable anesthetic with a wide margin of safety that is very similar in many ways to propofol (see Table 3.7 for a comparison of these two drugs). Alfaxalone has been available for many years in the United Kingdom, Australia, and New Zealand, as well as a number of other countries. As of August 2012, it was approved for distribution in the United States under the trade name Alfaxan (Jurox Inc.). This product, which had a shelf-life of 6 hours after first puncture of the vial, was replaced in 2018 by Alfaxan Multidose, a product with a longer shelf life due to the addition of preservatives.

Alfaxan Multidose is labeled for IV induction of anesthesia in dogs and cats and can be used to maintain anesthesia for at least 1 hour by administration of repeat boluses or CRI. In addition, it can also be given to cats by the IM route (of-label) to produce deep sedation or light anesthesia. Alfaxalone is a Schedule IV controlled substance in the United States.

TABLE 3.7 Comparison of Propofol and Alfaxalone

Characteristic	Propofol	Alfaxalone
Drug class	Phenol derivative	Neuroactive steroid
Mode of action	Binding to GABA receptors	Same
Compatibility with other drugs	Should not be mixed with other agents (according to label). Some extralabel protocols involve mixing with other agents, including ketamine	Should not be mixed with other agents (according to label).
Appearance	Milky (macroemulsion)	Clear and colorless
Route of administration for anesthesia	IV	IV
IV administration	Over 1–2 min-to effect	Same
Speed and quality of IV induction	Intubation in 1–2 min. May cause pain on injection, muscle twitching, rigidity of limbs, opisthotonos	Intubation in 1–2 min. Smooth, rapid induction. No pain on injection.
Duration of action and quality of recovery following single dose	Dog: 5–10 min following single dose/Cat: 5–10 min following single dose Generally rapid and smooth	Dog: 5–10 min following single dose/Cat: 15–30 min following single dose Excitement may occur, with agitation, muscle fasciculations, paddling, and sensitivity to external stimuli.
Use for anesthetic maintenance	IV repeat injections/CRI (up to 20 min or longer). Note that longer periods of maintenance or administration over consecutive days may be associated with slow recovery and significant adverse effects in cats.	IV repeat injections/CRI for 1 h or more or over consecutive days typically well tolerated.
Use as a sedative	Possible but not used clinically this way	Possible but not practical in medium to large dogs due to volume required/Given IM or SC for sedation of cats (extralabel)
Hypotension	Dose dependent—may be significant	Usually mild at clinical doses.
Respiratory depression	Significant (dependent on dose and speed of injection)	Significant but slightly less than propofol
Storage after vial puncture	6 h (PropoFlo)/28 days after vial puncture (Propoflo28)	28 days after vial puncture (Alfaxan Multidose)/56 days after vial puncture (Alfaxan Multidose IDX)
Approved for use	Dogs only	Dogs and cats *(Indexed for use in minor species)*
Controlled status	Not by the DEA at time of writing	Class IV in United States

CRI, Constant rate infusion; *GABA,* gamma-aminobutyric acid; *IM,* intramuscular; *IV,* intravenous; *SC,* subcutaneous.

This agent was originally marketed in the 1970s but was ultimately taken off the market in most countries because of adverse effects caused by the solubilizing agent in the formulation. The currently available formulation contains a different solubilizing agent that does not cause these undesirable effects.

Mode of Action and Pharmacology

Alfaxalone is a steroid molecule with anesthetic properties that appears to work in a similar manner to other hypnotics such as propofol and etomidate by binding to GABA receptors. Like propofol, it is rapidly metabolized and consequently is noncumulative.

> **TECHNICIAN NOTE** Major effects and adverse effects of alfaxalone are as follows:
> - CNS depression ranging from sedation to general anesthesia
> - Minimal cardiovascular depression at clinical doses, which may become severe in the event of rapid administration or overdose
> - Tachycardia
> - Hypotension, especially when used with inhalant anesthetics
> - Respiratory depression including apnea, especially after rapid injection or high doses
> - Muscle relaxation
> - Excitement may occur during recovery

Effects and Adverse Effects

Alfaxalone produces similar effects to propofol, including dose-dependent CNS depression; respiratory depression including apnea; hypotension, especially if used with inhalant anesthetics; and muscle relaxation. It is not an analgesic. Unlike propofol, cardiovascular system depression is minimal at clinical doses and in some circumstances, the heart rate may increase. However, overdosages or rapid IV injection can cause severe cardiorespiratory depression. Inductions are usually smooth, with no excitement, muscle twitching, or pain on IV injection. Inadvertent perivascular injection does not result in tissue irritation.

Use of Alfaxalone

Alfaxalone is given in a similar way to propofol. Rapid injection is more likely to cause apnea and vasodilation, so IV injection should be slow, with one-quarter of the calculated dose given every 15 seconds to effect. Owing to the risk of respiratory depression, the patient should be intubated and oxygen should be administered after induction. The duration of action is about 5 to 10 minutes in dogs and 15 to 30 minutes in cats after a single injection but may be longer when preanesthetic medications are used. General anesthesia may be maintained with repeat boluses to effect every 3 to 8 minutes, although the amount needed and frequency of administration for each case is influenced by the species, preanesthetic medications used, and a number of other factors. Excitement may occur during recovery (which can include disorientation, paddling, muscle twitching, and violent movements), so the patient should be monitored and should not be disturbed during that time.

The manufacturer states that alfaxalone should not be mixed with other injectable anesthetics prior to administration. Alfaxan Multidose contains three preservatives (ethanol, benzethonium chloride, and chlorocresol) and, like PropoFlo 28, may be stored at room temperature for 28 days following vial puncture.

A closely related product, Alfaxan Multidose IDX, was added to the FDA Index of Legally Marketed Unapproved New Animal Drugs for Minor Species, in February, 2020 (see https://www.fda.gov/animal-veterinary/minor-useminor-species/index-legally-marketed-unapproved-new-animal-drugs-minor-species). The FDA Index is a list of new animal drugs intended for use in species other than dogs, cats, horses, cattle, pigs, chickens, and turkeys which have gone through an alternative FDA review process to affirm safety and effectiveness for specific indications. Through this process, Alfaxan Multidose IDX is "indexed" and therefore can be marketed and sold for sedation, anesthesia, and/or immobilization of over 50 nonfood-producing minor species, including various reptiles, fish, birds, nonhuman primates, chinchillas, and ferrets. According to the manufacturer, Alfaxan Multidose IDX can be used for 56 days following initial vial puncture.

Etomidate

Etomidate is a noncontrolled, sedative–hypnotic imidazole drug that is occasionally used for induction of anesthesia in dogs, cats, and exotics. Because of its minimal effect on the cardiovascular and respiratory systems, etomidate is very useful in high-risk patients. However, it is not routinely used owing to its high cost and significant adverse effects, including pain on IV injection, nausea, and vomiting. This short-acting drug has a wide margin of safety, is noncumulative, and has a duration of action that is about 3 to 5 minutes but that is somewhat dependent on the dose.

Mode of Action and Pharmacology

Although the mode of action of etomidate is not completely understood, it appears to affect GABA receptors in a similar manner to propofol and alfaxalone. The duration of effect is short because, like propofol, the drug is redistributed away from the brain and rapidly metabolized.

TECHNICIAN NOTE Major effects and adverse effects of etomidate are as follows:
- Hypnosis with minimal analgesia
- Anticonvulsant effect
- Minimal effect on cardiopulmonary function
- Good muscle relaxation
- Myoclonus during induction and recovery
- Pain after IV injection
- Hemolysis in cats after rapid injection
- Decreased cortisol levels
- Nausea, vomiting, and excitement during induction and recovery

---

Effects and Adverse Effects Involving Major Organ Systems

Central nervous system
- Anesthesia with etomidate is characterized by hypnosis but little analgesia. The drug decreases brain oxygen consumption, maintains brain perfusion better than most other injectable agents, and has anticonvulsant properties. It is therefore a good choice for patients with brain trauma or those undergoing brain or spinal surgery.

Cardiovascular system
- After a brief period of hypotension, etomidate has little effect on heart rate, rhythm, blood pressure, and cardiac output. It is therefore the induction agent of choice for animals with moderate to severe heart disease or shock.

Respiratory system
- This drug minimally affects respiratory rate and tidal volume; however, a brief period of apnea may be seen after induction. Although it crosses the placental barrier, it is rapidly eliminated and causes little neonatal respiratory depression and so is a good choice for (C-section).

Other Effects and Adverse Effects
- Etomidate produces good muscle relaxation, but myoclonus (spontaneous muscle twitching) may occur during induction and recovery.
- IV injection is reported to be painful and may produce phlebitis, particularly if given in a small vein. Some authors recommend administration through a running IV fluid line to decrease pain. Perivascular injection may be associated with the development of sterile abscesses.
- Rapid injection of etomidate may cause RBC hemolysis in cats due to the propylene glycol vehicle. This is clinically insignificant unless the cat has an extremely low hematocrit or the drug is given repeatedly.
- Adrenal cortical function may be depressed for several hours after etomidate administration, decreasing levels of cortisol (a natural cortisone-like hormone). This is not harmful unless the drug is given for several hours or repeated over several days. For this reason, CRI is not recommended for sedation or anesthesia of patients with serious illnesses.
- Nausea, vomiting, and involuntary excitement may occur during induction or recovery, particularly in patients that have not been adequately premedicated.
- This agent should be used cautiously for eye surgery patients due to miosis, eye movements, and increases in intraocular pressure that may occur, and is undesirable in patients with glaucoma or corneal injury.

Use of Etomidate

Etomidate is administered only by the IV route. As with other induction agents, it is given to effect, starting with one-quarter to one-half of the calculated dose, depending on how rapid an induction is desired. Adverse effects including vomiting and muscle twitching are minimized by premedication with an opioid, midazolam or diazepam (0.5 mg/kg of midazolam or diazepam given intravenously 30 seconds before etomidate). Some authors also recommend premedication with dexamethasone to counteract suppression of the adrenal gland.

Like propofol, etomidate can be administered in repeated boluses for short-term maintenance of anesthesia.

Barbiturates

The barbiturates are a large class of controlled drugs developed during the 1930s through the 1950s, some of which were commonly used general anesthetics for many decades because of their low cost, ease of use, and relative safety for healthy animals. Now, they are rarely used because of the development of newer injectable agents such as the short-acting injectable nonbarbiturate anesthetic propofol and inhalant agents such as isoflurane and sevoflurane, and because the ultrashort-acting injectable barbiturate anesthetics such as thiopental sodium and methohexital have become unavailable or difficult to obtain. Despite this decline in use for general anesthesia in small- and large-animal practice, a few barbiturates are still used for specific indications, including the short-acting agent pentobarbital sodium and the long-acting agent phenobarbital. Specifically, pentobarbital sodium is used as a euthanasia agent, as a general anesthetic for small laboratory animals, and for treatment of intractable seizures; phenobarbital is used primarily to control seizures; to treat intractable seizures in dogs, cats, and horses; and occasionally as a sedative in dogs and cats.

> **TECHNICIAN NOTE** Uses for barbiturates are as follows:
> - The short-acting barbiturate pentobarbital is used to induce and maintain general anesthesia in laboratory animals and to treat status epilepticus in small animals.
> - The long-acting barbiturate phenobarbital is used as a sedative and anticonvulsant.

Dissociative Anesthetics

In the late 1950s, the introduction of the injectable anesthetic phencyclidine made available a new class of injectable anesthetic drugs called the *dissociative anesthetics*. Although phencyclidine is not used in veterinary medicine because of its abuse potential, its derivative, ketamine hydrochloride, can be used alone to induce dissociative anesthesia in cats for minor procedures. It is commonly used in combination with a variety of tranquilizers and opioids to induce general anesthesia in a wide variety of species, and it is given in subanesthetic doses by CRI to provide analgesia. Tiletamine hydrochloride, another dissociative agent, is combined with the benzodiazepine zolazepam in a proprietary product called Telazol (Zoetis)—other names of this combination include Zoletil (Virbac) and Tilzolan (Dechra). This product is administered intravenously or intramuscularly, alone or in combination with other agents, to produce sedation and anesthesia. Both ketamine and Telazol are class III controlled drugs.

Mode of Action and Pharmacology

The mechanism of action of the dissociative anesthetics is complex. Unlike most general anesthetics, which cause general CNS depression, dissociative anesthetics cause disruption of nerve transmission in some parts of the brain and selective stimulation in others. Dissociative agents also inhibit NMDA

(*N*-methyl-D-aspartate) receptors in the CNS that are responsible for "windup." Windup is an exaggerated response to low-intensity pain stimuli that results in worsening of postoperative pain. This NMDA inhibition is believed to be responsible for the analgesic effects and many of the other primary effects of these drugs (see Chapter 8).

The unusual combination of actions result in a distinctive trancelike state termed *dissociative anesthesia* (so called because it dissociates various regions of the brain), in which the animal appears awake but is immobile and unaware of its surroundings (Fig. 3.9). Dissociative anesthesia is described in the section on effects on the CNS. The effects of dissociative agents on the cardiovascular and pulmonary systems are also unique and different than effects produced by most other anesthetic agents.

The peak action of ketamine occurs about 1 to 2 minutes after IV injection and about 10 minutes after IM injection. The duration of effect is about 20 to 30 minutes. A higher dose increases duration but does not increase the anesthetic effect. Dissociatives are redistributed and metabolized by the liver; they may also be excreted unchanged in the urine and so should be used cautiously in patients with liver or kidney disease. As with propofol, redistribution is largely responsible for the initial decrease in effect.

> **TECHNICIAN NOTE** Major effects and adverse effects of dissociatives are as follows:
> - Cataleptoid state
> - Intact reflexes
> - Eyes open, pupils central and dilated
> - Normal or increased muscle tone
> - Analgesia (primarily somatic)
> - Sensitivity to sound, light, or other sensory stimuli, seizurelike activity, or bizarre behavior, especially during recovery
> - Nystagmus
> - Increased heart rate, cardiac output, and mean arterial pressure (MAP) secondary to SNS stimulation
> - Decreased inotropy
> - Apneustic respiration at higher doses
> - Increased salivary and respiratory tract secretions
> - Pain after IM injection

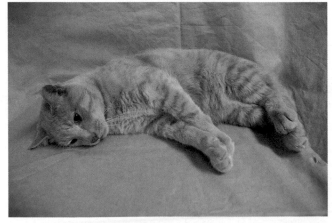

FIG. 3.9 A cat under dissociative anesthesia. Note the central dilated pupils, open eyes, and muscle rigidity. The patient appears awake but unaware of its surroundings.

Effects and Adverse Effects Involving Major Organ Systems

Central nervous system. The primary effect on the CNS is dissociative anesthesia. Dissociatives do not induce Stage III anesthesia. Characteristics of dissociative anesthesia include the following:

- Cataleptoid state. Catalepsy is a state in which a patient does not respond to external stimuli and has muscle rigidity in which the limbs will remain in the position in which they are placed. In humans, this state may be drug induced or may occur with conditions such as schizophrenia and epilepsy. A cataleptoid state (the suffix *-oid* means "like") is similar to catalepsy but with a variable degree of muscle rigidity.

- *Intact reflexes.* Palpebral, corneal, and pedal reflexes, PLR, and laryngeal and swallowing reflexes remain intact. Because reflex activity is preserved even at moderate anesthetic depth, it may be difficult to determine anesthetic depth in patients under dissociative anesthesia. Anesthetic depth in patients that show signs of purposeful movement is likely inadequate, whereas in those with very depressed respiration, it is likely excessive. When using these agents, the anesthetist may find it challenging to determine where an individual patient lies between these two extremes.

- *Ocular effects.* Unlike conventional anesthesia, dissociative anesthesia does not usually result in partial closure of the eyelids or eyeball rotation. The eye normally remains fully open, with a central and dilated pupil. Ophthalmic lubricant should be applied every 2 to 3 hours to prevent corneal drying.

- *Normal or increased muscle tone.* In some animals, muscle tone is retained, whereas in others, it is increased almost to the point of rigidity. The animal may assume a stiff posture, with outstretched front limbs and extended neck. During recovery or light anesthesia, spontaneous, random movements of the head and neck may be seen. This is in marked contrast to the muscle relaxation that is seen with most other anesthetics. The concurrent use of a tranquilizing agent such as midazolam, diazepam, acepromazine, dexmedetomidine, or xylazine helps prevent excessive muscle rigidity, improves ease of intubation, and produces a state more characteristic of general anesthesia.

- *Analgesia.* Because of inhibition of the NMDA receptor, dissociative agents provide significant analgesia to the skin and limbs (somatic analgesia) but limited visceral analgesia (that is, involving the organs). A patient given a dissociative anesthetic may be able to perceive pain but is unable to respond to it. It is the veterinarian's obligation to ensure that pain is not perceived through the use of supplementary anesthetic agents and/or analgesics.

- *Amnesia.* Human patients anesthetized with dissociative agents do not recall the procedure afterward, even though they do not appear unconscious at the time.

- *Sensitivity to sensory stimuli.* Animals anesthetized with these agents may show marked sensitivity to sound, light, and other sensory stimuli. These agents are used in combination with other drugs, particularly midazolam or diazepam, to avoid excitement and improve muscle relaxation.

- Animals recovering from dissociative anesthesia often show an exaggerated response to touch, light, or sound, and seizurelike activity may be observed. Reduction of light, sound, and other stimuli or administration of benzodiazepines may reduce this activity. Because CNS stimulation is seen with dissociatives, these drugs are contraindicated in animals with a history of epilepsy or other seizure disorders. Dissociative anesthetics should be avoided in animals that have ingested strychnine, street drugs, organophosphates, and other toxins that affect the CNS. Dissociative anesthetics should also be used with caution in animals undergoing procedures involving the neurologic system, including cerebrospinal fluid (CSF) taps and myelograms, because such animals are at increased risk for postoperative seizures immediately after these procedures.

- Some animals recovering from dissociative anesthesia may attempt to paw their faces or demonstrate other bizarre behavior, possibly resulting from hallucinations. Recovering patients should be closely monitored in the hospital to prevent self-injury. Personality changes that can persist for several days have been reported in animals after recovery from ketamine anesthesia. Fortunately, these usually resolve spontaneously after a few days or weeks.

- Dissociative anesthetics may induce nystagmus, a repetitive side-to-side motion of the eyeball. Ketamine-induced nystagmus is more commonly seen in cats than in dogs. This condition is harmless and resolves on recovery from anesthesia.

Cardiovascular system

- Unlike most other anesthetics, dissociative anesthetics do not decrease heart rate or decrease cardiac output in patients with normal heart function. In fact, most animals exhibit increased heart rate, cardiac output, and mean arterial blood pressure due to stimulation of the SNS. These cardiovascular effects are not usually harmful to the animal but can be if the patient has preexisting heart disease (e.g., cats with hyperthyroidism or cardiomyopathy) because cardiac work and oxygen consumption increase.

- Dissociative agents may decrease inotropy—an effect that is normally counteracted by SNS stimulation. This decrease in the strength of heart muscle contraction can become problematic in patients with preexisting heart disease, leading to sudden development of congestive heart failure, even if the heart disease is not evident. For this reason, it is important to screen patients for preexisting heart disease (such as hypertrophic cardiomyopathy caused by hyperthyroidism in cats) as these patients are at increased risk for serious complications if given dissociative agents.

- Dissociatives also slightly increase the risk that cardiac arrhythmias will develop in response to epinephrine release.

Respiratory system

- Dissociative anesthetics do not affect the respiratory system in the same way as most other anesthetics. Respiratory rate and tidal volume may change, but respiratory depression is usually insignificant at usual doses. At higher doses, animals exhibit apneustic respiration, a breathing pattern in which there is a pause for several seconds at the end of the inspiratory phase, followed by a short, quick expiratory phase. These animals appear to hold their breath.

- Although not usually a problem at conventional doses, overdoses may cause severe respiratory depression or respiratory arrest.
- Dissociatives also significantly increase salivation and respiratory tract secretions. Care must be taken to ensure that the airway is protected to prevent aspiration. Anticholinergics can be used to control these signs but may further predispose the patient to cardiac arrhythmias.

Other Effects and Adverse Effects

Dissociative anesthetics have many other effects, including the following:

- *Tissue irritation.* Ketamine and tiletamine are irritating to tissues, and many animals show transitory pain after IM injection. However, these agents do not cause tissue necrosis.
- *Increased intracranial and intraocular pressure.* Dissociative anesthetics are contraindicated in patients with cranial trauma, conditions that cause elevated CSF pressure, and some ocular surgeries.

Use of Dissociative Anesthetics

Unlike propofol, alfaxalone, and etomidate, dissociatives may be given by either the IM or IV route for anesthetic induction. The versatility and wide margin of safety of dissociatives has led to their widespread acceptance in veterinary anesthesia, particularly for use in cats and horses. When given in combination with a tranquilizer (e.g., diazepam, midazolam, xylazine, dexmedetomidine, acepromazine, or zolazepam), they are useful for brief procedures such as castration or as a means of induction before intubation and inhalation anesthesia. They are also useful for chemical restraint of intractable cats, allowing examinations and minor treatments without endangering hospital personnel. In dogs, dissociative–tranquilizer combinations (ketamine–diazepam or tiletamine–zolazepam) are also commonly used as induction agents. Dissociative agents are also used in combination with tranquilizers in an extremely wide variety of large-animal and exotic species for sedation, immobilization, and anesthesia. In addition to the uses listed above, ketamine is an NMDA antagonist-class analgesic used in combination with other analgesics for pain control.

One limitation of dissociatives is the lack of an effective reversal agent.

Ketamine. Ketamine is among the most commonly used agents in North American small-animal practice and can be used to anesthetize not only cats and dogs but also birds, horses, and exotic species. Currently, ketamine is licensed only for use in cats and nonhuman primates and is most commonly supplied as a 100 mg/mL solution.

Ketamine has a rapid onset of action after IV or IM administration. This is a result of its high lipid solubility, which allows quick entry into brain tissue. Cats may lose their righting reflex within 90 seconds of IV administration and within 2 to 4 minutes of an IM injection of ketamine. IV administration has several advantages over IM administration, including more rapid induction and recovery and a lower dose. The anesthetist

must ensure that the dose of ketamine is correct for the route of administration used: if the IM dose is inadvertently given by the IV route, serious overdose and death could result. Ketamine is given only by the IV route in dogs because IM ketamine may cause excitement and seizure activity.

In the past, ketamine was also administered orally to facilitate restraint of feral or aggressive cats. However, during recent years, increased availability of restraint devices such as the EZ Nabber (Campbell Pet Company) and Wild Child cat chamber (Har-Vet) has rendered this practice unnecessary in most cases.

Although ketamine can be administered repeatedly to maintain anesthesia, this should be done with caution. After repeated injections, large amounts of the drug accumulate in the tissues, increasing the risk of seizure activity during recovery and significantly prolonging recovery.

Recovery from ketamine anesthesia normally occurs within 2 to 6 hours in healthy patients, depending on the dose given and the route of administration. Dogs appear to have faster recoveries than cats, probably because of differences in ketamine metabolism and excretion. Elimination of ketamine depends on hepatic metabolism in the dog, but in the cat, the drug is primarily excreted through the kidneys. It follows that ketamine should be used with caution in dogs with hepatic disease and in cats with compromised renal function or urinary obstruction.

Ketamine is commonly used in combination with acepromazine, benzodiazepines, alpha$_2$-agonists, opioids, propofol, and other agents to produce a wide variety of mixtures. Although most of these mixtures will be covered in the species chapters, it is fitting to mention midazolam and ketamine, which is one of the most commonly used combinations in small and large animal practice.

Ketamine–midazolam combination. A mixture of ketamine and midazolam is popular for IV induction of cats and dogs and is formulated by combining equal volumes (a 1:1 ratio) of ketamine (100 mg/mL) and midazolam (5 mg/mL) or by combining these drugs in a 1:2 ratio. The drugs are commonly mixed in the same syringe, although there is a small risk of precipitate formation. The calculated dose of ketamine–midazolam is 1 mL/20 lb (9.1 kg). This is equivalent to doses of 5.5 mg/kg of ketamine and 0.28 mg/kg of midazolam when given at a 1:1 ratio, and 3.6 mg/kg of ketamine and 0.36 mg/kg of midazolam when given at a 1:2 ratio. After premedication with an opioid and/or tranquilizer, the calculated dose of ketamine–midazolam is given intravenously to effect. The animal loses consciousness within 30 to 90 seconds and remains sufficiently deeply anesthetized for intubation or minor procedures for 5 to 10 minutes. This is followed by a 30- to 60-minute recovery period.

This combination of ketamine and midazolam has several advantages, including minimal cardiac depression, good muscle relaxation, superior recovery, and some analgesia. Respiratory depression, however, may be greater than that seen with ketamine alone. Diazepam may be used in combination with ketamine in place of midazolam. It is available in the same concentration as midazolam (5 mg/mL) and is combined with ketamine using the same ratio. The clinical effects of these two combinations are almost indistinguishable. Consequently, they are used essentially in the same way.

Ketamine–diazepam does not work well when given by the IM route in either cats or dogs, because diazepam is poorly absorbed after IM injection. However, midazolam is well absorbed and may be given IM in place of diazepam for minor procedures (midazolam 0.28 mg/kg and ketamine 5.5 mg/kg).

Tiletamine. Tiletamine is a dissociative agent with effects similar to those of ketamine. Tiletamine is sold only in combination with zolazepam, which is a benzodiazepine closely related to diazepam. The use of zolazepam in combination with tiletamine reduces the risk of seizures during recovery and helps promote skeletal muscle relaxation. The product (Telazol) is sold as a powder, which contains 50 mg of each drug per milliliter. It is reconstituted with sterile water and is stable for 4 days at room temperature and 14 days if refrigerated. Telazol is a Class III controlled substance in the United States.

Tiletamine–zolazepam is used alone or in combination with other tranquilizers and with ketamine for immobilization, sedation, restraint, and anesthetic induction in a wide variety of domestic and exotic species. It is useful as an induction agent in healthy dogs and cats, particularly in animals with aggressive temperaments. It can be used alone (after premedication) or supplemented with inhalation anesthetics. The dose used is frequently lower than that recommended by the manufacturer.

The combination of tiletamine and zolazepam is similar in effect to ketamine–midazolam but offers the following advantages:
- Tiletamine appears to cause less pronounced apneustic respiration than ketamine. However, respiratory depression may be significant, particularly if a high dose is used or tiletamine is used in combination with other sedatives or anesthetics.
- Tiletamine–zolazepam may be administered intramuscularly, intravenously, or subcutaneously, although currently in the United States, Telazol is approved for IV and IM use in dogs and IM use only in cats, whereas Zoletil and Tilzolan are labeled for IM use only in dogs and cats.
- Tiletamine–zolazepam is effective in many species of wild, and in some species, it is the drug of choice for capture and immobilization.

Many reflexes are maintained throughout tiletamine–zolazepam anesthesia (including the palpebral, corneal, laryngeal, and pedal reflexes), and depth of anesthesia may be difficult to judge. As with ketamine, there is some analgesia, but visceral analgesia is inadequate for major abdominal surgery unless supplemented with other agents. Tachycardia and cardiac arrhythmias may be present under light anesthesia, and cardiac output is significantly reduced at high doses (more than 20 mg/kg IM). Like ketamine, tiletamine induces a marked increase in salivation and respiratory secretions unless the patient is premedicated with an anticholinergic.

One disadvantage of tiletamine–zolazepam is the long and difficult recovery seen in some animals, particularly dogs. This may be because in dogs, zolazepam is metabolized more rapidly than tiletamine, resulting in the loss of the tranquilizing effect, whereas the opposite is true of cats, resulting in smoother recoveries in this species.

As with ketamine, ataxia and increased sensitivity to stimuli are commonly observed during the recovery period. Tremors, muscle rigidity, seizure activity, and hyperthermia can also be seen, especially in dogs given tiletamine–zolazepam at labeled doses by the IM route. Administration of IV midazolam or diazepam may be helpful in affected animals. In cats, recovery may be prolonged (up to 5 hours after IM injection), particularly if high doses are administered. Because the drug is metabolized by the liver and excreted via the kidneys, prolonged recovery should be expected in animals with liver or kidney dysfunction.

Tiletamine–zolazepam should be avoided in patients with an American Society of Anesthesiologists (ASA) physical status class of P3 or greater and in animals with CNS signs, hyperthyroidism, cardiac disease, pancreatic or renal disease, pregnancy, glaucoma, or penetrating eye injuries.

Guaifenesin

Guaifenesin (aka: glyceryl guaiacolate or GG; and previously known as *glyceryl guaiacolate ether,* or GGE) is a noncontrolled muscle relaxant that is sometimes given to large animals to increase muscle relaxation, facilitate intubation, and ease induction and recovery. It is not an anesthetic or analgesic by itself and so is given in combination with other agents. At the time of writing, this drug can only be purchased from compounding pharmacie and is therefore less commonly used now than it once was.

Mode of Action and Pharmacology

Although the mechanism of action is not fully known, GG is felt to block nerve impulses in the CNS.

> **TECHNICIAN NOTE** Major effects and adverse effects of guaifenesin are as follows:
> - Skeletal muscle relaxation
> - Minimal cardiopulmonary effects
> - Few adverse effects at therapeutic doses
> - Thrombophlebitis after IV injection
> - Tissue reaction after perivascular injection

Effects and Adverse Effects Involving Major Organ Systems
- GG affects the cardiovascular and respiratory systems minimally, causing transient, mildly decreased blood pressure and tidal volume and mildly increased respiratory rate and GI motility.
- GG causes skeletal muscle relaxation, including the pharyngeal and laryngeal muscles but minimally affects the diaphragm.
- At therapeutic doses, few adverse effects are seen. Excessive doses can cause muscle rigidity and apneustic breathing.

Other Effects and Adverse Effects
- GG is irritating to the tissues, so IV injection can cause thrombophlebitis and perivascular injection may lead to tissue reaction.

- Use of concentrated solutions of this agent above 7% in ruminants and above 12% in horses can cause RBC hemolysis. Therefore a 5% or 10% solution in dextrose is preferred, and GG should be used with caution in anemic patients.

Use of Guaifenesin

GG in combination with ketamine is given IV to induce general anesthesia in horses (after premedication with an alpha$_2$-agonist) or ruminants (with or without premedication). GG is also used to maintain anesthesia for short periods (less than 1 hour) in horses as part of a total IV anesthetic mixture commonly known as "triple drip" (GG combined with ketamine and an alpha$_2$-agonist, typically xylazine).

For anesthetic induction of horses, GG is administered rapidly intravenously after premedication until the patient shows signs of ataxia ("knuckling" at the fetlock), after which the induction agent (most commonly ketamine) is given. GG can be used to induce anesthesia in ruminants in a similar way (except that they will sway or even lie down after receiving the GG) or by adding ketamine to the bag of GG (at a concentration of 1mg ketamine/mL of GG solution) and administering the mixture to effect. Recovery is usually smooth. *(Detailed instructions regarding preparation of GG for anesthetic induction and maintenance may be found in Chapters 10 and 11.)*

Guaifenesin should not be used without premedication or as the sole agent because excitement is likely to be seen during induction and large doses will be required for recumbency, which increases the risk of side effects. Sedation and analgesia are inadequate for surgery when this agent is used alone.

The 5% solution is prepared by adding 50 g of guaifenesin to 50 g of medical-grade dextrose, which is dissolved in 1 L of very hot sterile water. If a precipitate develops, it can be dissolved by rewarming the solution.

INHALATION ANESTHETICS

As mentioned in Chapter 1, the birth of modern anesthesia can be traced back to the mid-1800s, when inhalant anesthetics were first used clinically (diethyl ether in 1842, nitrous oxide in 1844, and chloroform in 1847). Before that time, surgery was performed under extreme and far less than ideal conditions. Surgeons often had to work at breakneck speed while conscious patients were restrained by attendants. Needless to say, surgery at that time involved fear, risk, and pain. Indeed, the introduction of inhalant agents marked one of the most significant advances of medical science by giving surgeons the ability to perform surgery safely and humanely.

The first inhalant anesthetics are no longer used because they have been gradually replaced by the halogenated agents, which continue to be among the safest and most commonly used anesthetics. In fact, their use is so commonplace for such a wide variety of routine veterinary procedures that it is difficult to imagine caring for patients without them.

The inhalation anesthetics in common use at present are the halogenated compounds isoflurane and sevoflurane. Desflurane and nitrous oxide are occasionally used in some practices and in academic and research settings. Enflurane is not used in veterinary patients owing to problematic adverse effects. Halothane became unavailable in the United States in 2008, and methoxyflurane has not been available for several decades. However, when learning about inhalation anesthetics, methoxyflurane and halothane remain useful points of comparison to the currently used agents isoflurane and sevoflurane. In addition, halothane is frequently mentioned in discussions about safe use of anesthetics because many of the early studies on exposure to waste anesthetic gases were done on this agent.

Many other inhalation agents that were used in the past (including diethyl ether, chloroform, divinyl ether, and trichloroethylene) are now of historical interest only.

Halogenated Organic Compounds

Isoflurane and sevoflurane, the most commonly used inhalation agents in veterinary practice, are classified as halogenated organic compounds. Other agents in this class include desflurane, halothane, methoxyflurane, and enflurane. Halogenated agents are liquids at room temperature (although the boiling point of desflurane is near room temperature). They are stored inside the vaporizer of the anesthetic machine and evaporate in the oxygen that flows through the vaporizer, with the exception of desflurane, which requires a special injection-type vaporizer. The resulting mixture of oxygen and anesthetic is delivered to the patient through a breathing circuit (discussed in detail in Chapter 4).

Mode of Action and Pharmacology

The mechanism of action of halogenated anesthetics in the CNS is not fully understood, although it has been suggested that these anesthetics inhibit nerve cell function in the brain and spinal cord.

The uptake, distribution, and elimination of these agents are very different from those of injectable agents. A basic understanding of these differences is necessary if the agents are to be used effectively and safely. What follows is a summary of the movement of these drugs within the body.

Within the anesthetic machine, liquid anesthetic is vaporized, mixed with oxygen, and delivered to the patient by mask or endotracheal tube. The anesthetic travels via the air passages to the lungs, where it diffuses across the alveolar cell membranes and enters the bloodstream. The rate of diffusion is controlled by the concentration gradient between the alveolus and the bloodstream, as well as the lipid solubility of the drug. During the induction period, the concentration of the agent in the alveolus is high and the concentration in the blood is low. This creates a steep concentration gradient, and diffusion of anesthetic from the alveolus into the blood is rapid during this period.

As with injectable agents, inhalation agents are carried to the body tissues in the blood. Consequently, tissues with high blood flow (brain, heart, kidney) are more quickly saturated with anesthetic than tissues with lower blood flow such as skeletal muscle and fat. Because of their relatively high lipid solubility, most inhalation agents readily leave the circulation and enter the brain, inducing anesthesia. The depth of anesthesia is determined by the partial pressure of the anesthetic agent in the brain. This in turn is related to the partial pressure of anesthetic in the blood and alveoli. Anesthesia is maintained as long as sufficient quantities of inhalation agent are delivered to the alveoli so that the alveolar, blood, and brain concentrations are maintained (Fig. 3.10).

When the concentration of the inhalation agent administered is reduced or discontinued by adjustment of the anesthetic machine vaporizer, the amount of anesthetic in the alveoli is reduced. Because the blood level is still high, the concentration gradient now favors the diffusion of anesthetic from the blood into the alveoli. The blood levels of the anesthetic are quickly reduced, provided the animal continues to breathe and eliminate anesthetic from the alveoli. The anesthetist can hasten

the elimination of anesthetic by periodically bagging the animal with 100% oxygen. This removes anesthetic from the alveoli and reestablishes a steep concentration gradient between the blood and the alveoli. As the concentration of the anesthetic in the blood falls, the agent leaves the brain and the patient wakes up.

Isoflurane, sevoflurane, and desflurane undergo minimal liver metabolism and renal excretion because they are eliminated from the body chiefly through the lungs. Some of the older halogenated compounds (in particular, methoxyflurane) have very high lipid solubility and accumulate in body fat. Unlike isoflurane, sevoflurane, and desflurane, older agents rely to a significant degree on liver metabolism and renal excretion for their complete elimination from the body.

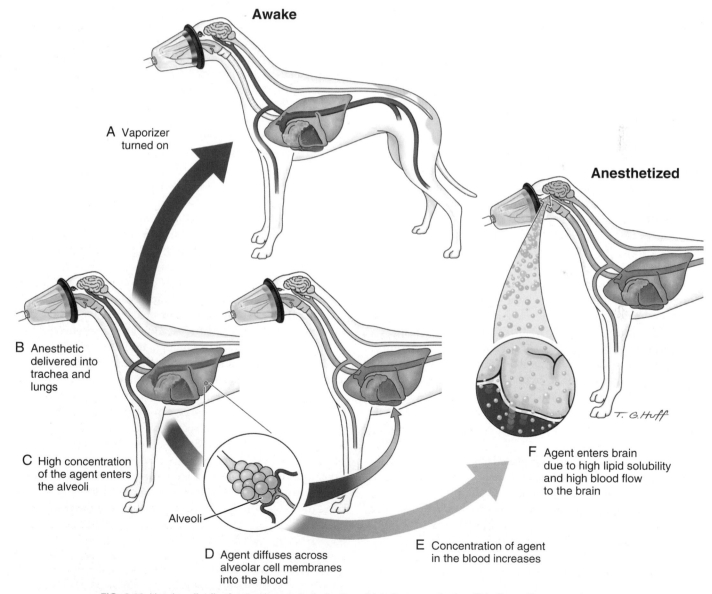

Awake

A Vaporizer turned on

Anesthetized

B Anesthetic delivered into trachea and lungs

C High concentration of the agent enters the alveoli

Alveoli

D Agent diffuses across alveolar cell membranes into the blood

E Concentration of agent in the blood increases

F Agent enters brain due to high lipid solubility and high blood flow to the brain

T. G. Huff

FIG. 3.10 Uptake, distribution, action, and elimination of inhalant anesthetics. This figure illustrates the process by which inhalation anesthetics enter the body and produce general anesthesia. This process is reversed when the anesthetic vaporizer is turned off. **1,** The concentration of the anesthetic in the alveolus is reduced. **2,** The concentration gradient favors movement from the blood into the alveoli and from the brain into the blood. **3,** The patient wakes up as the level of anesthetic in the brain falls.

Effects and Adverse Effects Involving Major Organ Systems

Although halogenated inhalation agents vary somewhat in their effects, the following characteristics are common to all (see Tables 3.1 to 3.4).

Central nervous system
- Halogenated agents cause a dose-related, reversible depression of the CNS.
- These agents also depress the temperature-regulating center, leading to hypothermia.
- Halogenated agents have little or no analgesic effect at sub-hypnotic doses. This, combined with the rapid recoveries seen with these agents, may lead to pain and excitement during recovery unless the animal is treated with analgesics.
- Paddling, excitement, and muscle fasciculations have been reported, primarily during the recovery period.
- Animals anesthetized with inhalation agents may develop increased intracranial pressure, especially if carbon dioxide levels in the blood are allowed to increase. This necessitates caution when anesthetizing patients with head trauma or brain tumors, and the use of controlled ventilation to keep carbon dioxide levels low.

Cardiovascular system
- Inhalation agents depress cardiovascular function. Although the effect on heart rate is variable, all of these agents cause dose-related vasodilation, hypotension, decreased cardiac output, and decreased tissue perfusion. The hypotension associated with these agents is a common and problematic adverse effect that may be profound, especially when using higher concentrations.
- Because inhalation anesthetics may decrease blood pressure, they have the potential to decrease renal blood flow. This can be clinically significant in animals with preexisting renal disease or in animals receiving nephrotoxic drugs such as gentamicin or nonsteroidal antiinflammatory drugs (NSAIDs) (see Chapter 8).
- Neither of the inhalation agents in common use (isoflurane and sevoflurane) sensitizes the heart muscle to epinephrine-induced arrhythmias.

Respiratory system
- In general, inhalation agents depress ventilation in a dose-dependent manner by decreasing tidal volume and respiratory rate.
- Hypoventilation is a possible adverse effect of all inhalation agents. Hypoventilation predisposes the animal to carbon dioxide retention and respiratory acidosis. A concentration of two to three times the MAC causes respiratory arrest in common domestic species.

Other Effects and Adverse Effects
- The commonly used halogenated inhalant agents induce adequate to good muscle relaxation.
- Halogenated agents readily cross the placenta and may depress respiration in neonates.
- Nearly all of the commonly used halogenated inhalant agents administered to a patient is eliminated through the lungs once the vaporizer is turned off. These agents have low fat solubility; consequently, little retention in body fat stores, little hepatic metabolism (0.2% of isoflurane, 2% to 5% of sevoflurane, and 0.02% of desflurane), and very little renal excretion of metabolites occur. For this reason, these agents are well suited to animals with liver or kidney disease and for neonatal and geriatric animals, where hepatic metabolism and renal excretion mechanisms may be less efficient than in the healthy adult animal.
- When exposed to desiccated (dried-out) CO_2 absorbent, these agents can produce carbon monoxide, which has over 200 times greater affinity for hemoglobin binding sites than oxygen. Desflurane has the greatest tendency to do this, followed by isoflurane. Carbon monoxide displaces oxygen from its binding sites, causing hypoxemia. This is not always easily detected, however, because animals with carbon monoxide poisoning may be asymptomatic, and oxygen saturation as measured by a conventional pulse oximeter will often be normal due to an inability to differentiate oxyhemoglobin (hemoglobin that is bound to oxygen) from carboxyhemoglobin (hemoglobin bound to carbon monoxide). Cherry red blood and mucous membranes suggest carbon monoxide exposure, which must be treated promptly.
- These agents, particularly sevoflurane, can also produce an exothermic (heat-producing) reaction when used with desiccated CO absorbers. This can lead to damage to the airway due to exposure to excess temperatures, or even fire. To prevent this, oxygen flowmeters should not be left on when the machine is not in use, and carbon dioxide absorbent should be changed regularly.

Despite the potential adverse effects of halogenated anesthetics, they are considered safe for most patients relative to other anesthetics. However, safety depends to a large degree on the care with which these agents are administered and the vigilance of the anesthetist in monitoring their effect on the patient.

Physical and Chemical Properties

Inhalant anesthetics differ considerably in their anesthetic effects, in part because of differences in their physical and

TABLE 3.8 Physical Properties of the Common Inhalation Anesthetics						
	Desflurane	**Sevoflurane**	**Isoflurane**	**Halothane**	**Methoxyflurane**	**Nitrous Oxide**
Approximate date of first and last clinical use in United States	1992 in use	1994 in use	1981 in use	1956 to 2008	1959 to approximately 1990	1845 in use
Saturated vapor pressure at 750 mmHg and 20°C	700	160	240	243	23	(N_2O is a gas at room temperature)
Blood–gas partition coefficient	0.42	0.68	1.46	2.54	15	0.47
Fat solubility	27	48	45	51	902	1.08
Rubber solubility	19	29	49	190	630	1.2
MAC in dogs (%)	7.2	2.34	1.3	0.87	–	188–297
MAC in cats (%)	9.8	2.58	1.63	1.19	–	255
MAC in horses (%)	7.23	2.34	1.31	0.88	–	190
Metabolism (%)	0.02	2–5	0.2	20–46	50–75	0.004

MAC, Minimum alveolar concentration.

Data from Grimm KA, Lamont LA, Tranquilli SA: *Lumb & Jones' veterinary anesthesia and analgesia,* ed 5, Ames, IA, 2015, John Wiley & Sons, Inc.; except for the MAC values, which are from Muir WW, Hubbell JA, Bednarski RM: *Handbook of veterinary anesthesia,* ed 5, St Louis, MO, 2013, Elsevier. Note that the figures above may not be the same as those published in other sources, as they vary from text to text.

chemical properties. The properties of chief importance to the anesthetist include vapor pressure, partition coefficient, minimum alveolar concentration (MAC), and rubber solubility. These agents also vary in their pharmacologic properties, including their effects on the cardiovascular, respiratory, and other vital systems. The agent-specific physical properties and pharmacology of commonly used inhalation anesthetic agents are summarized in Table 3.8.

> **TECHNICIAN NOTE** Vapor pressure is a measure of the tendency of a liquid anesthetic to evaporate and is significant to the anesthetist because it determines the type of vaporizer required to administer it safely.

Vapor pressure. When a liquid is in a closed container, some of the molecules evaporate from the liquid to form a gas. With time, the number of molecules leaving the liquid equals the number of molecules reentering the liquid—a state called *equilibrium.* Vapor pressure is the amount of pressure exerted by the gaseous form of a substance when the gas and liquid states are in equilibrium. In other words, the vapor pressure of an inhalation anesthetic is a measure of its tendency to evaporate. Vapor pressure is both agent and temperature dependent and is commonly measured at 20°C (68°F), which is considered to be room temperature. Vapor pressure is significant to the way these agents are used because it determines how readily the anesthetic liquid evaporates in the anesthetic machine vaporizer and thus the type of vaporizer required to administer it safely.

Agents with a high vapor pressure, such as isoflurane, sevoflurane, and desflurane, are described as volatile because they evaporate readily. For example, the maximum useful level of isoflurane in the fresh gas delivered to a patient is 5%. However, because isoflurane evaporates so readily, if not controlled, it can reach a concentration of over 30%—a level that would cause a fatal anesthetic overdose (Fig. 3.11). This is why volatile agents must be delivered from a precision vaporizer, which precisely controls the amount of anesthetic delivered and therefore allows them to be used safely.

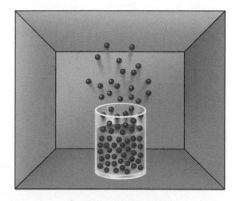

Container just opened

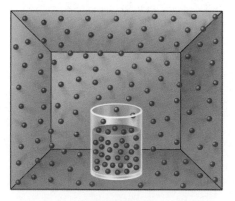

At equilibrium

FIG. 3.11 Volatility of high vapor pressure inhalation agents. High vapor pressure inhalation anesthetics such as isoflurane evaporate readily. When in equilibrium, they reach an unsafe concentration (>30% at room temperature in the case of isoflurane) if not controlled by a precision vaporizer.

For this reason, most precision vaporizers intended for use with isoflurane allow a maximum concentration of 5%, a level sufficient for clinical use. Volatile agents generally cannot be used in nonprecision vaporizers because they do not adequately control delivery of the agen, and there is an increased risk of overdose. Isoflurane is an exception because there is a nonprecision vaporizer called the Stevens Vaporizer that is intended for use with this agent. Close monitoring of the patient and anesthetic machine by a skilled anesthetist is required, however, if a nonprecision vaporizer is used (see Chapter 4).

In contrast with isoflurane, sevoflurane and desflurane, agents with low vapor pressure, do not require the use of a precision vaporizer (Fig. 3.12). For instance, the discontinued agent methoxyflurane can only attain a maximum concentration of 4% at room temperature, a safe level for this agent. Consequently, a nonprecision vaporizer, such as a glass jar with a wick (see Chapter 4, Fig. 4.35), would be adequate for vaporizing methoxyflurane.

All precision vaporizers are designed to deliver one specific halogenated agent (e.g., isoflurane, sevoflurane, or desflurane) because they are designed and calibrated for the vapor pressure unique to that agent. Each agent should therefore be used only in a vaporizer calibrated specifically for delivery of that agent, and two different agents should never be combined in the same vaporizer.

Although it is unacceptable to combine agents, it is acceptable to switch from one anesthetic to another during the course of surgery if the patient demonstrates an adverse reaction to an anesthetic. In this case, separate vaporizers must be available for each anesthetic, and either the vaporizers must be connected in series or the inlet and outlet hoses must be rapidly changed from one vaporizer to the other when it is time to make the change.

> **TECHNICIAN NOTE** The blood–gas partition coefficient is a measure of the solubility of an inhalant anesthetic in blood as compared with alveolar gas. It is significant because it indicates the speed of induction and recovery one should expect for a given inhalant anesthetic. The lower the blood–gas partition coefficient, the faster the expected induction and recovery.

Partition coefficient. Many of the physiologic effects of inhalant anesthetics can be explained by their solubility characteristics (how easily they dissolve) in various substances such as air within the alveoli, blood, lipids, and tissue. Solubility is usually expressed as a partition coefficient, which is a ratio of the concentration of an agent in two substances.

The blood–gas partition coefficient is a ratio of the concentration of an inhalation agent in the blood and in the alveolar gas. It is therefore a measure of the solubility of an inhalant anesthetic in blood as compared with alveolar gas. A blood–gas partition coefficient of 0.5 (a low coefficient) indicates that an anesthetic is half as soluble in the blood as it is in the alveolar gas. So-, at equilibrium, two-thirds of the anesthetic are in the alveolar gas and one-third is in the blood. In contrast, a blood–gas partition coefficient of 2 (a high coefficient) indicates that the anesthetic is twice as soluble in the blood as in the alveolar gas. In this case, at equilibrium, one-third is in the alveolar gas and two-thirds are in the blood. So an anesthetic with a low blood–gas partition coefficient is less soluble in blood than an anesthetic with a high blood–gas partition coefficient.

This is of importance to the anesthetist because the blood–gas partition coefficient indicates the speed of induction and recovery one should expect for a given inhalant anesthetic. The lower the blood–gas partition coefficient for an inhalant anesthetic, the faster the expected induction and recovery. This is because the relative concentration of the agent in the alveoli will remain high, creating a wide concentration gradient between the alveolar gas and the blood. Therefore when the agent enters or leaves the blood, it does so at a rapid rate. An example of an agent with a low blood–gas partition coefficient is sevoflurane, an anesthetic with very rapid induction and recovery characteristics.

In contrast, an agent with a high partition coefficient is highly soluble in the blood and tissues. Because the anesthetic is readily absorbed into the blood and tissues (called the *sponge effect*), high levels of the anesthetic do not build up within the alveoli. This low concentration gradient causes the agent to enter the blood slowly and gradually. As a result, agents with high partition coefficients induce anesthesia less rapidly than do agents with low partition coefficients. Similarly, agents with

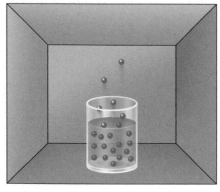

Container just opened

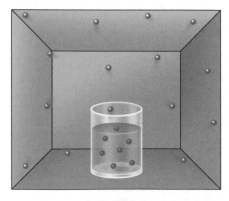

At equilibrium

FIG. 3.12 Volatility of low vapor pressure inhalation agents. Low vapor pressure inhalation anesthetics such as methoxyflurane have low volatility. When in equilibrium, methoxyflurane does not exceed a safe concentration (about 4% at room temperature) and so can be delivered by a nonprecision vaporizer.

high partition coefficients are slow to leave tissues, especially fat, and this gradual release results in a slow recovery. The discontinued agent methoxyflurane is an example of an agent with a high partition coefficient and, as expected, it demonstrates relatively slow induction and recovery rates.

The blood–gas partition coefficient of an inhalant agent strongly influences the clinical use of the agent in the following ways:

- *Induction.* Agents with a low blood–gas partition coefficient (isoflurane, sevoflurane, and desflurane) may be used for mask and chamber inductions because inductions are rapid enough to induce the patient safely and in a reasonable length of time. Methoxyflurane, an agent with a high partition coefficient, cannot be used this way.
- *Maintenance.* Agents with low blood–gas partition coefficients also have the advantage of allowing a rapid patient response to changes in anesthetic concentration during anesthesia. Patients anesthetized with isoflurane or sevoflurane may respond within a few minutes to changes in the vaporizer setting. If an agent with a higher partition coefficient (such as methoxyflurane) was used, the anesthetist would observe a slower patient response to changes in the vaporizer setting.
- *Recovery.* Patients anesthetized with agents with low blood–gas partition coefficients have a relatively fast recovery. Patients anesthetized with sevoflurane or isoflurane are often fully awake within a relatively short time after the vaporizer is turned off. Patients anesthetized with methoxyflurane often sleep quietly for 30 to 60 minutes after anesthesia.

> **TECHNICIAN NOTE** The MAC of an anesthetic agent is the lowest concentration at which 50% of patients show no response to a painful stimulus such as a surgical incision. It is significant because it is a measure of the potency of the agent and is used to determine the average vaporizer setting that must be used to produce surgical anesthesia.

Minimum alveolar concentration. The MAC of an anesthetic agent is the lowest concentration at which 50% of patients show no response to a painful stimulus (e.g., a hemostatic forceps applied to the base of the tail or creation of a surgical incision). For example, isoflurane has a MAC of 1.3% in the dog. This means that if 10 dogs were anesthetized with isoflurane delivered at a setting of 1.3%, five of them would respond to a painful stimulus and five would not. Thus the MAC is used to determine the average setting that must be used to produce surgical anesthesia and is a measure of the potency of the agent (see Fig. 3.13 for an illustration of the association of MAC, vaporizer dial settings, and clinical responses). An agent with a low MAC is a more potent anesthetic than an agent with a high MAC. For example, sevoflurane, which has a higher MAC than isoflurane, is less potent than isoflurane. A lower concentration of isoflurane will therefore be necessary to maintain a similar anesthetic depth.

For any inhalation anesthetic, a vaporizer setting of approximately 1 × MAC will maintain light Stage III anesthesia, 1.5 × MAC will maintain surgical anesthesia, and 2 × MAC will maintain deep Stage III anesthesia in most patients. These figures are useful only as a rough guide: MAC varies with the age, metabolic activity, and body temperature of the patient. Factors such as disease, pregnancy, and obesity may also alter the potency of an anesthetic agent in a given patient. Furthermore, the use of other agents prior to or concurrently with inhalant anesthetics, such as premedications and injectable anesthetics, typically decrease the amount of the inhalation anesthetic required (often involving upwards of a 30% to 50% reduction in concentration). This must be kept firmly in mind when using balanced anesthesia to prevent anesthetic overdose. The anesthetist should also be aware that the response to an anesthetic depends on the concentration of the anesthetic in the patient's brain, which is not necessarily the same as that indicated by the anesthetic machine vaporizer dial setting, particularly early in the induction period (see Chapter 4). Notwithstanding the many factors just discussed, based on the MAC of 1.3% in the dog, a concentration of approximately 2% isoflurane (~1.5% × 1.3%) can be expected to maintain surgical anesthesia in most dogs. Sevoflurane has a high MAC (approximately 2.4), and the maintenance level can be expected to be close to 3.5% (~1.5% × 2.4%). This is only a rough guideline and the anesthetist must, of course, monitor each animal's response to the anesthetic to determine the optimum setting for that individual.

Use of Halogenated Organic Compounds

Isoflurane. Isoflurane, a halogenated organic compound, is an inhalant agent used for induction and maintenance of general anesthesia. Although it is approved for use only in dogs and horses, it has gained widespread use in a wide variety of species including other domestic animals, exotic animals, and zoo animals. Despite the introduction of other agents such as sevoflurane and desflurane, it has remained the most commonly used inhalant agent in North America owing to its competitive cost, safety, and ease of use.

Physical and chemical properties. Isoflurane has a relatively high vapor pressure (240 mmHg) and therefore a precision vaporizer is normally used to deliver this agent.

The blood–gas partition coefficient of isoflurane is extremely low (1.46). This, combined with the relatively low tissue solubility of this agent, results in extremely rapid induction and recovery. Isoflurane is therefore well suited to mask or chamber induction. Unfortunately, some animals appear to be irritated by isoflurane vapors and resist mask induction. Recovery from anesthesia is also rapid, and the anesthetist must refrain from turning off the anesthetic machine vaporizer until the end of surgery because return of consciousness may commence as rapidly as a few minutes after isoflurane is discontinued. Because of the low partition coefficient, the anesthetist can change the patient's depth of anesthesia rapidly during the course of anesthesia. An animal under anesthesia that appears too deep or too light usually responds rapidly (within a few to several minutes) after adjustment of the vaporizer dial.

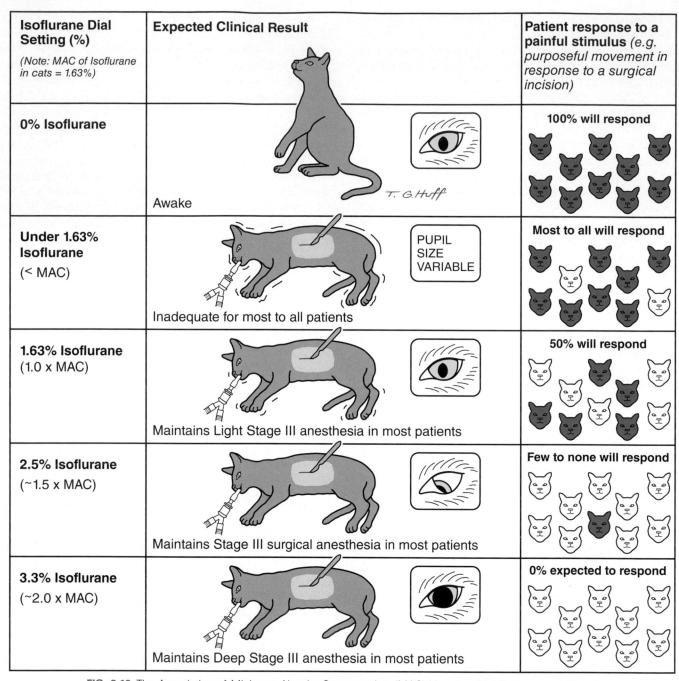

Isoflurane Dial Setting (%) *(Note: MAC of Isoflurane in cats = 1.63%)*	Expected Clinical Result	Patient response to a painful stimulus *(e.g. purposeful movement in response to a surgical incision)*
0% Isoflurane	Awake	**100% will respond**
Under 1.63% Isoflurane (< MAC)	PUPIL SIZE VARIABLE — Inadequate for most to all patients	**Most to all will respond**
1.63% Isoflurane (1.0 × MAC)	Maintains Light Stage III anesthesia in most patients	**50% will respond**
2.5% Isoflurane (~1.5 × MAC)	Maintains Stage III surgical anesthesia in most patients	**Few to none will respond**
3.3% Isoflurane (~2.0 × MAC)	Maintains Deep Stage III anesthesia in most patients	**0% expected to respond**

FIG. 3.13 The Association of Minimum Alveolar Concentration *(MAC)*, Vaporizer Dial Settings, and Clinical Responses for Isoflurane. Illustration of the percentage of patients expected to show a response (i.e., purposeful movement) to a painful stimulus, such as a surgical incision, and the expected clinical result (anesthetic depth) at various vaporizer dial settings. Note that the eye position (central or ventromedial) and the pupil size varies with anesthetic depth. The MAC of isoflurane = 1.63% in the cat. *(Note that each graphic of a cat's face in the column on the right represents 10% of patients anesthetized. Red face = patient response to a stimulus; White face = no patient response.)*

The MAC of isoflurane is 1.30% to 1.63% in the common domestic species. This means that anesthesia is maintained in most patients at a concentration of 1.5% to 2.5%. The rubber solubility of isoflurane is relatively low, and there is little absorption of this anesthetic into rubber components of the anesthetic machine and breathing circuit. Isoflurane is stable at room temperature and requires no preservative.

TECHNICIAN NOTE Of the volatile anesthetics commonly used in veterinary anesthesia, isoflurane is considered to have the fewest adverse cardiovascular effects and is therefore considered to be the inhalation agent of choice for patients with cardiac disease.

Sevoflurane. Sevoflurane is the second most commonly used inhalant anesthetic for induction and maintenance of

TABLE 3.9 Comparison of Isoflurane and Sevoflurane

Characteristic	Isoflurane	Sevoflurane
Potency in common domestic species:	Relatively more potent (induction 3%–5%, maintenance 1.5%–2.5%)	Relatively less potent (induction 4%–5%, maintenance 2.5%–4.0%)
Useful for mask induction?	Yes but irritating to airways	Best suited for mask induction; not irritating and more pleasant odor
Speed of induction (dogs/cats)	Induction: fast, 6–8 min	Induction: somewhat faster (as little as 3–7 min)
Quality of induction (if no premedication)	May struggle if given alone	Generally, somewhat less struggling (due to decreased irritation)
Change in anesthetic depth (dependent on oxygen flow rate)	Rapid (a few to several minutes)	More rapid than isoflurane (a few minutes)
Speed and quality of recovery	Usually rapid; may be rough if given alone	Usually very rapid; may be rough if given alone
Hypotension	Causes significant dose-dependent hypotension	Same
Respiratory depression	Dose dependent up to and including respiratory arrest	Same
Vascular resistance	Decreased	Same
Intracranial pressure and cerebral blood flow	Increased esp. in the presence of hypercapnia (high blood CO_2 level)	Same

general anesthesia (isoflurane being the most commonly used agent). Chemically, it is a halogenated organic compound closely related to isoflurane and has many of the same characteristics (see Table 3.9 for a comparison of these two drugs). Sevoflurane is labeled for use in dogs but has been used in a wide variety of species including exotic and zoo animals.

TECHNICIAN NOTE Sevoflurane is the inhalant agent best suited to mask and chamber inductions. The high controllability of anesthetic depth associated with sevoflurane has made this agent popular in equine anesthesia, despite its relatively high cost.

Physical and chemical properties. The vapor pressure of sevoflurane, although somewhat lower than that of isoflurane, is relatively high (160 mmHg). Therefore a precision vaporizer is required to deliver this agent.

The blood–gas partition coefficient (0.68) is even lower than that of isoflurane, allowing even more rapid induction and recovery. Observed time to intubation has been reported as little as 3 to 7 minutes after mask induction (compared with 6 to 8 minutes for isoflurane). Mask induction with sevoflurane is typically associated with less struggling than with isoflurane because this agent is nonirritating and has a more pleasant odor than isoflurane. Given these characteristics, sevoflurane is the agent best suited to mask and chamber inductions. The high controllability of anesthetic depth associated with sevoflurane has made this agent popular in equine anesthesia despite its relatively high cost.

The MAC of sevoflurane is 2.34% to 2.58% in common domestic species. Sevoflurane is therefore a less potent agent than isoflurane, and higher concentrations are required to induce and maintain anesthesia. A concentration of 4% to 5% is required for mask induction (compared with 3% to 5% for isoflurane) and 2.5% to 4% is the normal maintenance range (compared with 1.5% to 2.5% for isoflurane).

Sevoflurane can react with the potassium hydroxide (KOH) or sodium hydroxide (NaOH) in desiccated carbon dioxide absorbents to produce a chemical (compound A) that can cause renal damage in rats. This effect is most pronounced in full rebreathing systems, in low-flow systems, and at high sevoflurane concentrations. Renal damage has not been reported in dogs or cats anesthetized with sevoflurane. The potential for nephrotoxicity appears to be low in these species and in any case, it can be minimized by the use of carbon dioxide absorbents without KOH and lower amounts of NaOH.

Desflurane. Desflurane is a halogenated organic inhalant anesthetic closely related to isoflurane. It can be used for induction and maintenance of anesthesia, although its expense and some adverse effects currently preclude common use in veterinary patients.

Desflurane vapor is very pungent and may induce coughing and breath holding. This makes mask induction with this agent difficult unless the patient is premedicated. The effects on the nervous, cardiovascular, and respiratory systems are similar to those of isoflurane with the following exception: desflurane is reported to cause transient increases in heart rate and blood pressure in humans. This phenomenon (called a *sympathetic storm*) has not been reported in domestic animals.

Physical and chemical properties. Desflurane has the lowest blood–gas partition coefficient (0.42) of any of the currently used agents and therefore produces inductions and recoveries that are approximately twice as fast as those of isoflurane (sometimes referred to as "one-breath anesthesia" because it can seem as though a patient is anesthetized or wakes up after taking one breath).

The vapor pressure of desflurane is extremely high (700 mmHg), and the boiling point is near room temperature (23.5°C). Because of these properties, this agent requires a special electronic heated vaporizer that keeps the agent under pressure to prevent it from boiling off. The high cost of desflurane and the vaporizer is a significant factor limiting the use of this agent in veterinary medicine.

This agent is the least potent of any of the halogenated agents used in veterinary patients, as evidenced by a MAC of 7.2% to 9.8% in common domestic species. A concentration of 10% to 15% is required for mask induction (compared with 3% to 5% for isoflurane), and 8% to 12% is needed for maintenance (compared with 1.5% to 2.5% for isoflurane).

Like isoflurane, very little desflurane is metabolized by the liver (0.02%).

> **TECHNICIAN NOTE** Desflurane has the lowest blood–gas partition coefficient of any of the currently used agents and therefore produces inductions and recoveries that are approximately twice as fast as those of isoflurane (sometimes referred to as "one-breath anesthesia" because it can seem as if a patient is anesthetized or wakes up after taking one breath).

Nitrous Oxide

Nitrous oxide, introduced as an anesthetic more than 150 years ago, is still used in human anesthesia and, to a much lesser extent, in veterinary anesthesia. Unlike other inhalation anesthetics, nitrous oxide is a gas at room temperature, is stored in blue compressed gas cylinders, and does not require a vaporizer. Like oxygen, it is administered with a flowmeter, and it is mixed in concentrations of 40% to 67% with oxygen before being delivered to the patient.

When used with other agents, nitrous oxide (N_2O) speeds induction and recovery and provides additional analgesia. Nitrous oxide also reduces the MAC (and therefore the vaporizer setting) of other anesthetics by 20% to 30%. This reduces the risk of adverse effects on the cardiovascular, pulmonary, and other systems.

The advantages of nitrous oxide were significant when older agents such as methoxyflurane and halothane were in use. The advantages are much less important since the advent of newer agents such as isoflurane and sevoflurane because of the rapid inductions and recoveries characteristic of these agents and the availability of a wide variety of effective injectable analgesics. For these reasons, nitrous oxide is now rarely used in veterinary practice.

MISCELLANEOUS ANESTHETIC ADJUNCTS

Most anesthetic agents and many adjuncts are respiratory system depressants, so respiratory depression is commonly seen during anesthesia. This complication is usually managed by precise control of anesthetic depth and, if needed, manual or mechanical-assisted or mechanical-controlled ventilation. In emergency situations, severe respiratory depression associated with opioids and alpha₂-agonists can be treated with reversal agents, but the beneficial effects of the corresponding agonist, including sedation, analgesia, and hypnosis, will also be lost. When complete reversal is not desirable or when agents that cannot be reversed are used, the anesthetist may need to use other methods to manage respiratory depression. The pharmacologic agent most commonly used for this purpose is doxapram.

Doxapram

Doxapram is a noncontrolled injectable analeptic agent used in small animals to stimulate respiration and speed awakening during recovery or in emergency situations. It is also commonly used to stimulate respiration in neonates after dystocia or C-section (although use for this purpose is controversial due to adverse effects on the brain and heart), and may be used to assess laryngeal function in small animals. It is most commonly administered intravenously to adult animals. In neonates, it is often administered by placing a few drops under the tongue (sublingual administration), although it can be given subcutaneously or into the umbilical vein.

Mode of Action and Pharmacology

Although the mode of action is not completely known, doxapram stimulates the CNS, including the respiratory centers in the brainstem.

Effects and Adverse Effects

Within 2 minutes of IV injection, doxapram will temporarily increase respiratory rate and depth.

Although doxapram has a relatively wide margin of safety, it may cause hyperventilation, hypertension, and arrhythmias in some patients. It must not be used in patients with a history of seizures because the drug lowers the seizure threshold. Doxapram must be used only in the presence of adequate oxygen levels in the brain; otherwise, CNS damage may result. Several other cautions are detailed in pharmacology references.

> **TECHNICIAN NOTE** One drop of doxapram solution contains approximately 1 mg of doxapram. To stimulate respiration in neonates, 1–5 drops can be dripped under a neonatal puppy's tongue and 1–2 drops under a kitten's tongue, depending on the patient's size and degree of depression, although use for this purpose is controversial.

Use of Doxapram

After an initial injection, if CNS and respiratory stimulation is inadequate, a second injection can be given 15 to 20 minutes later. The dose of doxapram may vary widely depending on the situation. For instance, in small animals, the dose is much lower when used to reverse respiratory depression from inhalant agents (1.1 mg/kg IV) than when used to reverse respiratory depression from barbiturates (5.5 to 11 mg/kg IV).

Because this agent is supplied as a 20 mg/mL solution and there are approximately 20 drops in 1 mL, 1 drop of the solution contains approximately 1 mg of doxapram. For neonatal puppies, 1 to 5 drops can be dripped under the tongue (1 to 2 drops for kittens), depending on the animal's size and degree of depression, or 1 to 5 mg (1 to 2 mg for kittens) can be given subcutaneously to stimulate respiration.

KEY POINTS

1. All anesthetic agents and adjuncts have unique effects that are determined by several pharmacologic properties, including mode of action, protein binding, lipid solubility, redistribution, metabolism, and excretion. Knowledge of these properties guides the anesthetist regarding safe and effective handling and use of each drug.

2. Anesthetic agents and adjuncts classified as controlled substances by the Drug Enforcement Administration (DEA), including the benzodiazepines, dissociatives, alfaxalone, most opioids, and barbiturates, require strict adherence to special procedures regarding ordering, handling, storage, administration, disposal, and record keeping.

3. The anesthetic adjuncts gabapentin and trazodone are anxiolytics frequently administered at home to minimize the negative effects of stress, anxiety, and fear prior to undergoing anesthetic procedures.

4. Preanesthetic agents reduce the required dose of general anesthetics, minimize adverse effects, ease induction and recovery, provide muscle relaxation, and reduce patient stress and discomfort.

5. Although not anesthetics, the anticholinergics atropine and glycopyrrolate are used to prevent bradycardia, bronchoconstriction, excessive salivation, and other parasympathetic effects. These agents must be used sparingly and with caution, as they can produce serious adverse effects.

6. Tranquilizing agents include phenothiazines, benzodiazepines, and alpha$_2$-agonists. Phenothiazines have a wide margin of safety but may cause hypotension in some patients. Benzodiazepines have a calming effect on geriatric and debilitated animals and are excellent for prevention and treatment of seizures. Alpha$_2$-agonists are potent sedatives and produce excellent muscle relaxation but may cause serious cardiovascular and respiratory complications in some patients.

7. Opioid agonists, partial agonists, and agonist–antagonists may be used as preanesthetic agents, analgesics, and (in combination with tranquilizers) neuroleptanalgesics and induction agents. Many of the best analgesics available are in this group. With few exceptions, their use is subject to government regulation regarding purchase, handling, and dispensing.

8. Opioids, alpha$_2$-agonists, and benzodiazepines have corresponding reversal agents that can be used sequentially to sedate or anesthetize and then wake patients when a procedure or surgery is completed.

9. Although commonly used injectable and inhalation anesthetics have a relatively good safety profile, they have the potential to produce significant cardiovascular, respiratory, and thermoregulatory system depression.

10. Injectable anesthetics include propofol, alfaxalone, etomidate, dissociatives (ketamine and tiletamine), and neuroleptanalgesic combinations.

11. Barbiturates are a class of anesthetic drugs that have largely been replaced in recent years by newer general anesthetics such as propofol, alfaxalone, isoflurane, and sevoflurane. Of the drugs in this class, the short-acting agent pentobarbital is used to stop seizures and for laboratory animal anesthesia, and the long-acting agent phenobarbital is used for seizure control.

12. Propofol is a short-acting general anesthetic that is commonly used to induce and maintain general anesthesia in a wide variety of species. High lipid solubility, tissue redistribution, and rapid metabolism are associated with a number of its most desirable characteristics.

13. Most intravenous (IV) anesthetics are administered by titration (or "to effect") to achieve the minimum effective dose.

14. Injectable anesthetics are eliminated by redistribution, liver metabolism, and renal excretion, whereas commonly used inhalation anesthetics are eliminated primarily by exhalation from the lungs.

15. Dissociatives such as ketamine and tiletamine produce a state of dissociative anesthesia characterized by intact reflexes, central nervous system (CNS) excitement, apneustic respiration, tachycardia, and intact or increased muscle tone. Concurrent use of a tranquilizer is recommended to promote muscle relaxation and to prevent excitement during recovery.

16. Neuroleptanalgesia is a profound hypnotic state produced by the simultaneous administration of an opioid and a tranquilizer. These agents provide relatively safe induction in debilitated patients.

17. Propofol, alfaxalone, and etomidate are induction agents that can be given by repeat injection to maintain anesthesia. These agents have many properties in common but differences that make each uniquely suited for specific indications.

18. The inhalation agents in common use are isoflurane and sevoflurane. Both agents are administered by means of an anesthetic machine and either a mask or an endotracheal tube.

19. Inhalation anesthetic agents vary in their blood–gas partition coefficient, vapor pressure, and minimum alveolar concentration (MAC). These properties affect the speed of induction and recovery, the type of vaporizer that should be used, and the vaporizer setting that is required for anesthetic induction and maintenance.

20. All inhalation anesthetics may cause respiratory depression and decrease cardiac output and blood pressure. The commonly used agents isoflurane and sevoflurane are considered to have very favorable margins of safety and have among the shortest induction and recovery times.

21. Reversal agents for opioids, alpha$_2$-agonists, and benzodiazepines may be given after anesthesia to hasten anesthetic recovery. Maropitant and doxapram are anesthetic adjuncts used to mitigate adverse effects of anesthetic agents in the perioperative period.

REVIEW QUESTIONS

1. Which of the following statements about the anxiolytics trazodone and gabapentin is incorrect?
   a. When used for anxiolysis, these agents are most frequently given by the owner at home prior to travel.
   b. Both agents are FDA approved for relief of anxiety and stress in dogs and cats.
   c. Gabapentin is most often used in cats whereas trazodone is most often used in dogs.
   d. Adverse effects of these agents are generally mild and temporary.

2. A neuroleptanalgesic is a combination of:
   a. An opioid and an anticholinergic
   b. An anticholinergic and a tranquilizer
   c. An opioid and a tranquilizer
   d. An anticholinergic and a benzodiazepine

3. Dogs with an MDR1(ABCB1-1delta) gene mutation have increased sensitivity to which of the following drugs?
   a. Butorphanol and acepromazine
   b. Fentanyl and xylazine
   c. Atropine and diazepam
   d. Trazodone and gabapentin

4. Most preanesthetics will not cross the placental barrier.
   True
   False

5. It is recommended that atropine not be given to an animal that has tachycardia.
   True
   False

6. Which of the following drugs is used in the preanesthetic period to reduce perioperative nausea and vomiting?
   a. Dexmedetomidine
   b. Maropitant
   c. Doxapram
   d. Gabapentin

7. Anticholinergic drugs such as atropine block the release of acetylcholine at the:
   a. Muscarinic receptors of the parasympathetic system
   b. Nicotinic receptors of the parasympathetic system
   c. Muscarinic receptors of the sympathetic system
   d. Nicotinic receptors of the sympathetic system

8. High doses of opioids can cause bradycardia and respiratory depression.
   True
   False

9. Severe bradycardia caused by dexmedetomidine is best treated with:
   a. Atropine
   b. Naloxone
   c. Epinephrine
   d. Atipamezole

10. Opioids may be reversed with:
    a. Atipamezole
    b. Naloxone
    c. Atropine
    d. Yohimbine

11. Which one of the following drugs will precipitate when mixed with most other drugs or solutions?
    a. Atropine
    b. Acepromazine
    c. Diazepam
    d. Butorphanol

12. Which of the following signs is not characteristic of dissociative anesthesia?
    a. Normal to increased muscle tone
    b. Dilated pupils
    c. Increased heart rate
    d. Prolapsed third eyelid

13. Etomidate is particularly well suited for induction of dogs with which of the following conditions?
    a. Severe cardiac disease
    b. Renal failure
    c. Orthopedic disease
    d. Pediatric (younger than 4 weeks)

14. Which of the following is an example of a dissociative anesthetic?
    a. Thiopental sodium
    b. Pentobarbital sodium
    c. Ketamine hydrochloride
    d. Propofol

15. One of the disadvantages of the drug alfaxalone is that animals that are anesthetized with it may demonstrate excitement during recovery.
    True
    False

16. Compared with methoxyflurane, isoflurane is considered to have a:
    a. Higher vapor pressure
    b. Similar vapor pressure
    c. Lower vapor pressure

17. Use of an anesthetic agent that has a low blood-gas partition coefficient will result in _____ induction and recovery time.
    a. Slow
    b. Moderate
    c. Rapid

18. Which of the following has the lowest blood–gas partition coefficient?
    a. Desflurane
    b. Isoflurane
    c. Methoxyflurane
    d. Sevoflurane

19. As a rough guideline, to maintain surgical anesthesia safely, the vaporizer should be set at about:
    a. $0.5 \times MAC$
    b. $1 \times MAC$
    c. $1.5 \times MAC$
    d. $2 \times MAC$

20. Propofol sometimes causes transient apnea. To avoid this, the anesthetist should:
    a. Give it by infusion only
    b. Premedicate with opioids
    c. Administer it intravenously only
    d. Titrate this drug in several boluses
21. One problem frequently associated with recovery from tiletamine–zolazepam in dogs is:
    a. Excitement
    b. Bradycardia
    c. Hypotension
    d. Laryngospasm

For the following questions, more than one answer may be correct.

22. The concentration of propofol entering the brain is affected by a variety of factors such as:
    a. Blood flow to the brain
    b. Lipid solubility of the drug
    c. Plasma protein levels
    d. The rate at which it is given
23. Which of the following drugs is/are not full opioid agonists?
    a. Fentanyl
    b. Hydromorphone
    c. Nalbuphine
    d. Meperidine
24. Effects that are commonly seen after administration of a dissociative include:
    a. Increased blood pressure
    b. Increased heart rate
    c. Increased CSF pressure
    d. Increased intraocular pressure

25. Adverse effects common with isoflurane include:
    a. Hypotension
    b. Accumulation in body fat stores
    c. Depression of respiration
    d. Seizures during recovery
26. MAC will vary with:
    a. Body temperature of the patient
    b. Age of the patient
    c. Concurrent use of other drugs
    d. Anesthetic agent
27. Factors that may affect the speed of anesthetic induction with a volatile gaseous anesthetic include:
    a. Partition coefficient of the agent
    b. Vaporizer setting
    c. MAC of the agent
    d. Concurrent use of atropine
28. Which of the following are alpha$_2$-agonists?
    a. Atipamezole
    b. Xylazine
    c. Acepromazine
    d. Dexmedetomidine
29. Effects that atropine may have on the body include:
    a. Decreased salivation
    b. Increased vagal tone
    c. Decreased gastrointestinal motility
    d. Mydriasis
30. Characteristic effects of the benzodiazepines include:
    a. Pronounced sedation in healthy young animals
    b. Muscle relaxation
    c. Significant decrease in respiratory function
    d. Minimal effect on cardiovascular system

SELECTED READINGS

Berry SH: Injectable anesthetics. In Grimm KA, Lamont LA, Tranquilli SA, editors: *Lumb & Jones' veterinary anesthesia and analgesia*, ed 5, Ames, IA, 2015, John Wiley & Sons, Inc., pp 277–296.

Bill RL: *Clinical pharmacology and therapeutics for the veterinary technician*, ed 4, St. Louis, 2017, Elsevier.

DEA: *Drugs of abuse—A DEA resource guide/2020 edition*. https://www.dea.gov/sites/default/files/2020-04/Drugs%20of%20Abuse%202020-Web%20Version-508%20compliant-4-24-20_0.pdf. Accessed August, 2021.

Doherty T, Valverde A: *Manual of equine anesthesia and analgesia*, Ames, IA, 2022, Blackwell Publishing, Ltd.

KuKanich B, Wiese AJ: Opioids. In Grimm KA, Lamont LA, Tranquilli SA, editors: *Lumb & Jones' veterinary anesthesia and analgesia*, ed 5, Ames, IA, 2015, John Wiley & Sons, Inc., pp 207–226.

Lemke KA: Anticholinergics and sedatives. In Tranquilli WJ, Thurmon JC, Grimm KA, editors: *Lumb & Jones' veterinary anesthesia and analgesia*, ed 4, Ames, IA, 2007, Blackwell, pp 225–227.

Lerche P: Anticholinergics. In Grimm KA, Lamont LA, Tranquilli SA, editors: *Lumb & Jones' veterinary anesthesia and analgesia*, ed 5, Ames, IA, 2015, John Wiley & Sons, Inc., pp 178–282.

Love L: *Oral sedatives and anxiolytics for veterinary visits*, Posted July 26, 2019, North American Veterinary Anesthesia Society. https://www.mynavas.org/post/oral-sedatives-and-anxiolytics-for-veterinary-visits. Accessed August 4, 2021.

Muir WM, Hubbell JAE: *Equine anesthesia*, ed 2, St. Louis, MO, 2008, Saunders Elsevier.

Muir WW, McDonnel WN, Kerr CL, et al: Anesthetic physiology and pharmacology. In Grimm KA, Tranquilli WJ, Lamont LA, editors: *Essentials of small animal anesthesia and analgesia*, ed 2, Ames, IA, 2011, Blackwell, pp 240–273, 126–191.

Norkus C: *All things considered: "Balancing act—combining inhalant anesthetics and injectable drugs*, March 9, 2019, VetFolio. https://www.vetfolio.com/learn/article/all-things-considered-balancing-actcombining-inhalant-anesthetics-and-injectable-drugs. Accessed August 4, 2021.

Plumb DC: Plumb's Veterinary Drugs. https://plumbs.com/solutions/plumbs-veterinary-drugs/.

Rankin DC: Sedatives and tranquilizers. In Grimm KA, Lamont LA, Tranquilli SA, editors: *Lumb & Jones' veterinary anesthesia and analgesia*, ed 5, Ames, IA, 2015, John Wiley & Sons, Inc., pp 196–206.

Steffey EP, Mama KR, Brosnan RJ: Inhalation anesthetics. In Grimm KA, Lamont LA, Tranquilli SA, editors: *Lumb & Jones' veterinary anesthesia and analgesia*, ed 5, Ames, IA, 2015, John Wiley & Sons, Inc., pp 297–331.

Tranquilli WJ, Lamont LA, editors: *Essentials of small animal anesthesia and analgesia*, ed 2, Ames, IA, 2011, Blackwell, pp 240–273.

United States Department of Justice: *Practitioner's manual. An informational outline of the Controlled Substances Act, 2023 Edition*, Washington, 2023, United States Department of Justice Drug Enforcement Administration Diversion Control Division.

4

Anesthetic Equipment

LEARNING OBJECTIVES

When you have completed this chapter, you will be able to:

- Identify equipment that is used for anesthetic induction, endotracheal intubation, and anesthetic maintenance.
- Choose and prepare an appropriate endotracheal tube for a dog, cat, horse, or cow.
- List the reasons for and advantages of endotracheal intubation.
- Describe the four basic anesthetic machine systems and identify the parts of each system.
- Describe the basic operation of an anesthetic machine.
- Trace the flow of oxygen through an anesthetic machine and patient breathing circuit for rebreathing and non rebreathing systems.
- Describe the function and use of each component of an anesthetic machine, anesthetic masks, and anesthetic chambers.
- Explain the use of the oxygen supply of an anesthetic machine, including safety concerns associated with compressed gas cylinders.
- Explain the differences between a rebreathing and a nonrebreathing system with regard to equipment, gas flow, advantages, disadvantages, and indications for use.
- Identify the function and use of each component of commonly used rebreathing and nonrebreathing circuits.
- Differentiate between a precision and a nonprecision vaporizer and recognize the rationale for using a precision vaporizer to deliver commonly used halogenated inhalant anesthetics.
- Compare and contrast vaporizer-out-of-circuit (VOC) and vaporizer-in-circuit (VIC) configurations and explain why commonly used halogenated inhalant anesthetics are delivered using a VOC configuration.
- Identify factors that affect anesthetic vaporizer output.
- Explain the impact of oxygen flow rates on anesthetic concentration within the breathing circuit, changes in anesthetic depth, patient safety, and waste gas production.
- List oxygen flow rates for each common domestic species, breathing system, and period of an anesthetic event.
- Compare and contrast full rebreathing, partial rebreathing, minimal rebreathing, and nonrebreathing systems, and explain the rationale for using each.
- Explain the procedure that should be followed to prepare an anesthetic machine for use.
- Describe the proper maintenance procedures for anesthetic machines and associated equipment.

KEY TERMS

Adjustable pressure limiting (APL) valve	Compressed gas cylinders	Oxygen flush valve
Alveolar dead space	Compressed gas supply	Partial rebreathing system
Alveolar ventilation	Dead space	Physiologic dead space
Anatomic dead space	Endotracheal tube	Pressure manometer
Anesthetic chambers	Flowmeter	Pressure-reducing valve
Anesthetic masks	Fresh gas inlet	Rebreathing system
Anesthetic vaporizer	Full rebreathing system	Reservoir bag
APL occlusion valve	Gas exchange	Respiratory minute volume
Asphyxiation	High-pressure alarm	Safety pressure relief valve
Atelectasis	Jackson–Rees circuit	Scavenging system
Ayre's T-piece	Lack circuit	Supraglottic airway device
Bain block (see Universal control arm)	Laryngoscope	Tank pressure gauge
Bain coaxial circuit	Line pressure gauge	Tidal volume (V_T)
Barotrauma	Magill circuit	Unidirectional valves
Breathing circuit	Mapleson classification system	Universal control arm (aka: Bain block)
Breathing tubes	Mechanical dead space	Vaporizer-in-circuit
Carbon dioxide absorber canister	Minimal rebreathing system	Vaporizer-out-of-circuit
Common gas outlet	Nonrebreathing system	
	Norman elbow	

Before the introduction of anesthetic machines, the administration of inhalant anesthetics was a hazardous undertaking. Up until well into the 20th century, liquid anesthetics such as ether or chloroform were administered using open systems ("open cone," "open drop," or chamber) (Fig. 4.1). When these systems were used, control of anesthetic depth was crude at best and the anesthetist was not able to protect the airway, give supplemental oxygen, or assist ventilation. The development of modern anesthetic

equipment in the 1950s and 1960s greatly increased the safety and effectiveness of inhalation anesthesia by allowing the administration of precise concentrations of anesthetic and oxygen under controlled conditions. This chapter describes the purpose, function, use, and maintenance of equipment used to administer inhalant anesthetics, including machines, vaporizers, breathing circuits, endotracheal tubes, masks, and chambers. As anesthetic accidents and complications are frequently associated with

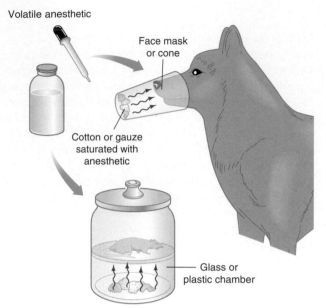

FIG. 4.1 Open systems. With the open cone technique, a mask containing liquid anesthetic-soaked gauze is held over the patient's muzzle until the patient is anesthetized. The position of the mask in relationship to the muzzle is altered to change anesthetic depth. The open drop technique is similar, but liquid anesthetic is dripped onto a cloth held over the patient's nose and mouth. Very small patients are anesthetized by dripping liquid anesthetic onto a cloth placed inside a chamber.

machine and equipment malfunctions and misuse, a comprehensive knowledge of and familiarity with this equipment are essential to the anesthetist's ability to deliver anesthetic gases safely.

ENDOTRACHEAL TUBES AND ASSOCIATED EQUIPMENT

An endotracheal tube (ET tube) is a flexible tube, placed inside the trachea of an anesthetized patient, that is used to transfer anesthetic gases directly from the anesthetic machine into the patient's lungs, bypassing the oral and nasal cavities, pharynx, and larynx. ET tubes are commonly used for patients undergoing general anesthesia because they maintain an open airway; decrease anatomic dead space; allow precise administration of inhalant anesthetics and oxygen; prevent pulmonary aspiration of stomach contents, blood, and other material; enable rapid response to respiratory emergencies; and allow the anesthetist accurately to monitor and control patient respiration. Given these benefits, many veterinarians use ET tubes for most or all patients, even if they are not receiving inhalant anesthetics.

ET tubes are available in several different types and materials and in a wide variety of diameters and lengths. Although the tubes are similar in basic design, this variety in size and type gives the anesthetist the ability to choose a tube uniquely suited to the needs of any particular patient.

There are two basic types of conventional ET tubes. The most commonly used type, Murphy tubes (Fig. 4.2 A, C, D, and E), have a beveled end and a side hole called the *Murphy eye* and may or may not have a cuff (a balloonlike structure on the patient end of the tube). Magill tubes (the second type) lack a side hole.

ET tubes are made of polyvinyl chloride (PVC), red rubber, or silicone. PVC tubes (see Fig. 4.2 C and E) are transparent and

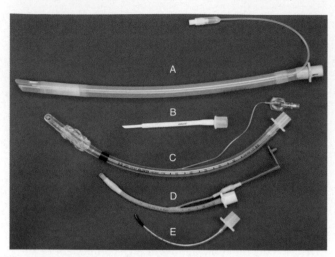

FIG. 4.2 Endotracheal tube type, material, and size comparison. **(A)** Cuffed 11-mm, silicone Murphy tube. **(B)** 2.5-mm Cole tube. **(C)** Cuffed 8-mm polyvinyl chloride (PVC) Murphy tube. **(D)** Cuffed 4-mm red rubber Murphy tube. (E) Uncuffed 2-mm PVC Murphy tube.

are somewhat stiffer than other types. This stiffness minimizes the risk of tube collapse but increases the risk of trauma to the tracheal mucosa during tube placement (referred to as *intubation*), when turning the patient, and during patient transfer. Red rubber tubes (see Fig. 4.2 D) are more flexible and less traumatic but have several disadvantages. They are more prone to kinking or collapse, especially if small. They may absorb disinfectant solutions, resulting in irritation from contact with the patient's oropharynx or trachea, and tend to dry and crack after prolonged use. Specialized tubes, called *spiral* or *anode tubes* (Fig. 4.3), contain a coil of metal or nylon embedded in the wall that is designed to resist kinking or collapse from external pressure.

Silicone tubes (see Fig. 4.2 A), although more expensive, combine strength with pliability and are consequently resistant to collapse and less irritating to tissues than either rubber or vinyl tubes.

ET tubes come in standard lengths. On most, with the exception of very small tubes, a scale printed on the side (Fig. 4.4 F) marks the distance from the patient end in centimeters. Before the tube is placed, this scale can be used to estimate the appropriate distance to advance the tube.

Tube size is most commonly expressed as the internal diameter (ID) in millimeters. The ID of each tube is written on its surface (see Fig. 4.4 G). ET tubes range in size from as small as 1 mm for exotic animals to 30 mm for mature large domestic animals. (See Chapters 9–11 for common sizes used in the common domestic species.)

Endotracheal Tube Parts

The patient end of the tube (see Fig. 4.4 I) is passed through the mouth or nose and into the trachea. The Murphy eye (see Fig. 4.4 J), if present, minimizes the risk of patient asphyxiation in the event that the end hole is blocked with mucus. The machine end (see Fig. 4.4 C) protrudes from the mouth or nose and is connected to the breathing circuit of the anesthetic machine via the connector (see Fig. 4.4 D). If present, the cuff (see Fig. 4.4 H) is inflated to create a seal between the tube and trachea. The cuff is connected via a small tube (the *pilot line*) to

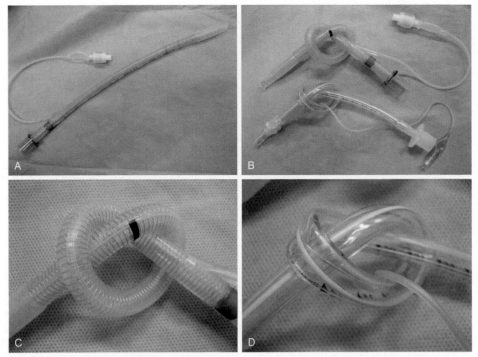

FIG. 4.3 (A) Silicone spiral imbedded tube. **(B)** Comparison of ability of a spiral imbedded tube and a conventional tube to resist kinking when bent. **(C and D)** The spiral imbedded tube remains patent when bent, whereas the conventional tube collapses.

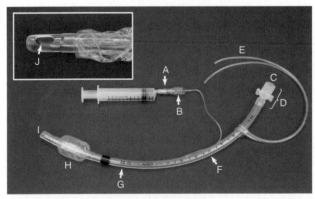

FIG. 4.4 Endotracheal tube parts. **(A)** Valve with syringe attached. **(B)** Pilot balloon. **(C)** Machine end. **(D)** Connector. **(E)** Tie. **(F)** Measurement of length from the patient end (cm). **(G)** Measurement of internal diameter (mm). **(H)** Inflated cuff. **(I)** Patient end. **(J)** Murphy eye.

a pilot balloon (see Fig. 4.4 B) and a valve (see Fig. 4.4 A) that is used to inflate the cuff. The valve opens to permit air to enter or exit the cuff when a syringe is seated firmly in the valve opening and automatically closes when the syringe is removed. The pilot balloon allows the anesthetist to monitor cuff inflation visually or manually.

During the intubation of mammals, use of a cuffed tube should be used whenever possible for the following reasons:

1. The inflated cuff helps prevent leakage of air and gases around the tube and therefore reduces waste gas pollution in the operating room.
2. Use of a cuffed tube minimizes the risk of aspiration of blood, saliva, vomitus, and other material into the lungs.
3. Cuffed tubes prevent the animal from breathing room air, which may otherwise flow around the outside of the tube

and dilute anesthetic gases. Adequate depth of anesthesia is difficult to maintain in animals breathing significant amounts of room air.

ETT cuffs come in two general types. They may be high volume/low pressure or low volume/high pressure (Fig. 4.5). Although either type can be used for short-term intubation, high volume/low pressure cuffs distribute pressure evenly along the entire length of the cuff, whereas low pressure/high volume cuffs tend to exert high pressure on a relatively small area, potentially increasing the risk of damage to the tracheal mucosa.

Despite the advantages of using a cuffed tube, any cuffed tube, whether or not the cuff is high or low pressure, should be used with caution, especially in small patients, because the cuff of the tube may exert significant pressure on the tracheal mucosa and cause local inflammation or necrosis if not appropriately inflated, particularly during long procedures, and in extreme cases, can even cause tracheal rupture. For this reason, tubes without a cuff or with the cuff not inflated are often used in very small patients to minimize the risk of tracheal damage.

The placement and management of ET tubes is reviewed in detail in Chapters 9–11; however, the following points should be noted:

- ET tubes should not bind during placement. Although some materials, such as silicon, are naturally slippery, all tubes should ideally be lubricated with a small amount of sterile commercial water-soluble lubricant, not only to facilitate passage but also to help to create a seal between the cuff and the trachea. If lubricant is not available, water or the patient's saliva may also be used.

- When correctly used, ET tubes reduce anatomic dead space (*see Box 4.1 for a discussion of dead space*). For this to be

Text continued on page 114

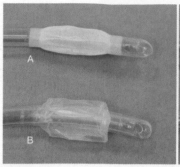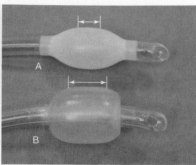

FIG. 4.5 Endotracheal tube cuff types (deflated-left and fully inflated-right). **(A)** Low volume/high pressure cuff. This cuff holds a relatively small volume of air and the pressure exerted on the trachea is concentrated over a relatively small surface area *(see double-ended arrow on top)*. **(B)** High volume/low pressure cuff. Note that this cuff holds a relatively large volume of air but distributes the pressure over a larger surface area than a low volume/high pressure cuff *(see double-ended arrow on bottom)*.

BOX 4.1   The Concept of Dead Space

During anesthesia, effective ventilation is required to supply the cells of the body with oxygen and to remove carbon dioxide. During inhalation, oxygen travels from its source (the inspiratory tube of a rebreathing circuit or the fresh gas inlet of a non rebreathing circuit) to the alveoli, where gas exchange occurs. Oxygen diffuses from the alveoli into the capillaries and is exchanged with carbon dioxide, which diffuses from the capillaries into the alveoli. Carbon dioxide is then removed from the body during exhalation. Dead space refers to the equipment tubes, bronchi, and other spaces through which these gases travel but in which no gas exchange occurs. The patient's tidal volume must be considerably more than the dead space volume in order for oxygen and anesthetic gas to reach the alveoli and for carbon dioxide to be eliminated, and thus prevent oxygen deprivation or carbon dioxide toxicity.

Types of Dead Space

There are three sources of dead space: anatomic, alveolar, and mechanical. Anatomic dead space refers to the respiratory passages in the animal's body through which the gases move (including the bronchi, trachea, larynx, pharynx, and nasal cavity). Alveolar dead space refers to alveoli that are inadequately perfused with pulmonary blood and therefore do not participate in gas exchange. Together, anatomic and alveolar dead space comprise physiologic dead space, which represents the total volume of dead space in the body.

Mechanical dead space refers to parts of the anesthetic equipment through which the gases travel from the oxygen source to the patient's body. This includes the length of the ETT that extends beyond the incisors, the ET tube connector, the Y-piece of a rebreathing circuit, swivel and right-angle adapters, spacers or probes for respiratory monitors, heat and moisture exchangers, the terminal end of a Universal F circuit or nonrebreathing circuit, and the volume within a face mask. Mechanical dead space can be considerable and can significantly reduce gases available for exchange, especially in smaller patients. Said another way, when more dead space is present, less oxygen is available to the body and less carbon dioxide is eliminated. At a certain point, this will lead to hypoxemia and difficulty keeping the patient anesthetized if inhalant anesthetics are used, and rebreathing of carbon dioxide and resulting hypercarbia. Therefore the anesthetist must strive to keep dead space to a minimum in every patient, especially those that are small.

The volume of gas available for exchange in the alveoli in a typical patient may be estimated based on the patient's body weight, although it is important to realize that several factors may influence the volume in any given animal including body condition score, respiratory rate and depth, degree of respiratory depression, and disease factors.

In an average patient, when awake, normal tidal volume is estimated to be approximately 10–15 mL/kg. In a normal nonanesthetized patient, physiologic dead space makes up approximately one-third of the patient tidal volume (~3.5–5 mL/kg), leaving approximately two-thirds of the gas available for exchange (~6.5–10 mL/kg). During anesthesia, tidal volume decreases by approximately 30% (to ~7–10.5 mL/kg), but physiologic dead space stays the same. This leaves only approximately one-half of inhaled air (~3.5–5 mL/kg) available for alveolar ventilation (the volume of air that makes it to the alveoli for exchange). Therefore the volume of gas left for gas exchange may become dangerously low if mechanical dead space becomes excessive.

Recommendations of the AAHA Anesthesia and Monitoring Guidelines for Dogs and Cats and the AAFP Feline Anesthesia Guidelines are that mechanical dead space should not exceed 2–3 mL/kg (~20% of normal tidal volume).

Terms and Definitions Relating to Dead Space

Tidal volume:	The total volume of gas inhaled during a normal breath.
Gas exchange:	The diffusion of oxygen from the alveoli to the blood and carbon dioxide from the blood to the alveoli during ventilation.
Dead space:	Equipment, tubes, bronchi, and other spaces through which inhaled and exhaled gases travel, but in which no gas exchange occurs. In these areas, airflow is bidirectional (it travels toward the alveoli during inspiration and away from the alveoli during expiration). Consists of the sum total of anatomic dead space, alveolar dead space, and mechanical dead space.
Anatomic dead space:	Dead space in anatomic structures such as the nose, pharynx, larynx, trachea, and bronchi through which inhaled air travels on its way to the alveoli. *(Note that the endotracheal tube extending from the patient end of the tube to the point even with the patient's incisors is considered part of anatomic dead space because it is occupying space through which oxygen would normally travel in the animal's body [the trachea, larynx, pharynx, and oral cavity]).*
Alveolar dead space:	Dead space in alveoli that are inadequately perfused with pulmonary blood and therefore in which no gas exchange occurs.
Physiologic dead space:	Spaces within the body through which inhaled and exhaled gases travel but in which no gas exchange occurs. In these areas, airflow is bidirectional (it travels toward the alveoli during inspiration and away from the alveoli during expiration). The sum total of anatomic dead space and alveolar dead space.

BOX 4.1 The Concept of Dead Space—cont'd

Mechanical dead space: Dead space in equipment such as the Y-piece, ETT connector, portion of the ETT extending beyond the incisors, respiratory monitor adaptors, moisture and heat exchangers, right angle adaptors, and the patient connector of nonrebreathing circuits.

Alveolar ventilation: The portion of the tidal volume that travels from the source of fresh gas to the alveoli and that participates in gas exchange.

Source of fresh gas: The point at which fresh gas enters an area occupied by dead space: (1), the patient end of the inspiratory tube of a rebreathing circuit; (2), the fresh gas inlet of a nonrebreathing circuit; or (3), the nostrils or mouth of a nonanesthetized patient.

For more information on dead space, the reader is directed to the following article: Stein B, Wilson, D: Veterinary anesthesia and analgesia support group: dead space-cause, effect, & management basics, 2005. Available from https:// www.vasg.org/dead_space.htm. Accessed March 25, 2022.

Mechanical Dead Space of Anesthetic Equipment

Note that mechanical dead space associated with each piece of equipment will vary among manufacturers depending on the details of design. It cannot be assumed that dead space in equipment designed for pediatric use is always less than that of equipment designed for adult use, so it is incumbent on the anesthetist to determine dead space prior to choosing equipment. The volumes listed in association with Figs. 1–3 are examples of measurements for commonly used equipment.

Mechanical Dead Space Typically Associated With Rebreathing Circuits (Fig. 1):

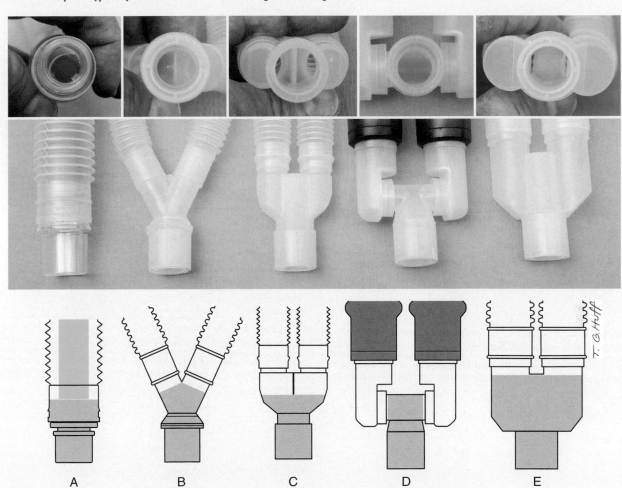

A   B   C   D   E

(Note: The pink area on each diagram delineates mechanical dead space.)

Rebreathing Circuit	Dead Space
Universal F-circuit (see Fig. 1A):	Typically 8–15 mL
Pediatric Y-piece/patient connector:	Typically 5–6 mL
Fig. 1B = pediatric Y-piece:	~6 mL
Fig. 1C = pediatric patient connector with septum	~5 mL
Adult Y-piece/patient connector:	(May vary from 5 to 15 mL or more)
Fig. 1D = adult swivel-type patient connector	~5 mL
Fig. 1E = adult patient connector without septum	15–18 mL

Continued

BOX 4.1   The Concept of Dead Space—cont'd

Mechanical Dead Space Typically Associated With Nonrebreathing Circuits (Fig. 2):

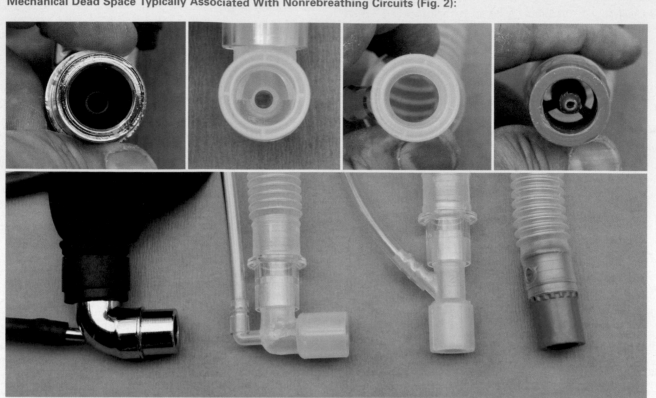

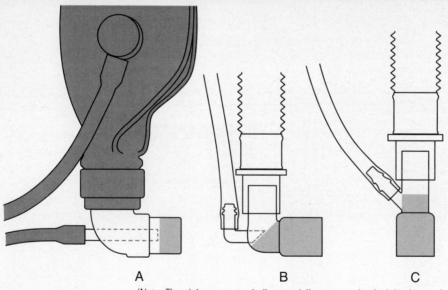

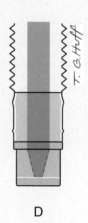

A	B	C	D

(Note: The pink area on each diagram delineates mechanical dead space.)

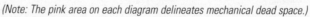

Nonrebreathing Circuit	Dead Space
Modified Norman elbow (see Fig. 2A):	Typically 1–2 mL
Modified Jackson-Rees or Ayre's T-piece (see Fig. 2B and C):	Typically 3–5 mL
Bain coaxial (see Fig. 2D):	Typically 1–4 mL

BOX 4.1 The Concept of Dead Space—cont'd

Mechanical Dead Space Typically Associated with Monitor Spacers and Misc. Equipment (Fig. 3)

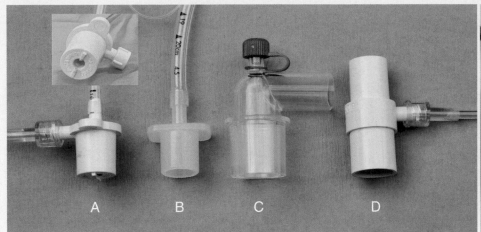
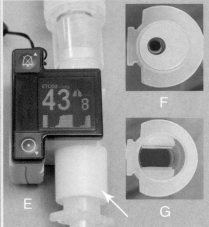

Monitor Spacers and Misc. Equipment:	Dead Space:
Sidestream ETco$_2$ dead space reducer/ETT connector (see Fig. 3A):	Typically ~ 0.5–2 mL
Traditional endotracheal tube connector (see Fig. 3B):	Typically ~2 mL
4 mm ETT: dead space/cm extending beyond incisors:	~0.1 mL/cm
11 mm ETT: dead space/cm extending beyond incisors:	~1 mL/cm
Elbow connector (see Fig. 3C):	Typically ~7–8 mL
Side-stream ETco$_2$ spacer (see Fig. 3D):	Typically ~5 mL
Mainstream capnograph (see Fig. 3E): *(arrow pointing to interchangeable adult chamber)*	
Pediatric chamber (see Fig. 3F): *(view from open end)*	Typically ~ 1–2 mL
Adult chamber (see Fig. 3G) *(view from open end)*	Typically ~7–8 mL

Comparison of the Effects of Low Mechanical Dead Space Versus Excessive Mechanical Dead Space on Patient Well-Being

The following scenarios illustrate a comparison of the effect on an anesthetized patient of mechanical dead space that is within the recommended allowable amount versus mechanical dead space that is excessive. The scenarios are based on a 3-kg (6.6-lb) cat receiving general anesthesia that is induced with an IV anesthetic and intubated with a 4.0 mm Murphy endotracheal tube prior to being maintained with inhalant anesthetic. This patient is assumed to have a tidal volume, physiologic dead space, and alveolar ventilation typical of an anesthetized patient as previously discussed.

Although these scenarios represent an extreme comparison, excessive dead space, even if it does not exceed the patient's V$_T$, will lead to hypoxemia and rebreathing of carbon dioxide-a situation, which, at the least, compromises patient wellbeing, and at worst, endangers the patient. Therefore in all anesthetized patients, dead space must be carefully considered, and equipment must be chosen that keeps mechanical dead space to a minimum, especially in very small patients.

Continued

BOX 4.1 The Concept of Dead Space—cont'd

Scenario #1: the Effects of Low Mechanical Dead Space

In Scenario #1, the ETT is connected to a modified Norman elbow nonrebreathing circuit by a low dead space sidestream capnograph spacer/ETT connector instead of a conventional ETT connector (see Fig. 4).

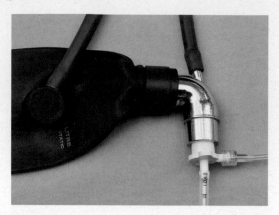

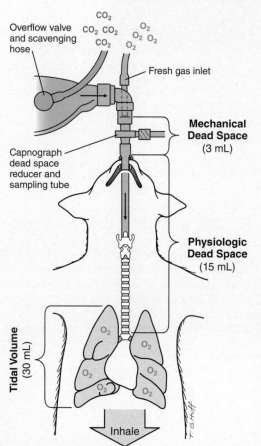

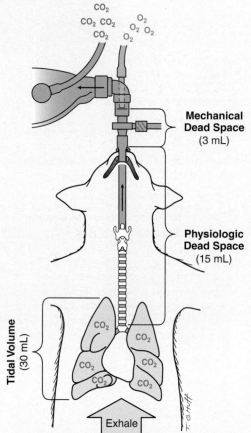

Using this equipment, assumptions are as follows:

Maximum anticipated tidal volume (V_T) during anesthesia: ~30 mL (10 mL/kg)

Physiologic dead space: ~15 mL (~½ of the V_T)

Mechanical dead space using this equipment: ~3 mL total (~½ of the recommended maximum of 6 mL [or 20% of V_T]):
- Norman elbow connector: ~1.5 mL
- Capnograph dead-space reducer/ETT connector: ~1.5 mL

Total dead space (physiologic and mechanical): ~18 mL (15 mL + 3 mL)

Alveolar ventilation (air available for exchange): 12 mL (30 mL V_T minus 18 mL dead space).

In this scenario, mechanical dead space is approximately one-half the recommended allowable maximum of 2–3 mL/kg, and the tidal volume is significantly higher than the total dead space volume. Consequently, during inhalation, fresh oxygen from the fresh gas inlet reaches the alveoli and during exhalation, carbon dioxide reaches the breathing bag, where it will be forced out of the overflow valve by fresh gas flow during the pause between exhalation and the next inhalation. Therefore, as long as recommended fresh gas flow is used, the exchange of oxygen and carbon dioxide is adequate for this patient's needs.

BOX 4.1   The Concept of Dead Space—cont'd

Scenario #2: the Effects of Excessive Mechanical Dead Space
In Scenario #2, the ETT is connected to the Y-piece of a rebreathing circuit with pediatric breathing tubes, with a conventional sidestream capnograph spacer and an elbow connector in between *(see Fig. 5)*.

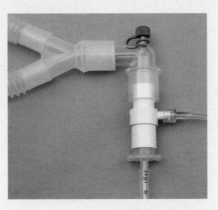

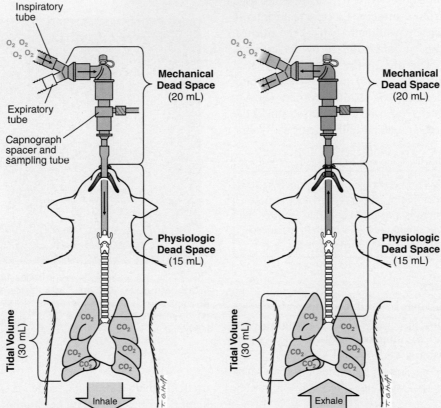

Using this equipment, assumptions are as follows:
Anticipated tidal volume (V_T) during anesthesia: ~30 mL (10 mL/kg)
   Physiologic dead space: ~15 mL (~½ of the V_T)
   Mechanical dead space using this equipment: ~20 mL total (over three times the recommended maximum of 6 mL [or 20% of V_T]):
   • Pediatric Y-piece: ~6 mL
   • Elbow connector: ~7 mL
   • Side-stream capnograph spacer: ~5 mL
   • Endotracheal tube connector: ~2 mL
   Total dead space (physiologic and mechanical): ~35 mL (15 mL + 20 mL, which is more than the patient V_T)
Alveolar ventilation (air available for exchange): None—because dead space volume exceeds tidal volume by ~5 mL (35 mL dead space minus 30 mL V_T).

In this scenario, tidal volume is insufficient to overcome the excess mechanical dead space associated with this combination of equipment. Consequently, during inhalation, V_T is insufficient to draw fresh gas into the alveoli, and during exhalation, V_T is insufficient to move exhaled carbon dioxide to the exit point (the opening of the expiratory breathing tube). This results in a "shuttle effect" in which oxygenated fresh gas is shuttled from the inspiratory breathing tube to the distal large airways during inhalation and back to the expiratory tube during exhalation, whereas carbon dioxide is shuttled from the alveoli to approximately the level of the elbow connector during exhalation and back to the lungs during the subsequent inhalation. In this situation, no fresh oxygen reaches the alveoli and carbon dioxide is rebreathed. This will result in an anesthetic fatality within minutes of attaching the patient to the breathing circuit.

achieved, the ET tube should be no longer than the distance between the most rostral aspect of the mouth and the thoracic inlet. If longer, there are two possible risks. First, if the tube extends an excessive distance inside the trachea, the patient end may enter one mainstem bronchus. Only one lung will then be supplied with oxygen and anesthetic gas, leading to hypoventilation, hypoxemia, and possibly difficulty keeping the patient anesthetized. Second, if the tube extends beyond the rostral aspect of the mouth, it will increase mechanical dead space, resulting in hypoventilation, especially in small patients. A guideline is that if the tube is more than 2.5 cm longer than the distance between the most rostral aspect of the mouth and the thoracic inlet, it is too long and should be cut shorter or replaced with a shorter tube. To cut the tube, remove the ETT connector, use a sharp box cutter blade to cut off an appropriate length of the machine end of the tube, taking care to avoid the pilot line, and then firmly reattach the connector.

- Special cautions must be observed when ET tubes are used in conjunction with laser surgery. Lasers create intense heat; in a high-oxygen environment such as the trachea, there is a risk of fire and if compromised by the laser, the ET tube may ignite. The anesthetist should use special laser-resistant tubes or adapt regular tubes by wrapping them with US Food and Drug Administration (FDA)–approved materials. It may also be advisable to shield the tube with saline-soaked sponges and fill the cuff with saline instead of air.

> **TECHNICIAN NOTE** The ET tube should be no longer than the distance between the most rostral aspect of the mouth and the thoracic inlet. If longer, there is a risk that only one lung will be supplied with oxygen and anesthetic gas or that mechanical dead space will be increased, leading to hypoxemia.

Endotracheal Tube Ties

A wide variety of materials may be used to secure endotracheal tubes including roll gauze, cut lengths of IV administration set tubing, shoelaces, and commercial products (Fig. 4.6). It is important that the material selected will securely hold the tube when wet without constricting the lumen, and that it is either disposable or can be easily and effectively disinfected between uses.

Laryngoscopes

A laryngoscope is a device used to increase visibility of the larynx while placing an ET tube. Laryngoscopes have a handle, a blade, and a light source. The handle contains batteries to power the light source, the blade is used to depress the tongue below the epiglottis, and the light source illuminates the throat (Fig. 4.7). Small-animal blades are available in many sizes, ranging from 0 (small) to 5 (large). Custom large-animal blades up to 18 inches in length are available for use in swine, small ruminants, camelids, and some exotics. Miller blades are straight (see Fig. 4.7 A and C), and McIntosh blades are curved (see Fig. 4.7 B and D). Laryngoscopes are often

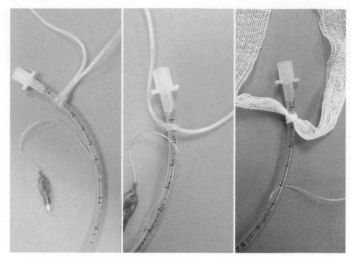

FIG. 4.6 Endotracheal tube ties: IV administration set tubing tied with a lark's head knot (left) and single throw (center); and roll gauze tied with a single throw (right).

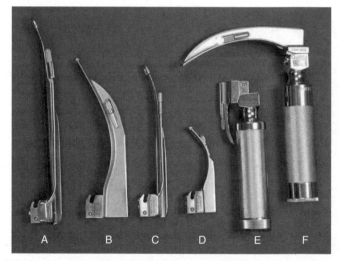

FIG. 4.7 Laryngoscope handles and blades. **(A)** Size 4 Miller blade. **(B)** Size 4 McIntosh blade. **(C)** Size 2 Miller blade. **(D)** Size 1 McIntosh blade. **(E)** Laryngoscope handle with size 00 Miller blade in unlocked position. **(F)** Laryngoscope handle with size 3 McIntosh blade in locked position (note that the light turns on when the blade is locked).

used in small ruminants, camelids, and swine and may be helpful in dogs and cats. They are not generally used in adult cattle, which are intubated by digital palpation, and horses, which are intubated blindly.

Endotracheal Tube Cuff Pressure Manometers

After placing a conventional cuffed ET tube, it is very important that the cuff be inflated to a level that will ensure a tight seal but that will not damage the trachea from application of excessive pressure to the tracheal wall. An inadequate seal increases the risk of pulmonary aspiration secondary to regurgitation or reflux of gastric fluids, increases pollution of the surgery suite with waste anesthetic gases, and may make it more difficult to keep the patient at an appropriate plane of anesthesia. Excessive inflation can cause decreased blood perfusion of the tracheal

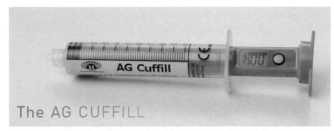

FIG. 4.8 Anapnoguard (AG) Cuffill Device.(Courtesy Hospitech Respiration Ltd.; https://www.cuffill.com/.)

FIG. 4.9 Safe-Seal endotracheal tube.(Courtesy Jorgensen Labs; https://jorvet.com/product/safe-seal-endotracheal-tube/.)

mucosa, necrosis of the tracheal wall, or in an extreme case, tracheal wall rupture.

In general, the cuff pressure in small and large animals should be in the range of 18 to 20 cm of H_2O *(note that the AAFP Feline Anesthesia Guidelines recommends 16 to 18 cm of H_2O for cats)*. Most methods of determining the appropriate amount of air to place in the cuff (such as palpating the pilot balloon or inflation of the cuff until leakage can no longer be heard are not always accurate indicators of appropriate cuff pressure and are subject to variations in operator technique. An alternative technique that more accurately assesses inflation is direct measurement of cuff pressure using a manometer (a device used to measure pressure). A variety of products are available for this purpose including the Posey Cufflator (TIDI Products, LLC, Neenah, WI) and the TLF Cuff (ICST Corporation, Saitama, Japan). The Anapnoguard (AG) Cuffill Device (Hospitech Respiration Ltd., Petah Tikva, Israel) (Fig. 4.8) is one example of several less expensive alternatives that can be used to guide the anesthetist in determining an appropriate level of cuff inflation. Regardless of the method used to determine appropriate cuff inflation, the anesthetist must endeavor to achieve as close to the target inflation pressure as possible and recheck the pressure frequently throughout the procedure in order to protect the well-being of the patient.

ALTERNATIVES TO CONVENTIONAL ENDOTRACHEAL TUBES

Cole Tubes

Cole tubes (see Fig. 4.2 B) have no cuff or side hole but are designed with an abrupt decrease in diameter near the patient end of the tube. Cole tubes are used for species that have complete tracheal rings such as birds and some reptiles to prevent damage to the trachea that would be caused by a cuffed tube. A seal is created by seating the neck of the tube (the point of transition between the larger- and smaller-diameter portions of the tube) at the tracheal opening.

Safe-Seal Endotracheal Tubes

The Safe-Seal Endotracheal Tube (Jorgensen Labs, Loveland, CO) (Fig. 4.9) is a proprietary silicone tube that is designed with six baffles that replace a conventional cuff for the purpose of creating a seal with the wall of the trachea. Safe-Seal tubes come in several sizes for dogs within a specific weight range (e.g., 7 to

25 lb (short and long), 26 to 60 lb, 40 to 60 lb, 61 to 200+ lb) and one size for small dogs and cats 4 to 12 lb in body weight. Each tube has a collar near the machine end that can be used to secure the tube. Some reported advantages of this tube are (1) the flexibility of the baffles allows the release of airway pressure over 20 to 30 cm H_2O, thus reducing the risk of barotrauma in the event that excess pressure builds up in the breathing circuit; (2) less trauma to the tracheal mucosa due to the limited area of contact with the baffles; and (3) a sweeping motion created by the baffles that helps carry liquids out of the trachea during extubation. Because there are not as many size options as there are for Murphy and Magill tubes, resistance to breathing may be higher for some animals, especially those at the higher end of each weight range, and dead space may be greater in some patients due to an inability to cut the tubes to length. In any case, these tubes offer an alternative to conventional cuffed tubes, which may be desirable under some circumstances.

Supraglottic Airway Devices

A supraglottic airway device (SGAD) (also known as laryngeal mask airway or LMA) is a device used to maintain an open airway in an anesthetized patient that connects with the opening of the glottis and thus unlike a conventional ET tube, allows the anesthetist to manage the airway without invading the tracheal lumen. SGADs have been used for many years in human patients but have relatively recently become available in the veterinary market. Although significantly more expensive than conventional ET tubes, SGADs have several reported advantages, including the decreased likelihood of laryngospasm, decreased resistance to breathing due to maintenance of a large airway channel, decreased risk of airway trauma during intubation, and no postoperative coughing and other effects related to tracheal irritation. As with a conventional ET tube, the anesthetist must follow a prescribed set of steps to ensure proper placement. A tight seal between the SGAD and the patient's airway is confirmed by observing a normal waveform on a capnograph (carbon dioxide monitor). SGADs offer an alternative to conventional ET tubes in species such as the cat and rabbit, in which endotracheal intubation is challenging and often results in a higher incidence of complications.

The v-gel ADVANCED Cat, v-gel ADVANCED Rabbit (Fig. 4.10), and v-gel ADVANCED Dog (docsinnovent) are veterinary-specific SGADs for cats, rabbits, and dogs, respectively, available in several sizes for each species. The v-gel

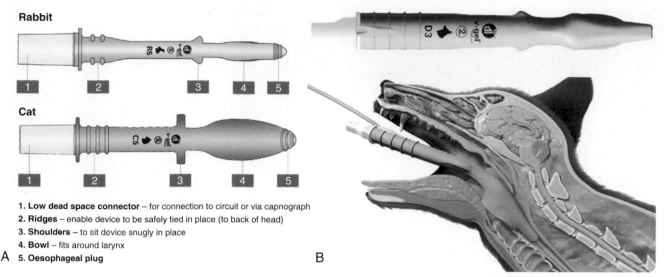

Rabbit

Cat

1. **Low dead space connector** – for connection to circuit or via capnograph
2. **Ridges** – enable device to be safely tied in place (to back of head)
3. **Shoulders** – to sit device snugly in place
4. **Bowl** – fits around larynx
5. **Oesophageal plug**

A   B

FIG. 4.10 (A) Key features of v-gel ADVANCED Rabbit *(top)* and v-gel Advanced Cat *(bottom)* supraglottic airway device (SGAD). **(B)** Anatomical cutaway of dog showing position of v-gel when properly placed over the glottis. (Courtesy Docsinnovent Ltd; www.docsinnovent.com.)

ADVANCED has an enlarged patient end designed to create a seal around the opening of the larynx and concurrently seal the opening of the esophagus to prevent gastric reflux. In 2020, v-gel ADVANCED Cat and Rabbit replaced the original v-gel products that were available from 2012 to 2020. Although both products are similar, the new products have several improvements designed to improve the fit and seal and simplify placement. They are also designed for single use as opposed to multiple use as was the case with the original product. The v-gel ADVANCED Dog was introduced in March 2022.

The manufacturer of v-gel ADVANCED also makes a device known as the d-grip flexible circuit support, designed to hold breathing circuits and monitoring devices in the precise positions necessary to protect the patient airway and ensure a tight seal, which is key to correct and safe function of the v-gel ADVANCED. Because SGADs may dislodge and compromise the airway, especially when moving the patient, capnography should be used to monitor the patient continuously during any procedure in which an SGAD is used. Detailed information about v-gel and d-grip devices, including training information and videos, can be found on the manufacturer's website (https://docsinnovent.com/).

ANESTHETIC MASKS

Anesthetic masks are cone-shaped devices used to administer oxygen and anesthetic gases to nonintubated patients via the nose and mouth (Fig. 4.11). Masks may be used for both anesthetic induction and maintenance and are often used exclusively to administer anesthetic gases to very small patients such as birds, rats, mice, and other laboratory and exotic species in which intubation is difficult. They may also be used to administer pure oxygen to dyspneic, hypoxic, or other critically ill patients requiring supplemental oxygen.

Masks are usually made of plastic or rubber and come in a variety of diameters and lengths. They have a rubber gasket over the open end, designed to create a seal around the patient's muzzle.

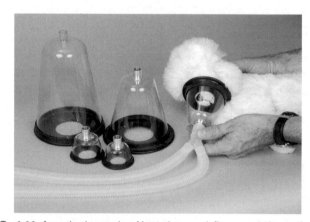

FIG. 4.11 Anesthetic masks. Note the good fit around the patient's muzzle to minimize leakage.

Masks allow the anesthetist to administer oxygen rapidly to a fully conscious patient, sedated patient, or anesthetized patient that cannot be intubated or in which tube placement is delayed. Masks have several disadvantages, however. They do not maintain an open airway as ET tubes do, so airway obstruction is possible, particularly in brachycephalic animals and other patients prone to obstruction. There is no protection against pulmonary aspiration as there is with a tube, nor is the anesthetist able to ventilate the patient when necessary. The technique for mask induction is described and illustrated in Procedure 9.4, Chapter 9.

ANESTHETIC CHAMBERS

Anesthetic chambers are clear, aquarium-like boxes used to induce general anesthesia in small patients that are feral, vicious, or intractable, or that cannot be handled without undue stress (see Fig. 9.7, Chapter 9).

They are often made of acrylic or Perspex, and have a removable top with two ports, one of which serves as a fresh gas source and the other which allows exit of waste gas.

Chambers are very useful for any patient that would be a danger to the anesthetist or itself if physically restrained. They prevent close monitoring of the patient, however, thus necessitating extreme care when patients are anesthetized using this method. The technique for chamber induction is described in Procedure 9.5.

ANESTHETIC MACHINES

The primary function of any anesthetic machine is to deliver precise amounts of oxygen and volatile anesthetic under controlled conditions to patients undergoing general anesthesia. Over the course of a career, the veterinary technician or nurse will likely encounter a wide variety of machines in terms of brand, age, size, and sophistication (Fig. 4.12). For example, machines in common use may be new or more than 30 years old. New anesthetic machines can cost from $2000 to $5000 for a basic model to more than $100,000 for a machine with state-of-the-art features such as built-in monitors and multiple vaporizers. Despite this diversity, all machines have the same basic design, which has changed surprisingly little over the past several decades, and principles of operation which are universal. Underlying these similarities, however, is an inherent complexity which may result in anesthetic accidents if not thoroughly understood. So the technician or nurse must devote much study and practice to achieving the mastery required to use an anesthetic machine safely.

The basic principle of operation of any anesthetic machine can be described as follows. A liquid anesthetic (such as isoflurane or sevoflurane) is vaporized in a carrier gas (oxygen with or without medical air or nitrous oxide), which delivers the anesthetic to the patient via a breathing circuit. To achieve this result, the anesthetic machine and breathing circuit must perform several important functions:

- The carrier gases must be delivered at a controlled flow rate. Oxygen (O_2) is the primary carrier gas used in all anesthetic machines.

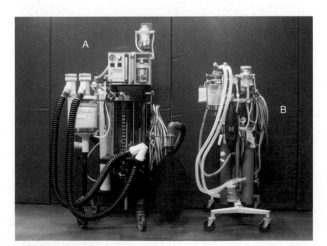

FIG. 4.12 Comparison of large-animal and small-animal anesthetic machines. (A) Large-animal machine with precision isoflurane and sevoflurane vaporizers, a built-in ventilator, and a 30-L reservoir bag. (B) Small-animal machine with an isoflurane precision vaporizer and a 5-L reservoir bag. This picture illustrates differences in size and sophistication among anesthetic machines.

- A precise concentration of liquid inhalant anesthetic (most commonly isoflurane or sevoflurane) must be vaporized, mixed with the carrier gases, and delivered to the patient.
- Exhaled gases containing carbon dioxide (CO_2) must be moved away from the patient and either removed through a scavenging system or recirculated to the patient. If the gases are recirculated, the machine must remove the CO_2 before returning them to the patient.

Anesthetic machines are used not only for inhalation anesthesia but also as a means of delivering oxygen to critically ill patients. In these situations, the vaporizer (i.e., the anesthetic source) is turned off and the breathing circuit is used to deliver oxygen directly to the patient via an ET tube or a mask held over the patient's muzzle.

COMPONENTS OF THE ANESTHETIC MACHINE

The anesthetic machine consists of four distinct systems that can best be understood by following the flow of gases from the oxygen source to the vaporizer, through the breathing circuit to the patient, and finally to the scavenging system (Figs. 4.13 and 4.14).

- The compressed gas supply supplies carrier gases (oxygen and sometimes medical air or nitrous oxide) (Fig. 4.15 A).
- The anesthetic vaporizer (see Fig. 4.15 B) vaporizes liquid inhalant anesthetic and mixes it with the carrier gases. Vaporizers are classified as precision or nonprecision, and vaporizer-out-of-circuit (VOC) or vaporizer-in-circuit (VIC).
- The breathing circuit conveys the carrier gases and inhalant anesthetic to the patient and removes exhaled carbon dioxide. Breathing circuits are classified as rebreathing circuits or nonrebreathing circuits (see Fig. 4.15 C).
- The scavenging system disposes of excess and waste anesthetic gases (see Chapter 5 for a detailed discussion of scavenging systems).

The parts of each system are listed in Box 4.2.

Anesthetic machines can be configured in several ways. They may have either a precision or a nonprecision vaporizer and may be fitted with a rebreathing or nonrebreathing circuit. The most common machine configuration, used for all but the smallest patients, is one with a precision vaporizer and a rebreathing circuit (see Fig. 4.15). A machine configured with a precision vaporizer and a nonrebreathing circuit is used for patients under 3 kg and may be used for patients up to 7 kg in body weight (Fig. 4.16).

Compressed Gas Supply

Oxygen is necessary to sustain normal cellular metabolism and must be continuously supplied to every patient throughout anesthesia. Room air has an oxygen concentration of about 21%. In a healthy, conscious patient breathing room air with 21% oxygen, the approximate concentration in the alveolus is 13%, in arterial blood 12%, in capillary blood at tissue level 5%, and in the tissues only 2%.

Anesthetized patients breathing room air often have lower tissue oxygen concentrations because most anesthetics decrease both the respiratory rate and tidal volume (VT). Consequently, the total volume of inspired oxygen is lower. It is therefore desirable to increase the concentration of oxygen in inspired air to at least 30% to

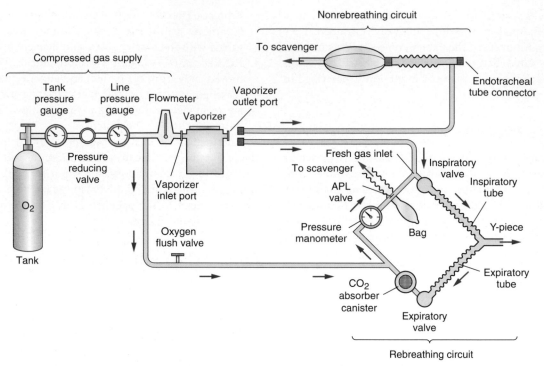

FIG. 4.13 Schematic of an anesthetic machine without a common gas outlet, configured with a vaporizer-out-of-circuit (VOC) precision vaporizer. Both rebreathing and nonrebreathing circuits are illustrated.

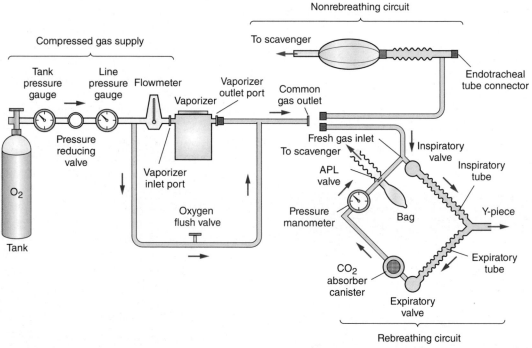

FIG. 4.14 Schematic of an anesthetic machine with a common gas outlet, configured with a vaporizer-out-of-circuit (VOC) precision vaporizer. Both rebreathing and nonrebreathing circuits are illustrated.

compensate for this decrease. Anesthetic machines are designed to provide up to 100% oxygen, thus fulfilling this requirement.

Note that the oxygen has a second function. Not only does it meet metabolic requirements, but it also passes through the vaporizer and carries vaporized anesthetic to the patient. Therefore no anesthetic is delivered to the patient unless oxygen is present to act as a carrier gas.

Compressed Gas Cylinders

Description and function. Compressed gas cylinders (also called "tanks") contain a large volume of carrier gas in a highly pressurized state (as much as 2200 psi or 15,000 kilopascals [kPa]). This enables large amounts of gas to be stored in a space small enough to be of practical use. Oxygen, nitrous oxide, and medical air are three gases used for anesthesia that are stored in compressed

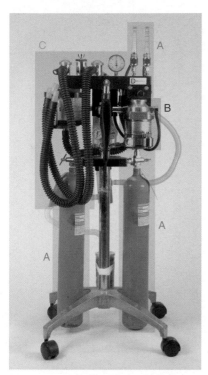

FIG. 4.15 Anesthetic machine systems. *A*, Compressed gas supply: note the two size E compressed gas oxygen cylinders beside the *A*'s at the bottom of this image. *B*, Precision anesthetic vaporizer. *C*, Breathing circuit. Note that the scavenging system (see Fig. 5.1) is not visible in this view.

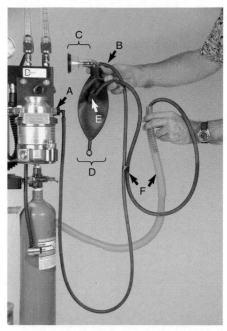

FIG. 4.16 Parts of a nonrebreathing circuit. **(A)** Outlet port of the vaporizer with keyed fitting. **(B)** Fresh gas inlet. **(C)** Connector with mask attached. **(D)** Reservoir bag. **(E)** Pressure relief valve. **(F)** Scavenging hose.

BOX 4.2   Parts of Anesthetic Machine Systems

A. Compressed gas supply
  Compressed gas cylinders
  Tank pressure gauge
  Pressure-reducing valve
  Line-pressure gauge
  Flowmeter(s)
  Oxygen flush valve
B. Anesthetic vaporizer
  Vaporizer inlet port
  Vaporizer outlet port and common gas outlet
C. Breathing circuit—rebreathing (R) or nonrebreathing (N-R)
  Fresh gas inlet (R and N-R)
  Unidirectional valves (R only)
  Adjustable pressure limiting (APL) valve (R and N-R if so equipped) or overflow valve (N-R)
  Reservoir bag (R and N-R)
  Carbon dioxide absorber canister (R only)
  Pressure manometer (R and N-R if so equipped)
  Air intake valve (R only)
  Breathing tubes and Y-piece (R) or corrugated tube (N-R)
D. Scavenging system
  Waste gas port
  Transfer tubing
  Interface
  Gas evacuation system

gas cylinders. Nitrous oxide is a carrier gas that although used in the past in conjunction with older inhalant anesthetics, is seldom used in the current practice of anesthesia. Although medical air is not commonly used in veterinary anesthesia, it is mixed with oxygen in human patients to provide an optimal concentration of oxygen in the breathing circuit. Therefore when using a machine originally manufactured for human use, a medical air flowmeter, yoke, and/or quick-release connector may be present. In contrast to nitrous oxide and medical air, oxygen is used for all anesthetic procedures involving inhalant anesthetics and therefore will be the focus of the discussion that follows.

In the United States (US) and Canada, compressed gas cylinders most commonly used are either small (E tanks, which are 26 inches × 4.5 inches) (Fig. 4.17 B) or large (H tanks, which are 51 inches × 9.25 inches) (see Fig. 4.17 A). K tanks, which are very similar to and equal in capacity and size to an H tank may also be encountered. In the United Kingdom (UK), and the European Union (EU), E (34 inches × 4 inches, but of similar capacity to E tanks used in North America), F (36 inches × 5.5 inches with approximately twice the capacity of an E tank), and J (56.5 inches × 9 inches and similar in capacity to H tanks) are more commonly used. In many hospitals, H, J, or K tanks are the primary source of oxygen, and E tanks are used as a backup supply. In locations where piped-in gas is unavailable, E tanks may be used as both the primary and the secondary supplies.

The specific tank types differ not only in size but also in the valve type. Each valve has a specific way it opens and a specific attachment to the pressure regulator that prevents the wrong gas type (oxygen, nitrous oxide, medical air, etc.) from being attached to the yoke or distribution system.

E tanks supply gas by direct attachment to the yoke of an anesthetic machine and may be stored on a cart when not in use

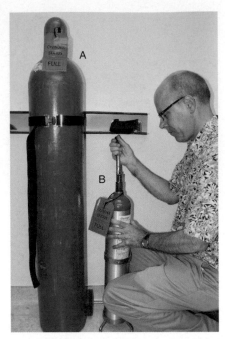

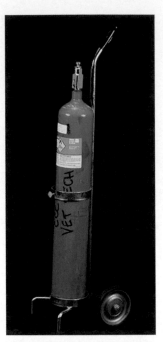

FIG. 4.17 (A) Size H compressed gas cylinder. **(B)** Size E compressed gas cylinder.

FIG. 4.18 E tank in a cart, which is used to store or transport the tank safely.

(Fig. 4.18) or in a rack (Fig. 5.11, Chapter 5). When attached to a machine, gas is conveyed by the yoke directly to a pressure-reducing valve.

H, K, and J tanks, which are considerably larger than E tanks, are usually stored on a cart or chained to the wall and supply gas via a distribution system of intermediate-pressure gas lines that carry gas throughout the hospital. The gas distribution system with large tanks is usually in the form of a cylinder manifold (Fig. 4.19) consisting of two banks of two or more cylinders, one of which is used as the primary source and the

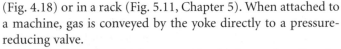

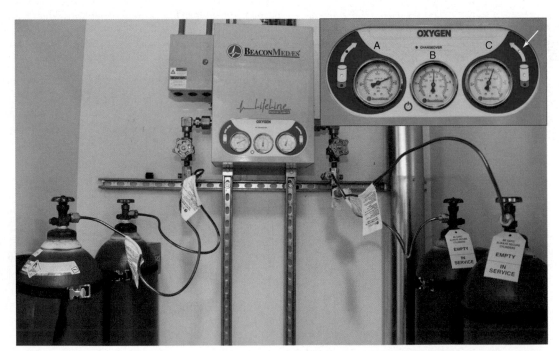

FIG. 4.19 Cylinder manifold with two banks of H tanks (one bank of two tanks on the left and a second bank of two tanks on the right), used as a primary oxygen supply for the entire hospital via intermediate-pressure gas lines hidden in the ceiling. The control box in the center controls the flow of the gas. Inset—The tank pressure gauges on left *(A)* and right *(C)* sides of the control box indicate pressure in the bank on each respective side (2250 psi on the left and just under 1800 psi on the right in this photo), and the line pressure gauge in the middle *(B)* indicates pressure in the intermediate-pressure lines (52 psi). The green light on the right arrow is lit (see *red arrow*), indicating that oxygen is currently flowing from the right bank. (Courtesy Beacon-Medaes; https://www.beaconmedaes.com/.)

other which serves as a secondary supply when the pressure in the primary bank falls below a minimally acceptable level. The gas from the bank in use is conveyed directly to a pressure regulator that reduces the gas pressure to a usable level (40 to 58 psi) and subsequently into intermediate pressure lines. Switchover between banks is usually automatic and the user is warned about the change by an alarm control panel (Fig. 4.20) so that arrangements are made to refill the empty bank.

An alternative to a cylinder manifold is to attach a pressure regulator and associated gauges directly to the primary cylinder (Fig. 4.21). This type of system is much less costly and simple in comparison to a cylinder manifold but has the disadvantage of requiring careful monitoring of the supply and manual changeover to a full backup cylinder when the primary cylinder is empty. This may result in interruption of the supply in the event that the status of the tanks is not frequently and adequately checked by personnel.

Gas lines of the distribution system may take the form of flexible hoses or pipes mounted within the ceiling or wall. These hoses terminate in gas-specific, quick-release diameter-index safety system (DISS) outlets mounted in the ceiling (Fig. 4.22 A) or in the wall (see Fig. 4.22 B); or terminating in ceiling drops (gas lines hanging from the ceiling with DISS connectors—Fig. 4.23). Quick-release connectors are attached to these outlets and convey the gas via intermediate lines directly to the machine.

The capacities of cylinders are given in Table 4.1. Cylinders are often owned by the company that supplies the oxygen but may be purchased by the user. In either case, empty cylinders are periodically picked up by the oxygen supplier, refilled, and returned to the user.

All compressed gas cylinders have a valve on the top to control the flow of gas. The valve on an H tank or K tank has a threaded outlet port through which the gas flows (see Fig. 4.21 A). In contrast, the valve on an E tank and J tank has three holes—one outlet port and two pin index safety system holes (Fig. 4.24). The outlet port is connected to a pressure-reducing valve (see Figs. 4.21 B and 4.29 C) (directly or via a pipeline in the case of an H, J, or K tank, or via the yoke in the case of an E tank), which

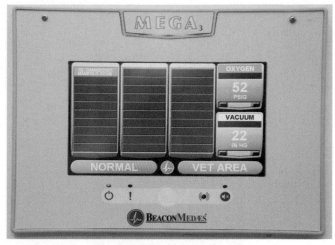

FIG. 4.20 Alarm control panel for a central oxygen supply. An audible alarm will sound and a visual indicator will appear on the screen when oxygen tanks need to be refilled.(Courtesy BeaconMedaes; https://www.beaconmedaes.com/.)

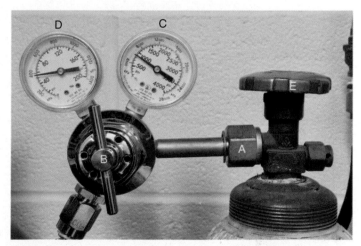

FIG. 4.21 Size H compressed gas cylinder with two-stage pressure regulator. *A,* Threaded outlet port. *B,* Pressure-reducing valve. *C,* Tank pressure gauge. *D,* Line pressure gauge. *E,* Knurled knob.

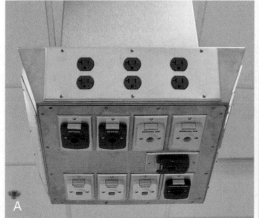
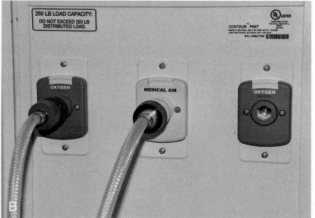

FIG. 4.22 **(A)** Ceiling-mounted quick-release diameter-index safety system (DISS) outlets for oxygen *(green)*, nitrous oxide *(blue)*, medical air *(yellow)*, and vacuum *(white)*. **(B)** Wall-mounted quick-release DISS connectors used to couple intermediate-pressure gas lines to the anesthetic machine. Note that the diameter of each outlet port type is unique to prevent attachment of the wrong connector. (B, Courtesy Hill-Rom; https://www.hillrom.com.)

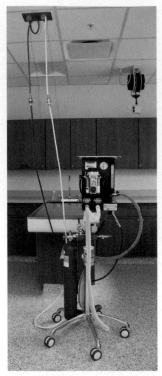

FIG. 4.23 Primary central oxygen supply attached to an anesthetic machine via ceiling drop. The green line on the left is oxygen supply and the white line on the right is waste gas scavenging.

reduces the outgoing pressure to a usable level before conveying it to the machine through intermediate-pressure gas lines.

> **TECHNICIAN NOTE** At the beginning of the day, it is vital that the anesthetist check the primary oxygen supply to be sure it is turned on as well as the secondary oxygen supply to be sure it is full and operational. A failure to do this may result in a patient not receiving oxygen, a dangerous error that if not recognized may be fatal!

Use. At the beginning of the day, it is vital that the anesthetist check the primary oxygen supply to be sure it is turned on as well as the secondary oxygen supply to be sure it is full and operational. A failure to do this may result in a patient not receiving oxygen, a

dangerous error that if not recognized may be fatal. Because pressurized gas remains in the high- and intermediate-pressure lines even if the tank is turned off, a failure to turn a tank back on may easily go unnoticed unless double-checked by the anesthetist.

Oxygen flows from the outlet port of the valve when the stem is turned in a counterclockwise direction (i.e., to the left) (see Fig. 4.24 B). The stem should be turned slowly a minimum of two full turns or ideally until it is fully open. H, F, and K-tank valve stems often have a knurled knob (see Fig. 4.21 E) that is turned by hand. E-tank valve stems are opened and closed with a special wrench or via a lever that can be turned by hand (Fig. 4.25). The flow stops when the valve stem is turned completely clockwise (i.e., to the right) until firmly closed. The mnemonic "left loose, right tight" (*loose* meaning open and *tight* meaning closed) has been used by several generations of anesthesia students as an aid in remembering the direction to turn the stem. When opening and closing these valves, you should not have to use excessive force. Difficulty in turning the valve stem may indicate a malfunction. In this case, the valve should be professionally serviced before use is continued.

After use, the outlet valve of each tank should be closed. Failure to turn off the gas valve can create danger if anyone attempts to remove the tank while it is open, and over a long period, it may result in leakage of gas from the tank.

Oxygen pressure remaining in the intermediate-pressure lines after the valve is closed (called *line pressure*) should be released by depressing the oxygen flush valve or by turning the flowmeter to a high rate of flow until all the gas is vented. This process is referred to as purging the system. Failure to evacuate line pressure may give the anesthetist the false impression that the oxygen is turned on when in fact it is not. (Information on removing and replacing cylinders may be found in the section on anesthetic machine maintenance on page 154.)

> **TECHNICIAN NOTE** When handling compressed gas cylinders:
> - Avoid contact with flames, sparks, or other sources of ignition
> - Turn the tank on *only* when it is attached to a yoke or pressure regulator
> - Store tanks *only* attached to a yoke, secured in a cart or rack designed for this purpose, or chained to the wall
> - Never attempt to attach a tank to a yoke that does not fit, and never tamper with the safety system on a tank, line, or pressure-reducing valve

TABLE 4.1   Compressed Gas Cylinder Characteristics, Capacity, and Pressure

Gas and Symbol	State Within Cylinder	Cylinder Color	Pressure When Full (psi/kPa) at 21°C	Minimum Pressure at Which to Change (psi/kPa)	Cylinder Dimensions (Inches)		Empty Weight (kg)	Capacity (L)
Oxygen (O_2)	Gas	White with white shoulder (ISO) Green (US)	1900–2200/ 13,000–15,000	100–200/ 690–1380	E	4.25 OD; 26 High	6.4	660
					H	9.25 OD; 51 High	54	600
Nitrous oxide (N_2O)	Liquid and gas	White with blue shoulder (ISO) Blue (US)	745/5140	500/3400	E	4.25 OD; 26 High	6.4	1590
					H	9.25 OD; 51 High	54	15,800

OD, Outside diameter.

Modified from Tranquilli WJ, Thurmon JC, Grimm KA: *Lumb and Jones' veterinary anesthesia and analgesia,* ed 4, Ames, IA, 2007, Blackwell.

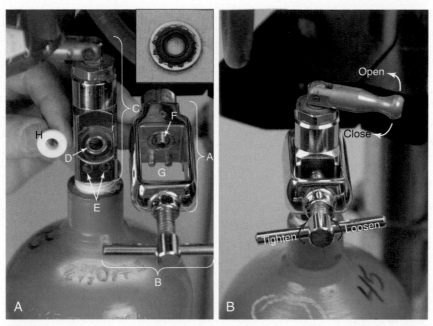

FIG. 4.24 **(A)** Parts of a size E compressed gas cylinder and yoke. *A*, Yoke. *B*, Wing nut. *C*, Outlet valve. *D*, Outlet port. *E*, Pin–index safety system holes. *F*, Nipple of yoke. *G*, Index pins. *H*, Nylon washer. Inset: Bodok seal. **(B)** Opening and closing the outlet valve; loosening and tightening the wing nut.

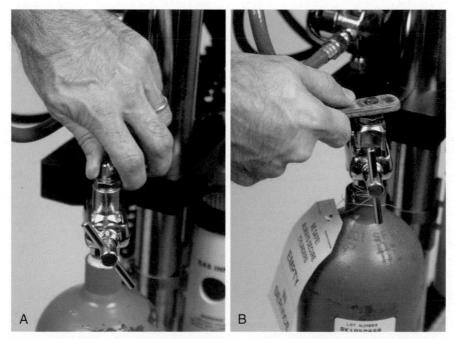

FIG. 4.25 **(A)** Turning on an E tank with a built-in lever. **(B)** Turning on an E tank using a wrench.

Safety. There are four potential risks from compressed gas cylinders:
1. Both oxygen and nitrous oxide support combustion. Contact with flames, sparks, and other sources of ignition must therefore be avoided.
2. A forceful release of gas from an unprotected outlet port may tear the skin or injure an eye. To avoid this type of injury, turn the tank on *only* when it is attached to a yoke or

pressure regulator. The only exception to this rule is when opening the valve to clean dust and dirt from the outlet port before attaching it to a machine or pressure regulator. In this case, turn the valve on *slowly* and only enough to expel the dirt from the port.
3. If a cylinder is dropped and the valve breaks off, the cylinder may cause serious personal injury! High-pressure gas exiting a cylinder through a broken valve will cause the cylinder to

fly at high velocity in the opposite direction to the released gas, becoming in effect a torpedo, the force of which is sufficient to penetrate concrete and injure or kill anyone in its path. Therefore these tanks must be stored *only* attached to a yoke, secured in a cart designed for this purpose, or chained to the wall. *Never drop a compressed gas cylinder and never leave it standing alone with no support or lying on its side.*

4. If a cylinder is inadvertently attached to a valve, yoke, or hose intended for a different type of gas, the wrong gas will be delivered to a patient. For example, if a nitrous oxide cylinder were attached to an oxygen yoke, the patent would receive nitrous oxide instead of oxygen, resulting in asphyxiation. To safeguard against this, all compressed gas supplies have safety systems and features designed to prevent the wrong type of gas cylinder from being attached to the machine connections.

   a. First, all cylinders, flowmeters, pressure-reducing valves, gas lines, and quick-release connectors are color-coded to prevent inadvertent use of an incorrect gas. The United States (US) uses a color-coding system that is different from that set by the International Organization for Standardization (ISO), which is an entity that sets standards to be used worldwide. However, in some countries, conformation with the ISO standard is not mandatory, so colors encountered may differ from those indicated here. In any case, the ISO standard stipulates that all cylinders holding medical gases should have a white body and the specific gas is indicated by the color of the shoulder (the portion of the cylinder right below the valve). In the US, the entire cylinder is painted with a solid color corresponding to the gas. Oxygen cylinders are green (US) or white body and shoulder (ISO), nitrous oxide cylinders are blue (US) or white with blue shoulder (ISO), and medical air cylinders are yellow (United States) or white with a white and black shoulder (ISO) (see Table 4.1). Carbon dioxide is designated by the color gray (US) or white with a gray shoulder (ISO). Although not used for anesthesia, carbon dioxide is used as a euthanasia agent for specific applications such as meatpacking plants and research facilities.

   b. E tank and J tank yokes are equipped with a pin–index safety system (PISS; see Fig. 4.24) which, unless tampered with, physically prevents the wrong gas from being connected to the yoke. For example, a carbon dioxide cylinder cannot be put on an oxygen yoke (Fig. 4.26), an error that would result in a fatality.

   c. H tank and K tank pressure-reducing valves are threaded to accept only one gas. Quick-release connectors are protected with a diameter-index safety system (DISS). In this system, the diameter of the male and female parts of the connector is specific to one gas (see Fig. 4.22).

Attempting to defeat a safety system by removing the pins on a pin–index safety system of an E tank or J tank, stacking several washers in a yoke of a machine, or using a thread converter on an H tank or K tank will create a life-threatening situation. Never attempt to attach a tank that does not fit or to tamper with the safety system on a tank, line, or pressure-reducing valve.

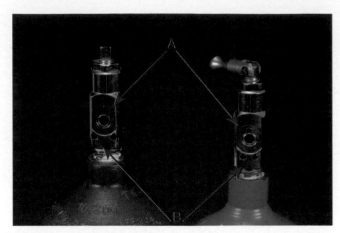

FIG. 4.26 *A,* Outlet port. *B,* Pin–index safety system holes. Note that the pin holes on the carbon dioxide tank *(left)* are farther apart than the pin holes on the oxygen tank *(right).* The unique pin hole position for each gas prevents a tank containing the wrong gas from being attached to the yoke.

Alternate Oxygen Sources

The anesthetist will encounter situations in which the primary oxygen supply is a bulk tank of liquid oxygen or an oxygen concentrator instead of compressed gas cylinders. A bulk tank is most likely to be encountered primarily in large hospitals, whereas oxygen concentrators may be encountered in a hospital of any size.

Oxygen concentrator. An oxygen concentrator is a device that uses a compressor and special adsorbent to extract nitrogen from room air. The remaining gas, containing over 90% oxygen, is transferred into a storage tank and pressurized for medical use. Because the final concentration of oxygen produced by concentrators is less than the USP standard of at least 99% for compressed gas, the product produced by a concentrator is often referred to as oxygen-enriched air. Oxygen concentrators are available either as large stationary units designed to supply an entire hospital or as small mobile units that attach directly to an anesthetic machine via a standard DISS connector (Fig. 4.27).

Oxygen concentrators work by taking ambient air (containing ~78% nitrogen gas, ~21% oxygen, and ~1% argon gas) into the unit via a compressor and passing it through filters designed to remove airborne particles and bacteria. The air is then passed in a cyclical fashion into one of two or more sieve beds (an aluminum tube containing a substance called zeolite that binds nitrogen gas to its surface). Nitrogen in the air is removed by the zeolite as oxygen passes through. As one sieve bed is adsorbing nitrogen from the incoming air, the previously used sieve bed is being purged of adsorbed nitrogen to ready it for the next cycle. The remaining gas (which is approximately 90% to 96% oxygen) flows into a small storage tank and into a flow control system that delivers it at the correct pressure required to operate the anesthetic machine. Since a relatively small volume of oxygen is stored even when the machine is running, a backup system, usually in the form of an E tank, should be available at all times to use in the event of a power failure or malfunction of the unit.

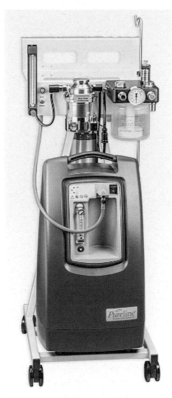

FIG. 4.27 Pureline 8000 Series Oxygen Concentrator. (Courtesy Supera. https://products.shor-line.com/pureline-oc8000-series-oxygen-concentrators.)

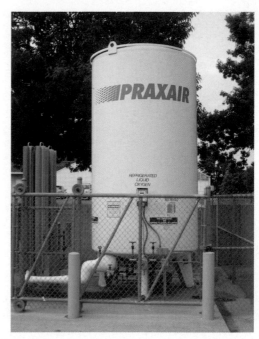

FIG. 4.28 A bulk oxygen tank. These are used in some large hospitals as a primary oxygen source in place of compressed gas cylinders.

Concentrators are generally very efficient and reliable if properly cared for and once purchased, have the advantage of resulting in considerable cost savings over time when compared to the cost of refilling conventional compressed gas cylinders. The units most commonly used are portable and, if mounted on a stand that can also accommodate an anesthetic machine, will provide the convenience of serving as a primary source of oxygen that does not need to be refilled. Although they require little regular maintenance, oxygen concentrator filters must be cleaned or replaced periodically. In addition, over time, the zeolite adsorbent may become contaminated and require replacement, especially if operated in an area where there are significant air pollutants.

Oxygen concentrators do have limitations of which the anesthetist must be aware. The maximum flow rate many are capable of producing is often in the range of 4 to 5 L/min, so the flow may not be adequate for some situations, such as large-animal anesthesia or a supply of gas-driven ventilators. They require an electrical source to function and so cannot be used when an outlet is not in the immediate vicinity. Oxygen output can be reduced under certain conditions including operation at high altitudes or high ambient humidity. Argon, which is not removed by the unit, may accumulate in the concentrated gas, especially when using a full rebreathing circuit. Therefore it is generally recommended to use a minimum fresh gas flow of 0.5 L/min when using a concentrator, and inspired oxygen fraction (Fio_2) should be monitored to ensure an adequate supply

of oxygen to the patient.[a] As with any other piece of equipment, before using a concentrator, the technician or nurse should consult the owner's manual to ensure familiarity with recommendations regarding safe setup, operation, and maintenance.

Bulk Tank. A bulk tank contains a large quantity of oxygen in liquid form (Fig. 4.28). Liquid oxygen is stored in an insulated tank at a temperature of -150 to -170°C and a pressure of 5 to 10 atoms (~73 to ~147 psi).[b] One liter of liquid oxygen will liberate approximately 860 L of oxygen gas at room temperature. This is in contrast to approximately 150 L that are liberated from 1 L of oxygen gas stored in a compressed gas cylinder at 2200 psi.

Tank Pressure Gauge

Description and function. A tank pressure gauge is a device attached to the yoke of a machine or the pressure regulator of an H or K tank, or that is part of the control box of a manifold; that indicates the pressure of gas remaining in a compressed gas cylinder or bank of cylinders, measured in pounds per square inch (psi) in the United States or kilopascals in Europe and Canada (see Figs. 4.19 A and C, 4.21 C, and 4.29 B). See Appendix D for a conversion formula from pounds per square inch to kilopascals.

Use. When the tank valve is opened, the gauge indicates the gas pressure inside the tank. This gauge must be checked before commencing of any procedure to ensure that enough gas remains in the tank to safely complete it. The pressure in a full

[a]Cooley KG, Johnson RA: *Veterinary anesthetic and monitoring equipment*, ed 1, Ames, IA, 2018, John Wiley & Sons, Inc., p 18.
[b]Cooley KG, Johnson RA: *Veterinary anesthetic and monitoring equipment*, ed 1, Ames, IA, 2018, John Wiley & Sons, Inc., p 8.

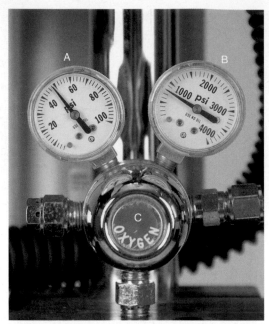

FIG. 4.29 *A*, Line pressure gauge (registering 48 psi). *B*, Tank pressure gauge (registering 800 psi). *C*, Pressure-reducing valve.

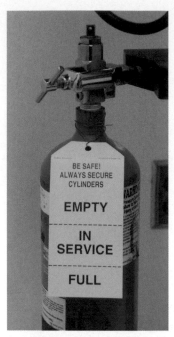

FIG. 4.30 Label for compressed gas tanks. The current status of the tank is shown by the wording at the bottom of the label. The label shown is from a newly acquired tank and reads "FULL." When the tank is first opened, the lower portion of the label is removed so that the remaining label reads "IN SERVICE." When the tank is empty, the "IN SERVICE" stub is removed, leaving the label that reads "EMPTY."

oxygen tank is about 2200 psi (about 15,000 kPa). As gas is used, the pressure in the tank will gradually fall, reaching zero when the tank is empty. The gauge also reads zero if the tank is not empty but is turned off and the remaining gas in the intermediate-pressure line has been evacuated (i.e., purged or "bled off") (see page 127 for a description of this procedure). This gauge functions passively and therefore requires no action on the part of the anesthetist.

> **TECHNICIAN NOTE** The volume in liters of oxygen present in a compressed gas cylinder can be calculated by multiplying the pressure (in psi) in an E tank by 0.3 or by multiplying the pressure in an H tank by 3.

The approximate volume in liters (L) of oxygen present in an E tank can be calculated by multiplying the pressure (in psi) by 0.3 (see Table 4.1). For example, a full E tank at a pressure of 2200 psi contains about 660 L of oxygen (i.e., 0.3 × 2200 psi). A reading of 1100 psi indicates the tank is approximately half full and therefore contains approximately 330 L of oxygen. The approximate volume in liters for the larger H tank can be calculated by multiplying the pressure (in psi) by 3. For example, a full H tank at a pressure of 2200 psi contains approximately 6600 L of oxygen (i.e., 3 × 2200 psi).

The volume of oxygen in the tank indicates how much longer the tank can be used. For example, if the anesthetist selects an oxygen flow rate of 1 L per minute (L/min), a full E tank containing 660 L of oxygen will last approximately 11 hours (i.e., 660 minutes), whereas at a flow rate of 2 L/min, the same full tank will last approximately 5.5 hours (i.e., 330 minutes). In contrast, a full H tank at a flow rate of 1 L/min contains enough oxygen to last 110 hours (6600 minutes).

Tanks should be marked "full," "in service," or "empty" to indicate their status (Fig. 4.30), and a full backup tank must always be kept on the machine as a spare in case the primary tank runs out. The anesthetist may notice a considerable drop in pressure during a lengthy anesthetic procedure. If not detected in time, oxygen flow to the patient will cease and this will put the patient in danger because most veterinary anesthetic machines have no alarm to warn of inadequate flow unless so equipped. The anesthetist must therefore periodically monitor the oxygen tank pressure gauge during each procedure and change the tank when the gauge indicates that the tank is close to empty. As an example, an E tank with 600 psi should give the anesthetist enough gas to last at least 1 hour, assuming that an oxygen flow of no more than 3 L/min is used and the oxygen flush valve is not activated frequently. In any case, a tank should be changed when the pressure drops below 500 psi (about 3400 kPa), indicating only 150 L of oxygen remaining in the tank.

Pressure-Reducing Valve (Pressure Regulator)

Description and function. Immediately after exiting the tank, the gas flows through a pressure-reducing valve (see Figs. 4.21 B and 4.29 C), which is located near the tank pressure gauge, and then into an intermediate gas line. The pressure-reducing valve reduces the pressure of the gas to a constant safe operating pressure of 40 to 58 psi (about 276 to 400 kPa) regardless of the pressure changes within the tank. Pressure-reducing valves all look slightly different but are usually round and have a color-coded insignia on the outside to identify the gas flowing through them.

H and K tanks, if not attached to a cylinder manifold, may be fitted with a two-stage pressure regulator, which is a device attached to the outlet valve that serves as a pressure-reducing valve, a tank pressure gauge, and a line-pressure gauge (see Fig. 4.21), and ensures correct delivery pressure regardless of the pressure remaining in the tank.

Use. The pressure-reducing valve functions passively and therefore requires no action on the part of the anesthetist. The line pressure gauge (if present) should be checked before every procedure, however, to verify the correct pressure in the intermediate pressure gas lines (40 to 58 psi).

Line Pressure Gauge

Description and function. The line pressure gauge indicates the pressure in the intermediate-pressure gas lines between the pressure-reducing valve and the flowmeters (see Figs. 4.19 B, 4.21 D, and 4.29 A). It is not present on all machines but when present is immediately downstream from the pressure-reducing valve.

Use. Like the tank pressure gauge and pressure-reducing valve, this gauge functions passively and so requires no action on the part of the anesthetist. When the oxygen is turned on, this gauge should read 40 to 58 psi. A pressure higher or lower than this indicates a malfunction of or a need to adjust the pressure-reducing valve. After the oxygen tank has been turned off, the line pressure gauge will continue to register line pressure until it is evacuated or purged. This is accomplished by depressing the oxygen flush valve until the gauge reads 0 psi.

Flowmeter

Description and function. After leaving the pressure-reducing valve, the carrier gas flows through an intermediate-pressure gas line into the flowmeter. A flowmeter is a vertical glass cylinder of graduated diameter with a valve attached to the bottom. When the valve knob is turned, gas enters the cylinder at the bottom and exits at the top. An indicator within the cylinder rises to indicate the gas flow expressed in liters of gas per minute (L/min) (Fig. 4.31).

The flowmeter also further reduces the pressure of the gas in the intermediate-pressure line from about 50 psi (about 345 kPa) to 15 psi (about 100 kPa). This pressure is only slightly above atmospheric pressure (about 14.7 psi) and is the optimum pressure for entry into the breathing circuit and ultimately the patient's lungs.

If a machine is set up to use oxygen as well as another carrier gas such as nitrous oxide or medical air, there will be separate flowmeters so that the flow rates of the two gases can be monitored and adjusted separately (Fig. 4.32). To prevent the controls for oxygen and nitrous oxide from being confused, they are touch- and profile-coded (they feel and look different), color-coded (green or white for oxygen, blue for nitrous oxide, and yellow or white and black for medical air), and are labeled according to the gas they regulate. Some machines provide two flowmeters for oxygen, one for flow rates greater than 1 L/min (coarse adjustment) and one to adjust flow rates accurately at less than 1 L/min (fine adjustment).

Use. The flowmeter is opened by turning the valve knob counterclockwise (to the left), and the flow is then adjusted to the appropriate level for the patient (see page 149 for a discussion of oxygen flow rates). All flowmeters have a ball or bobbin indicator that rises to a height proportional to the flow of gas. The scale on the cylinder indicates the gas flow. The meter is read at the center of a ball indicator or the top of a bobbin indicator (Fig. 4.33).

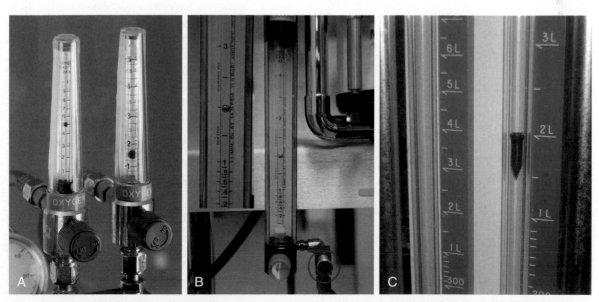

FIG. 4.31 (A) Oxygen flowmeters with ball indicators. The fine adjustment flowmeter on the left is adjusted to 0.5 L/min and the coarse adjustment flowmeter on the right is adjusted to 1.5 L/min for a total oxygen flow of 2 L/min. (B) Single oxygen flowmeter with both coarse and fine adjustment, adjusted to a flow rate of 2.0 L/min. Inset: Note that below 1 L/min, the scale is marked in 0.2 L increments. At flows higher than 1 L/min, the scale is marked in 0.5 L increments. The oxygen flush valve is circled in red. (C) Flowmeter with bobbin-type indicator adjusted to 2 L/min. (From Warren RG: *Small animal anesthesia*, St Louis, MO, 1983, Mosby.)

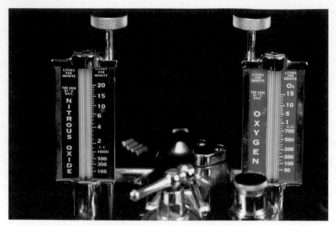

FIG. 4.32 An anesthetic machine with two flowmeters, one for nitrous oxide and one for oxygen.

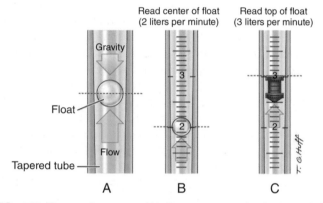

FIG. 4.33 Oxygen flowmeter. **(A)** Oxygen enters the bottom of the tube, flows past the indicator, and exits the top of the tube. Therefore the height of the indicator in the tube is proportional to the rate of flow. **(B)** Read a ball-shaped indicator at the center (see *dotted line*). **(C)** Read a bobbin-shaped indicator at the top (see *dotted line*).

Flowmeters must be treated gently when turning them off. The valve stem inside the flowmeter is delicate and can be damaged by rough handling. Therefore when turning off a flowmeter, turn it clockwise (to the right) just until the ball or bobbin drops to 0 L/min. Even though the knob can still be turned on most machines, do *not* turn it any further to the right. Failure to turn off the flowmeter may result in a sudden rush of air into the meter when the oxygen tank is opened, which may jam the bobbin or ball at the top of the tube. Note that some machines, such as Vetland machines, are equipped with a stop to prevent overtightening of the flowmeter.

TECHNICIAN NOTE When turning off a flowmeter, turn clockwise (to the right) just until the ball or bobbin drops to 0 L/min. Even though the knob can still be turned on most machines, do *not* turn it any further to the right or you will damage the valve!

Safety. The flowmeter must be turned on if the patient is to receive oxygen. Therefore a tank pressure gauge or line pressure gauge that registers oxygen pressure does not ensure that the patient is receiving oxygen unless the flowmeter is also on.

Oxygen Flush Valve

Description and function. The oxygen flush valve is a button or lever that when activated rapidly delivers a large volume of pure oxygen at a flow rate of 35 to 75 L/min directly from the line exiting the pressure-reducing valve into the common gas outlet or directly into the breathing circuit of a rebreathing system, bypassing the anesthetic vaporizer and oxygen flowmeters. This feature is used to rapidly fill a depleted reservoir bag. It is also used to deliver oxygen to a critically ill patient or, at the end of the anesthetic period, to dilute out the anesthetic gas remaining in the circuit (Fig. 4.34 F). Note that oxygen flush valves may be positioned differently and look very different among machines so before using a new machine, always check carefully for its location (see Fig. 4.31 B for an example of the appearance and location of the flush valve on a different machine than the one shown in Fig. 4.34).

Use. The high oxygen flow generated by activation of an oxygen flush valve can quickly lead to pressures within the breathing circuit and the patient's respiratory tree that greatly exceed a safe level (generally 20 cm H_2O for SA patients or 40 cm H_2O for LA patients). This is especially true for very small patients because small reservoir bags used with these patients (500 mL to 1 L) can become dangerously full within activation of the oxygen flush valve for less than one second. If this happens, increased intrathoracic pressure, hypotension, and damage to the lungs due to barotrauma can easily result. Therefore most experts recommend

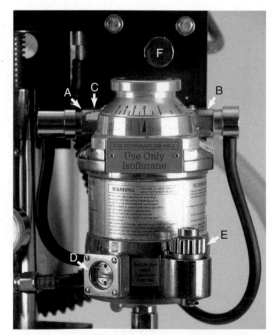

FIG. 4.34 Precision anesthetic vaporizer for isoflurane set at 2%. *A,* Inlet port with keyed fitting leading from the flowmeters. *B,* Outlet port with keyed fitting leading to the fresh gas inlet or common gas outlet. *C,* Safety lock (outlined in red). *D,* Indicator window. *E,* Fill port. *F,* Oxygen flush valve (part of the compressed gas supply).

activation only after the patient is temporarily removed from the circuit.

When activating the flush valve to refill a collapsed reservoir bag, first disconnect the ET tube from the breathing circuit, occlude the connector, then press the flush valve briefly using short bursts, while watching the reservoir bag and pressure manometer to ensure that the bag does not overfill and the pressure in the circuit does not exceed 3 cm H_2O. Then reconnect the patient. When using the oxygen flush valve for this purpose, remember that the gas flowing into the breathing circuit from the valve will contain no inhalant anesthetic. Thus the gas delivered by this valve will dilute the concentration of inhalant anesthetic in the breathing circuit and in the patient's lungs, leading to a decreased plane of anesthesia. A preferable way to fill a collapsed bag without affecting the plane of anesthesia is to temporarily turn up the oxygen flow until it refills.

When using the valve to deliver fresh oxygen to a critically ill patient or to flush inhalant anesthetic out of the circuit during anesthetic recovery or during a crisis, first turn off the vaporizer. Next, force the gases out of the reservoir bag and into the scavenging system using gentle hand pressure. Finally, disconnect the patient, occlude the connector, press the flush valve to refill the bag with fresh oxygen, and reconnect the patient.

Safety. Some anesthetic machines are configured such that the oxygen flush valve discharges into the common gas outlet instead of the rebreathing circuit. In these cases, the oxygen flush valve must never be used with a nonrebreathing system attached because a high flow rate of oxygen into this type of circuit can seriously damage the animal's lungs.

Anesthetic Vaporizer
Description and Function
After exiting the flowmeter, oxygen enters the vaporizer through the inlet port (see Fig. 4.34 A). The function of the vaporizer is to convert a liquid anesthetic such as isoflurane or sevoflurane to a gaseous state and to add controlled amounts of this vaporized anesthetic to the carrier gases (O_2, and medical air or N_2O if used). After exiting the vaporizer through the outlet port, the oxygen and anesthetic mixture (known as *fresh gas*) enters the breathing circuit through a connection referred to as the *fresh gas inlet*. Vaporizers are designed for use with only one specific anesthetic agent, which is purchased in liquid form and poured into the vaporizer.

The vaporized anesthetic can exit the vaporizer only by traveling in carrier gas, which transports it from the vaporizer into the breathing circuit. In other words, no anesthetic is delivered to the patient if the flowmeter reads zero because there is no flow of carrier gas to deliver the anesthetic.

Most newer vaporizers are classified as *agent-specific, variable-bypass, and flow-over*. Agent-specific because they are designed and calibrated for use with one specific anesthetic (i.e., isoflurane, sevoflurane, or desflurane); variable-bypass because they regulate the anesthetic output by routing a portion of the carrier gas through the vaporization chamber where the liquid anesthetic is located, while the remainder of the carrier gas bypasses the vaporization chamber; and flow-over because the portion of the carrier gas that enters the chamber flows over the surface of the liquid anesthetic and picks up vaporized anesthetic. Therefore the more carrier gas that is routed through the vaporization chamber (as opposed to bypassing it) by turning the dial to a higher percentage, the higher the concentration of the anesthetic delivered to the patient.

Types of Anesthetic Vaporizer
Anesthetic vaporizers are also classified as either precision or nonprecision. This differentiation separates those that allow precise control of the amount of anesthetic delivered to the patient (expressed as the percentage of the total gases exiting the vaporizer) from those that allow only an estimation of the amount delivered. Nonprecision vaporizers (Fig. 4.35) were used in the past to deliver low vapor pressure anesthetics—such as methoxyflurane—which are no longer available.

Although nonprecision vaporizers can be used to deliver isoflurane or sevoflurane, as long as specific procedures are carefully followed, this practice is rare and not advised. In contrast, precision vaporizers (see Fig. 4.34) are used to deliver all commonly used liquid anesthetics including isoflurane, sevoflurane, and desflurane, and are the main type the anesthetist is likely to encounter in clinical practice. Therefore the discussion that follows refers specifically to precision vaporizers.

The commonly used liquid anesthetics (isoflurane, sevoflurane, and desflurane) are classified as high vapor pressure liquids. The designation "high vapor pressure" means that these anesthetics readily evaporate and may reach concentrations of 30% or greater within the anesthetic circuit if the amount of vapor being delivered to the breathing circuit is not controlled. Because the maximum useful concentration for isoflurane and sevoflurane is 5% and 8%, respectively, uncontrolled delivery of anesthetic vapor will result in excessively high levels that could be dangerous for the patient. It is therefore necessary to use a

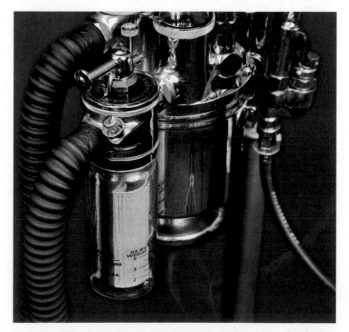

FIG. 4.35 Nonprecision vaporizer (Ohio No. 8 vaporizer), designed for delivery of methoxyflurane.

precision vaporizer to deliver these agents, affording the anesthetist more exact control of the concentration of anesthetic in the circuit.

Vaporizer-out-of-circuit versus vaporizer-in-circuit. The abbreviations *VOC* and *VIC* are used to describe two different ways anesthetic machines are configured based on the location of the vaporizer in relation to the breathing circuit. The letters *VOC* are an abbreviation for *vaporizer-out-of-circuit* (Fig. 4.36 A) and indicate that the vaporizer is not located within the breathing circuit. In this case, oxygen from the flowmeters flows into the vaporizer before entering the breathing circuit. Precision vaporizers are positioned in a VOC configuration.

Similarly, the letters *VIC* are an abbreviation for *vaporizer-in-circuit* (see Fig. 4.36 B). In this type of machine, carrier gases enter the breathing circuit directly from the flowmeter without first entering the vaporizer. Instead, the vaporizer is located in the breathing circuit, most often between the expiratory breathing tube and the expiratory unidirectional valve. Exhaled gases enter the vaporizer each time the patient breathes. Nonprecision vaporizers, which are rarely used, are positioned this way.

The location of the vaporizer in relationship to the breathing circuit (VOC vs. VIC) is governed by the resistance to the flow of gases through it. This is because the patient's respiratory drive (the force exerted by contraction and relaxation of the patient's respiratory muscles) during normal breathing is the force that moves gases around the breathing circuit. When resistance to gas flow is high, as is the case with precision vaporizers, the respiratory drive is insufficient to push gases through

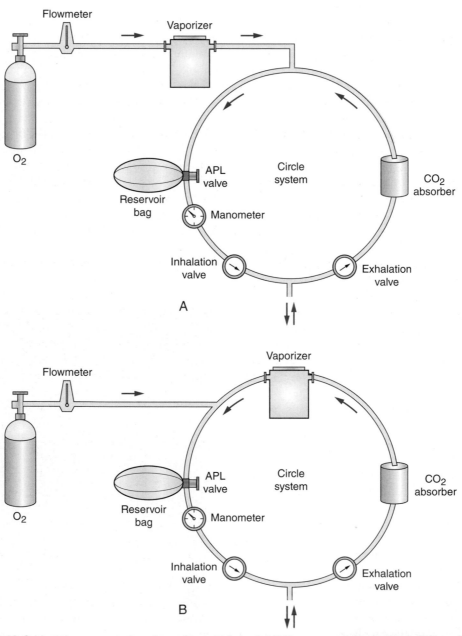

FIG. 4.36 Schematic representation of vaporizer-out-of-circuit (VOC) versus vaporizer-in-circuit (VIC) configurations. **(A)** VOC. **(B)** VIC. (From Warren RG: *Small animal anesthesia*, St Louis, MO, 1983, Mosby.)

the vaporizer. Consequently, precision vaporizers must be placed outside the breathing circuit. In contrast, nonprecision vaporizers offer little resistance to gas flow and therefore can safely be placed in the breathing circuit.

Factors Affecting Vaporizer Output

The concentration of anesthetic delivered by any vaporizer depends not only on the vaporizer setting but also on a variety of other factors including temperature, carrier gas flow rate, respiratory rate and depth, and back pressure. Newer precision vaporizers are compensated and deliver a precise concentration independent of each of these factors with relatively little error or variation. However, older precision vaporizers and nonprecision vaporizers do not automatically compensate for these factors. Regardless of the type of vaporizer the anesthetist is using, a complete knowledge of proper use requires an understanding of the potential effect of each of these factors on vaporizer output.

Temperature. Volatile anesthetics, like all liquids, vaporize more readily at high temperatures than at low temperatures. Vaporization directly affects vaporizer output. In a vaporizer that is not temperature compensated, vaporization would vary with changes in ambient (room) temperature because room temperature affects the temperature of the anesthetic. For example, if a noncompensated vaporizer was used in a cold room, vaporization of the gas would decrease and the anesthetic output would be lower than that indicated on the dial. Conversely, in a warm room, the output would be greater than the dial setting.

The temperature of the anesthetic is also affected by carrier gas flow. This is because gas exiting a compressed gas cylinder is cold. At high carrier gas flow rates, the temperature of the liquid anesthetic falls, leading to decreased vaporization and lower anesthetic output than that indicated on the dial when a noncompensated vaporizer is used.

Most recently manufactured precision vaporizers are temperature compensated and so may be used without concern about variations in ambient temperature.

Carrier gas flow rate. The amount of carrier gas that flows through the vaporization chamber (primarily controlled by the vaporizer dial setting) determines the anesthetic output. In a vaporizer that is not flow compensated, flow through the chamber is also affected by the carrier gas flow rate (determined by the flowmeter setting). Higher flowmeter settings result in increased flow through the chamber, and lower settings result in decreased flow through the chamber. For example, if a noncompensated vaporizer was used, the output would be higher at a flowmeter setting of 3 L/min than at a flowmeter setting of 500 mL/min.

Most modern precision vaporizers compensate for carrier gas flow and will deliver the amount of anesthetic indicated on the dial over a wide range of oxygen flow rates. Even in a flow-compensated vaporizer, compensation is not unlimited, however. Flows that are very high (i.e., in excess of 10 L/min) or very low (i.e., below 500 mL/min) may affect the output of flow-compensated vaporizers. Consequently, the vaporizer setting will not accurately reflect the concentration of anesthetic released at these extreme flow rates.

In precision vaporizers, whether compensated or uncompensated, carrier gas flow rate also influences the concentration of the anesthetic in the breathing circuit (and consequently in the air that the patient breathes). An oxygen flow rate that approaches the patient's respiratory minute volume (RMV) (the total amount of gas a patient inhales or exhales in 1 minute) will produce a concentration in the circuit close to the dial setting. At a lower flow rate, although the anesthetic concentration in the carrier gas delivered to the circuit does not change, the total amount delivered to the patient is lower. This is because as an anesthetic is absorbed in the patient's lungs and diluted by expired gases, the concentration within the circuit decreases. For example, if a 20-kg dog is connected to an anesthetic machine with an oxygen flow rate of 200 mL/kg/min (in this case, 4 L/min) and a vaporizer setting of 2%, the actual concentration of anesthetic being inhaled by the animal is close to 2%. If the oxygen flow rate is reduced to 100 mL/kg/min (in this case, 2 L/min), then to 50 mL/kg/min (1 L/min), and finally to 10 mL/kg/min (200 mL/min), the percentage of anesthetic in the circuit may drop to 1.8%, 1.2%, and 0.8%, respectively. In each case, the vaporizer is delivering a 2% concentration to the circuit, but the concentration within the circuit varies as a result of dilution and absorption. This is why precision vaporizer settings may need to be increased if low oxygen flow rates are used.

Respiratory rate and depth. Respiratory rate and depth will also affect anesthetic delivery if using a VIC nonprecision vaporizer. This is because the respiratory rate and effort affect the flow of carrier gas through the vaporization chamber. Consequently, high and low respiratory rates and depths will have the same effect on vaporizer output as high and low carrier gas flow. This is not an issue with VOC precision vaporizers because in this circumstance, the patient's respiratory drive has no influence on the amount of carrier gas passing through the vaporization chamber.

Back pressure. Back pressure refers to an increase in pressure at the vaporizer outlet port caused by manual ventilation (bagging) or activation of the oxygen flush valve. A vaporizer that is not back pressure compensated will deliver more anesthetic under these circumstances. Most precision vaporizers are pressure compensated so that bagging or flush valve activation does not affect the amount of anesthetic released.

Use

As previously mentioned, each precision vaporizer is designed to be used with a specific inhalant anesthetic such as sevoflurane, isoflurane, or desflurane. So that the anesthetist can easily identify the agent being used, vaporizers are color-coded (purple, isoflurane; yellow, sevoflurane; blue, desflurane).

The vaporizer is turned on by depressing the safety lock and turning the dial to the desired level. The safety lock is present as a lever on some vaporizers and is incorporated into the dial on others (Fig. 4.37). Inhalant anesthetic levels are measured in percentage concentration. For common domestic species, the induction rate of isoflurane is approximately 3% to 5%. The maintenance rate is about 1.5% to 2.5%. The induction rate of sevoflurane is approximately 4% to 5%, and the maintenance rate is about 2.5% to 4%. The induction rate of desflurane is

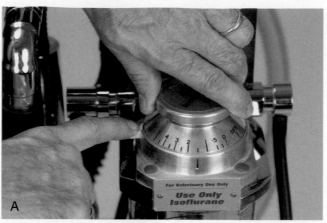

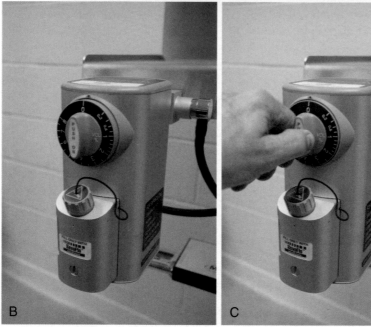

FIG. 4.37 **(A)** Tec 3 vaporizer. The dial lock (white lever) must be pressed down to turn the vaporizer on. **(B)** Penlon Sigma Delta vaporizer. The dial must be pressed in to turn the vaporizer on. **(C)** Vaporizer with the dial unlocked.

approximately 10% to 15%. The maintenance rate is about 8% to 12%. Patients should receive rates at the lower end of these ranges if preanesthetic medications have been administered and may even need less depending on a variety of patient factors as well as the influence of other analgesic and anesthetic agents used as a part of a balanced anesthesia protocol.

The dial of a precision vaporizer (see Fig. 4.34) is graduated in percentage concentration (e.g., 1%, 2%). Throughout any anesthetic procedure, the anesthetist must control the amount of inhalant anesthetic delivered to the patient by periodically adjusting the vaporizer dial in response to careful and frequent evaluation of monitoring parameters. Appropriate and safe use of the vaporizer requires knowledge, experience, and detailed observation. Specifics regarding the safe use of the vaporizer are discussed in detail in Chapters 9–11.

Vaporizers must be checked before each procedure to make sure that enough anesthetic remains in the vaporization chamber. Most vaporizers have an indicator window at the base that allows the anesthetist to inspect the amount of liquid anesthetic

remaining. In order for the vaporizer to function properly, the liquid anesthetic level must be between the upper and lower lines of the window (Fig. 4.38). The vaporizer should be refilled as needed but should be kept at least half full at all times. Overfilling a vaporizer will result in an anesthetic overdose, and underfilling will result in an inability to keep the patient anesthetized.

> **TECHNICIAN NOTE** Vaporizers must be checked before each procedure to make sure the liquid anesthetic level is between the upper and lower lines of the indicator window. The vaporizer should be refilled as needed but should be kept at least half full at all times.

Safety

Vaporizers are subject to excess output if the anesthetic machine is tipped over, shaken vigorously, or overfilled. Under these circumstances, liquid anesthetic enters bypass channels of the

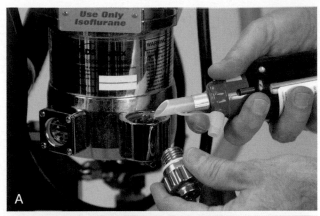

FIG. 4.38 The indicator window of an anesthetic vaporizer. The level of the liquid anesthetic must be kept between the upper and lower lines.

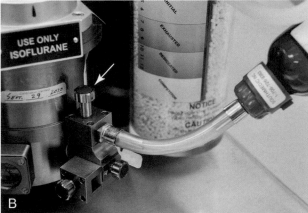

FIG. 4.39 Devices intended to prevent spills when filling a vaporizer. **(A)** Note the purple pouring spout attached to the top of the liquid anesthetic bottle. This filling device will only fit on a corresponding bottle (isoflurane device on an isoflurane bottle). **(B)** Keyed adapter. This adapter is locked in the fill port by (1) loosening the purple knob on top (see *arrow*), (2) inserting the keyed end of the adapter (which can only be inserted in one orientation so that the holes through which the liquid flows into the vaporizer line up), then tightening the knob. This adapter seals the system and prevents contamination of room air with evaporated liquid anesthetic during the filling process. It can only be used for a single agent (isoflurane in this case) and in a vaporizer equipped with a special fill port.

vaporizer, and a potentially lethal dose of anesthetic may be delivered to the next patient. If an anesthetic machine is tipped, shaken, or overfilled, the liquid anesthetic should be drained out, and oxygen should be run through the machine at the maximum flow rate (with the vaporizer dial turned on) until no agent remains in the machine. Emptying anesthetic machine vaporizers before transport is the best way to avoid this problem.

> **TECHNICIAN NOTE** If a bottle of liquid inhalant anesthetic accidentally breaks, vacate the room immediately and allow the room to air out until the anesthetic is completely evaporated and evacuated from the room.

Volatile anesthetics readily evaporate when exposed to air. Precautions must therefore be taken to avoid inhaling the gas. First, take care not to drop or break the bottle. When refilling the vaporizer, make sure other personnel are not in the immediate vicinity, place a scavenging hose near the bottle while it is open to evacuate evaporated gas, cap the bottle promptly when finished, and close the vaporizer fill chamber immediately after filling. A pouring spout (Fig. 4.39 A) or keyed fill adapter (see Fig. 4.39 B) designed for use with these bottles is a valuable aid in preventing spills.

Vaporizer Inlet Port

Description and function. The vaporizer inlet port is the point where oxygen and any other carrier gases enter the vaporizer from the flowmeters (see Fig. 4.34 A).

Use. The vaporizer inlet port is connected to the flowmeters by a hose with a female keyed connector. This keyed connector prevents the operator from inadvertently attaching the outlet hose to the inlet port. Check that this connector is securely attached to the vaporizer before the commencement of any procedure.

Vaporizer Outlet Port and Common Gas Outlet (Fresh Gas Outlet)

Description and function. Both the vaporizer outlet port and the common gas outlet are fittings to which a hose connects. The vaporizer outlet port (see Fig. 4.34 B) is the point where oxygen, inhalant anesthetic, and other carrier gases (if used) exit the vaporizer on the way to the breathing circuit. On some machines, this port connects directly to the breathing circuit via a hose or other tubing. On other machines, it connects instead to the common gas outlet. The common gas outlet (Fig. 4.40) then connects directly to the breathing circuit via a second hose

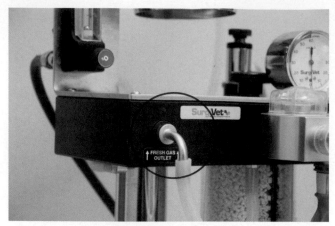

FIG. 4.40 This 15-mm port is the common gas outlet with the hose leading to the breathing circuit attached. It is present on some machines as an additional connection between the vaporizer outlet port and the fresh gas inlet.

or piece of tubing. Therefore, on a machine with a common gas outlet, there are two lengths of hose or tubing between the vaporizer outlet port and the breathing circuit instead of one (see Fig. 4.14).

Use. The vaporizer outlet port is connected to the common gas outlet or directly to the breathing circuit by a hose with a male keyed connector. This keyed connector prevents the operator from inadvertently attaching the inlet hose to the outlet port. It is important to check that this fitting is securely attached to the vaporizer before the commencement of any procedure.

Safety. When a nonrebreathing circuit on a machine without a separate common gas outlet is used, the male keyed connector of the rebreathing circuit is removed from the outlet port, and the male keyed connector for the nonrebreathing circuit is attached to the vaporizer outlet port (see Fig. 4.13) in its place. When a machine with a separate common gas outlet is used, the connector for the nonrebreathing circuit is attached to the common gas outlet instead. Regardless of which type you are using, after any procedure in which a nonrebreathing circuit is used, the connector of the rebreathing circuit must be reattached to the outlet port or common gas outlet before the next patient is anesthetized. It may, however, be inadvertently left unattached. When this happens, anesthetic gas will discharge into the room instead of into the circuit. This will result in an inability to keep the patient anesthetized and exposure of personnel to anesthetic gas. Checking the machine for leaks before each procedure can prevent this error.

> **TECHNICIAN NOTE** After the use of a nonrebreathing circuit, the connector of the rebreathing circuit must be reattached to the outlet port or common gas outlet before the next patient is anesthetized. A failure to do this results in an inability to keep the patient anesthetized and exposure of personnel to anesthetic gas.

Breathing Circuit

The breathing circuit consists of a group of components that carry anesthetic and oxygen from the fresh gas inlet to the patient and convey expired gases away from the patient. The breathing circuit may be incorporated into the anesthetic machine (as is the case with a rebreathing system), or it may be a separate unit (as is sometimes the case with a nonrebreathing system).

Scavenging System

The scavenging system is discussed in detail in Chapter 5.

REBREATHING SYSTEMS

A rebreathing system is an anesthetic machine fitted with a rebreathing circuit. Rebreathing systems are also called *circle systems* because exhaled gases minus carbon dioxide are recirculated and rebreathed by the patient, along with variable amounts of fresh oxygen and anesthetic. These systems are appropriate for almost all patients except those that are very small (under 3 kg in body weight).

When a rebreathing system is used, the gases exhaled by the patient travel through the expiratory breathing tube and the expiratory unidirectional valve, then enter the CO_2 absorber canister. They are then directed past the reservoir bag, adjustable pressure limiting (APL) valve, and pressure manometer, and back toward the patient through the inspiratory unidirectional valve and inspiratory breathing tube. Exhaled gases include O_2, anesthetic vapor, CO_2, nitrogen (at the beginning of anesthesia), water vapor, and other carrier gases (if used). Fresh oxygen and anesthetic enter the circuit from the fresh gas inlet and mix with the patient's exhaled gases. The flow of gas through the anesthetic machine therefore is circular (inspiratory unidirectional valve, inspiratory tube, animal, expiratory tube, expiratory unidirectional valve, carbon dioxide canister, past the reservoir bag, APL valve, and pressure manometer, and back to the inspiratory unidirectional valve) (see Fig. 4.13). When correctly adjusted, the flowmeters, vaporizer, reservoir bag, and APL valve work in concert to maintain a constant flow of gas to the patient.

Rebreathing systems are further subdivided based on carrier gas flow into full rebreathing systems (also known as complete, closed, or total rebreathing systems), partial rebreathing systems (also known as semiclosed rebreathing systems), and minimal rebreathing systems. The main differences among these systems lie in the amount of carrier gas that is delivered to the breathing circuit (the flow rate) and in some circumstances, the position of the APL valve. A full rebreathing system is one in which the flow of oxygen is very low, providing only the volume necessary to meet the patient's metabolic needs (~5 to 10 mL/kg/min). When using this system, the APL valve may sometimes be kept nearly or completely closed. When the system is operating optimally, it is not necessary to vent gases from the circuit because the same volume of gas is added to the circuit as is consumed by the patient. In reality, however, this delicate balance of input and consumption is difficult to achieve and requires constant monitoring and adjustment. For this reason, full rebreathing systems are seldom used in small-animal practice but are used for large-animal anesthesia to conserve gas.

In contrast, a partial rebreathing system (also called a semi-closed rebreathing system) is one in which more oxygen is added than the patient requires (usually in the range of 20 to 200 mL/kg/min). In this system, the APL valve is positioned partially or completely open and a portion of the gases is recirculated, but the amount beyond the volume that is used by the patient exits through the APL valve into the scavenging system. This type of system is relatively easy to use and meets the needs of the majority of patients. For this reason, it is the most common machine configuration used in clinical practice.

Rebreathing Circuits

A rebreathing circuit consists of the following parts:

- Fresh gas inlet
- Unidirectional (or one-way) valves
- APL valve
- Carbon dioxide absorber canister
- Pressure manometer
- Air intake valve
- Breathing tubes
- Y-piece

A nonrebreathing circuit is less complex and is discussed on page 144.

Fresh Gas Inlet

Description and function. The fresh gas inlet is the point at which the carrier and anesthetic gases enter the breathing circuit. This inlet is usually located near the inspiratory unidirectional valve. The vaporizer outlet port or common gas outlet and the fresh gas inlet are connected by a hose (which is often black or clear) (see Fig. 4.34 B).

Use. The fresh gas inlet is permanently attached to the breathing circuit whether rebreathing or nonrebreathing, so no action needs to be taken by the anesthetist.

Unidirectional Valves

Description and function. The two unidirectional valves, also known as one-way valves (Fig. 4.41 A and C), control the direction of gas flow through the rebreathing circuit as the patient breathes. The inspiratory (inhalation) unidirectional valve is the attachment point for the inspiratory breathing tube, and the expiratory (exhalation) unidirectional valve is the attachment point for the expiratory breathing tube. The valves are located inside the housing with a clear plastic dome on top that allows the anesthetist to observe the action of the valves, which open and close as the patient breathes to allow anesthetic gases to flow past.

When the patient inhales, the inspiratory valve opens, allowing the oxygen and anesthetic gas to enter the inspiratory breathing tube and travel toward the patient. The gases then pass through the Y-piece and into the ET tube or mask. On reaching the patient's lungs, oxygen and anesthetic molecules are absorbed and enter the bloodstream. At the same time, carbon dioxide and anesthetic molecules are released from the bloodstream, enter the alveoli, and are exhaled on the next breath.

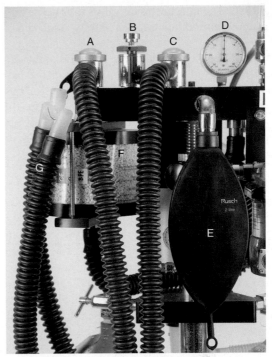

FIG. 4.41 Parts of a rebreathing circuit. *A,* Expiratory unidirectional valve. *B,* Adjustable pressure limiting (APL) valve. *C,* Inspiratory unidirectional valve. *D,* Pressure manometer. *E,* Two-liter reservoir bag. *F,* Carbon dioxide absorber canister. *G,* Small-animal corrugated breathing tubes.

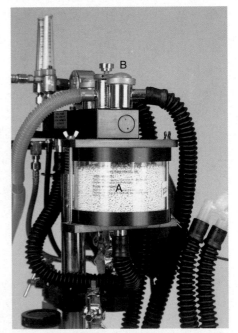

FIG. 4.42 *A,* Carbon dioxide absorber canister. Note that exhaled air is directed by the expiratory valve *(B)* directly into the canister.

Exhaled gases travel through the ET tube or mask and the Y-piece, enter the expiratory breathing tube, pass through the expiratory valve, and pass directly into the carbon dioxide absorber canister (Fig. 4.42). This ensures that carbon dioxide is removed from the expired gas before the expired gas returns to the patient. The unidirectional valves thus cause the gases to travel a one-way modified circular path through the breathing circuit.

Use. The unidirectional valves function passively as the patient breathes and so require no action on the part of the anesthetist. These valves may be used to monitor the patient respiratory rate and depth, and as an aid to check for the proper placement of the ET tube. If the tube is not properly placed, the valves will move sluggishly or not at all despite normal respiratory volume and rate.

Adjustable Pressure Limiting Valve

Description and function. The adjustable pressure limiting valve (APL) valve (also known as the popoff valve, pressure relief valve, or overflow valve) is the point of exit of anesthetic gases from the breathing circuit (see Fig. 4.41 B). APL valves have different appearances but, in all cases, have a knob that can be turned to open or close them.

The main function of the APL valve is to allow excess carrier and anesthetic gases to exit from the breathing circuit and enter the scavenging system. By venting excess gas, the APL valve prevents the buildup of excessive pressure or volume of gases within the circuit. If allowed to occur, this excess pressure could damage the animal's lungs by causing the alveoli to overdistend and rupture. Excess intrathoracic pressure also dramatically decreases the return of blood to the heart, resulting in severely decreased cardiac output.

Use. In a similar way to a water tap, the APL valve can be set anywhere from fully closed by turning the ring clockwise to fully open by turning it counterclockwise, allowing varying amounts of gas to exit from the system and maintaining optimum volume in the reservoir bag (Fig. 4.43 A). When fully open, an APL valve that is working properly releases when the gas pressure in the circuit exceeds 1 to 3 cm H_2O. As the valve is tightened, more pressure is required for release.

When a partial rebreathing system is used, the valve is kept fully open or in some cases, partially open when the patient is spontaneously breathing. During anesthesia, it is closed only when providing manual ventilation so that gases may be forced into the patient's lungs using hand pressure. After each breath provided by manual ventilation, it must be opened again to allow the escape of gases. This rule does not always apply to the use of a full rebreathing system (see Appendix A).

> **TECHNICIAN NOTE** When manual ventilation is provided, the APL valve is closed before the bag is pressed. After each breath, the APL valve *must* be opened again to allow the escape of gases.

A failure to keep the APL valve open at all times when a patient is spontaneously breathing is one of the most frequent causes of serious anesthetic complications and fatalities. Therefore a number of devices designed to prevent such an error are available and should be considered as an add-on feature for any anesthetic machine.

Adjustable pressure limiting occlusion valve. The APL valves on some machines are outfitted with an APL occlusion valve. An APL occlusion valve temporarily prevents air escaping

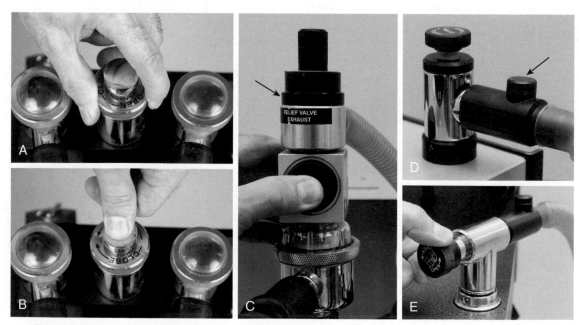

FIG. 4.43 (A) The adjustable pressure limiting (APL) valve on any machine can be closed by turning it clockwise and opened by turning it counterclockwise. **(B)** On machines equipped with an APL occlusion valve, the APL valve can also be closed by pressing the occlusion valve button firmly as shown and opened by releasing pressure. (C) On a different machine, the APL valve (see arrow) is mounted on the expiratory unidirectional valve dome with an APL occlusion valve in between (which is shown being pressed). **(D)** Vertically mounted APL valve with an APL occlusion valve (see arrow) in between the APL valve and the pink scavenging hose. **(E)** Horizontally mounted APL valve with an APL occlusion valve in between the APL valve and pink scavenging hose.

from the APL valve as long as a button on the occlusion valve is pressed. An APL valve thus outfitted can be closed either by turning it, as with other valves, or by pressing firmly on the APL occlusion valve button (see Fig. 4.43 B). This allows the patient to be manually ventilated quickly and easily by pressing the reservoir bag. The valve is opened again by releasing pressure on the button. Use of the occlusion valve minimizes the likelihood of barotrauma resulting from inadvertently leaving the APL valve closed.

Several styles of these occlusion valves are available. Some are placed between the outlet port of the APL valve and the scavenging system and others are built into the APL valve (*see* Fig. 4.43 C–E for other examples of APL valves and APL occlusion valves).

For nonrebreathing circuits, the Safe-Sigh occlusion valve and In-Circuit Patient Pressure Manometer (JD Medical Dist. Co., Inc.; Phoenix, AZ) (Fig. 4.44) provide a pressure manometer and APL occlusion valve that can be placed between the breathing tube and reservoir bag of a nonrebreathing circuit. This gives the anesthetist pushbutton control of the waste gas release and measurement of the pressure applied to the circuit, which provides similar protection against barotrauma when using nonrebreathing circuits.

Safety pressure relief valve. A safety pressure relief valve is a device designed to passively limit the maximum pressure in the breathing circuit and by extension, the patient's lungs, with no action required on the part of the anesthetist. The valve is generally placed between the expiratory breathing tube and the expiratory unidirectional valve of a rebreathing circuit, or between the breathing tube and reservoir bag of a nonrebreathing circuit, or it may be built into the APL valve. It allows gas release when pressure exceeds a safe maximum (usually 20 cm H_2O) and conveys the waste gas to the scavenging system. The Safety Pressure Relief Valve (Supera Anesthesia Innovations, Estacada, OR) (Fig. 4.45) is one example of a valve of this type that allows venting of gas when airway pressure exceeds a safe level.

High Pressure Alarm

A high pressure alarm is a monitoring device that can be added to the breathing circuit to detect and warn the anesthetist of the buildup of excess pressure in the circuit. These devices have a spacer that is placed between the expiratory tube and expiratory unidirectional valve and are often powered by a standard 9-volt battery. The unit emits an audible alarm if pressure exceeds a safe level (usually 20 cm H_2O). The High Patient Pressure Alarm (Surgivet) (Fig. 4.46) is one example of this type of alarm.

The APL valve should be checked for proper operation and adjusted before the commencement of any procedure. In most cases, this will be the fully open position. This should be done at the beginning of every day as a part of the low-pressure system leak test (see Procedure 4.1). It should also be checked periodically during the anesthetic procedure to maintain optimum gas volume within the circuit as indicated by the size of the reservoir bag.

The flowmeter setting, the size of the reservoir bag, and the position of the APL valve (fully open, partially open, or closed) are related in the following way. The flowmeter setting determines the rate at which gas enters the breathing circuit, and the APL valve setting determines the rate at which waste gas leaves the breathing circuit. The size of the bag reflects the net volume of gas in the breathing circuit at any given time. Therefore by adjusting the carrier gas flow rate and APL valve setting, the anesthetist can keep the reservoir bag optimally inflated but not pressurized. Note that the adjustment of the interface of an active scavenging system (see Chapter 5, p 171) can also influence venting of waste gas if too far closed (by preventing escape of waste gas) or too far open (by exerting excess vacuum on the breathing circuit). So proper adjustment of the scavenging system interface is also necessary for appropriate reservoir bag inflation.

Reservoir Bag

Description and function. The reservoir bag (also called the *breathing bag* or *rebreathing bag*) is a rubber bag, often black,

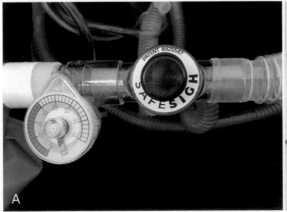
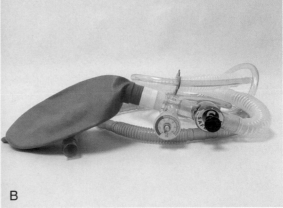

FIG. 4.44 (A) Safe-Sigh occlusion valve *(upper right)* and In-circuit Patient Pressure Manometer *(lower left)* (JD Medical Dist. Co., Inc.; Phoenix, AZ) allows the anesthetist to temporarily close the waste gas outlet of a nonrebreathing system and monitor breathing circuit pressure as the patient is bagged. The valve automatically reopens when released. (B) Note that both the valve and manometer are inserted between the clear breathing tube on the right and the reservoir bag on the left. (Courtesy JD Medical; http://jdmedical.com/veterinary-anesthesia-machines-products/anesthesia-accessories/circuit-patient-pressure-manometer-safe-sigh-circuit.)

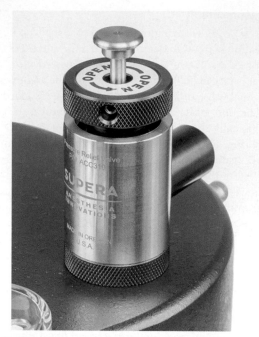

FIG. 4.45 Safety Pressure Relief Valve (Supera Anesthesia Innovations). This device serves as a conventional adjustable pressure limiting (APL) valve. When the button is pressed, the patient can be bagged, but the relief valve will automatically allow release of gas when pressure exceeds 20 to 25 cm H₂O. (Courtesy Supera Anesthesia Innovations; https://www.superavet.com/ACC311.)

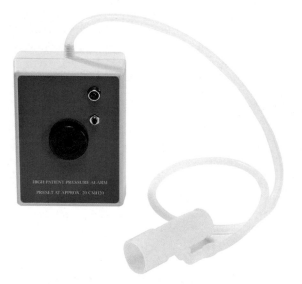

FIG. 4.46 High Patient Pressure Alarm (Surgivet) The white spacer is generally placed between the expiratory tube and expiratory unidirectional valve, and the alarm sounds if pressure in the breathing circuit exceeds a safe level. (Courtesy © 2023 Copyright ICU Medical Inc. or its Affiliates. All rights reserved)

blue, or green (see Fig. 4.41 E), which serves a number of functions, including the following:

- *It serves as a flexible storage reservoir.* Because the breathing circuit is essentially a system of tubes and parts with a fixed volume, a space is necessary to accept expired air and provide air needed to fill the lungs during inspiration.

- *It allows the anesthetist to observe the animal's respiration.* The bag expands as the patient exhales and contracts as the patient inhales. Both the respiratory rate and the respiratory depth can be estimated by observing the movement of the bag. A lack of movement of the bag indicates apnea, a disconnected Y-piece, or blockage of the airway. Inadequate movement indicates a leak in the system, a partial airway blockage, or a decreased V_T. Either situation will alert the anesthetist to a need for intervention.

- *It may be used as one indicator of proper ET tube placement.* Movement of the bag in concert with patient respiratory movements indicates that the ET tube is correctly placed within the trachea.

- *It allows the delivery of anesthetic gases to the patient.* By application of light pressure to the bag (also known as *manual ventilation* or *bagging*), oxygen with or without anesthetic gas can be forced into the patient's lungs. Manual ventilation is used for a variety of purposes including management of apnea, prevention of atelectasis, and provision of ventilation to patients undergoing any surgical procedure in which the chest cavity is open, and to patients given neuromuscular blockers.

There are three reasons why bagging is beneficial for all anesthetized patients:

1. A condition known as **atelectasis** occurs to some degree in most anesthetized patients and compromises **gas exchange**. Bagging helps to reinflate the collapsed alveoli. Many experts recommend bagging all anesthetized patients every 5 to 10 minutes to inflate the lungs gently with fresh oxygen and anesthetic. Use of this technique is further described in Chapter 7.

2. Most anesthetics depress respiratory drive and decrease V_T to as little as 50% of the volume seen in a normal awake patient. This may lead to hypercarbia and hypoxemia. Bagging forces fresh gas into the alveoli, normalizing gas exchange.

3. Anesthetized patients frequently experience decreased respiratory rate or apnea. Bagging allows the anesthetist to normalize the respiratory rate.

Use. Reservoir bags are available in various sizes, from 500 mL (for very small patients) to 30 L (intended for use in adult horses and cattle) (see Figs. 4.12 and 4.47). Ideally, the bag should hold a volume of at least 50 mL/kg of patient weight (approximately five times the patient's V_T during anesthesia), but this is not always practical or necessary. From a practical perspective, the bag should contain enough gas to fill the patient's lungs during an inhalation but should not be so large as to prevent visualization of respiratory movements (Box 4.3).

If the bag is undersized or oversized, a number of complications may arise. If the reservoir bag is too small, the patient may be unable to fill its lungs completely during inspiration. An undersized bag may also become overinflated during exhalation, increasing air pressure in the patient's airways. On the other hand, movement of an oversized bag is hard to see, impairing the ability of the anesthetist to monitor respiration and judge the amount of gas delivered to the patient when providing manual ventilation. A bag that is too large also increases the overall volume of a rebreathing circuit, which will slow the rate of change of the concentration of inhalant anesthetic in the breathing circuit when the vaporizer dial is adjusted.

PROCEDURE 4.1

Low-Pressure System Leak Test and Adjustable Pressure Limiting (APL) Valve Adjustment for Rebreathing Systems (used to test the integrity of the lines and machine parts between the flowmeter[s] and the Y-piece or other patient connector)

1. Turn the oxygen supply on.
2. Close the APL valve and place one hand (or preferably a stopper) over the Y-piece or patient connector. (This closes off all avenues of gas escape from the machine.) (Fig. 1.)

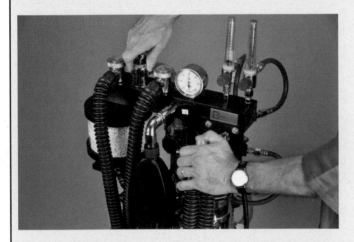

3. Turn the flowmeter on to 3–5 L/min and/or use the oxygen flush valve to fill the reservoir bag. If the reservoir bag does not fill, this is a sign that the machine is not assembled correctly or that there is a large leak in the system. When the bag is full and tight and the pressure manometer registers 30 cm H_2O, turn the flowmeter off (Fig. 2).

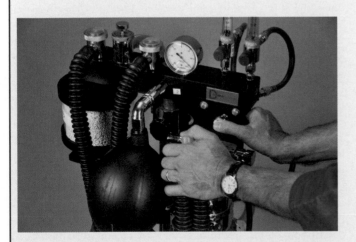

4. Pressure should be maintained at 30 cm H_2O for at least 10 sec. If the pressure begins to drop in that time, slowly turn the flowmeter on until a constant pressure of 30 cm H_2O is maintained for at least 30 sec. No more than 200 mL/min (0.2 L/min) of flow should be necessary to maintain the pressure in the system (Fig. 3). *(If more flow is needed to maintain pressure, there is a significant leak in the system. The connections, hoses, bag, unidirectional valves, the CO_2 absorber canister, and all other parts of the breathing circuit should be checked for leaks. Common locations for leaks are the neck of the reservoir bag, the Y-piece, hoses, and CO_2 absorber canister (see Chapter 5, Fig. 5.9). Others include the air intake valve and the APL valve.)*

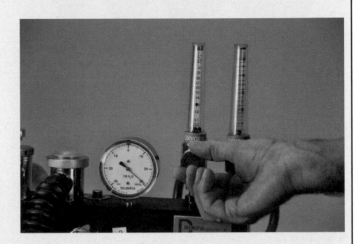

5. Keep the APL valve closed and continue to occlude the Y-piece or patient connector with your thumb or hand. *(If the Y-piece/patient connector is released prior to opening the APL valve, dust from the carbon dioxide absorbent may enter the breathing circuit and cause a variety of problems, including damage to the patient's respiratory tree.)*
6. Turn the oxygen flow on to the anticipated maximum for that procedure (about 1–3 L/min for patients <30 kg, about 3–5 L/min for small animal patients ≥30 kg, and 10 L/min for large animal patients).
7. Without delay, gradually open the APL valve until the pressure manometer indicates a pressure of 1–3 cm H_2O (Fig. 4. On most machines, provided the APL valve is working properly, this should happen when the valve is fully open.

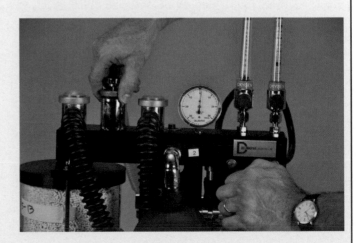

8. During the anesthetic procedure, periodically check that the bag is not collapsed or too full and readjust the APL valve accordingly. (The goal is for the bag to remain about three-quarters full at peak expiration.)

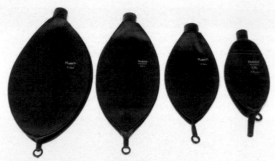

FIG. 4.47 The comparative size of 5-, 3-, 2-, and 1-L reservoir bags.

BOX 4.3

Guidelines for Selecting a Bag
- 500 mL for patients up to 3 kg
- 1 L for 4–7 kg
- 2 L for 8–15 kg
- 3 L for 16–50 kg
- 5 L for 51–150 kg
- 30 to 35 L (on a LA machine) for large animals over 150 kg

Modified from Muir WW, Hubbell JA, Bednarski RM, Lerche, P: *Handbook of veterinary anesthesia*, ed 5, St Louis, MO, 2013, Mosby.

The anesthetist should ensure that the reservoir bag is properly inflated during anesthesia. Inflation is determined by two factors: (1) the rate at which gas is entering the breathing circuit through the fresh gas inlet, which in turn is regulated by the flowmeter setting, and (2) the rate at which gas is exiting the breathing circuit through the APL or overflow valve. During any procedure, the bag should be approximately three-quarters full at peak expiration. If the fresh gas flow is in excess of the patient's demand (as is most often the case), the bag will tend to remain relatively full. If the bag becomes overfilled, excess gas will be vented through the APL valve (see the next section), provided it is left partially or fully open.

> **TECHNICIAN NOTE** During any procedure, the reservoir bag should be approximately three-quarters full at peak expiration.

Safety. Unless a full (total) rebreathing system is being used (which is seldom the case in practice, except for large-animal patients), the APL valve should always be left open when the patient is breathing spontaneously. In the event that it is not left at least partially open, the pressure in the breathing circuit will exceed safe limits and make it difficult or impossible for the animal to exhale. When this happens, the reservoir bag will assume the appearance of an inflated beach ball. If not corrected, the pressure will eventually exceed the maximal safe level (see the discussion of pressure manometers on page 141) and may lead to dangerously decreased cardiac output, ruptured alveoli, and pneumothorax from barotrauma, which are life-threatening complications. Although most commonly caused by a failure to open the APL valve adequately, overinflation of the reservoir bag can also be caused by an obstruction in the scavenging system.

On the other hand, the bag should not be allowed to empty completely when the animal inhales because the patient will be unable to fill its lungs completely with anesthetic gases. Complete emptying of the bag indicates that the fresh gas flow is inadequate, the bag is too small, the APL valve is open too far, or the scavenging system is improperly adjusted.

Carbon Dioxide Absorber Canister

Description and function. All exhaled gases are directed by the expiratory unidirectional valve to the carbon dioxide absorber canister (see Fig. 4.42) before being returned to the patient. Gas may enter the canister through the bottom or the top, depending on the design. The canister contains absorbent granules. The carbon dioxide absorbent and primary ingredient in these products is calcium hydroxide ($Ca[OH]_2$) along with 12% to 20% water, depending on the product. Traditional absorbents, often referred to as soda lime-based absorbents, also contain small amounts of sodium hydroxide (NaOH) and potassium hydroxide (KOH), which activate the chemical reaction. Newer absorbents, such as Amsorb Plus (Armstrong Medical Ltd.; Derry/Londonderry, United Kingdom), Carbolyme (Allied Healthcare Products, Inc.; St. Louis, MO), Sodosorb LF (ICU Medical Global; San Clemente, CA), and Litholyme (Allied Healthcare Products, Inc.; St. Louis, MO) contain no KOH and smaller amounts of NaOH or no NaOH. All of these agents react with exhaled carbon dioxide to form calcium carbonate ($CaCO_3$) and small amounts of other chemicals. During this reaction, heat and water are produced and the pH decreases.

When significant amounts of carbon dioxide are absorbed, the heat released by this reaction may cause the carbon dioxide absorber canister to become warm during use. The water produced by this reaction may serve to humidify the fresh gas entering the breathing circuit from the fresh gas inlet.

The chemical reaction has several steps and varies slightly depending on the activator but results in the following overall reaction:

$$CO_2 + Ca(OH)_2 \rightarrow CaCO_3 + H_2O + Heat$$

Carbon dioxide absorbents are supplied as loose granules or in a prepackaged cartridge. The granules are of a size (4 to 8 mesh) large enough to allow gases to pass though without excessive resistance, but small enough to provide adequate surface area for the absorption of carbon dioxide.

Use. The carbon dioxide absorber canister must be filled in a particular way to ensure efficient absorption (see page 156 for a description of this technique) so that channels do not form, which will decrease absorption efficiency. Carbon dioxide absorbents do not last indefinitely. After absorption of an amount of CO_2 which varies among absorbents, the granules become exhausted. The use of depleted granules will result in rebreathing of carbon dioxide, leading to hypercapnia. There are several ways in which the anesthetist may become aware of granules that are exhausted and must be replaced, including the following:
- Fresh granules, containing mainly calcium hydroxide, can be chipped or crumbled with finger pressure, whereas granules saturated with carbon dioxide (containing mainly calcium carbonate) become hard and brittle.

- Most granules contain a pH indicator that will cause the granules to change color when exhausted, usually from white to violet (in those that contain ethyl violet dye) or, in some cases, from white to pink (in those containing phenolphthalein dye), depending on the brand (Fig. 4.48). The color reaction does not always occur, however, especially when smaller patients are anesthetized, and the color change may not be visible when looking at the outside of the canister in the event that the exhaled gases flow through channels in the granules at the center of the canister. In addition, some brands of absorbent granules that have changed color (indicating saturation with carbon dioxide) may return to the original color after a few hours, although they are still saturated with carbon dioxide. Thus it is important that the anesthetist change the absorbent in the event that a color change is noted as soon as possible after using an anesthetic machine.
- When a capnograph is used to monitor the patient, the concentration of carbon dioxide during peak inspiration should be at or near 0 mmHg if the absorbent is working correctly. A higher carbon dioxide level at peak inspiration indicates possible exhaustion of the absorbent (although there are other causes of elevated inspired CO_2 such as a nonfunctional expiratory unidirectional valve).
- The presence of visible moisture in the canister and warmth noted when touching the canister suggests possible exhaustion of the absorbent.

Regardless of whether or not any of the previously mentioned indicators are evident, the granules should always be changed after 6 to 8 hours of use, or after 30 days (some experts recommend 2 weeks) even if the machine has not been used. They should also be changed in the event that the oxygen flowmeter was inadvertently left on overnight or during any other equivalent period the machine was not in use.

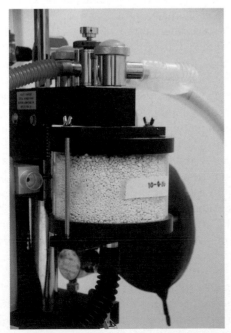

FIG. 4.48 The color change to violet indicates exhaustion of the carbon dioxide absorbent and a need to change the granules. Note that some granules turn from white to pink.

> **TECHNICIAN NOTE** Signs that CO_2 granules must be changed are as follows:
> - Hard, brittle granules
> - Color change of one-third to one-half of the granules
> - A carbon dioxide (CO_2) level greater than 0 during peak inspiration as measured with a capnograph
> - The presence of moisture and heat generation in the canister
> - After 6–8 hr of use
> - After 14–30 days, even if (1) the maximum of 6–8 hr has not been reached or (2) the machine has not been used
> - If the oxygen flowmeter was inadvertently left on overnight or for any equivalent period

Safety. Studies have shown that some absorbents, particularly soda lime-based absorbents, may react with sevoflurane to produce a potentially nephrotoxic substance known as *compound A*. The production of this substance has been found to have no clinically significant adverse effects in veterinary patients, however.

After use, absorbents may also become desiccated (dried out) and produce a variety of adverse effects. This most commonly happens when oxygen continues to flow through the machine when not in use, such as would happen if the oxygen flowmeter was inadvertently left on. The absorbent may also become desiccated if the bag or other container is left open to room air for a prolonged period. When desiccated, absorbents containing KOH or NaOH can react with some anesthetics (including isoflurane, sevoflurane, and desflurane) to produce excessive heat and carbon monoxide, formaldehyde, and various other toxins that are harmful to the patient. These effects are minimized, however, by using absorbents without KOH and with lower concentrations of or no NaOH. For this reason, newer agents containing no KOH and little or no NaOH are available (such as Amsorb Plus, Carbolyme, Sodasorb LF, and Litholyme). In any case, when purchasing an absorbent, check with the manufacturer to be sure that it is compatible with the inhalant anesthetic you are using.

Pressure Manometer

Description and function. The pressure manometer (not to be confused with the tank pressure gauge or line pressure gauge) (see Fig. 4.41 D) indicates the pressure of the gases within the breathing circuit and by extension, the pressure in the animal's airways and lungs. This pressure is most often expressed in centimeters of water (cm H_2O) although on some machines, the pressure may be expressed in millimeters of mercury (mmHg) or kilopascals.

Use. The pressure manometer is used when bagging an animal to determine the pressure being exerted on the animal's lungs when the anesthetist squeezes the reservoir bag (Fig. 4.49). The pressure manometer should read 0 to 3 cm H_2O when the patient is breathing spontaneously. It should read no more than 20 cm H_2O (15 mmHg) in small animals, or 40 cm H_2O (30 mmHg) in large animals when positive pressure assisted or controlled ventilation is provided unless the chest cavity is open, in which case the pressure can be somewhat higher. Excessive pressure in the circuit

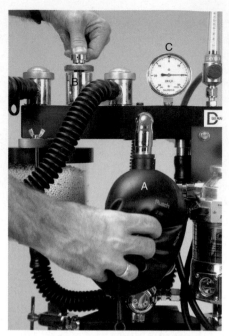

FIG. 4.49 Providing manual ventilation, or "bagging" the patient. The adjustable pressure limiting (APL) valve or APL occlusion valve *(B)* is closed and the bag *(A)* is squeezed while the pressure manometer *(C)* is watched to ensure that safe pressure is not exceeded. The APL valve or APL occlusion valve is immediately opened as soon as pressure on the bag is released.

can result in dyspnea, lung damage, or pneumothorax. Therefore as previously mentioned, the pressure must be watched closely during any anesthetic procedure.

Higher pressure may be needed in an animal with pulmonary dysfunction, such as a dog with gastric dilatation–volvulus or a colicky, bloated horse. In the case of a dog with gastric dilatation–volvulus, pressures of 30 to 35 cm H_2O may be needed to deliver a reasonable tidal volume, and in bloated horses, pressures up to 50 to 55 cm H_2O may be necessary.

TECHNICIAN NOTE Maximum safe pressure manometer readings (when the chest is closed) are as follows:
- 0–3 cm H_2O when the patient is breathing spontaneously
- 20 cm H_2O in small animals when positive-pressure ventilation is provided
- 40 cm H_2O in large animals when positive-pressure ventilation is provided

---

Air Intake Valve (Negative Pressure Relief Valve)

Description and Function. An air intake valve is present on some machines, either as a separate part or incorporated into the inspiratory unidirectional valve or the APL valve (Fig. 4.50). This valve admits room air to the circuit in the event that negative pressure (a partial vacuum) is detected in the breathing circuit, a situation indicated by a collapsed reservoir bag. If a partial vacuum develops, the patient will be unable to fill its lungs and will develop hypoxemia because of inadequate oxygen levels. This may happen when the machine is incorrectly assembled or when an active scavenging system is exerting excessive suction.

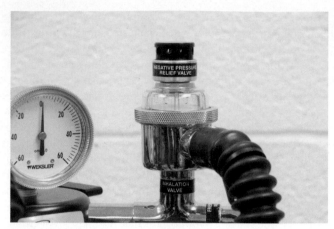

FIG. 4.50 Air intake valve. The valve labeled "Negative Pressure Relief Valve," which on this machine is positioned on top of the inspiratory unidirectional valve, will open and admit room air into the breathing circuit in the event that negative pressure develops within the circuit.

Negative pressure may also develop in the circuit if the oxygen flow rate is too low or if the tank runs out of oxygen. The air intake valve ensures that the patient always receives some oxygen by admitting room air (which contains 21% oxygen) into the circuit. Even though this situation is not ideal, it is preferable that the patient breathes room air rather than none at all, as would be the case if the air intake valve were not present.

Breathing Tubes and Y-Piece

Description and function. The inspiratory and expiratory breathing tubes (corrugated breathing tubes) complete the breathing circuit by carrying the anesthetic gases to and from the patient. Each tube is connected to a unidirectional valve at one end and to the Y-piece or other patient connector at the other end. They are made of rubber or plastic and come in three sizes: (1) large-animal 50-mm diameter tubes (designed for animals weighing 150 kg or more), (2) small-animal 22-mm diameter tubes (designed for medium to large patients), and (3) small-animal pediatric 15-mm diameter tubes (designed for small animals weighing 7 kg or less) (Fig. 4.51 A and B). An alternative configuration known as a *Universal F-circuit* is a type of breathing tube in which the inspiratory tube is located within the expiratory tube. This arrangement is designed to decrease the overall bulk of the breathing tubes and also to conserve body heat as cold-inspired gases traveling through the inner turquoise tube are warmed by expired gases traveling through the outer transparent tube (see Fig. 4.51 C). The degree to which this effect is realized is controversial and, in any case, is dependent on the carrier gas flow and other factors.

Use. Before using the machine, select the appropriate breathing tubes for the patient. Standard small-animal tubes are used on small-animal machines for patients over 7 kg body weight, whereas pediatric tubes are recommended for patients weighing 3 to 7 kg, primarily to reduce mechanical dead space. Large-animal tubes are designed for use only on large-animal machines. One end of each tube must be firmly attached to the inspiratory and expiratory unidirectional valves and the other

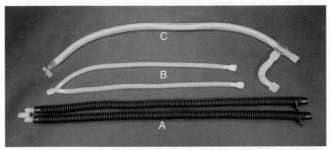

FIG. 4.51 Corrugated breathing tubes. **(A)** Standard 22-mm small animal breathing tubes, **(B)** 15-mm pediatric tubes, **(C)** Universal F-circuit.

end of each tube to the Y-piece, which connects the two tubes together. The remaining port of the Y-piece is then connected to a mask or to an ET tube.

The tubes used must be large enough to minimize resistance to airflow as the patient breathes. In a practical sense, this means that they should be no smaller in diameter than the size of the ET tube. On the other hand, larger tubes are associated with greater mechanical dead space in the patient connector, which has many negative consequences and which must be minimized in all patients, particularly those that are very small.

> **TECHNICIAN NOTE** Standard small animal tubes are used on small animal machines for patients over 7 kg body weight, whereas pediatric tubes are recommended for patients weighing 3–7 kg to reduce mechanical dead space. Large animal tubes are designed for use only on large animal machines.

NONREBREATHING SYSTEMS

Although the rebreathing systems just discussed are well suited to many patients, very small patients (those under 3 kg body weight) require the use of an alternative machine configuration called a nonrebreathing system. The main difference in the design of a nonrebreathing system is that there is no carbon dioxide absorbent and there are no unidirectional valves. Exhaled carbon dioxide is instead pushed out of the circuit by high fresh gas flow. In a nonrebreathing system, little or no exhaled gas is returned to the patient, assuming there is adequate fresh gas flow; it is instead evacuated through an APL or overflow valve, or an exit port. The main advantages of nonrebreathing circuits are that they (1) decrease resistance to breathing that is associated with the movement of air through some unidirectional valves and carbon dioxide absorber canisters, and (2) decrease equipment dead space in most cases. Both of these advantages are beneficial for the safety of small patients (those weighing <7 kg) and necessary for very small patients (those weighing <3 kg) due to the very low respiratory drive and tidal volume in patients of this size. The characteristics of rebreathing and nonrebreathing systems are compared in Table 4.2.

When a nonrebreathing system is used, the rebreathing circuit is disabled by detaching the fresh gas hose connector from the vaporizer outlet port or the common gas outlet if present. Then a nonrebreathing circuit is attached in its place. As with a rebreathing system, the nonrebreathing system can best be understood by tracing the path of the oxygen from the compressed gas cylinder to the patient and ultimately to the scavenging system.

Just as in a rebreathing system, oxygen (and other carrier gases, if used) flows from the tank, through a flowmeter, and into the vaporizer. After exiting the vaporizer, however, the gases follow a different path. Instead of routing the fresh gas into the circle as occurs with a rebreathing system, the fresh gas is routed directly to the patient via a fresh gas inlet that is most often positioned very near the patient connector. Exhaled gases pass through another hose, often a clear corrugated tube, then in most systems, enter a reservoir bag and ultimately are released into the scavenging system through an overflow valve or other exit port. In this system, carbon dioxide absorbent is unnecessary because exhaled gases are vented from the system immediately after exhalation.

TABLE 4.2	**Comparison of Rebreathing and Nonrebreathing Systems**	
Parameters	**Nonrebreathing System**	**Rebreathing System (Partial or Full)**
CO_2 absorption	Not required	Must have CO_2 absorber canister
Changes in depth of anesthesia	Fast	Slow
Oxygen flow rates	High-flow rates: generally must equal or exceed the respiratory minute volume	Low-flow rates: considerably less than the respiratory minute volume
Cost of operation (per unit body weight)	High because of the amount of oxygen and anesthetic used	Low because less oxygen and anesthetic used
Amount of waste gas produced	High	Low
APL valve position	Fully open	Fully to partially open
Heat and moisture conservation (from exhaled gases)	Poor	Good
Vaporizer position	Outside the breathing circuit (no circle present)	VOC (when using precision vaporizers)
Size of animal	Any size: limited only by the total gas flow that is delivered; generally recommended for animals under 7 kg	Only for animals over 7 kg (if pediatric hoses are used, can be used for animals 3–7 kg also)

VOC, Vaporizer-out-of-circuit.

Nonrebreathing Circuits

Nonrebreathing circuits are available in several configurations with a confusing variety of names, including (1) Magill circuit, (2) Lack circuit, (3) Bain coaxial circuit, (4) Ayre's T-piece, (5) Jackson–Rees circuit, and (6) Norman elbow. Most of these circuits are lightweight, easy to move and position, and comparatively inexpensive to purchase.

Common parts of each of these circuits include a patient connector, a fresh gas inlet, a reservoir bag, an overflow valve or exit port, and an associated scavenger tube to connect the overflow valve or exit port to the scavenging system. Most also have a corrugated breathing tube joining the patient connector

and reservoir bag. The overflow valve may function like an expiratory unidirectional valve, may be opened and closed in a similar manner to the APL valve of a rebreathing system, or may effectively function as an "on-off switch," meaning a lever that opens or closes but does not allow fine adjustment. Where these circuits differ is in the position of the fresh gas inlet, reservoir bag, and overflow valve or exit port. Nonrebreathing circuits are grouped using the Mapleson classification system into classes A though F based on the position of these parts (Fig. 4.52). Note that only class A, modified A, modified D, E, and F are in common use for veterinary patients.

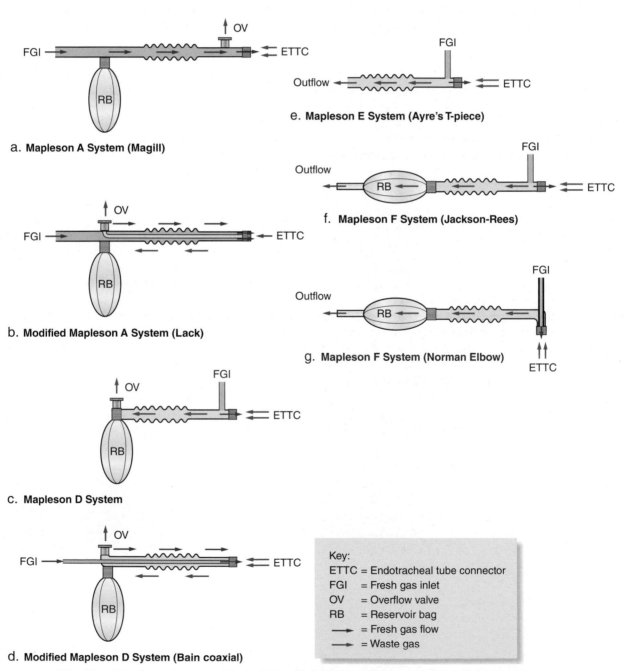

FIG. 4.52 (a) Mapleson A system (Magill). (b) Modified Mapleson A system (Lack). (c) Mapleson D system. (d) Modified Mapleson D system (Bain coaxial). (e) Mapleson E system (Ayre's T-piece). (f) Mapleson F system (Jackson–Rees). (g) Mapleson F system (Norman elbow).

Mapleson A and Modified Mapleson A Systems

The Mapleson A and modified Mapleson A systems, although somewhat different in construction, are functionally the same in that they both generally require lower fresh gas flow during spontaneous ventilation and are more efficient than other Mapleson designs when the patient is spontaneously breathing (as opposed to being manually ventilated). These systems are more commonly used in Europe and the UK than in North America.

Magill Circuit (Mapleson A System). The Magill circuit (see Fig. 4.52 A) has an overflow valve at the patient end of the breathing tube. Both the fresh gas inlet and the reservoir bag are located away from the patient at the opposite end of the breathing tube. Fresh gas flow pushes exhaled gases through the overflow valve. The chief advantage of this system is the relatively low fresh gas flow required during spontaneous ventilation (0.7 to 1.0 × the RMV). It is therefore feasible to use this system for medium or large patients. When a patient is manually ventilated, some rebreathing of expired gases may occur with this system and for that reason, it is not recommended for providing controlled ventilation.

Lack circuit (modified Mapleson A system). The Lack circuit (see Fig. 4.52 B) is similar to the Magill circuit except that it has an expiratory tube that runs from the ET tube connector to an overflow valve near the bag. In this system, the fresh gas inlet, the overflow valve, and the reservoir bag are located away from the patient at the opposite end of the breathing tube. This system is used in a similar way as the Magill circuit.

Mapleson D, E, and F Systems

Mapleson D, E, and F systems are structurally similar in that they all have a fresh gas inlet near the patient connector and a breathing tube that conducts exhaled gases away from the patient to an overflow valve or exit port, and functionally similar in that they require higher fresh gas flows to prevent rebreathing. These systems are the only systems in common use in North America.

Bain coaxial circuit (modified Mapleson D system). The Mapleson D system (see Fig. 4.52 C) has a fresh gas inlet near the patient connector. Both the overflow valve and the reservoir bag are located away from the patient at the opposite end of the breathing tube. The overflow valve may be built into the bag or near the bag. The Bain coaxial circuit (see Fig. 4.52 D) is a modification of the Mapleson D system in which the tube supplying fresh gas is surrounded by the larger, corrugated tubing (which conducts gas away from the patient). In this respect, it looks like a Universal F-circuit (previously discussed under rebreathing systems), but the two must not be mistaken for one-another because they are very different in terms of function and use. This "tube within a tube" arrangement allows the incoming gases to be warmed slightly by the exhaled gases that surround them before reaching the patient. This beneficial effect is minimal, however, due to high fresh gas flow rates that are used with nonrebreathing systems.

When this system is used, some rebreathing of waste gases will occur unless an oxygen flow rate of approximately two to three times the RMV is used (up to a maximum of 3 L/min for patients under 7 kg) although when the patient is breathing spontaneously, minimal rebreathing may occur at lower flow rates, depending on other factors such as the respiratory rate and the length of the pause between expiration and inspiration.

Universal control arm. Many nonrebreathing circuits have design characteristics that can be problematic when providing manual assisted or controlled ventilation. Most do not have a pressure manometer. In addition, many of these systems either do not have an APL valve or have an overflow valve that functions like an on-off switch and consequently is not easy to adjust. These characteristics make it challenging to control the size of the reservoir bag and to make sure appropriate pressure is applied when bagging a patient. When using a Modified Mapleson D System (Bain coaxial circuit), these disadvantages can be overcome by using a universal control arm (also known as a Bain block). A universal control arm is a device that when attached to a Bain coaxial circuit, provides a conventional APL valve and manometer, increasing the ease and accuracy with which manual ventilation can be provided. It is usually attached to the stand of a conventional anesthetic machine (Fig. 4.53). The breathing tube of the Bain coaxial circuit is attached to the breathing tube port of the universal control arm instead of to the bag and overflow valve that is provided with the circuit. The breathing tube port communicates with a reservoir bag, pressure manometer, and conventional APL valve, allowing manual ventilation with similar ease to that obtained with a rebreathing system.

Ayre's T-piece (Mapleson E system). The Ayre's T-piece (see Fig. 4.52 E) is a T-shaped tube with a fresh gas inlet entering the patient end of the breathing tube at a 45- to 90-degree angle (like the base of the letter *T; thus the name "T-piece"*). Unlike other circuits, the Ayre's T-piece does not have a reservoir bag at the opposite end of the breathing tube. The fresh gas flow with this system should be two to three times the RMV.

Jackson–Rees circuit and Norman elbow (Mapleson F systems). The Jackson–Rees circuit and the Norman elbow (see Fig. 4.52 F and G) have a fresh gas inlet at the patient end of the

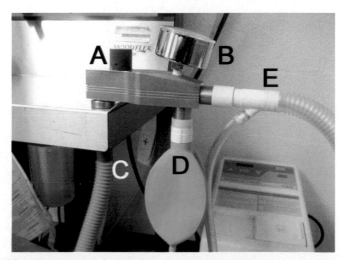

FIG. 4.53 Universal Control Arm. *A,* Adjustable pressure limiting (APL) valve *(black knob); B,* pressure manometer; *C,* transfer hose to the scavenging system; *D,* reservoir bag; *E,* the breathing tube of the Bain coaxial circuit is attached to the port of the universal control arm instead of to the bag and overflow valve that comes with the circuit.

breathing tube and a reservoir bag at the opposite end. The fresh gas inlet of a Jackson–Rees circuit enters the patient connector at a 45- to 90-degree angle. The Norman elbow is almost identical to a Jackson–Rees circuit except that the fresh gas inlet travels inside the patient connector and discharges fresh gas very near the ET tube. This circuit is intended to reduce mechanical dead space when compared with an Ayre's T-piece or Jackson–Rees but otherwise is used in a similar manner to these circuits. The fresh gas flow with both the Norman elbow and the Jackson–Rees should be two to three times the RMV.

Heat and Moisture Exchangers

Under normal circumstances, in an awake animal, the temperature and humidity of inhaled air is increased by the nose and nasopharynx (from approximately 22°C and 30% humidity to 32°C and 100% humidity) before entering the lower respiratory passages and the alveoli. This natural heating and humidification support normal lung functions such as mucociliary clearance. During an anesthetic event, anesthetic gases in a breathing circuit are relatively cool (close to room temperature) and dry (<10% humidity) and bypass the nose and nasopharynx when traveling through an ETT or supraglottic airway device. Consequently, natural heating and humidification does not occur. This may lead to a variety of negative effects including hypothermia, dehydration, damage to respiratory epithelium, thickening of respiratory mucus, bronchospasm, and inflammation.[a]

Several steps can be taken to minimize these effects, including leak testing the machine before use, using a rebreathing circuit as opposed to a nonrebreathing circuit when possible, avoiding excessive fresh gas flow, and ensuring that carbon dioxide absorbent is fresh (which adds heat and moisture to the system as products of the chemical reaction associated with carbon dioxide removal). Other ways to mitigate these effects involve the use of a passive or active humidification device.

A heat and moisture exchanger (HME) (Fig. 4.54) is a single-use, disposable device designed to passively heat and humidify the gases by capturing exhaled warmed water vapor and releasing it back into the inhaled air when placed between the airway and the patient connector of the breathing circuit. HMEs consist of a plastic housing containing a substance such as foam, paper, or cellulose that captures and condenses moisture. Many include a filter designed to remove bacterial and viral particles from exhaled gases as well. These devices are small, easy to use, and inexpensive, and help to conserve moisture that would ordinarily be lost. It is important to keep in mind that HMEs will increase mechanical dead space and increase resistance to breathing when wet, both of which may be problematic, especially when anesthetizing very small patients.

Electronic Anesthesia Machines

A relatively recent development in the veterinary market is the introduction of electronic anesthesia machines. The Vetland EX3000 Electronic Veterinary Anesthesia Machine (Vetland Medical Sales and Services, LLC, Louisville, KY) is an example of this technology (Fig. 4.55). This machine is electronically controlled and thus requires connection to an electrical outlet. An isoflurane vaporizer and a sevoflurane vaporizer are incorporated into the body of the machine with only the fill ports exposed. Major machine functions such as oxygen flow and the vaporizer setting are electronically controlled by the use of a touchscreen. It includes internal monitors that track several parameters related to patient safety to warn of impending problems before they become critical. These are (1) pressure of the primary oxygen supply, (2) pressure in the breathing circuit, (3) audible breath sounds, (4) level of liquid anesthetic in the vaporizer, and (5) the percentage of inhalant anesthetic in the breathing circuit.

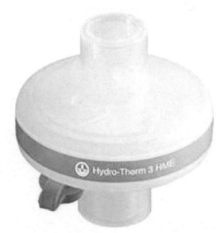

FIG. 4.54 Heat and moisture exchanger (HME). (Courtesy Intersurgical ltd.)

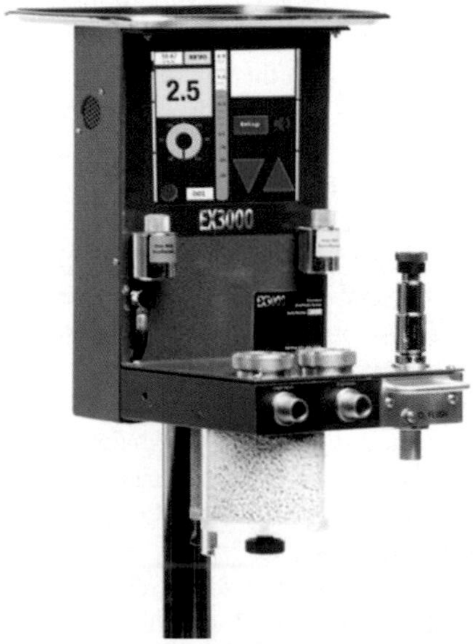

[a]From Cooley KG, Johnson RA: *Veterinary anesthetic and monitoring equipment*, Ames, IA, 2018, John Wiley & Sons, Inc, pp 91–93.

FIG. 4.55 An example of an electronically controlled anesthesia machine with touchscreen controls.

OPERATION OF THE ANESTHETIC MACHINE

Daily Setup

At the beginning of each day, before using an anesthetic machine, the anesthetist must assemble the machine or machines to be used and check the oxygen and liquid anesthetic levels. Before each case, the anesthetist must also choose between a small-animal and a large-animal machine, determine what type of breathing circuit to use (rebreathing or nonrebreathing), and choose carrier gas flow rates. Finally, the low-pressure system must be checked for leaks and the APL or overflow valve must be appropriately set. (See Procedure 4.1 for rebreathing systems and Procedure 4.2 for nonrebreathing systems.

Procedure 4.3 is a checklist to be followed when setting up anesthetic equipment.)

> **TECHNICIAN NOTE** The appropriate choice of a machine (large animal vs. small animal), reservoir bag, breathing tubes, oxygen flow rates, and breathing circuit type is based on the patient's body weight.

Choosing a Machine

The decision of whether to use a small-animal or large-animal machine is based on the patient's weight. A small-animal machine is intended for patients under 150 kg (about 350 lb) and

---

PROCEDURE 4.2

Low-Pressure System Leak Tests and Overflow Valve or Adjustable Pressure Limiting (APL) Valve Adjustment for Nonrebreathing Systems (used to test the integrity of the lines and machine parts between the flowmeter[s] and the patient connector)

1. Turn the oxygen supply on.
2. Close the overflow valve or APL valve and place one hand (or preferably a stopper) over the patient port. (This closes off all avenues of gas escape from the machine.) (Fig. 1.)

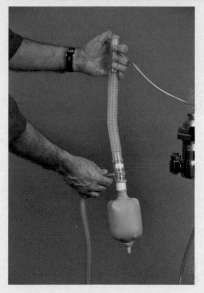

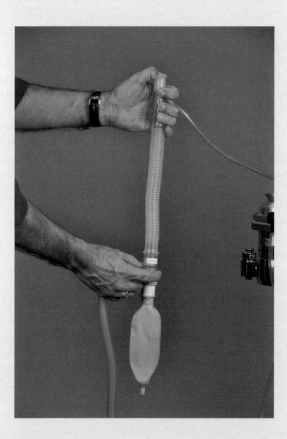

3. Turn the flowmeter on to 1–3 L/min to fill the reservoir bag (Fig. 2). If the reservoir bag does not fill, this is a sign that the machine is not assembled correctly or there is a large leak in the system.

4. When the bag is full and tight, turn the flowmeter off. If the circuit is attached to a universal control arm or other pressure manometer, the pressure in the circuit should register 30 cm H_2O. The bag should remain fully inflated and pressure should be maintained for at least 10 sec. *(A significant decrease in pressure indicates that a leak is present. The connections, hoses, bag, and all other parts of the breathing circuit should be checked for leaks.)*
5. The APL valve or overflow valve should always be fully open when this system is used except when positive-pressure manual ventilation is being provided.

*Testing a Bain Coaxial System for integrity of the Fresh Gas Inlet (used to test the integrity of the inner fresh gas tube)

1. For a test of the internal hose (fresh gas tube) of a Bain circuit, turn the oxygen flowmeter on to 2–4 L/min.
2. Occlude the fresh gas inlet (visible within the patient end of the breathing hose) with a 3-mL syringe plunger while the flowmeter is observed for 2–5 sec.
3. If there is no leak, the ball or bobbin indicator in the oxygen flowmeter should drop slightly, indicating adequate back pressure.
4. When the plunger is removed, the release of pressurized gas should make a hissing sound. To avoid damage to the flowmeter, avoid occluding the inner tube any longer than necessary.
5. A test failure indicates that the inner tube may be disconnected or leaky, resulting in a large increase in mechanical dead space, in which case the patient will be in danger of rebreathing exhaled gases.
   Note: This test will not work if there are side holes at the end of the fresh gas flow tube.

PROCEDURE 4.3

Equipment and Machine Setup Checklist
1. Assemble all needed supplies.
2. If using an active scavenging system, turn on the scavenging system exhaust fan or vacuum pump.
3. Identify and weigh the patient.
4. Choose appropriately sized endotracheal tubes based on patient signalment and body weight.
5. Check the endotracheal tubes for integrity and inflate the endotracheal tube cuffs to check for leaks.
6. If a laryngoscope is used, choose an appropriately sized blade and check the light.
7. Choose an appropriate machine (large animal [LA] versus small animal [SA]) based on the patient's body weight.
8. Choose an appropriate breathing circuit (rebreathing or nonrebreathing) based on the patient's body weight.
9. If using a rebreathing system, choose appropriate corrugated breathing tubes (LA, SA, or pediatric) and a reservoir bag based on the patient's body weight (see Box 4.3).
10. Assemble the machine(s):
    a. Connect the vaporizer inlet port hose.
    b. Connect the fresh gas inlet hose of the breathing circuit to the vaporizer outlet port or common gas outlet if present.
    c. If using a rebreathing system, attach an appropriately sized reservoir bag and breathing tubes.
    d. Connect the scavenging system hoses.
11. Check that all compressed gas cylinders are correctly mounted in the yokes (E or J tanks) or connected to the pressure regulator (H or K tanks).
12. Turn on the oxygen supply, check the primary and secondary oxygen supply pressure, and replace empty tanks as necessary.
13. Attach DISS connectors to oxygen outlets or drops if using a hospital distribution system.
14. Check the flowmeter controls to ensure proper function.
15. Check the amount of anesthetic in the vaporizer and replenish as necessary. Ensure that the vaporizer and flowmeter are off before filling the vaporizer.
16. Rotate the vaporizer dial to ensure smooth function. Turn to "off."
17. Check the carbon dioxide absorbent and change it if necessary.
18. Check the low-pressure system for leaks and set the APL or overflow valve (see Procedures 4.1 and 4.2).

BOX 4.4   Time Constants

The concept of time constants helps explain why a change in the vaporizer dial setting takes time to be reflected in the circuit (and in the patient's lungs), and also gives the anesthetist a rough idea as to how long they can expect to wait for a change in anesthetic concentration to occur. *The time constant (in minutes) is calculated by dividing the total volume of the breathing circuit (in L) by the carrier gas flow rate (in L/min).* When the vaporizer dial setting is changed, it takes five time constants to effect a 95% change in circuit concentration.

Consider a circuit that has a total volume of about 5 L (2 L for the reservoir bag, 1.5 L for the carbon dioxide absorber, and 1.5 L in the inspiratory and expiratory hoses). If the fresh gas flow rate is 2 L/min, the time constant is 2.5 min (5 L ÷ 2 L/min). In this example, if the vaporizer dial setting is changed, it will take 12.5 min (five time constants, i.e., 2.5 min × 5) before the anesthetic concentration in the circuit reaches 95% of the new dial setting. In contrast, if the anesthetist is using a low-flow technique (e.g., an oxygen flow rate of 500 mL or 0.5 L) with a circuit volume of 5 L, the time constant is 10 min (5 L ÷ 0.5 L/min). This amounts to a total of 50 min (10 min × 5) for the anesthetic concentration in the circuit to reach 95% of the new dial setting! This explains why there is such a time lag between making a vaporizer dial change and seeing a change in the anesthetic depth if low flows are used. There are two ways to change the concentration more rapidly: turn up the fresh gas flow rate and shorten the time constant for the circuit being used, or make a large change in the vaporizer dial setting.

Anesthetic vaporizers must also be checked to make sure that enough anesthetic remains in the vaporization chamber. Most vaporizers have an indicator window at the base that allows the technician to inspect the amount of liquid anesthetic remaining. In order for the vaporizer to function properly, the liquid anesthetic must be between the full and empty lines of the window. The vaporizer should be refilled as needed but kept at least half full at all times. A pouring spout or keyed adapter (see Fig. 4.39) should be used for this purpose. Overfilling a vaporizer will result in an anesthetic overdose, and underfilling will result in an inability to keep the patient anesthetized. The vaporizer should also be turned off when the machine is not in use.

Choice of Rebreathing Versus Nonrebreathing System

The decision of whether to use a rebreathing system or a nonrebreathing system is generally made on the basis of the patient's size. This is because the patient's respiratory drive—the force generated by the respiratory muscles during breathing—is directly related to body weight. The respiratory drive of very small patients is insufficient to move gas through areas of resistance to air movement (primarily the unidirectional valves, carbon dioxide canister, and breathing tubes).[a] In contrast, nonrebreathing systems offer little resistance to air movement, a significant advantage for these patients. The choice of system to be used is important in terms of machine setup and use because it will determine the following:

- The type of equipment required (a conventional anesthetic machine, with or without a nonrebreathing system such as a Bain coaxial circuit)

a large-animal machine is intended for patients weighing 150 kg or more.

Machine Assembly

Before assembling the machine, choose the breathing circuit and, if using a rebreathing circuit, choose appropriately sized breathing tubes and reservoir bag. These decisions are based on patient weight. Once the equipment has been chosen, connect all necessary parts, including the vaporizer inlet and outlet port hoses, the breathing circuit if using a nonrebreathing system, and the reservoir bag and breathing tubes if using a rebreathing system. Finally, connect the scavenging system hoses and any other parts required for the machine you are using, such as the common gas outlet.

Checking Oxygen and Anesthetic Levels

The oxygen supply must be checked to be sure enough oxygen remains to complete the procedure. Guidelines regarding oxygen supply may be found in the discussion of the tank pressure gauge.

---

[a]Note that the size of the ET tube has a greater effect on resistance than does the type of circuit used. The use of an ET tube that is too small results in far greater resistance to air movement than that offered by the remainder of the anesthetic circuit, even in a rebreathing system.

- The position of the APL valve (closed, partially open, or open)
- Oxygen flow rates

Rebreathing systems may be safely used on all larger patients but as mentioned, are not safe for very small patients. For this reason, most anesthetists recommend a rebreathing system for patients weighing 7 kg (15 lb) or over unless the system is fitted with pediatric hoses (and assuming the unidirectional valves are of a lightweight and nonstick design), in which case it may also be used on patients as small as 3 kg. Patients smaller than 3 kg should be placed on a nonrebreathing system.

Although patient weight is the primary determining factor in making a decision concerning which system to use, other advantages and disadvantages of each of these systems must be considered including the following:

- *Cost:* Full rebreathing (closed) systems are the most economical because the very low gas flow rates used with these systems conserve carrier and anesthetic gases. Partial and minimal rebreathing systems use higher gas flow rates and so are not as economical as full rebreathing systems. Nonrebreathing systems are the least economical because they use the highest gas flow of all the systems and consequently use more carrier and anesthetic gas per unit body weight.
- *Control of anesthetic depth:* The speed at which the anesthetist can change anesthetic depth depends in part on the type of system used. Changes take longer with a rebreathing system because the flow of fresh oxygen and anesthetic into the system is low compared with the volume of the circuit. Therefore when the vaporizer setting is changed, it will take longer for the concentration of anesthetic in the breathing circuit to reach the desired level. A nonrebreathing system allows a much faster turnover of gases because flow rates of fresh gas are higher relative to the volume of the circuit. Because of this higher flow and because the fresh gas is often delivered very close to the patient, changes in the anesthetic concentration breathed in by the patient occur more rapidly. This means that the anesthetic concentration breathed by the patient is very close to that indicated by the dial with a nonrebreathing system soon after a change is made. In contrast, with a rebreathing system, the concentration of anesthetic breathed in by the patient will not be the same as that indicated on the dial for several to many minutes after the setting has been changed.[a] The time required for the anesthetic concentration in the circuit to approximate that on the dial can be determined by calculating the time constant. (See Box 4.4 for information on time constants.)
- *Conservation of heat and moisture:* Fresh gas entering a breathing system from the vaporizer is relatively cool and dry compared with the patient's exhaled gases, which are warm and moist. Inspired fresh anesthetic gases are delivered at or near room temperature (23°C [~73°F]) and have a relative humidity of less than 10%, whereas exhaled gases have significantly higher temperature and humidity. Rebreathing systems

automatically warm and humidify fresh gas that enters the circuit as it mixes with the patient's expired gases. In nonrebreathing systems, the warmed and humidified gases exhaled by the patient exit through the scavenger, and the patient breathes only the cool, dry fresh gas. Nonrebreathing systems are therefore associated with significant loss of heat and water from the patient. In addition, the dry anesthetic gases may impair tracheobronchial ciliary function and dry the airways.

- *Production of waste gas:* Full rebreathing systems release little waste anesthetic gas because oxygen flow rates are low and exhaled gases are recirculated rather than vented through the APL valve. Partial and minimal rebreathing systems vent some waste anesthetic gas, which varies depending on the carrier gas flow rates used. In contrast, nonrebreathing systems vent nearly all exhaled gas.

Checking the Low-Pressure System for Leaks and Adjusting the Adjustable Pressure Limiting Valve

Once the anesthetic machine has been set up and prepared for use, the low-pressure system must be checked for leaks. The low-pressure system includes the breathing circuit, the vaporizer, and all the tubing between the flowmeters and the Y-piece or patient connector. Checking this system for leaks helps to ensure that the machine is properly assembled and has no damaged or missing parts (Case Presentation 4.1 illustrates the importance of leak testing any anesthetic machine before use).

On both rebreathing and nonrebreathing systems, the APL valve or outlet valve should be adjusted immediately after the leak test is performed. The action ensures that the APL or outlet valve has not been inadvertently left closed and is set at the right level for the patient.

The procedure for performing a low-pressure system leak test and adjusting the APL valve on a rebreathing system can be found in Procedure 4.1. If using a Bain coaxial nonrebreathing circuit, in addition to the low-pressure system leak test, the inner tube (the fresh gas inlet) must be checked for integrity because such a leak between this tube and the exhalation tube will significantly increase rebreathing of exhaled gases, and such a defect will not be revealed by a simple low-pressure leak test. The method for performing a low-pressure system leak test, setting the APL or outlet valve on a nonrebreathing system, and testing for integrity of the fresh gas inlet of a Bain circuit may be found in Procedure 4.2.

Choice of Carrier Gas Flow Rates

At various times during any anesthetic procedure, the anesthetist must determine the appropriate carrier gas flow. Usually, oxygen is used alone, but if other carrier gases are used as well, flow rate determinations must take into consideration the total flow of all gases as well as the individual flow rates of each gas.

The carrier gas flow rates for each anesthetic procedure are calculated using the patient body weight and the V_T or RMV. The V_T is considered to be approximately 10 mL/kg in most anesthetized animals. The RMV is V_T multiplied by the respiratory rate in breaths per minute (an average of 10 to 20 breaths/min in most patients). Therefore the RMV is considered to be about 100 to 200 mL/kg/min (10 mL/kg × 10 to 20 breaths/min).

[a]The type of volatile anesthetic used will also determine how quickly anesthetic depth can be changed, regardless of oxygen flow rates or the type of circuit used. (See discussion of blood-gas solubility coefficients in Chapter 3.)

CASE PRESENTATION 4.1   The Importance of Machine Testing

Molly, a 1-year-old, 3.5-kg female domestic shorthair (DSH) cat, was anesthetized in preparation for a routine ovariohysterectomy. Based on preanesthetic assessment, she was classified as a physical status class PS1 patient. Molly was premedicated with 0.05 mg/kg of hydromorphone and 0.01 mg/kg of dexmedetomidine intramuscularly (IM) 15 min before anesthetic induction and was induced with a mixture of 5.5 mg/kg of ketamine and 0.28 mg/kg midazolam intravenously (IV) to effect. She was intubated, connected to a Bain coaxial nonrebreathing circuit, placed on isoflurane, and prepared for surgery. During the preparation of the surgical site, oxygen saturation was 97% and Molly was in a surgical plane of anesthesia and remained stable.

After being transferred to the operating room, Molly was connected to a different machine and maintained with 1.5% isoflurane and 1 L/min oxygen. The final surgical preparation was completed, the patient was draped, and preparations were made to make the incision. As the monitoring probes were being attached, the attending

veterinarian noticed that Molly's respiratory efforts seemed somewhat labored, and she appeared to be in a light plane of anesthesia. She asked the circulating nurse to lift the drapes and assess Molly more closely. The circulating nurse determined that the lung sounds were normal, but the mucous membrane color had a mild gray tint and oxygen saturation was found to be 82%. In addition, the heart and respiratory rates were elevated, but other vital signs were normal. The oxygen flow rate was 1 L/min and the endotracheal tube was correctly placed. The oxygen flow was increased to 2 L/min in response to the doctor's order.

During this time, the patient's color deteriorated, at which point the attending veterinarian ordered that the patient be removed from the breathing circuit. The mucous membrane color improved immediately after removal.

1. *What are three possible causes of the abnormalities observed in this patient?*
2. *What steps would you take to identify the cause?*
3. *What actions would you take to maximize the likelihood of a successful outcome?*

Flow rates also depend on the type of breathing system (full rebreathing, partial rebreathing, minimal rebreathing, or nonrebreathing) and the period of anesthesia (i.e., induction, maintenance, or recovery, or when changing the anesthetic depth). Relatively high rates are used for nonrebreathing systems at all times regardless of the period of anesthesia. With full rebreathing systems, flow rates are very low (only enough to meet the metabolic needs of the patient). With partial rebreathing systems, flow rates vary from relatively low rates when maintaining a patient at a desired anesthetic depth to relatively high rates during induction and recovery and when changing anesthetic depth. This is because higher flows cause the concentration of

anesthetic within the breathing circuit to change more rapidly and consequently cause the patient's anesthetic depth to change more quickly. This is desirable when a rapid change in anesthetic depth is necessary, such as during induction and when the patient's anesthetic level is excessive. With minimal rebreathing systems, flow rates meet or exceed the RMV, resulting in a system that functions in a similar way to a nonrebreathing system. These very high rates may be used to speed anesthetic recovery or during response to a complication or emergency in which high oxygen flow is desirable. See Box 4.5 for recommended flow rates and Box 4.6 for examples of flow rate calculations. Tables 9.2, 9.3, and 10.1 in the species chapters are quick reference

---

BOX 4.5   Recommended Oxygen Flow Rates

Oxygen Flow Rates for Small Animals, Foals, Calves, and Small Ruminants (<150 kg [350 lb])

Chamber and Mask Inductions
Chamber induction:
• **5 L/min**
Mask induction: *(Approximately 300 mL/kg/min or 30 times V_T)*
• **1–3 L/min for patients 10 kg or less**
• **3–5 L/min for patients more than 10 kg**

Rebreathing Systems
Partial rebreathing system after induction, during a change in anesthetic depth, or during recovery: *(Approximately ¼ to ½ of the RMV.)*
• **50–100 mL/kg/min up to a maximum of 5 L/min.**
  (Note: Flows at the higher end of this range will result in faster changes in anesthetic depth.)
Partial rebreathing system during maintenance:
• **20–40 mL/kg/min with a minimum of 500 mL/min regardless of patient size**
  (Note: The use of a maintenance rate of 20 mL/kg/min is sometimes referred to as "low flow.")
Minimal rebreathing during maintenance:
• **200–300 mL/kg/min up to a maximum of 5 L/min.**
  (Note: At this flow rate, the machine functions in a manner similar to a nonrebreathing system.)
Full rebreathing system during maintenance:
• **5–10 mL/kg/min** *(Note: Oxygen flow rates below 0.5 L/min may decrease the accuracy of vaporizer output, making the use of a full rebreathing system more challenging in many small animal patients.)*

Nonrebreathing Systems (*used only for patients weighing 7 kg or less*)
Mapleson A (Magill) and modified Mapleson A (Lack): *(~100 to 200 mL/kg/min. This is equal to approximately 0.75–1.0 times the RMV)*
• **Approximately 0.5–1.5 L/min**
Modified Mapleson D systems (Bain coaxial), Mapleson E systems (Ayre's T-piece), and Mapleson F systems (Jackson–Rees and Norman elbow): *(~200 to 400 mL/kg/min. This is equal to approximately two to three times the RMV)*
• **Approximately 1–3 L/min**

Oxygen Flow Rates for Large Animals (≥150 kg [350 lb])
Rebreathing Systems (Note: Only rebreathing systems are used for LA patients.)
Partial rebreathing system after induction, during a change in anesthetic depth, or during recovery:
• **Approximately 8–10 L/min.** *(This guideline represents approximately 20 mL/kg/min with a maximum of 10 L/min.)*
Partial rebreathing system during maintenance:
• **Approximately 3–5 L/min.** *(This guideline represents approximately 10 mL/kg/min with a maximum of 5 L/min.)*
Full rebreathing system during maintenance:
• **Approximately 1–2.5 L/min.** *(This guideline represents approximately 3–5 mL/kg/min.)*

LA, Large animal; *RMV,* respiratory minute volume; *V_T,* tidal volume.

BOX 4.6 Examples of Flow Rate Calculations

1. **Given a 5-kg cat and an anesthetic machine with a sevoflurane vaporizer, what type of circuit and oxygen flow rate would normally be used?**

Answer: Because the cat weighs less than 7 kg, a Bain coaxial circuit or other nonrebreathing system is preferred, although a rebreathing system with pediatric hoses could also be used for this patient. The flow rate recommended for the Bain system is 200–400 mL/kg/min during all periods of anesthesia (induction, maintenance, and recovery). Thus the anesthetist should select an oxygen flow rate of 1–2 L/min (200–400 mL × 5 kg). In a patient this small, choosing equipment that will minimize dead space should be a high priority, and the Bain system should be checked for low-pressure system leaks and integrity of the inner tube of the circuit before the procedure. Also, a pulse oximeter and capnograph should be utilized to ensure that oxygen saturation is adequate and that inspired CO_2 is less than 5 mmHg.

2. **Given a 25-kg dog and an anesthetic machine with an isoflurane vaporizer, what type of circuit and flow rate would be preferred during the maintenance period?**

Answer: Based on the body weight, this patient should be placed on a partial rebreathing system. The oxygen flow rate during the maintenance period is 20–40 mL/kg/min. Thus the anesthetist could select an oxygen flow rate between 500 mL/min and 1 L/min (20–40 mL/kg/min × 25 kg) as long as the anesthetic depth remains optimum. Using a rate this low during maintenance will conserve body heat and moisture as well as anesthetic gases and will produce less waste gas. This is advantageous to both the patient and the personnel involved.

3. **Given a 15-kg dog and an anesthetic machine with an isoflurane vaporizer, what would be the recommended flow rate if the patient's anesthetic depth is inadequate and needs to be increased?**

Answer: Based on the body weight, this patient should be placed on a partial rebreathing system. When trying to increase anesthetic depth, the flow rate should be between 50 and 100 mL/kg/min. For this animal, the flow rate therefore should be 750 mL–1.5 L/min (50–100 mL/kg/min × 15 kg). Although any flow in this range may be used, the higher the flow, the more rapidly the anesthetic depth will change. So if it is important that the anesthetic depth changes quickly, it is always preferable to choose a higher rate, even though more gas will be used. If the change can be more gradual, a lower rate (750 mL/min in this case) can be used to reduce heat and moisture loss and to conserve anesthetic gases. These rates are appropriate any time the anesthetic depth needs to be changed, including the induction and recovery periods.

---

charts for smal-animal rebreathing systems, nonrebreathing systems, and large-animal rebreathing systems, respectively.

TECHNICIAN NOTE With partial or minimal rebreathing systems, flow rates vary from relatively low when maintaining a patient at a desired anesthetic depth to relatively high during induction and recovery and when changing anesthetic depth. This is because higher flows cause the patient's anesthetic depth to change more quickly.

Flow Rates During Mask or Chamber Induction

During mask and chamber induction, very high flow rates are required. Use of high flow rates in the induction period saturates the anesthetic circuit with carrier gas and anesthetic vapor and dilutes the expired gases of the patient. Otherwise, expired nitrogen gas (N_2), which comprises almost 80% of the air in the patient's lungs and bloodstream at the start of the anesthetic period, will enter the circuit and dilute out the anesthetic vapor

and oxygen. If high flow rates are used, the nitrogen will be flushed out of the breathing circuit by fresh gas within a few minutes. The flow rate can be decreased to a maintenance level once the patient reaches the desired plane of anesthesia.

For mask induction, it is generally agreed that the flow rate per minute should equal 30 times the V_T (approximately 300 mL/kg/min) for cats and small dogs and somewhat less for larger dogs. This works out to a recommended total flow rate of 1 to 3 L/min for animals $\leqq$ 10 kg, and 3 to 5 L/min for animals over 10 kg. A flow rate of 5 L/min is recommended for chamber induction regardless of the patient body weight.

In large-animal anesthesia, mask induction is rarely used with the exception of neonates, when rates similar to those for cats and dogs can be used, and pigs, because of the difficulty in gaining venous access in conscious swine. Small- to medium-sized pigs (<50 kg) require oxygen flow rates of 3 to 5 L/min during mask induction. A flow rate of 5 L/min is rarely exceeded, even when larger pigs are masked to decrease pollution of the induction area with anesthetic gases because masks for this size of a pig are commonly homemade and may leak. The induction will, however, be much slower, so if faster induction time is required, flow rates of up to 10 L/min can be used.

Flow Rates When Using a Partial Rebreathing System

After induction with an injectable agent. For animals induced with an injectable anesthetic and subsequently intubated and connected to an anesthetic machine, the flow rate should be relatively high (50 to 100 mL/kg/min). This results in a flow rate of between 500 mL to 5 L/min depending on the patient's body weight for small animals and for large-animal patients connected to a small-animal anesthetic machine. Initial flow rates for large-animal patients on a large-animal machine range from 8 to 10 L/min.

Flow rates when making changes in anesthetic depth. It is also desirable to use a higher oxygen flow rate (50 to 100 mL/kg/min) when the patient's level of anesthesia is too deep or too light and a change in anesthetic depth is desired. Although not absolutely required, the use of flows at the higher end of this range will result in more rapid changes in the desired anesthetic concentration within the breathing circuit and ultimately, in the patient's anesthetic depth.

Flow rates during maintenance. Once the animal reaches a satisfactory level of anesthetic depth, the flow rate may be safely reduced to a maintenance level. Rebreathing systems require relatively low flow rates compared with nonrebreathing systems during this period because carbon dioxide is removed from the expired gases, which are then returned to the patient. Provided the carbon dioxide absorbent is effective and there are no leaks in the system, the carrier gas and anesthetic can be recycled continuously, and only a small amount of fresh gas is required. During this period flow rates of 20 to 40 mL/kg/min are recommended for small animals and 3 to 5 L/min for adult large animals.

Flow rates during anesthetic recovery. When the vaporizer is turned off, the patient enters the recovery period. During this time, even though the vaporizer is turned off, anesthetic gas is exhaled by the recovering patient and remains in the circuit until replaced by fresh oxygen. Recovery will be delayed if this waste anesthetic gas is allowed to remain in the circuit. Therefore it is to the patient's advantage to remove this waste gas as quickly as possible by taking the following actions.

Immediately after the vaporizer has been turned off, increase the flow to the same rate used during induction (50 to 100 mL/kg/min). Then, with the APL valve open and the patient detached from the circuit, use gentle pressure to evacuate the reservoir bag and refill it, using short bursts from the oxygen flush valve. These actions will flush out waste anesthetic gas, increase the oxygen concentration in the breathing circuit, and hasten patient recovery. Reattach the patient to the circuit and maintain this higher flow for 5 minutes or until the patient must be extubated.

This same procedure can be followed for patients connected to a large-animal anesthetic machine, using flow rates of up to 10 L/min to "flush" the system.

Flow rates when minimal rebreathing of anesthetic gases is desired. Note that when the oxygen flow rate matches or exceeds the patient's RMV (when it is set to a minimum of 200 to 300 mL/kg/min), a rebreathing system can be made to function in a manner similar to a nonrebreathing system. In emergency situations such as exhaustion of the carbon dioxide absorbent, these rates help to flush exhaled gases from the breathing circuit through the APL valve and may be necessary until the problem is rectified.

Flow Rates When Using a Full Rebreathing System

Full rebreathing systems are normally used only during anesthetic maintenance. When these systems are used, the oxygen flow must equal only the oxygen requirements of the animal. The minimum metabolic oxygen requirement for the anesthetized animal is 5 to 10 mL/kg/min (see Appendix A). The anesthetist should be aware that when flow rates of less than 250 to 500 mL/min are used, some precision vaporizers and flowmeters might not accurately deliver the dialed vaporizer concentration and oxygen flow. Large-animal patients, particularly adult horses and cattle, have lower metabolic oxygen requirements, and it is possible that oxygen flow rates as low as 3 to 5 mL/kg/min may be used during maintenance with a full rebreathing system.

Safety concerns with a full rebreathing system. Although full rebreathing systems are more economical than partial or minimal rebreathing systems, there are serious safety concerns that must be addressed when a full rebreathing system is used:
- *Carbon dioxide accumulation.* If the carbon dioxide absorber in a full system is not operating efficiently, exhaled carbon dioxide will build up within the circuit. This is less likely to happen in a partial rebreathing system, in which some CO_2 is vented to the scavenger.
- *Increased pressure in the anesthetic circuit.* In a full rebreathing system, the volume of gas in the system may increase as fresh gas enters the circuit, particularly if the fresh gas flow exceeds the patient's uptake of oxygen and anesthetic and the APL valve is closed. As a result, excessive pressure may build up in the circuit, making it difficult for the animal to exhale. This risk is lessened with a partial rebreathing system because the APL valve is partially or fully open and excessive gas is vented.

- These disadvantages must be balanced against the economic advantages of a full rebreathing system and the fact that little or no waste anesthetic gas is produced when flow rates are low. In most situations (e.g., where continuous monitoring of the patient and the anesthetic machine is not possible), the anesthetist may prefer to use a partial rather than a full rebreathing system for the safety reasons just outlined. The anesthetist may choose to err on the side of wasting some gas by using higher gas flow rates rather than risking the accumulation of carbon dioxide and depletion of oxygen within the circuit. A full rebreathing system can easily be converted to a partial rebreathing system by opening the APL valve (except when bagging the patient) and increasing the oxygen flow rate.

Procedures used in the operation of a full rebreathing system are listed in Appendix A.

Flow Rates When Using a Nonrebreathing System

Nonrebreathing systems require relatively high flow rates per unit body weight during all periods of general anesthesia (induction, maintenance, and recovery) because the removal of carbon dioxide from the circuit is dependent on fresh gas flow, which must be sufficient to ensure that there is minimal rebreathing of exhaled gases. Therefore close attention must be given to the selection of an appropriate flow rate. Recommended rates are based on body weight and the Mapleson classification of the circuit. Because these systems are generally used for patients weighing less than 7 kg, the maximum rates listed are based on this body weight.

With Mapleson A systems (Magill circuit) and modified Mapleson A systems (Lack circuit), carrier gas flow should be near the RMV (100 to 200 mL/kg/min) when the patient is spontaneously breathing. This equals about 0.5 to 1.5 L/min depending on patient size. Much higher flow rates are necessary during assisted or controlled ventilation to prevent rebreathing, so low efficiency makes them less useful when used under these circumstances.

Modified Mapleson D systems (Bain coaxial circuit), Mapleson E systems (Ayre's T-piece), and Mapleson F systems (Jackson–Rees circuit or Norman elbow circuit) require an oxygen flow rate of approximately two to three times the RMV, although recommendations vary widely. The authors of the AAHA Anesthesia and Monitoring Guidelines for Dogs and Cats recommend a rate of 200 to 400 mL/kg/min when using these systems. These recommended flow rates are high enough to prevent most exhaled gases from being rebreathed by the patient, although some rebreathing of gas can occur, particularly during peak inspiration; if the respiratory rate is rapid; or if the volume of the circuit is lower than it should be for the size of the patient. The anesthetist can partially control the amount of gas rebreathed by adjusting the oxygen flow rate. For example, when using a Bain coaxial circuit, if the anesthetist selects a high oxygen flow rate (e.g., 2 L/min for a 5-kg cat), there is little return of exhaled gases to the patient. The system is therefore truly nonrebreathing. At lower flow rates (e.g., 500 mL of oxygen per minute for the same 5-kg cat), significant rebreathing of exhaled gases may occur. So even though these systems are technically classified as nonrebreathing, the way they function is somewhat dependent on carrier gas flow. For this reason, it is recommended in the AAHA Guidelines that capnography be used on patients that are on a nonrebreathing system and that the oxygen flow rate be adjusted to keep the inspired CO_2 as measured by a capnograph under 5 mmHg.

Summary

Within the aforementioned guidelines, there is considerable leeway for the anesthetist's own judgment in determining the flow rate for any particular procedure. (See Boxes 4.5 and 4.6 for a summary of recommended oxygen flow rates and examples of flow rate calculations.) In many cases, the ultimate decision is based on the needs of the patient but may be influenced by economic factors and concerns about waste gas pollution. For instance, low gas flow rates are more economical and less polluting than high flow rates because less carrier gas and anesthetic are used, but higher rates may be necessary at certain times (such as induction, recovery, and during a change in anesthetic levels, or during the management of a crisis). On the other hand, if the patient is small, the cost and environmental impact of anesthetic gas use is less significant.

CARE AND MAINTENANCE OF ANESTHETIC EQUIPMENT

Routine Maintenance

As with any piece of equipment, the anesthetic machine requires periodic maintenance to ensure proper performance. In addition to routine maintenance procedures performed by hospital staff, a qualified repair professional should be contracted to examine and test all parts of each anesthetic machine every 4 to 12 months.

> **TECHNICIAN NOTE** In addition to routine maintenance procedures performed by hospital staff, a qualified repair professional should be contracted to examine and test all parts of each anesthetic machine every 4–12 months.

Compressed Gas Cylinders

Usually, compressed gas cylinders are regularly inspected and maintained by the company that fills them, and they require no regular maintenance by hospital staff. At times, however, tank valve stems become difficult to turn. If excessive force is needed, the tank should not be used again until it is sent in for inspection and maintenance. Petroleum products (e.g., grease and kerosene) should never be used to lubricate oxygen tanks or their connections because an explosion could occur when these materials contact oxygen released from the tank. When empty, compressed gas cylinders must be removed, refilled, and replaced as described in the following paragraphs.

Removing and replacing E tanks. When viewed from the front face, the E-tank valve has three holes—one outlet port, through which the gas exits the cylinder, and two receiving holes for the pin–index safety system. The outlet port fits on the nipple of the yoke with a single washer placed in between to prevent leakage. The pin–index holes fit onto the pins of the yoke (see Fig. 4.24). To remove an E tank from the machine, be sure the tank valve is closed and the oxygen is purged from the system. Place your foot under the tank to support it. Loosen the wing nut and back the valve port off the yoke. Carefully remove your foot and lower the tank until the valve clears the yoke. The tank should be stored in an upright position, on a cart, or chained to the wall until it is picked up by the company for refilling.

When replacing a tank on a machine, first inspect the valve port for cleanliness, then place a single washer between the valve port and the nipple. There are two types of washers. Flanged washers have a flange on one side that fits inside the outlet port (see Fig. 4.24 *H*). A flat washer, which has no flange, fits on the nipple of the yoke. A Bodok seal is a specialized synthetic rubber flat washer with a metal collar that is very effective in minimizing leaks in gas cylinder connections (see Fig. 4.24, inset). Either type (flanged or flat) may be used as long as it is clean, undamaged, and smooth, with no surface defects. After the washer has been placed, gently raise the tank into place, lining up the valve port and the pin holes with the corresponding structures on the yoke. Tighten the wing nut as securely as you are able to by hand. Open the tank slowly and listen for leaks. If the tank leaks, recheck the holes for proper alignment, tighten the wing nut further, or use a new washer. One of these maneuvers should resolve the problem.

Detaching and reattaching H or K tanks. Most remote oxygen sources have a bank of two or more H, J, or K tanks next to one another (see Fig. 4.19). J tanks are attached to a pipe via a yoke in a similar way to an E tank. H and K tanks are attached to a threaded connector of a cylinder manifold or pressure-reducing valve and a series of lines that pipe the gas to DISS connectors throughout the hospital (see Figs. 4.22 and 4.23). To change an H or K tank, first be sure that no patients are currently receiving oxygen. Then turn the empty tank or tanks off before attempting to remove the threaded connector. Use a hex wrench to loosen the nut attaching the line to the tank, and then remove the nut by hand. Immediately attach the manifold line or pressure-reducing valve to another full tank and turn the tank on.

At least weekly, or more often if a problem is suspected, a high-pressure leak test should be performed to check the integrity of the high- and intermediate-pressure lines of an anesthetic machine (between the oxygen source and the flowmeters). See Procedure 4.4.

Tank and Line Pressure Gauges, Pressure Manometer, and the Oxygen Flush Valve

Some parts of the anesthetic machine, including the tank pressure gauge, line pressure gauge, pressure manometer, and oxygen flush valve, require no regular maintenance. A repair professional should check these parts for proper function during a regular maintenance visit or when a problem is suspected, and they should specifically check that the pressure gauges and manometer register accurate pressures.

PROCEDURE 4.4 High-Pressure and Intermediate-Pressure System Leak Test

Method #1 (used to test the integrity of the lines and machine parts between the oxygen source and the flowmeter[s])

1. Turn the oxygen tank (if checking an E tank) on or attach the machine to a DISS connector (if checking a central supply).
2. Place a 1:1 solution of water and dishwashing liquid on all tank connections and joints between the compressed gas cylinder or DISS connector and the flowmeter(s) (Fig. 1).

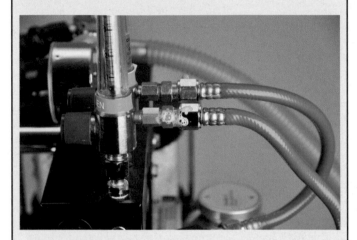

3. Observe each location for bubble formation, which indicates a leak (Fig. 2).

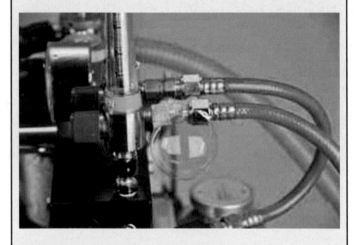

Method #2 (used to test the integrity of the lines and machine parts between a compressed gas cylinder and the flowmeter[s])

1. Turn the oxygen tank on.
2. Check that the flowmeters are off.
3. Note the reading on the tank pressure gauge.
4. Turn the tank off, but do not purge the lines.
5. Check the tank pressure gauge again in 1 hr. The pressure should have decreased by no more than 50 psi.

If the pressure is at or near zero, there is a leak somewhere between the cylinder and the flowmeter and oxygen is escaping into the room air. The most likely location of the leak is at the connection of the cylinder to the machine yoke. Although the escape of small amounts of oxygen poses little or no risk of health problems to the anesthetic machine operator, it may lead to premature emptying of the oxygen tank. In contrast, the escape of some other carrier gases, such as nitrous oxide, will result in exposure to this waste anesthetic gas.

Pressure-Reducing Valve

The pressure-reducing valve may need to be adjusted if the line pressure is not correct (40 to 58 psi). Many valves have an external adjusting screw that is turned left or right to increase or decrease the pressure. Consult the manufacturer's instruction manual for specific directions. The two-stage pressure regulator on an H or K tank is adjusted by turning the knob or thumbscrew attached to the valve (see Fig. 4.21 B).

Flowmeters

Although flowmeters require no regular maintenance, always treat them gently by not overtightening the valve when turning them off. If excessive hand pressure is necessary to stop oxygen flow, the valve is damaged and needs to be replaced.

Flowmeter accuracy can be assessed easily by performing the following test:

- Empty the reservoir bag completely
- Close the APL or overflow valve
- Occlude the Y-piece or patient connector
- Choose a flow setting that corresponds to the size of the reservoir bag in liters (e.g., 2 L/min for a 2-L bag or 3 L/min for a 3-L bag)
- The flowmeter is accurate if the bag fills completely in 1 minute

Vaporizer

Precision vaporizers must be serviced and maintained regularly to ensure accurate output. Because they are the most complex part of the anesthetic machine, they should be cleaned, tested, and recalibrated by the manufacturer or other qualified personnel every year or as indicated by the manufacturer. It may be necessary to remove the vaporizer from the anesthetic machine and send it away for servicing. Many companies provide a "loaner" vaporizer during the servicing period.

Vaporizer Inlet Port, Outlet Port, Common Gas Outlet, and Fresh Gas Inlet

The vaporizer inlet port, outlet port, common gas outlet, and fresh gas inlet are all components of the low-pressure system. The hoses commonly attached to these parts are subject to damage and may degrade over time, resulting in leaks, so check all hoses for holes or defects and replace them as necessary. A routine low-pressure leak test of the machine will usually uncover any damage.

Unidirectional Valves

Periodically, the unidirectional flow valves should be disassembled, cleaned, and inspected to prevent a buildup of water vapor, mucus, and dust from the carbon dioxide absorbent and other material. Valves that are not cleaned may become sticky and adhere to the machine housing, impeding airflow through the circuit or preventing closure.

To clean these valves, unscrew the valve collar and remove the valve parts. Clean the dome, collar, valve, valve seat, and gaskets with a low- or intermediate-level disinfectant (Table 4.3), although alcohol should not be used because it can cause plastic components to crack and leak over time. After drying the parts,

TABLE 4.3   CDC Guidelines for Equipment Disinfection and Sterilization[b]

Risk of Transmission	Examples of Equipment	Level of Treatment	Spectrum of Activity	Methods Used
High-risk (critical)	Items that contact sterile tissues and vasculature (such as IV catheters, surgical instruments, urinary catheters, and laparoscopes)	Sterilization	All microorganisms including spores killed	• Pressurized steam • Ethylene oxide (EO) gas • Hydrogen peroxide gas plasma • [a]Liquid chemical sterilants
Intermediate-risk (semicritical)	Items that contact mucous membranes and nonintact skin (such as ETTs, supraglottic airway devices, stylets, laryngoscope blades, esophageal probes, and face masks); note that detachable breathing circuit parts are usually included here	High-level disinfection	All microorganisms killed except for small numbers of bacterial spores	• [a]Liquid chemical sterilants (but with contact time of 12–30 min at temp. $\geq 20°C$) • 0.55% orthophthalaldehyde (OPA) (contact time of 12–30 min at temp. $\geq 20°C$)
Low-risk (noncritical) patient care items	Items that contact intact skin only (such as ECG leads, blood pressure cuffs, Doppler probes, and stethoscope parts); note that nondetachable breathing circuit parts are usually included here	Intermediate-level disinfection	Bacteria, including mycobacteria, most viruses, and fungi killed but no spores	• 70%–90% ethyl or isopropyl alcohol • Sodium hypochlorite (household bleach) 5.25%–6.15% (diluted 1:500) • Phenolic germicidal detergent solutions (at labeled dilution) • Iodophor germicidal detergent solutions (at labeled dilution)
Low-risk (non-critical) environmental surfaces	Tables, carts, floors, and the outside surfaces of anesthesia machines.	Low-level disinfection	Some bacteria, viruses and fungi killed, but other microbes are not, such as mycobacteria and spores	• Intermediate-level disinfectants (listed under low-risk patient care items) • Quaternary ammonium germicidal detergent solution (at labeled dilution)

[a]Chemical sterilants recommended by the CDC include $\geq 2.4\%$ glutaraldehyde-based formulations, 1.12% glutaraldehyde with 1.93% phenol/phenate, 7.5% stabilized hydrogen peroxide, 7.35% hydrogen peroxide with 0.23% peracetic acid, and 1.0% hydrogen peroxide with 0.08% peracetic acid with a contact time upwards of 3–10 hours.

[b]Note that when cleaning, disinfecting, or sterilizing equipment, manufacturer's instructions, if available, should always be consulted, and CDC guidelines should be reviewed for details regarding the safe use of these methods and agents before proceeding.

Adapted from Centers for Disease Control (CDC) publication "Guidelines for Disinfection and Sterilization in Healthcare Facilities, 2008, https://www.cdc.gov/infectioncontrol/guidelines/disinfection/index.html."

inspect the valve and valve seat to ensure they are not damaged or warped. An incompetent valve will allow reinhalation of expired carbon dioxide—a serious or potentially fatal complication. Finally, reassemble the valve, being sure that it is properly positioned on the valve seat.

The integrity of the unidirectional valves can be tested as follows:
- Put on a surgical mask
- Detach the *expiratory* breathing tube of a rebreathing circuit from the Y-piece
- Place the end of the tube up to your mouth with the surgical mask in between so that the air will pass through the mask
- Attempt to *inhale* through the tube
- Now detach the *inspiratory* breathing tube from the Y-piece and place the end up to your mouth as before
- Attempt to *exhale* through the tube

Any air movement through either tube indicates an incompetent valve, which must be serviced before the machine is used again.

Adjustable Pressure Limiting Valve

Although the APL valve does not require regular maintenance, it should be checked for proper operation and adjusted (see Procedure 4.1) before the commencement of any procedure. This should be done at the beginning of every day, immediately after the low-pressure system leak test. If working correctly, it should allow gas to exit the breathing circuit at 1 to 3 cm H_2O. The valve should also be checked periodically during the anesthetic procedure to maintain optimum gas volume within the circuit.

Reservoir Bag, Breathing Tubes, and Y-Piece

Before each case, the reservoir bag, breathing tubes, and the Y-piece or nonrebreathing circuit should be removed, cleaned, disinfected, and thoroughly rinsed to prevent interpatient transfer of infectious agents that may collect inside (more about this in the next section). After cleaning, hang these parts in a vertical position until they are completely dry because lingering moisture encourages the growth of microbes such as mold during storage.

Some of these detachable parts including some non-rebreathing circuits are intended for single use and so may not tolerate repeated hard use. In any case, before reattaching them, check each part for integrity. The neck of the bag is especially vulnerable, and holes commonly develop in this location.

Carbon Dioxide Absorber Canister

The carbon dioxide absorbent must be changed according to the guidelines indicated on pp 140–141. To change the absorbent, you must first remove the absorber canister and dispose of the absorbent granules. Next, disassemble the canister, clean, disinfect, and rinse each part thoroughly. Dry each part, check all gaskets for integrity, and reassemble the canister. Fill the clean canister loosely with fresh granules but leave at least 1 cm or ½-inch of air space at the top to allow unimpeded airflow. Gently shake the canister to distribute the granules evenly. This helps prevent channels from forming among the granules, which could reduce the efficiency of the absorbent. Following reassembly, the canister must be airtight. An airtight seal may be prevented if any granules inadvertently become lodged in a seal or gasket.

Absorbent granules should not be handled without gloves, and dust from the absorbent granules should not be allowed to enter the tubing or hoses of the machine or be breathed in by the technician because it is irritating to skin and corrosive to mucous membranes. Also, some machines have a water trap below the absorber canister. Any water that collects in this trap should be periodically drained.

Cleaning and Disinfecting Anesthetic Equipment

Like other medical equipment, anesthetic equipment requires regular cleaning and disinfection or sterilization between uses to prevent the transmission of microbes. This is of particular concern when equipment is used on a patient that is at risk of harboring highly infectious viruses or bacteria (such as feline upper respiratory viruses, *Bordetella,* and other respiratory pathogens) that may easily be transmitted between patients.

General Principles of Equipment Cleaning

When performing cleaning and disinfection or sterilization procedures, manufacturers' recommendations, if available, should be followed to ensure that agents and techniques are being used that are both effective and safe for the equipment. Such recommendations will usually be available for equipment that is intended for multiple uses but not for items intended for single use, such as ET tubes. Instructions that come with disinfectants and other agents, including appropriate concentrations, dilutions, and contact time, must be observed to ensure the agent will perform as expected, and general principles must be followed to ensure that items are appropriately cleaned prior to disinfection or sterilization.

As soon as possible after use, each device or part should be washed with warm water and mild detergent to remove any organic as well as inorganic material from both inside and outside surfaces, then rinsed thoroughly. This can be difficult when cleaning certain surfaces of anesthetic equipment such as the inside of ET tubes, the folds in ETT cuffs, corrugated tubes, and coaxial breathing circuits. Brushes and other specialized equipment, when available, should be used to reach these and other areas where microorganisms might hide. If not removed, residual organic material such as mucus and other respiratory secretions will inactivate many commonly used disinfectants. After washing, equipment should be thoroughly rinsed and dried to lessen the potential for dilution of disinfectants with residual rinse water, which may decrease effectiveness.

Equipment Disinfection or Sterilization

Evidence-based recommendations on how medical equipment should be disinfected or sterilized following cleaning are available from a number of sources, including the Centers for Disease Control (CDC) and the FDA. The CDC publication "Guideline for Disinfection and Sterilization in Healthcare Facilities (2008)" (May 2019 update) is one such set of recommendations that may be found at https://www.cdc.gov/infectioncontrol/guidelines/disinfection/index.html.

The CDC Guidelines are based on a system originally developed by Earle H. Spaulding that suggests that recommendations for disinfection or sterilization of medical equipment be based on the likelihood of microbial transmission. Under this system, medical devices are classified as high risk (critical), intermediate-risk (semicritical), or low risk (noncritical). The level of disinfection or sterilization required for each piece of equipment and therefore the procedures and agents that are appropriate is based on the risk level (see Table 4.3). For example, high-risk (critical) items must be sterilized which, by definition, means that all microorganisms and spores must be killed. Intermediate-risk (semi-critical) items must be subject to high-level disinfection (in which all microorganisms are killed except for small numbers of bacterial spores), and low-risk (non-critical) patient care items must be subject to intermediate-level disinfection (in which bacteria, including mycobacteria, most viruses, and fungi are killed but no spores). Low-level disinfection is used for low-risk (non-critical) environmental surfaces. With this level, some bacteria, viruses, and fungi are killed, but other microbes, such as mycobacteria and spores, are not.

High-risk (critical) items are those that contact sterile tissues and vasculature such as IV catheters, surgical instruments, urinary catheters, and laparoscopes. Sterilization of high-risk items can be accomplished by pressurized steam, ethylene oxide (EO) gas, hydrogen peroxide gas plasma, or liquid chemical sterilants. Chemical sterilants recommended by the CDC include ≥2.4% glutaraldehyde-based formulations, 1.12% glutaraldehyde with 1.93% phenol/phenate, 7.5% stabilized hydrogen peroxide, 7.35% hydrogen peroxide with 0.23% peracetic acid, and 1.0% hydrogen peroxide with 0.08% peracetic acid. These sterilants are effective if the equipment has been cleaned prior and requirements regarding concentration, contact time, temperature, and pH are observed. For instance, some of these chemical agents require prolonged contact time (upwards of 3 to 10 hours) to achieve sterilization.

Intermediate-risk (semicritical) items are those that contact mucous membranes and nonintact skin. This category includes many items used in anesthesia including ET tubes, supraglottic airway devices, stylets, laryngoscope blades, esophageal probes, and face masks. Although not directly in contact with mucous membranes, removable anesthetic breathing circuit parts including reservoir bags, breathing tubes, Y-pieces, adapters, capnograph spacers, and elbow connectors are usually included in this classification because they are exposed to gases coming from the patient airway. High-level disinfection necessary for this category of items can be achieved by the use of chemical disinfectants. Many of the same chemical sterilants previously mentioned, as well as 0.55% orthophthalaldehyde (OPA), can be used for this purpose but require a much shorter contact time (12 to 30 minutes at $\geq 20°C$) in order to achieve high-level disinfection.

Accelerated hydrogen peroxide (AHP) (Virox Technologies, Oakville, ON, Canada) is another agent that in adequate concentration may be useful for disinfection of most intermediate-risk items, based on its relatively short contact time, effectiveness against a wide range of microbes, and compatibility with many materials.[a] After disinfection with any agent, all equipment must be thoroughly rinsed with copious amounts of tap water to ensure adequate removal, as tissue irritation may occur.

Although not included in the CDC's list of recommended disinfectants, the biguanide, chlorhexidine solution, is used in many practices as a soak for disinfecting medical equipment (often as a 0.5% solution for 10 minutes). It is important to be aware that chlorhexidine is one of several disinfectants that have been shown to be subject to microbial contamination, so care must be taken to prevent this risk. Another concern is that cats have been shown to develop mouth ulcers, pharyngitis, and tracheitis from exposure to concentrated chlorhexidine if not adequately rinsed from ET tubes.

In addition to the CDC guidelines, another useful resource for agents that can be used for sterilization or high-level disinfection is the document entitled "FDA-Cleared Sterilants and High-Level Disinfectants with General Claims for Processing Reusable Medical and Dental Devices," available at https://www.fda.gov/medical-devices/reprocessing-reusable-medical-devices-information-manufacturers/fda-cleared-sterilants-and-high-level-disinfectants-general-claims-processing-reusable-medical-and.

Low-risk (noncritical) patient care items are those that contact intact skin only, such as ECG leads, blood pressure cuffs, Doppler probes, and stethoscope parts. Nonremovable parts of the anesthetic machine such as unidirectional valve parts, APL valves, and carbon dioxide absorber canisters are often grouped in this category for purposes of cleaning and disinfection. Intermediate-level disinfection required for these items may be accomplished by the use of intermediate-level disinfectants including 70% to 90% ethyl or isopropyl alcohol, sodium hypochlorite (household bleach) 5.25% to 6.15% (diluted 1:500), phenolic and iodophor germicidal detergent solutions diluted according to manufacturer's directions.

Low-risk (noncritical) environmental surfaces such as tables, carts, floors, and the outside of the anesthetic machine may be disinfected with the intermediate-level disinfectants listed in the previous paragraph as well as with quaternary ammonium germicidal detergent solution (at the labeled dilution), which is considered to be a low-level disinfectant.

Regardless of what level of risk an item is, it is important to choose a method of disinfection or sterilization that is available and practical to use, that is compatible with the equipment, and that will not harm the patient. Most of these methods and agents have the potential to harm the user, the patient, or the equipment being processed if not used appropriately. For instance, some items, such as plastics or ferrous metals, can be damaged by heat or moisture and therefore cannot be processed by steam sterilization (autoclaving). Ethylene oxide (EO) gas is an effective sterilizing agent for heat and moisture-sensitive items and is compatible with most equipment but requires special equipment and training to use it safely. This is because EO gas is extremely flammable, explosive, and toxic, and may cause severe tissue injury to hospital personnel and to the patient if the anesthetic equipment or supplies are not properly handled. For instance, when EO gas sterilizes intubation equipment, adequate venting, which is upwards of 8 to 12 hours, is necessary to prevent tracheal damage and organ damage that can occur if patient tissues are exposed to residual EO gas.

Specific recommendations for disinfecting and sterilizing veterinary anesthetic equipment may be found in de Miguel Garcia and Cooley.[a] Table 4.4 summarizes these recommendations for specific items used in anesthesia, including machine parts, monitoring probes, and miscellaneous equipment.

[a]de Miguel Garcia C, Cooley KG: Equipment cleaning and sterilization. In Cooley KG, Johnson RA, editors: *Veterinary anesthetic and monitoring equipment*, ed 1, Ames, IA, 2018, John Wiley & Sons, Inc., p 382.

[a]de Miguel Garcia C, Cooley KG: Chapter 28, Equipment cleaning and sterilization. In Cooley KG, Johnson RA, editors: *Veterinary anesthetic and monitoring equipment*, ed 1, Ames, IA, 2018, John Wiley & Sons, Inc., pp 377–389.

TABLE 4.4   Specific Recommendations for Disinfecting or Sterilizing Anesthetic Equipment

Equipment	Classification	Recommendations for Disinfection/Sterilization	Comments
Airway equipment—endotracheal tubes (ETTs)	Semicritical	• Steam sterilization for items that are heat tolerant, such as Safe-Seal ETTs and some silicone tubes (check with manufacturer) • Ethylene oxide (EO) sterilization or soaking in chemical sterilants for heat-sensitive items • High-level disinfectants (HLD) can also be used to soak these items (e.g., accelerated hydrogen peroxide, 8 min contact time at room temp), followed by thorough rinsing with copious amounts of water	Recommendations regarding processing of these items varies; some practices consider these items single use Sterilization of reused items preferred, although some practices process with HLD As with any processing, all items must be carefully cleaned prior to sterilization or high-level disinfection
Airway equipment—supraglottic airway devices (SGADs) OR laryngeal mask airways (LMAs)	Semicritical	• Steam sterilization (original v-gels manufactured 2012–2020) • Check with manufacturer for other SGADs or LMAs	v-gel Advanced is intended to be single use, whereas the original v-gel can be steam sterilized for a maximum of 40 uses. As with any processing, all items must be carefully cleaned prior to sterilization.
Monitoring equipment probes in contact with mucous membranes (e.g., esophageal stethoscope catheters, esophageal temperature probes, pulse-oximeter probes)	Semi-critical	Clean with mild detergent and warm water to remove all organic material in cracks and crevices Gently wipe down, including cords, catheters, tubing, etc. with manufacturer recommended HLD or 70% isopropyl alcohol *(note that alcohols are flammable and will damage rubber or plastic parts after repeated use and so should not be used on these items)*	Many of these items may not tolerate heat or immersion in liquids—check with manufacturer for recommendations regarding cleaning and disinfection
Monitoring equipment parts in contact with intact skin (e.g., Doppler probes, ECG clips, blood pressure cuffs, stethoscope parts)	Noncritical	If visibly soiled, clean with mild detergent and warm water; wipe down with manufacturer-recommended intermediate- or low-level disinfectant (LLD).	
Breathing hoses, breathing bags, and other detachable anesthesia machine parts	Often considered semicritical (even though most do not directly contact the patient)	Clean and disinfect with an HLD if contaminated with body fluids or blood Even if not contaminated, Y-pieces, patient end of hoses, and other parts exposed to mucous membranes should be routinely cleaned and disinfected with an HLD (Cooley)	Bags and hoses are difficult to clean and dry. Routine cleaning should be concentrated on portions of these items near to or exposed to mucous membranes.
Other anesthesia machine parts (e.g., unidirectional valve discs and domes, APL valve, CO_2 absorber canister)	Noncritical	Clean unidirectional valve parts with mild detergent and warm water; wipe down or soak parts with manufacturer recommended low or intermediate-level disinfectant. Clean carbon dioxide absorber canister with mild detergent and warm water; wipe down this and other parts such as APL valve with manufacturer-recommended low- or intermediate-level disinfectant.	When anesthetizing patients with known communicable bacterial or fungal infections, consider a bacterial-viral filter between the expiratory valve and breathing tubes to minimize contamination.
Anesthesia machine surfaces	Noncritical	Clean parts with mild detergent and warm water; wipe down with recommended LLD	
Misc. equipment (elbow connectors, $ETco_2$ spacers, mouth gags, speculums, stylets, face masks)	Semicritical	Clean, then soak in HLD for time recommended for disinfection or sterilization, then rinse thoroughly with copious amounts of water	Some HLDs may discolor or cloud clear plastics or damage rubber diaphragms on masks—check compatibility before use

Adapted from: de Miguel Garcia C, Cooley KG: Chapter 28, Equipment cleaning and sterilization. In Cooley KG, Johnson RA, eds.: *Veterinary anesthetic and monitoring equipment*, Ames, IA, 2018, John Wiley & Sons, Inc., pp 377–389.

KEY POINTS

1. ET tube or supraglottic airway device placement offers many advantages and increases patient safety for both injectable and inhalant anesthetic techniques.
2. Proper ET tube selection, preparation, placement, and monitoring are of primary importance in any general anesthetic procedure.
3. Anesthetic machines deliver precise amounts of carrier and anesthetic gases, remove carbon dioxide, and permit manual ventilation of anesthetized patients.
4. An anesthetic machine can be used as a source of oxygen in emergencies.
5. Compressed oxygen cylinders store carrier gases under high pressure. Cylinders come in various sizes and capacities, and the gas contained within is identified by the color of the cylinder.
6. The pressure-reducing valve decreases carrier gas pressure to a safe operating pressure of 40 to 58 psi before the gas enters the flowmeters.
7. The flow rate of each carrier gas is set by its respective flowmeter. Flows are generally expressed in liters per minute. The flow rate indicates to the anesthetist how much gas is being delivered to the patient at any given time.
8. Liquid anesthetic is vaporized and added to the carrier gas in the vaporizer. The combination of anesthetic vapor, oxygen, and medical air or nitrous oxide (if present) is called *fresh gas*.
9. Vaporizers may be precision or nonprecision based on their construction. Precision vaporizers are used to deliver inhalant anesthetics with high vapor pressures (including isoflurane and sevoflurane) and provide compensation for variations in temperature, carrier gas flow rate, respiratory rate and depth, and back pressure.
10. Precision vaporizers have high resistance to gas flow and are therefore positioned outside the anesthetic circuit (VOC).
11. The reservoir bag (breathing bag) serves as a reservoir to receive and provide gas during the respiratory cycle. It can be used to monitor the animal's ventilation and to deliver oxygen (with or without anesthetic) to the patient by a process called *bagging*.
12. Inspiratory and expiratory unidirectional valves permit only a one-way flow of gas through the breathing circuit and prevent rebreathing of CO_2.
13. Waste gas exits the machine at the APL valve and is removed by the scavenging system. In most cases (except when using a full rebreathing system), the APL valve must be kept open at all times during spontaneous breathing to prevent the risk of barotrauma.
14. Carbon dioxide is removed from a rebreathing circuit by absorbent granules. These granules must be replaced when saturated, or at least every 6 to 8 hours or every 14 to 30 days, regardless of hours of use, to prevent rebreathing of carbon dioxide and other adverse effects.
15. The pressure manometer measures the pressure of gases within the breathing circuit and the patient's lungs and must be monitored carefully during any anesthetic procedure.
16. Anesthetic circuits may be classified as rebreathing (full, partial, or minimal) or nonrebreathing. Rebreathing systems use lower oxygen flow rates but must provide for carbon dioxide absorption. Nonrebreathing systems, such as the Bain system, require relatively high flow rates and are commonly used in small patients.
17. Carrier gas flow rates vary with the period of anesthesia and type of anesthetic circuit used (i.e., rebreathing or nonrebreathing). With a rebreathing system, high flow rates are used during induction, recovery, and changing of anesthetic depth, and lower rates are used during maintenance. When a nonrebreathing system is used, high flow rates are used at all times.
18. Anesthetic equipment requires routine cleaning, inspection, and maintenance, including regular sterilization or disinfection based on the likelihood of microbial transmission.

REVIEW QUESTIONS

1. Which type of the following tubes or associated devices is designed specifically for use in birds and reptiles?
   a. Safe-Seal tube
   b. Murphy tube
   c. v-gel advanced
   d. Cole tube
2. When the oxygen tank is half full, the tank pressure gauge will read approximately:
   a. 1100 psi
   b. 2000 psi
   c. 500 psi
   d. 2200 psi
3. Oxygen is present in a compressed gas cylinder as a:
   a. Liquid
   b. Gas
   c. Liquid and a gas
4. The amount of oxygen an animal is receiving is indicated by the:
   a. Oxygen tank pressure gauge
   b. Flowmeter
   c. Pressure manometer
   d. Vaporizer setting
5. Which of the following does not contribute to mechanical dead space?
   a. Portion of ETT inside the patient's airways
   b. Y-piece connector
   c. Portion of ETT that extends beyond incisors
   d. Sidestream capnograph spacer
6. Flowmeters that have a ball for reading the gauge should be read from the _____ of the ball.
   a. Top
   b. Bottom
   c. Middle

7. Which of the following oxygen flow rates are within the recommended ranges for a 25-kg dog on a partial rebreathing system when you wish to increase anesthetic depth and when you wish to maintain the current anesthetic depth, respectively?
   a. 250 mL/min; 100 mL/min
   b. 500 mL/min; 250 mL/min
   c. 1 L/min; 500 mL/min
   d. 2 L/min; 1 L/min
   e. 4 L/min; 2 L/min

8. Which of the following parts of an anesthetic machine is specifically designed to increase the ease with which manual ventilation can be provided?
   a. APL valve
   b. Negative pressure relief valve
   c. APL occlusion valve
   d. Safety pressure relief valve

9. The minimum size for the reservoir bag can be calculated as:
   a. 20 mL/kg
   b. 50 mL/kg
   c. 80 mL/kg
   d. 100 mL/kg

10. The unidirectional valves on an anesthetic machine help to:
    a. Control the direction of movement of gases
    b. Maintain a full reservoir bag
    c. Regulate pressure
    d. Vaporize the liquid anesthetic

11. The APL valve is the part of the anesthetic machine that helps to:
    a. Vaporize the liquid anesthetic
    b. Prevent excess pressure from building up within the breathing circuit
    c. Keep the oxygen flowing in one direction only
    d. Prevent waste gases from reentering the vaporizer

12. In small-animal anesthesia, when the patient is bagged, the pressure manometer reading should not exceed:
    a. 5 cm H_2O
    b. 10 cm H_2O
    c. 15 cm H_2O
    d. 20 cm H_2O

13. Rebreathing systems, when used with standard small-animal corrugated breathing tubes, are best reserved for animals weighing more than
    a. 3 kg
    b. 7 kg
    c. 15 kg
    d. 50 kg

14. When using a rebreathing system, the amount of the expired gases that are rebreathed is determined primarily by the:
    a. Fresh gas flow
    b. Type of anesthetic
    c. Presence of a reservoir bag
    d. Position of the APL valve (i.e., open, partially open, closed)

15. Mapleson D, E, and F nonrebreathing systems should have maintenance flow rates that are:
    a. Low (20 to 40 mL/kg/min)
    b. Moderate (50 to 100 mL/kg/min)
    c. High (100 to 200 mL/kg/min)
    d. Very high (200 to 400 mL/kg/min)

16. The negative pressure relief valve is particularly important when:
    a. Nitrous oxide is being used
    b. There is no scavenging system
    c. There is a failure of oxygen flow through the system
    d. The carbon dioxide absorber is no longer functioning

17. The tidal volume of an anesthetized animal is considered to be approximately_____ mL/kg of body weight.
    a. 5
    b. 10
    c. 15
    d. 20

18. Physiologic dead space in an anesthetized patient is usually in the range of
    a. 2.0 to 3.0 mL/kg
    b. 3.5 to 5 mL/kg
    c. 7 to 10.5 mL/kg
    d. 10 to 15 mL/kg

19. A scavenging system is generally attached to:
    a. The pressure-reducing valve
    b. The expiratory unidirectional valve
    c. The APL valve
    d. The negative pressure-relief valve

   For the following questions, more than one answer may be correct.

20. A reservoir bag that is not moving well may indicate that:
    a. The ET tube is not in the trachea
    b. The animal has a decreased tidal volume
    c. There is a leak around the ET tube
    d. The vaporizer is empty

21. Which of the following signs indicate that the granules in the carbon dioxide absorber have been depleted?
    a. The anesthetist can smell the waste carbon dioxide
    b. The granules are hard and brittle
    c. The granules have changed color
    d. The patient's blood oxygen content is low

22. In a patient with a normal respiratory rate and tidal volume, an increase in the depth of anesthesia can be achieved quickly by:
    a. Using high oxygen flow rates
    b. Using high vaporizer settings
    c. Using a full rebreathing system
    d. Bagging the patient two to four times a minute

23. The concentration of anesthetic delivered from a compensated precision vaporizer may be affected by the:
    a. Temperature of the liquid anesthetic
    b. Flow rate of the carrier gas through the vaporizer
    c. Back pressure from manual ventilation
    d. Type of anesthetic in the vaporizer

24. According to CDC Guidelines for Equipment Disinfection and Sterilization, which of the following pieces of anesthetic equipment is/are considered semicritical items consequently should be treated using a high-level disinfectant?
    a. Carbon dioxide absorber canister
    b. Esophageal monitoring probe
    c. Doppler probe
    d. ET tube

25. When an anesthetic machine is operating correctly, the pressures in the machine are always:
    a. 40 to 58 psi between the pressure-reducing valve and the flowmeters
    b. 15 psi between the flowmeters and the breathing circuit
    c. 2200 psi between the compressed gas cylinder and the pressure-reducing valve
    d. 15 psi entering a VOC vaporizer

ANSWERS TO CASE PRESENTATION

Case Presentation 4.1

Question #1: The labored breathing that started when Molly was changed to the second machine suggests that Molly was having difficulty moving air into and/or out of her airways. This could be explained by (1) a blocked or partially blocked airway, (2) insufficient oxygen flow, or (3) an inability to move air around the breathing circuit due to a buildup of excess pressure or insufficient air volume in the circuit. The gray tint to the mucous membranes is most compatible with early cyanosis, which could also result from any of these causes.

Question #2: The technician would need to act rapidly by: (1) checking the patency of the ET tube by looking for obvious kinks or blockages, and listening or looking for evidence of airflow corresponding with respiratory movements; (2) checking that the oxygen tank is not empty, and that the flowmeter is on and registering oxygen flow; (3) checking the reservoir bag to be sure it is not either empty or overpressurized.

Question #3: When managing this case, the anesthetist must be aware of the extreme importance of a rapid response because cyanosis is a medical emergency that indicates a serious decrease in the oxygen content of the blood. Improvement associated with detachment from the breathing circuit points to a number of issues relating to inadequate fresh gas such as an empty oxygen tank, a lack of adequate oxygen flow, a blocked breathing circuit, or a closed APL valve. If a cause could not be identified quickly, the patient's airway should be checked for patency, and the patient should be changed to another anesthetic machine until the problem can be identified and corrected.

Outcome of This Case

For the reasons mentioned previously, the veterinarian asked that the patency of the airway be confirmed and, because it was patent, she suspected a machine malfunction and ordered that another machine be used for the rest of the procedure until the problem could be identified. After this change was made, the patient continued to improve and the oxygen saturation returned to normal (98%).

For the remainder of the procedure, the patient was continuously monitored. The patient was bagged as needed and kept on an oxygen flow of 2 L/min until vital signs were completely stable.

Later examination of the machine revealed the problem. The machine had both an isoflurane and a sevoflurane vaporizer. The day before, the previous user had used sevoflurane to anesthetize a bird but had not reconnected the inlet and outlet hoses to the isoflurane vaporizer after the procedure. The machine had not been leak tested before this procedure, and therefore the error in machine assembly was not identified. Because a nonrebreathing system was attached to the outlet port of the isoflurane vaporizer, but the carrier gas supply line was attached to the sevoflurane vaporizer inlet port instead of the isoflurane vaporizer inlet port, no oxygen was entering the vaporizer and thus was not being delivered to the patient. The patient was attempting to breathe against a partial vacuum in the breathing circuit.

This case illustrates the importance of careful examination of the machine before use. Anesthetic machines are complex and subject to a variety of malfunctions that must be identified and corrected before use. If this machine had been leak tested, the error in machine assembly would have been identified. Although this patient was not harmed, had rapid action not been taken, this error could have resulted in a variety of serious complications, including permanent central nervous system (CNS) damage or even an anesthetic fatality.

SELECTED READINGS

Clarke KW, Trim CM, Hall LW: *Veterinary anaesthesia*, ed 11, St. Louis, MO, 2014, Elsevier, pp 209–244.

Cooley KG, Johnson RA: *Veterinary anesthetic and monitoring equipment*, ed 1, Ames, IA, 2018, John Wiley & Sons, Inc.

Doherty T, Valverde A: *Manual of equine anesthesia and analgesia*, ed 2, Ames, IA, 2022, Blackwell.

FDA-cleared sterilants and high level disinfectants with general claims for processing reusable medical and dental devices, Food and Drug Administration. https://www.fda.gov/medical-devices/reprocessing-reusable-medical-devices-information-manufacturers/fda-cleared-sterilants-and-high-level-disinfectants-general-claims-processing-reusable-medical-and. Accessed August 31, 21.

Guideline for disinfection and sterilization in healthcare facilities, 2008, May, 2019 update, CDC. https://www.cdc.gov/infectioncontrol/guidelines/disinfection/index.html. Accessed August 31, 21.

Lerche P, Muir W, Bednarski RM: Rebreathing anesthetic systems in small animal practice, *J Am Vet Med Assoc* 217(4):485–492, 2000.

Mosley CA: Anesthesia equipment. In Grimm KA, Lamont LA, Tranquilli SA, editors: *Lumb & Jones' veterinary anesthesia and analgesia*, ed 5, Ames, IA, 2015, John Wiley & Sons, Inc., pp 23–85.

Muir WW, Hubbell JAE: *Equine anesthesia: monitoring and emergency therapy*, ed 2, St. Louis, MO, 2009, Elsevier.

Muir WW, Hubbell JA, Bednarski RM, Lerche P: *Handbook of veterinary anesthesia*, ed 5, St. Louis, MO, 2013, Elsevier.

Tranquilli WJ, Lamont LA, editors: *Essentials of small animal anesthesia and analgesia*, ed 2, Ames, IA, 2011, Blackwell, pp 158–196.

Workplace Safety

OUTLINE

LEARNING OBJECTIVES

When you have completed this chapter, you will be able to:
- Identify recommended exposure limits for waste anesthetic gases and list factors that affect waste gas levels in a veterinary hospital.
- Describe both the short-term and long-term effects of waste anesthetic gas on persons working in health care environments.
- Compare and contrast active and passive scavenging systems and describe the four components of a scavenging system.
- Explain how waste anesthetic gases are monitored.
- Describe procedures and practices used to minimize waste gas release.
- Identify hazards associated with use of compressed gas cylinders and potent injectable agents.
- Describe proper procedures for handling, storing, and transporting compressed gas cylinders.
- Outline the precautions necessary for handling potentially hazardous injectable agents.

KEY TERMS

Activated charcoal canister
National Institute for
   Occupational Safety and
   Health (NIOSH)

Occupational Safety and Health
   Administration (OSHA)
Passive dosimeter
Recommended exposure limit (REL)

Scavenging system
Ultrapotent opioids
Waste anesthetic gas (WAG)

When acting as anesthetist, the veterinary technician, veterinary nurse, or veterinarian must handle a wide variety of drugs, gases, substances, and equipment that have potential to cause personal harm. Over the course of a career, they may participate in the anesthetic management of several to many thousands of animals. It is therefore essential to develop familiarity with human safety considerations associated with veterinary anesthesia. These can be divided into three categories: (1) hazards of exposure to waste anesthetic gas, (2) safety considerations for handling compressed gas cylinders, and (3) hazards associated with potent injectable agents.

This chapter outlines the precautions that the anesthetist can take to reduce, as much as possible, the health risks of working with anesthetic equipment, inhalant anesthetics, injectable drugs, and compressed gases.

The authors and the publisher wish to acknowledge the contribution of Diane McKelvey, whose original work served as the foundation for this chapter.

WASTE ANESTHETIC GAS

The term waste anesthetic gas (sometimes referred to as "*WAG*") refers to anesthetic vapors that are breathed out by the patient or that escape from the anesthetic machine, including the volatile general anesthetics such as isoflurane, sevoflurane, and desflurane (see Chapter 3 for a discussion of these agents), and the gas anesthetic nitrous oxide (see Chapter 3 for a discussion of this agent). Isoflurane and sevoflurane are the most commonly used inhalant general anesthetics for both small and large animals. These agents are liquids at room temperature. When put in an anesthetic vaporizer, they evaporate to a gaseous form that is carried by oxygen into the patient's airways.

Nitrous oxide is a gas anesthetic that is primarily used in human medicine to provide sedation and analgesia for patients undergoing dental and medical procedures. In veterinary medicine, it is rarely used as an anesthetic adjunct but is sometimes used to produce the very cold temperatures required for cryogenic surgical procedures (those involving destruction of abnormal tissue, such as tumor cells, by freezing). When using nitrous oxide for this purpose, procedures must be in place to minimize exposure of personnel to the waste gas. The National Institute for Occupational Safety and Health (NIOSH) publication entitled "Control of Nitrous Oxide During Cryosurgery," available at https://www.cdc.gov/niosh/docs/99-105/pdfs/99-105.pdf, details procedures that should be followed.

WAGs such as isoflurane and sevoflurane are breathed inadvertently by all personnel working in areas where animals are anesthetized or are recovering from inhalation anesthesia. Significant exposure to these agents can also occur when emptying or filling anesthetic vaporizers. In addition, short-term exposure to high levels of anesthetic vapors can occur because of an accidental spill of liquid anesthetic. It is therefore imperative that the anesthetist be aware of steps that can be taken to keep exposure to a minimum.

> **TECHNICIAN NOTE** The National Institute for Occupational Safety and Health (NIOSH) recommends that the concentration of any volatile gas anesthetic (including isoflurane, sevoflurane, and desflurane) not exceed 2 parts per million (ppm) when used alone.

Measurement of Waste Anesthetic Gas

The concentration of waste anesthetic gas in the workplace is determined by air sample analysis (see p 174 for a discussion of waste gas monitoring) and is usually expressed in parts per million (abbreviated ppm). If the concentration of an anesthetic gas such as isoflurane is 30 ppm, this means that out of every 1 million molecules of room air, 30 are isoflurane. (The rest are chiefly nitrogen, oxygen, argon, and carbon dioxide.) Measurement of these levels is necessary to gather meaningful data regarding the risk of exposure to these agents, to provide meaningful recommendations regarding workplace limits, and to monitor exposure accurately in the workplace.

The National Institute for Occupational Safety and Health (NIOSH) recommends that the concentration of any volatile gas anesthetic (including isoflurane, sevoflurane, and desflurane) not exceed 2 ppm when used alone. If used with nitrous oxide, the concentration of these agents should not exceed 0.5 ppm, and the nitrous oxide concentration should not exceed 25 ppm. These recommended exposure limits (RELs) were chosen because they were the lowest concentrations that were detectable using the recommended analytic techniques, and these levels were found to be achievable at the time these recommendations were originally published in 1977. In contrast, the British Government Health Service Advisory Committee recommends a maximum of 50 ppm isoflurane, 100 ppm nitrous oxide, and 10 ppm halothane (average reading over an 8-hour period). Although much higher than the NIOSH recommendations, these levels were chosen in 1995 because evidence from available studies suggested that they "are well below the levels at which any significant adverse effects occurred in animals and represent levels at which there is no evidence to suggest human health would be affected." In any case, because levels of waste gases that are harmful have not been definitively determined and NIOSH-recommended levels are achievable when good workplace practices are followed, it is prudent and advisable to keep waste gases below NIOSH recommended levels to minimize the risk to workers. Even though the Occupational Safety and Health Administration (OSHA) has not set permissible exposure limits, it can (and does) issue citations for failing to meet the NIOSH standard.

It is important to note that the sense of smell is a very insensitive detector of levels of waste anesthetic gas exceeding recommended limits. For instance, according to the NIOSH publication *Waste Anesthetic Gases,* halothane cannot be detected by 50% of the general population until the concentration is more than 125 times the NIOSH REL. In other words, by smell alone, operating room personnel are unable to identify the point at which waste gases exceed the recommended limit. Furthermore, measurement of WAGs is not routine in most clinical situations. From a safety standpoint, this means that safe practices must be followed carefully and consistently when handling anesthetic gases to keep the levels of waste gas below the recommended limits.

> **TECHNICIAN NOTE** By smell alone, operating room personnel are unable to identify the point at which waste gases exceed the recommended limit. Furthermore, measurement of waste anesthetic gases is not routine in most clinical situations. From a safety standpoint, this means that safe practices must be followed carefully and consistently when handling anesthetic gases to keep the levels of waste gas below the recommended limits.

Waste Anesthetic Gas Levels in the Veterinary Hospital

Surveys of human and veterinary hospitals reveal a wide variation in the levels of waste anesthetic gas present in different locations within the clinic (see Table 5.1 for data from a study of waste anesthetic gas exposures from 10 practices in Manitoba, Canada). As reflected in the data from this study, the level of waste anesthetic gas that is present is influenced by a variety of factors such as the effectiveness of the endotracheal

TABLE 5.1 Waste Anesthetic Gas Exposures from 10 Practices in Manitoba, Canada

Specifics of Sample Collection[a] (e.g., gas collected, sampling location, workplace practices)	Real-Time Halogenated Gas Concentrations (ppm)
Isoflurane/halothane concentrations in eight small animal clinics[b] *(with inflation of ETT cuff and minimal equipment leaks)*	Isoflurane: 0.9–13.0 Halothane: 0.1–12.0
Halothane concentrations in one equine clinic[b] *(with a very secure ETT cuff seal and minimal equipment leaks)*	<1.3
Halothane concentrations in one small animal clinic[b] *(without inflation of ETT cuff and significant unidentified equipment leaks)*	1.1–65
Isoflurane/halothane concentrations in the animal's breathing zone during surgery (with cuffed ETT)	Isoflurane: 1–18 Halothane: 0.4–4.3
Isoflurane/halothane concentrations in the animal's breathing zone during recovery	Isoflurane: 1.6–80 Halothane: 0.4–152
Peak halothane concentrations in the vicinity of a chamber after opening the lid *(during induction only)*	≤100

[a]Samples were taken for the duration of one complete surgical procedure. Note that all 10 clinics had passive scavenging systems. Six of the clinics used isoflurane and the remaining four used halothane.
[b]The range listed includes results of personal sampling from the breathing zone of the veterinarian, personal sampling from the breathing zone of the assistant, and area sampling from the middle of the room at the level of the breathing zone.
ETT, Endotracheal tube.
Data from Korczynski RE: Anesthetic gas exposure in veterinary clinics, *Appl Occup Environ Hygiene* 14:384–390, 1999.

tube cuff seal, the presence or absence of machine leaks, exposure to exhaled air from the patient, and whether or not a chamber was used; however, it is primarily influenced by whether or not a scavenging system is used. A scavenging system is a device that is attached to the breathing circuit of an anesthetic machine to capture WAGs and discharge them outside the clinic (see p 168 for a detailed discussion of a scavenging system).

As expected, air samples taken from surgery suites, surgical preparation rooms, and anesthetic recovery rooms are more likely to contain waste gas than samples taken elsewhere in the clinic. During the anesthetic period itself, the level of waste gas is highest immediately adjacent to the anesthetic machine, but the actual level varies according to the following factors.

Duration of Anesthesia

The longer the anesthetic machine is in use, the higher the waste gas concentration in the air in the room. For example, if a surgery room is used for several procedures in one morning, the waste gas levels may slowly increase, reaching a peak at the end of the final surgery.

Flow Rate of Carrier Gas (i.e., oxygen and nitrous oxide if used)

Higher flow rates may lead to more waste gas pollution. For example, if the oxygen flow rate is 2 L/min, the room will contain more waste gas than if the flow rate were 500 mL/min unless a very effective gas scavenger is in use.

Anesthetic Machine Maintenance

Leak testing and periodic maintenance of the anesthetic machine are important in reducing the escape of anesthetic gas from the machine, which contributes to room air pollution.

Use of an Effective Scavenging System

When a circle system (rebreathing system) with no scavenging system is used, anesthetic gas mixed with oxygen is vented through an open adjustable pressure limiting (APL) valve at a rate approximately equal to the oxygen flow rate (usually 500 mL to 3 L/min for small-animal patients and 1 to 5 L/min for large-animal patients during maintenance). If a nonrebreathing system such as a Bain circuit is in use, the gas exits through the overflow valve or reservoir bag outlet. Either way, in the absence of a scavenging system, all of the waste gas enters the room air.

Anesthetic Techniques Used

Anesthetic masks and anesthetic chambers may release high levels of waste gas because a considerable quantity of air can leak around mask or chamber gaskets and is released when an anesthetic chamber is opened or when a mask is removed. There are also risks associated with use of an endotracheal tube. For instance, when repositioning a patient (such as turning the patient from side to side when performing a COHAT (dental cleaning), the breathing circuit must be detached from the endotracheal tube. During the time the two are disconnected, a significant quantity of waste gas can leak from the open endotracheal tube connector or from the patient end of the breathing circuit.

Room Ventilation

Room ventilation is the only means of eliminating waste gases that leak from anesthetic machines or are exhaled through or around an endotracheal tube or mask (scavengers are unable to retrieve these gases once they enter the air). It is therefore advised that all rooms in which anesthetic gases are released have a nonrecirculating ventilation system that provides at least 15 air changes per hour, 3 of which should be fresh air. (A rate of 21 air changes per hour is preferred.) Rooms with a ceiling fan, wall fan, or other ventilating device generally have lower levels of waste gas, and open windows and doors also reduce waste gas levels, although the use of these methods is not consistent with principles of hospital design and sterile technique in surgical suites and other related areas.

> **TECHNICIAN NOTE** It is advised that all rooms in which anesthetic gases are released have at least 15 air changes per hour, 3 of which should be fresh air. A rate of 21 air changes per hour is preferred.

Anesthetic Spills

The highest levels of waste gas contamination are associated with spills of anesthetic liquids. Liquid anesthetic evaporates rapidly when it is poured or spilled, and this produces a very large amount of concentrated anesthetic vapor that rapidly mixes with room air. Accidental spillage of only 1 mL of liquid halothane, for example, will evaporate to form 200 mL of vapor, with a concentration of 1,000,000 ppm. Liquid anesthetic spilled on the skin can also be absorbed into the circulation.

Hazards of Exposure to Waste Anesthetic Gas

The suspected health hazards associated with exposure to WAGs can be divided into two categories: (1) short-term problems that occur during or immediately after exposure to these agents and (2) long-term problems that may become evident days, weeks, or years after exposure.

Short-Term Effects

The short-term problems associated with breathing waste gas appear to arise from a direct effect of anesthetic molecules on brain neurons. Persons working in environments with a high level of waste gas have reported symptoms such as fatigue, headache, drowsiness, nausea, depression, and irritability. Although these symptoms usually resolve spontaneously when the affected person leaves the area, the frequent occurrence of these symptoms may indicate that excessive levels of waste gas are present and that a potential for long-term toxicity exists.

Long-Term Effects

Long-term inhalation of high levels of waste gas may be associated with serious health problems, including reproductive disorders, liver and kidney damage, bone marrow abnormalities, and chronic nervous system dysfunction. Although current evidence suggests that the risk of serious effects is low in normal veterinary practice settings in which WAGs are scavenged, every person working in an environment in which waste gas is present should be aware of the potential for adverse health effects and practices that must be followed to minimize this risk.

The mechanism of long-term anesthetic gas toxicity is not fully understood but is thought to be the result of toxic metabolites produced by the breakdown of anesthetic gases within the liver and their subsequent excretion by the kidneys. These metabolites include inorganic fluoride or bromide ions, oxalic acid, and free radicals, all of which are known to have harmful effects on animal tissues. It is widely accepted that anesthetic agents that are retained by the body and metabolized are likely to have greater long-term toxicity than those that are quickly eliminated through the lungs. The two most commonly used halogenated agents, isoflurane and sevoflurane, are thought to be among the inhalation agents least likely to cause long-term toxicity because the percentage of these agents that is metabolized (approximately 0.2% of inhaled isoflurane and 2% to 5% of sevoflurane) is very small. In contrast, a much higher percentage of the older halogenated agents administered to a patient or inhaled by the anesthetist (approximately 15% to 20% of halothane and 40% to 50% of methoxyflurane) is retained within the body fat to be metabolized in the liver and excreted

through the kidneys over the next few hours to days. Metabolites of halothane have been recovered from the urine of human patients as long as 20 days after anesthesia. In the same way, the anesthetist who inhales waste anesthetic gas may retain the gas or its metabolites for a considerable period. For example, anesthetists may show traces of halothane in their breath 64 hours after administering this gas to a patient.

> **TECHNICIAN NOTE** It is widely accepted that anesthetic agents that are retained by the body and metabolized are likely to have greater long-term toxicity than those that are quickly eliminated through the lungs.
>
> Isoflurane and sevoflurane are thought to be among the inhalation agents least likely to cause long-term toxicity because the percentage of these agents that is metabolized (approximately 0.2% of inhaled isoflurane and 2% to 5% of sevoflurane) is very small.

The hazards associated with exposure to WAGs are surprisingly difficult to determine with exactness. Since the first study of waste anesthetic gas was published in 1967, many investigators have attempted to define the adverse health effects of isoflurane, enflurane, halothane, sevoflurane, methoxyflurane, nitrous oxide, and other anesthetic agents on operating room personnel. Even with the information provided by the many studies conducted over the intervening years, neither the precise amount of gas exposure that is hazardous nor the adverse effects associated with each agent are fully known. It is difficult to arrive at definitive answers to these questions for several reasons, including the following:

- Caution must be used in interpreting the epidemiologic evidence provided by these studies. The evidence produced by various studies (or within one study) is sometimes contradictory. For example, some early studies showed a variety of adverse effects in animals and humans, including organ damage; reproductive effects including infertility, spontaneous abortion, and congenital abnormalities; and neurologic effects including decreased motor and cognitive function, but other studies suggested the opposite. This discrepancy may arise from inconsistencies in the way in which the studies were conducted.
- Studies vary widely in regard to the type of anesthetics to which personnel are exposed, the duration and level of waste gas exposure, and the control measures available (such as a scavenging system). Most anesthetists surveyed had been exposed to several different agents, and the investigators were unable to determine which agent(s) were responsible for the observed adverse health effects.
- Although many epidemiologic studies indicate an increased incidence of health problems in persons working in an environment where exposure to waste gas occurs, it does not necessarily follow that the anesthetic gases are the causative agents. Other chemicals such as ethylene oxide, exposure to x-rays, or other factors present in the operating room or dentist's office may contribute to an increased incidence of health disorders.

- Many of the early studies have been faulted for low response rates, lack of verification of reported outcomes, and the possibility of bias. Some commentators have observed that the increased risks observed are small and could be a result of uncontrolled variables.
- Most studies of the adverse effects of WAGs do not measure the level of waste gas present in the working environment. Epidemiologic studies do not always include information about the use of scavengers and procedures that reduce waste gas pollution. Without this information, interpretation of the findings of any study is difficult.

> **TECHNICIAN NOTE** The hazards associated with exposure to waste anesthetic gases are surprisingly difficult to determine with exactness. Neither the precise amount of gas exposure that is hazardous nor the adverse effects associated with each agent are fully known.

So what conclusions can be drawn regarding the risk of exposure to WAGs? Regulatory agencies and professional organizations to which the veterinary anesthetist can look for guidance include the American College of Veterinary Anesthesia and Analgesia (ACVAA), the American Society of Anesthesiologists (ASA), the American Association of Nurse Anesthesiology (AANA), OSHA, and NIOSH. Each of these agencies and organizations has reviewed the available literature on the topic, drawn conclusions regarding risks of exposure, and made recommendations regarding workplace practices designed to minimize that risk. Table 5.2 lists publications regarding management of WAGs available from each of these organizations.

Comparison of these publications reveals a strong consensus. Consequently, they bring clarity to the question of dangers posed by WAGs and serve as a useful guide to use of inhalant anesthetic agents by the practicing veterinary professional in a way that minimizes risk.

This consensus may be summarized as follows:

- Evidence suggests potential adverse health effects associated with long term exposure to high levels of waste anesthetic gas, especially in environments where scavenging is not used.
- Studies have failed to prove an association between the low levels of waste anesthetic gas normally found in scavenged hospitals and adverse effects on hospital employees.
- Since the amount of gas exposure that is hazardous is not definitively known, it is prudent to take steps to reduce exposure to the lowest practical level.
- A waste anesthetic gas scavenging system should always be used with any equipment used to deliver halogenated inhalant anesthetics or nitrous oxide.
- Specific workplace practices, including regular leak checks on all anesthetic machines and breathing circuits, should be followed to keep exposure to WAGs to a minimum.
- Each facility should develop a comprehensive hazard control and communication program that includes employee training regarding the hazards associated with WAG exposure as well as ways to minimize risk.

> **TECHNICIAN NOTE** Minimizing risks associated with exposure to WAGs:
> - Evidence suggests long-term exposure to high WAG levels, especially in environments where scavenging is not used, may lead to adverse health effects.
> - There is no proven connection between exposure to low WAG levels typically found in hospitals where scavenging is used and adverse effects.
> - Since the amount of WAG exposure that is hazardous is not known, all personnel should take steps to reduce exposure to the lowest practical level.
> - A waste anesthetic gas scavenging system should always be used with any equipment used to deliver anesthetic gases.
> - Specific workplace practices, including regular equipment leak checks, should be followed to keep WAG exposure to a minimum.
> - Each facility should have a comprehensive hazard control and communication program to minimize personnel exposure to WAGs.

TABLE 5.2 Publications Related to Risk From and Control of Waste Anesthetic Gases		
Agency or Professional Organization	**Publication**	**Date of Release**
American College of Veterinary Anesthesia and Analgesia (ACVAA) Ad Hoc Committee on Waste Anesthetic Gas Pollution and Its Control	Commentary and Recommendations on Control of Waste Anesthetic Gases in the Workplace Available at: https://acvaa.org/wp-content/uploads/2019/05/Control-of-Waste-Anesthetic-Gas-Recommendations.pdf	November 18, 2013[a]
American Association of Nurse Anesthesiology	Management of Waste Anesthetic Gases Available at https://issuu.com/aanapublishing/docs/2_-_management_of_waste_anesthetic_8c0745b2cdeda9	February 2018
American Society of Anesthesiologists (ASA) Task Force on Trace Anesthetic Gases	Information for Management in Anesthetizing Areas and the Postanesthesia Care Unit (PACU) Available at http://www.cdc.gov/niosh/docket/archive/pdfs/NIOSH-064/0064-010199-McGregor_Ref2.pdf	1999
Occupational Safety & Health Administration (OSHA)	Anesthetic Gases: Guidelines for Workplace Exposures Available at: https://www.osha.gov/dts/osta/anestheticgases/	July 20, 1999 (rev. May 18, 2000)
National Institute for Occupational Safety and Health (NIOSH)	Waste Anesthetic Gases: Occupational Hazards in Hospitals Available at: http://www.cdc.gov/niosh/docs/2007-151/pdfs/2007-151.pdf	September 2007

[a]Originally published in the Commentary and recommendations on control of waste anesthetic gases in the workplace. American College of Veterinary Anesthesiologists. *J Am Vet Med Assoc* 209(1):75–77, 1996.

Reducing Exposure to Waste Anesthetic Gas

The ACVAA recommends that any veterinary facility using inhalant anesthetics should institute and maintain a control program for WAGs. According to the findings of the ASA, when effective scavenging systems are used and appropriate workplace practices are followed, trace levels of WAGs have been shown to be within the exposure limits recommended by regulatory agencies. Therefore from the perspective of hospital employees working with these gases, minimizing one's risk is dependent on close adherence to these two important recommendations.

> **TECHNICIAN NOTE** According to the findings of the ASA, when effective scavenging systems are used and appropriate workplace practices are followed, trace levels of waste anesthetic gases have been shown to be within the exposure limits recommended by regulatory agencies. Therefore from the perspective of hospital employees working with these gases, minimizing one's risk is dependent on close adherence to these two important recommendations.

Use of a Scavenging System

A scavenging system is attached to the anesthetic machine APL valve or, in the case of a nonrebreathing system, to the overflow valve, outlet port, or tail of the reservoir bag. The function of a scavenging system is to collect waste gas from the machine and conduct it to a disposal point outside the building. The installation and consistent use of an effective waste gas scavenging system are the most important steps in reducing waste gas exposure. According to the ACVAA document Commentary and Recommendations on Control of WAGs in the Workplace, "an efficient scavenging system is capable of reducing ambient concentrations of waste gases by up to 90%."

> **TECHNICIAN NOTE** The installation and consistent use of an effective waste gas scavenging system are the most important steps in reducing waste gas exposure. According to the ACVAA document, Commentary and Recommendations on Control of Waste Anesthetic Gases in the Workplace, "an efficient scavenging system is capable of reducing ambient concentrations of waste gases by up to 90%."

From the regulatory perspective, OSHA's Hazard Chemical Standard (1910.1200) requires the employer to install adequate engineering controls to ensure that occupational exposure to any chemical never exceeds the permissible exposure limit. In the case of waste anesthetic gas, this is difficult or impossible to achieve in a veterinary clinic unless a waste anesthetic gas scavenging system is used on every anesthetic machine. Scavenging should include the waste gas exhaust not only from the anesthetic machine but also from ancillary equipment including ventilators, anesthetic chambers, cryosurgery devices, and sidestream capnographs.

Ideally, scavenging systems should be professionally installed when the veterinary clinic is built. However, it is not difficult to assemble and install an effective scavenging system in an established veterinary hospital. Scavenger parts may be purchased or can be readily assembled with simple materials. The hose or transfer tubing of the scavenging system may be constructed from plastic tubing, polyvinyl chloride (PVC) pipe, or other gas-impermeable material. Most modern anesthetic machines have fittings that allow easy connection to a scavenging system. Older machines can be retrofitted with adapters that can be connected to a scavenger hose. The international standard for scavenger system attachments for anesthetic machines is 30 mm.

Scavenging systems are classified as active (Fig. 5.1) or passive systems (Fig. 5.2). Although both active and passive scavenging systems appear to be effective when correctly assembled and operated, the most efficient is an active system with a dedicated vacuum generator. However, active scavenging systems are more costly to install than passive systems, require more maintenance, and the operator must remember to turn on the system each day.

Active scavenging system. An active scavenging system uses suction created by a vacuum pump or fan to draw WAGs from the APL valve or other discharge point into the scavenger. Active systems are subclassified according to whether they generate a relatively low or high flow of gas.

An active scavenging system has four basic components (see Fig. 5.3):
A. The waste gas port
B. Transfer tubing
C. The interface
D. Gas evacuation system

The waste gas port (component A) is the opening through which WAGs exit the APL valve on a rebreathing system or the overflow port on a nonrebreathing system. The transfer tubing (component B) conveys WAGs from the waste gas port to the interface (component C) (Fig. 5.4). The diameter of this tubing must fit tightly onto the waste gas port to produce an airtight seal. The gas evacuation system (component D) (Fig. 5.5) removes WAGs by conveying them from the interface to the atmosphere outside the building.

The interface (component C) provides storage for WAGs in a reservoir until they are removed by the evacuation system. This storage is often in the form of a flexible bag that looks a lot like a breathing bag (see Fig. 5.4 A) or a canister (see Fig. 5.4 B). The interface also protects the patient's lungs from excessive pressure or excessive vacuum from developing within the breathing circuit. Scavenging system interfaces are classified as open or closed based on how they provide positive pressure relief (release of gases into the room if there is an obstruction downstream from the interface) and negative relief (influx of room air into the interface in the event that there is excess vacuum).

A closed interface is one in which the communication with room air is via positive and negative pressure relief valves (Fig. 5.4 A). This type works best with low-flow active evacuation systems. In contrast, an open interface is one that is open to the room air and contains no valves or a simple butterfly valve (see Fig. 5.4 B). In this type, an open port communicating directly with the room air provides positive and negative pressure relief. This type works best with high-flow active evacuation systems.

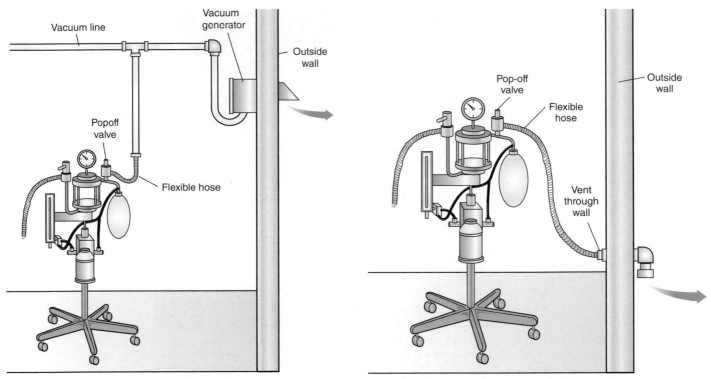

FIG. 5.1 Active scavenging system.

FIG. 5.2 Passive scavenging system.

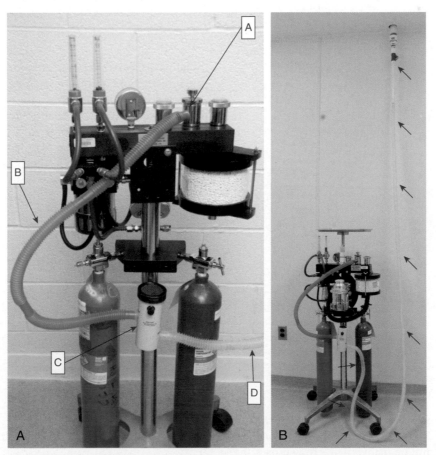

FIG. 5.3 Scavenging system. (A) Waste anesthetic gases exit the adjustable pressure limiting valve through the waste gas port (A), and travel through the flexible blue transfer tubing (B) into the interface (C). The gas is then conveyed to the gas evacuation system via the flexible white transfer tubing (D). (B) The flexible white transfer tubing is attached to the gas evacuation system ceiling outlet.

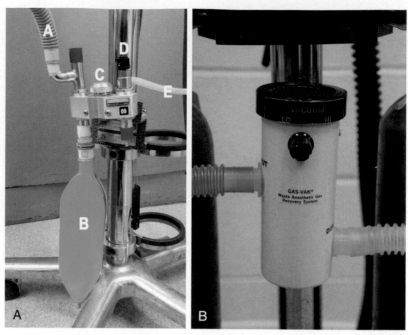

FIG. 5.4 Scavenging system interfaces. **(A)** Closed interface of a low-flow active scavenging system. *A*, Transfer tubing from breathing circuit; *B*, reservoir bag (holds waste gas until it is moved into the gas evacuation system); *C*, positive (mushroom-shaped) relief valve; *D*, adjustable needle valve (controls strength of vacuum); *E*, transfer tubing to hospital gas evacuation system. Note that the negative pressure relief valve is located beneath the positive pressure relief valve (not visible in this picture). **(B)** Open interface of a high-flow active scavenging system. The canister serves as the reservoir and communicates directly with the room air via an adjustable butterfly valve that serves as both positive and negative pressure relief. Waste gas is conveyed from the waste gas outlet to the interface by the blue transfer tubing and to the gas evacuation system by the white transfer tubing.

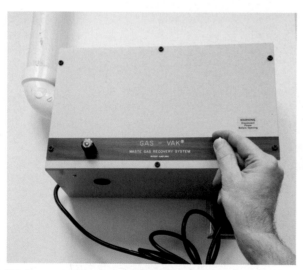

FIG. 5.5 Gas evacuation system. The fan inside this gas evacuation system housing (Gas Vac System) creates the vacuum that pulls the waste anesthetic gas from the interface reservoir, through pipes in the ceiling, and ultimately, out of the building. For this to work, the gas evacuation system must be turned on each day.

The waste gas collected by the scavenging system must be expelled outside the building, away from doors, windows, and air intakes, so that it will not be inadvertently drawn back into the building. Waste gas collected in the tubing should be totally confined within the scavenging system from the APL valve to the point of discharge and must not be recirculated into the building air. Scavenger hoses that discharge gas on the floor of the surgery room or into an attic or a basement, or that conduct the waste gas into a recirculating central vacuum system or recirculating ventilation exhaust, merely contaminate all rooms in the building with the waste gas and are not acceptable.

Passive scavenging system. A passive scavenging system uses the positive pressure of the gas in the anesthetic machine to "push" gas into the transfer hose of the scavenger unit and out of the building or into a charcoal canister. Passive systems usually do not have an interface because the gas does not have to be "stored" at any stage of the evacuation, and, because anesthetic agents are heavier than air, the transfer tubing should generally travel in a downward direction to the exit point. A conventional passive system discharges waste gas to the outdoors through a hole in the wall (Fig. 5.2). This system is best suited for rooms adjacent to the exterior of the building and is ineffective for interior rooms where the distance to the outlet outside of the building is more than 20 feet (7 m).

> **TECHNICIAN NOTE** A conventional passive scavenging system is best suited for rooms adjacent to the exterior of the building and is ineffective for interior rooms where the distance to the outlet outside of the building is more than 20 feet (7 m).

An activated charcoal canister (e.g., F/Air, AM Bickford, Inc; Breath Fresh, Jorgensen Laboratories, Inc.; VaporGuard, VetEquip; Enviropure, Smiths Medical) (Fig. 5.6) is an

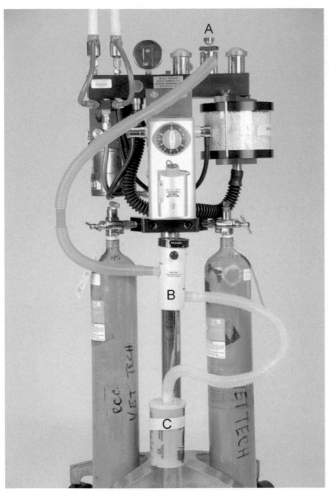

FIG. 5.6 Activated charcoal canister scavenging. The waste gas exits from the waste gas port of the adjustable pressure limiting valve (A) of this rebreathing system (or the overflow valve of a nonrebreathing system), flows through the interface (B), and finally flows into an activated charcoal canister (C). Note that when using this type of scavenger with an open interface as shown here, the butterfly valve must be adjusted fully closed to prevent the waste gas from venting into the room air before being scavenged.

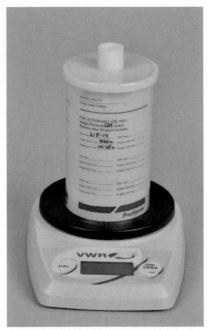

FIG. 5.7 Weighing an activated charcoal canister. In order to remain effective, F-air activated charcoal canisters must be replaced after 12 hours of use or after a weight gain of 50 g, whichever comes first. The canister pictured here weighs 234 g, and it will gain weight as waste halogenated volatile anesthetic is absorbed. Therefore, it will need to be replaced when it reaches a weight of 284 g. Note that the number of hours it has been used can also be tracked.

alternative passive scavenging device that may be used in situations in which a conventional scavenging system (i.e., either the active system or the passive system previously discussed) is not available. This may be the case when working in a specialized room such as an x-ray room, or during transport of an anesthetized patient from one location to another. The activated charcoal in these canisters is an adsorbent that binds halogenated gas anesthetics such as isoflurane and sevoflurane to its surface. Waste gas moves into an inlet port (usually on the top of the canister) through the charcoal (which binds to and removes the waste halogenated gas) and out of one or more exit ports (often holes on the bottom of the canister) back into the room air. As more waste gas in adsorbed, the canister gains weight until it is saturated.

Although activated charcoal canisters can remove these agents effectively under carefully controlled conditions, they are not able to adsorb nitrous oxide and do not provide the reliability of conventional active or passive systems. For instance, efficiency and capacity varies depending on the brand as well as the specific gas scavenged and carrier gas flow. These devices may absorb waste gas less efficiently at high carrier gas flow rates, and most are not as effective when mounted in a horizontal position and so should be mounted in an upright position unless indicated otherwise by the manufacturer (e.g., according to the manufacturer, Vapor-Guard canisters can be used in any position).

In order to remain effective, these canisters must be replaced after a specified maximum weight gain (e.g., 50 g in the case of F/air canisters). Some experts also recommend replacing them after a maximum number of hours of use regardless of the weight gain. So before using these devices, the canister must be weighed on a gram scale and the starting weight recorded on the canister (Fig. 5.7). Also, the manufacturer's instructions should be read and followed regarding details of proper use, including positioning, criteria used to determine when to change the canister, and maximum fresh gas flow if stipulated.

Checking and Adjusting a scavenging system. Normally, use of a scavenging system with an anesthetic machine does not alter the operation of the machine. The anesthetist should, however, be aware of two potential difficulties that can occur when a scavenging system is present:

1. When an active scavenging system is used, the anesthetist should prevent the negative pressure (vacuum) from the scavenger from being excessively applied to the breathing circuit. This is generally done by adjusting the vacuum regulator provided with the unit (Fig. 5.8 A) and by adjusting the valve on the interface according to the manufacturer's

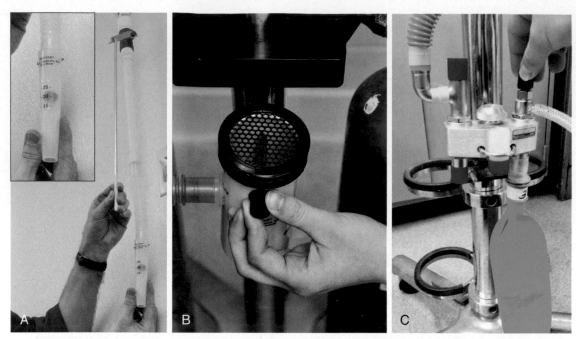

FIG. 5.8 Adjusting the vacuum on an active scavenging system. **(A)** Adjusting the vacuum regulator on a high-flow gas evacuation system with an open interface (Gas Vac System). With this particular system, the vacuum at each outlet in the hospital is adjusted to a flow recommended by the manufacturer (in this case, 20 L/min [see inset]). **(B)** Adjusting the butterfly valve on an open interface (Gas Vac System). Note that this valve is at the full open position. This valve prevents excess vacuum from being applied to the breathing circuit by admitting room air when the vacuum flow exceeds the production of waste gas and also prevents excess positive pressure from being applied to the breathing circuit. **(C)** Adjusting the needle valve on a closed interface. This prevents excess vacuum by limiting the flow of waste gas into the gas evacuation system. It should be adjusted so that the reservoir bag remains between empty and half full. (Fig. 5.8 A inset courtesy Jorgensen Labs; https://jorvet.com/product/gas-vak-multi-station-unit/)

recommendations (Fig. 5.8 B and C). If excessive vacuum is present due to a maladjusted valve, the reservoir bag will collapse. To prevent patient asphyxiation in the event that a vacuum develops, many anesthetic machines are equipped with an air intake valve, adjacent to the APL valve or inhalation unidirectional valve (see Chapter 4, Fig. 4.50), which opens automatically if negative pressure is detected in the circuit. The open valve admits room air into the circuit, thereby ensuring that a vacuum does not develop. When a machine is used that is not equipped with an air intake valve, it is especially important for the anesthetist to ensure that the reservoir bag is at least partially inflated at all times. Otherwise, the patient could be compromised or die of asphyxiation.

2. If either a passive or an active scavenging system is in use, the anesthetist must be aware that an obstruction may occur and block waste gas entry into the system. If this happens, gas will accumulate within the anesthetic circuit. This situation has the same effect as operating a machine with a closed APL valve and may result in excessive pressure developing within the circuit and the patient's lungs. To avoid this, the previously discussed positive pressure relief valve on the interface opens automatically if excessive pressure builds up within the circuit.

In view of these potential difficulties, scavenging systems must be checked daily for proper operation. Just because the light on the gas evacuation system box is illuminated does not mean the device is functioning properly. Consequently, it is prudent to check the status of the scavenger as part of the daily checks of the anesthetic machine.

> **TECHNICIAN NOTE** In order to remain effective, activated charcoal cartridges must be replaced after a specified maximum weight gain. Also, the manufacturer's instructions should be read and followed regarding details of proper use including positioning, criteria used to determine when to change the canister, and maximum fresh gas flow if stipulated.

Use of Respirators

For additional protection from WAG exposure, beyond using a scavenging system, respirators with activated charcoal filters can be worn by personnel who may be considered at special risk (such as pregnant workers). (Note: If respirators are worn by staff members, the practice must fully comply with all the requirements of the Respiratory Protection Standard-1910.134.) Like the activated charcoal canister for anesthetic machines, these are not effective in filtering out nitrous oxide vapors; however, organic vapor cartridges effectively absorb isoflurane, sevoflurane, and other anesthetic gases and vapors. Surgical masks or masks with cartridges designed for particulate matter do not absorb anesthetic vapors and should not be used for this purpose.

TECHNICIAN NOTE Gas leaks from anesthetic machines are a significant source of operating room pollution and are not captured by a scavenging system.

Effective Workplace Practices

As mentioned previously, in addition to scavenging waste gas, the anesthetist must adhere to workplace practices that minimize waste gas release. These practices include minimizing leaks in anesthetic delivery systems, following anesthetic techniques and procedures that minimize usage of anesthetic gases, avoiding spills of liquid anesthetic, capturing exhaled waste gas, and minimizing the use of anesthetic techniques that make effective scavenging difficult such as use of masks and chambers.

Equipment leak testing. Gas leaks from anesthetic machines are a significant source of operating room WAG pollution and are not captured by a scavenging system. Leakage is common and may occur from any part of the machine in which nitrous oxide or volatile gas anesthetic is present. (See Chapter 4 for a discussion of these parts and Fig. 5.9 for a diagram.)

The most common problems that can result in waste gas leakage are the following:
- Breathing hoses, the reservoir bag, or the endotracheal tube have holes or are not securely connected to the machine or breathing system.
- The carbon dioxide absorber canister is not securely sealed. Leaks are often caused by improper positioning of the canister or by the presence of absorbent granules on the seals around the canister.
- The covering over a unidirectional valve is not tightly closed.
- The connection between the APL valve and scavenger is not airtight.
- The vaporizer cap was not replaced or not tightly closed after the vaporizer was last filled.
- If using nitrous oxide, the connections for nitrous oxide gas lines were not tightly secured, or O-rings, washers, and other seals joining nitrous oxide gas tanks to machine hanger yokes or other equipment are missing, worn, or out of position.

In some cases the presence of a leak is obvious—there may be an audible hiss, the odor of anesthetic, or a jet of air coming out of the reservoir bag or hose. However, small leaks are often undetected unless the anesthetist regularly performs a leak test.

Two types of leak tests are commonly done in veterinary clinics: high-pressure tests and low-pressure tests.
1. High-pressure tests check for high-pressure leaks arising between the compressed gas cylinders and the flowmeters where the pressure is 40 to 58 pounds per square inch (psi) or greater. These leaks release only pure oxygen (and medical air or nitrous oxide, if used) without volatile anesthetic.
2. Low-pressure tests check for anesthetic gases that escape from the vaporizer, the breathing circuit, and the associated connections where the pressure of gas within the machine is

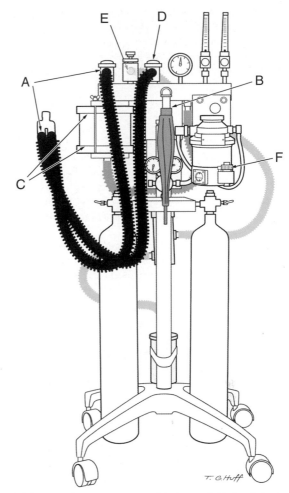

FIG. 5.9 Diagram of common areas of leakage. *A,* Ends of the breathing hoses and Y-piece; *B,* neck of the reservoir bag; *C,* seals of the carbon dioxide absorber canister, due to improper positioning of the canister or the presence of absorbent granules on the seals around the canister; *D,* the covering over a unidirectional valve; *E,* the connection between the adjustable pressure limiting valve and scavenger; and *F,* the vaporizer cap.

approximately 15 psi. Low-pressure leaks may arise in any parts of the vaporizer or breathing circuit that do not fit together tightly or a part that develops a hole. Low-pressure leaks release waste volatile anesthetic gas as well as oxygen (and medical air or nitrous oxide, if in use).

The type of leak test regularly performed on an anesthetic machine depends on the type of carrier gas used. If oxygen alone is used, it is necessary to perform only a low-pressure test because release of oxygen into the room through a high-pressure leak does not adversely affect the air quality, although it wastes oxygen and may empty the tank prematurely. If both nitrous oxide and oxygen are used, both a high-pressure and a low-pressure test should be performed.

Low-pressure tests should be completed before use of the machine each day. High-pressure tests on nitrous oxide tanks should be performed once weekly and whenever the nitrous oxide tank is changed. Details of high-pressure and low-pressure tests are given in Chapter 4, Procedures 4.1, 4.2, and 4.4.

See Case Presentation 5.1 for an example of the importance of leak testing.

Jennifer, a registered veterinary technician, was acting as anesthetist on a typical surgery day. Following her usual routine, Jennifer started by preparing all the necessary equipment and supplies. Among other things, this involved performing a low-pressure leak test on an anesthetic machine fitted with a rebreathing circuit.

Jennifer assembled the machine, turned on the oxygen, closed the adjustable pressure limiting valve, occluded the Y-piece, and attempted to perform the test, but she was unable to pressurize the breathing circuit. Even when using the oxygen flush valve, the pressure would not remain above 10 cm H_2O for more than a few seconds.

She confirmed that the machine was correctly assembled and looked in all the usual places, but the location of the leak was not readily apparent.

1. *What anesthetic machine parts commonly leak and should be checked?*
2. *Given that the leak was not coming from the usual areas, can you think of other possible sources of the leak?*
3. *What steps should be taken to locate and fix the leak?*

TECHNICIAN NOTE The type of leak test regularly performed on an anesthetic machine depends on the type of carrier gas used. If oxygen alone is used, it is necessary to conduct only a low-pressure test. Low-pressure tests should be completed before use of the machine each day.

For both nonrebreathing and rebreathing systems, the location of either high- or low-pressure leaks may be determined by listening for the hiss of escaping air or by using a detergent solution, as described in Procedure 4.4. It is important never to try to stop the flow of gas from a high-pressure leak by putting a hand over the leaking part. Once the source of a leak has been identified, it can often be fixed by tightening a connection or replacing a part. If the leak cannot be fixed, the machine should not be used until it has been serviced by qualified personnel. Frequent, routine servicing of the anesthetic machine and breathing circuit by qualified personnel every 4 to 12 months is helpful in detecting equipment problems that can lead to leaks but is not an adequate substitute for daily leak testing of the machine by the anesthetist.

TECHNICIAN NOTE Anesthetic machines including breathing circuits should be routinely serviced by qualified personnel every 4 to 12 months. Note that OSHA expects at least annual preventative maintenance checks by a trained service technician.

Anesthetic Techniques and Procedures

The anesthetist, by their choice of anesthetic techniques, has considerable control over the amount of waste gas released into the room air. One survey of human hospitals found that faulty work practices accounted for 94% to 99% of waste anesthetic gas released in scavenged operating rooms.

The steps Procedure 5.1 in are recommended to minimize waste gas release. Box 5.1 shows a summary of these procedures.

Monitoring Waste Gas Levels

It is advisable to monitor waste anesthetic gas levels periodically to ensure that the NIOSH-recommended levels are not exceeded.

PROCEDURE 5.1 Procedures for Minimizing Waste Gas Release

1. Anesthetic induction chambers are a significant source of anesthetic waste gas pollution in veterinary facilities. Unless a scavenging system is connected to the chamber, significant amounts of waste gas are released when the chamber is opened. In addition, the fur of the patient is saturated with anesthetic during the induction and gives off waste gas vapor when the animal is removed from the chamber. Chambers should be used only in a well-ventilated room with a nonrecirculating ventilation system or under a fume hood. They must be tightly sealed to avoid leaks. The chamber should have two inlet holes to which the breathing hoses from the anesthetic machine can be attached once the Y-piece has been removed (see Chapter 9, Fig. 9.7). With this setup, the anesthetic machine scavenger will be able to remove the exhaust vapors. Alternatively, the patient connector from a nonrebreathing circuit can be attached to one inlet, and a scavenger system transfer hose can be directly attached to the other inlet (either of which may require a special connector to create an airtight seal). Either way, the chamber should be closed immediately after the patient has been removed, and the oxygen flow should be continued for several minutes to purge waste gas into the scavenger rather than releasing waste gas into the room air. Anesthetic chambers should be washed with soap and water after each use to remove residual anesthetic and contaminants from the animal.
2. Avoid using masks to maintain anesthesia. Significant amounts of anesthetic gas may escape from around the diaphragm of the mask and enter the room air. It has been suggested that waste gas concentrations around the patient's head can be reduced by 50% if an endotracheal tube is used instead of a mask. If the situation dictates the use of a mask, it should be fitted tightly over the animal's face. Face masks are available in a variety of sizes and should be chosen to fit the patient snugly but comfortably (see Fig. 1 from Procedure 9.4). When a mask is used, the sequence of events is the same as for an endotracheal tube: turn the oxygen on, place the mask on the patient, then turn the vaporizer on. This order should be reversed when ending the procedure. If mask induction is required, ideally, the animal should be intubated when it reaches an appropriate depth.
3. Use cuffed endotracheal tubes when possible. To be effective, the tube must be of adequate size and the cuff must be inflated and in good repair. Before use, inflate cuffs with air to check for leaks. After intubation of the patient, check the fit of the endotracheal tube within the trachea by closing the adjustable pressure limiting (APL) valve and gently squeezing the reservoir bag. The cuff should not leak up to an airway pressure of 16–20 cm H_2O (see Chapter 4 for specific recommendations) but should leak at higher pressures. Note that the leakage at pressures over 20 cm H_2O is necessary to reduce the risk of barotrauma in case the APL valve is closed and accidentally forgotten. (Note: To prevent overinflation of the patient's lungs, ensure that the circuit pressure displayed on the manometer does not exceed 20 cm H_2O when applying pressure to the bag to check the cuff.)
4. When using a rebreathing system, ensure that the reservoir bag inflates and deflates synchronously with the patient's respiration (in other words, inflates on expiration and deflates on inspiration, with the volume of movement approximately equal to the animal's tidal volume). If this does not occur, one should suspect either air leakage around the endotracheal tube or esophageal intubation. Significant release of waste gas can occur in either case. (It is also likely that the patient will wake up because a significant amount of room air enters the lungs in either case.)

PROCEDURE 5.1   Procedures for Minimizing Waste Gas Release—cont'd

5. Keep oxygen flow rates as low as can safely be used. The safe level is determined by patient need, flowmeter and vaporizer design, and the breathing circuit in use. The "low-flow" technique (see Chapter 4, Box 4.5) can be safely used during anesthetic maintenance in most circumstances when using a partial rebreathing system but should never be used with nonrebreathing systems because these systems require use of a higher oxygen flow rate during all phases of an anesthetic procedure. The use of full rebreathing systems may also help minimize waste gas pollution. Use of partial, minimal, or nonrebreathing systems and high gas flow (i.e., >3 L/min) is associated with greater release of waste gas, particularly if effective scavenging is unavailable.

6. When working with an anesthetic machine designed for use with dogs and cats, do not turn the vaporizer on until the breathing circuit is connected to the endotracheal tube and the cuff is inflated. The practice of filling the machine and reservoir bag with anesthetic gas before connecting the machine to a dog or cat should be discouraged. This practice is acceptable when working with large animals, and in this case, the Y-piece should be occluded with a rubber plug. When it is time to attach the circuit to the intubated patient, the connection should be made quickly. Once the anesthetic procedure is under way, avoid disconnecting the patient from the breathing circuit unnecessarily. If the patient is to be disconnected from the machine, the vaporizer setting and flowmeters should temporarily be turned to zero.

7. Do not release the contents of the reservoir bag into the room air. If it is necessary to empty the reservoir bag, leave it attached to the machine, leave the endotracheal tube attached to the breathing circuit or occlude the Y-piece, and evacuate the contents into the scavenger by gently pressing the bag.

8. After the vaporizer has been shut off, maintain the connection between the animal and the machine, having the animal breathe pure oxygen at a rate of 50–100 mL/kg/minute for several minutes. Periodically flush anesthetic gas out of the system by emptying the reservoir bag through the APL valve and allowing it to refill with pure oxygen. If possible, leave the patient attached to the machine until extubation occurs. This allows expired anesthetic to enter the scavenging system rather than the room air.

9. Ensure that all rooms in which anesthetic gases are released (e.g., surgical preparation room, operating room, recovery room, and radiography room) have adequate ventilation that provides at least 15 air changes per hour, 3 of which should be fresh. A properly designed ventilation system helps eliminate residual waste gases not collected by the scavenging system (e.g., those that arise from leaks or improper work practices).

10. One study found that concentrations of waste anesthetic gases were higher in recovery areas than in scavenged operating rooms. For the reduction of waste gas levels, it is usually necessary to have an exhaust fan or nonrecirculating ventilation system operating in the room where patients are recovering from anesthesia. Whenever possible, avoid being closer than 3 feet (1 m) to the nose of an animal recovering from anesthesia.

11. Have anesthetic machines serviced every 4–12 months by a qualified service technician to ensure minimal leakage through machine components. A log of evaluation and maintenance procedures and leak testing should be maintained for each anesthetic machine, ventilator, and vaporizer.

12. Inspect equipment (anesthetic machine AND scavenger) often and perform necessary maintenance. The routine maintenance procedures for machines are usually outlined in the operating manual. Hoses, reservoir bags, and endotracheal tubes that are cracked or worn should be discarded. Endotracheal tubes with nonfunctional or leaking cuffs should not be used.

13. After use, wash hoses, reservoir bags, masks, endotracheal tubes, and all other detachable rubber components of the anesthetic circuit with soap and water; flush well with water; and allow them to air dry. These components may absorb significant amounts of anesthetic during use. Washing not only removes absorbed waste gas, but also reduces transfer of microorganisms between patients.

14. Emptying and filling vaporizers may release significant amounts of anesthetic vapor into the surrounding air. If possible, pregnant personnel should not be involved in this task. Anesthetics may also be spilled onto the technician's hands and clothing. Ideally, vaporizers should be filled at the end of the workday when personnel are leaving the hospital. Use a filling device (a specialized attachment that transfers anesthetic directly into the vaporizer) rather than pouring from a bottle to replenish liquid anesthetic in the machine. Agent-specific keyed filler systems are preferred (see Chapter 4, Fig. 4.39 B). If no filling device is available, use a bottle adapter with a pouring spout to prevent spillage (see Chapter 4, Fig. 4.39 A) and. if possible, place a scavenger hose near the fill port to evacuate evaporated anesthetic. Fill vaporizers in a well-ventilated area and, after filling a vaporizer, ensure that the filling port is properly closed. Use of an approved organic cartridge respirator (a device that fits over the mouth and nose and filters anesthetic gas out of incoming air), vinyl or plastic gloves, a lab coat or plastic apron, and other protective equipment will also minimize exposure to anesthetic liquid or vapors. The gloves should be removed and hands washed immediately after the vaporizer has been filled because liquid anesthetics are readily absorbed through intact skin.

15. Vaporizers and flowmeters should be turned off when not in use.

16. If liquid anesthetic is spilled, high concentrations of anesthetic vapor will be present in the immediate area of the spill. If a spill occurs, increase ventilation as much as possible during the cleanup by opening windows or using fans. Close doors to the rest of the building and turn off the central vacuum system to avoid spreading the fumes throughout the building. For anything other than a small spill, all personnel not involved in the cleanup should leave the area, and the remaining staff should wear approved protective clothing, vinyl or plastic (not latex or rubber) gloves, and organic cartridge respirators. Remove all contaminated articles, including lab coats. Pour absorbent material such as cat litter on the spill so that the liquid is completely absorbed. Dispose of the litter in an airtight container outside the clinic. If the spill is large or if protective equipment is unavailable, all personnel should leave the building and the local fire department should be notified.

17. Cap empty anesthetic bottles before discarding them because residual anesthetic in the bottle may evaporate into the room air. For the same reason, store vaporizer filling devices in a sealed plastic bag between uses.

Monitoring waste gas levels is particularly important if a hospital employee becomes pregnant and is still working around anesthetized animals. Waste gas monitoring is also advisable if hospital employees frequently detect the odor of anesthetic gas or if there are special concerns about waste gas levels (e.g., if the clinic is using induction chambers). If professional monitoring is required, an accredited industrial hygiene laboratory can be contacted for assistance. (Industrial hygienists may be found by going to the American Industrial Hygiene Association [AIHA] website at https://www.aiha.org and performing a search.) An occupational hygienist will usually visit the hospital to evaluate ventilation and scavenging techniques and to interview the anesthetist regarding procedures used to minimize waste gas release. Air samples should be collected from all areas in which anesthetics are used, and the level of waste gas in the collected air should be determined with an infrared spectrometer.

Professional monitoring services are not always necessary. Clinic employees can inexpensively monitor waste gas levels using detector badges. Badges may detect only one chemical, such as halothane, isoflurane, or nitrous oxide, or may be

BOX 5.1   Summary of Procedures for Minimizing Waste Gas Release

- Minimize use of anesthetic induction chambers. When necessary, use anesthetic chambers in a well-ventilated room and close the anesthetic chamber immediately after the patient has been removed.
- Minimize the use of anesthetic masks for induction or maintenance. When use is necessary, ensure that the mask fits snugly but comfortably around the face.
- Use cuffed endotracheal tubes and check the cuff for leaks before use.
- Choose the lowest fresh gas flow rates that can be safely used.
- Connect the patient to the breathing circuit and cuff the endotracheal tube before turning on the vaporizer.
- Avoid disconnecting the patient from the breathing circuit unnecessarily and occlude the Y-piece or turn off the flowmeters and vaporizer when it is necessary to do so.
- When it is necessary to empty the breathing bag, gently evacuate the contents into the scavenging system instead of into the room.
- At the end of a procedure, turn the vaporizer off and have the animal breathe pure oxygen for several minutes before detaching the endotracheal tube connector.

- In all rooms in which anesthetic waste gas is released, ensure ventilation at a rate of at least 15 air changes per hour, 3 of which should be fresh.
- Keep at least 3 feet (1 m) distant from recovering animals when possible and use an exhaust fan in recovery areas, if available.
- Service anesthetic machines regularly.
- Inspect equipment often and perform routine maintenance.
- Discard damaged or nonfunctional equipment.
- Wash, rinse, and dry hoses, reservoir bags, masks, endotracheal tubes, and all other detachable rubber components after use.
- Fill vaporizers at the end of the workday. If possible, place a scavenger hose near the fill port to evacuate evaporated anesthetic, wear gloves and an apron, and use a filling spout or keyed adapter to minimize spills. Cap empty liquid anesthetic bottles, wash hands, and launder protective clothing immediately after.
- Turn vaporizers and flowmeters off when not in use.
- If liquid anesthetic is spilled, use approved methods to clean up, cap empty bottles, and store vaporizer filling devices in a sealed plastic bag.

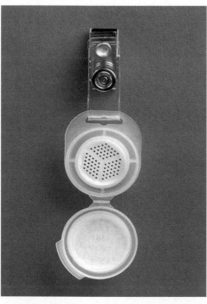

FIG. 5.10 Passive dosimeter. To measure waste anesthetic gases (WAGs), the passive dosimeter is uncapped, as shown here, clipped to the clothing near the anesthetist's breathing zone (for personal monitoring) or placed in the room at the level of the breathing zone (for area monitoring), recapped at the end of the exposure period (usually 2 to 8 hours), and returned to the supplier for analysis. (Courtesy Assay Technology; https://assaytech.com)

sensitive to all halogenated anesthetics. The badges (called **passive dosimeters;** Fig. 5.10) are uncapped at the beginning of the exposure period, then worn by personnel in the surgical preparation room, operating room, or recovery area for a timed period when anesthetic gases are being used (usually, an exposure time of 2 to 8 hours is chosen). Alternatively, the badge may be placed in a room for area monitoring. This method does not correlate well with exposure of individual employees, however, because staff members typically move in and out of the area during the test period. For this reason, individual monitoring is preferred. After exposure, the badge is recapped and returned to the supplier (usually an industrial health and safety supply house or a company specializing in OSHA

compliance) for analysis. Results are given as a time-weighted average in parts per million. The cost, including analysis, is approximately $50 to $75 per badge.[a]

OSHA expects practices to conduct ongoing exposure monitoring of WAGs with tests conducted at least every 4 to 12 months. If a test reveals exposure levels above the permissible limits (2 ppm), then corrective actions must be taken, followed by retesting to confirm compliance.

> **TECHNICIAN NOTE** It is advisable to monitor waste anesthetic gas levels periodically to ensure that the NIOSH-recommended levels are not exceeded, especially if a hospital employee becomes pregnant and is still working around anesthetized animals. Waste gas monitoring is also advisable if hospital employees frequently detect the odor of anesthetic gas or if there are special concerns about waste gas levels (e.g., if the clinic is using induction chambers).

HAZARDS ASSOCIATED WITH COMPRESSED GASES

Carrier and anesthetic agents that are gases at room temperature (such as oxygen, medical air, and nitrous oxide) are stored in compressed gas cylinders (see Chapter 4, Fig. 4.17). These cylinders store large volumes of gas under high pressure. Although not flammable, both oxygen and nitrous oxide support combustion and cause fuels to burn more readily. For these reasons, there are several hazards associated with compressed gas cylinders of which the anesthetist must be aware: (1) fire, (2) injury caused by rapid release of gas, (3) injury caused by damage to the cylinder, and (4) physical injury from the weight of the tanks falling on one's feet or legs.

Fire Safety Precautions When Using Compressed Gas Cylinders

There is a potential for fire in any room where oxygen or nitrous oxide is used. Even static electricity can cause fires in

---

[a]Current suppliers include Assay Technology (1-800-833-1258) and Vetamac (1-800-334-1583).

areas in which oxygen and flammable materials are used together. (This is one of the reasons why diethyl ether, which is extremely flammable, is no longer used in veterinary anesthesia.) It is recommended that no flames or sources of ignition (e.g., matches, lighters, or Bunsen burners) be present in any room in which oxygen or nitrous oxide cylinders are stored or used. For obvious reasons, smoking also must be prohibited in all rooms in which oxygen is stored or used.

A risk of fire also exists when cautery or medical lasers are used in proximity to oxygen sources. Fires can occur when the spark caused by a cautery unit or a laser beam contacts an airway containing a high concentration of oxygen or penetrates an endotracheal tube. These fires can burn the patient externally or can burn the interior of the airway, resulting in devastating complications. For this reason, great care must be used when using cautery or a laser beam in the vicinity of the head and neck of a patient that is receiving oxygen. The use of a special shielded endotracheal tube and adherence to practices that minimize the risk of fire are essential to prevent this complication when performing laser surgery or using electrocautery in this location.

> **TECHNICIAN NOTE** A risk of fire exists when cautery or medical lasers are used in proximity to oxygen sources. These fires can burn the patient externally or can burn the interior of the airway, resulting in devastating complications. For this reason, great care must be used when using cautery or a laser beam in the vicinity of the head and neck of a patient that is receiving oxygen.

Use and Storage of Compressed Gas Cylinders

Tanks of compressed gas can be viewed as storehouses of tremendous amounts of energy waiting for release. This is because the gas in a cylinder is pressurized to up to 150 times atmospheric pressure. When a cylinder is turned on, gas will forcefully exit the outlet port unless it is connected to an anesthetic machine yolk or pressure-regulating valve. The force of this gas is sufficient to tear skin or the cornea of the eye or cause the operator to lose their grip and drop the cylinder. For these reasons, a cylinder should never be turned on unless it is connected to an anesthetic machine or a pressure-reducing valve.

To prevent these injuries, persons connecting compressed gas cylinders to an anesthetic machine or gas piping system should wear impact-resistant goggles to protect their eyes from jets of gas. If a cylinder leak occurs, never use your hand to try to stop the leak. When turning on a compressed air tank that is connected to the anesthetic machine, use the appropriate wrench and turn the valve slowly to the open position. Keep your head and face away from the valve outlet, pressure gauge, and pressure relief device.

Cylinders can also pose a danger if dropped or damaged. If a cylinder or cylinder neck is damaged, the sudden release of gas can have catastrophic consequences. If, for example, a cylinder is punctured or is knocked over and the pressure regulator (the metal attachments at the top of an H, J, or K tank) or cylinder neck is broken off the tank, the force of the gas suddenly escaping from the tank may cause it to spin like a pinwheel or move like a rocket through a wall or roof and injure or kill any persons

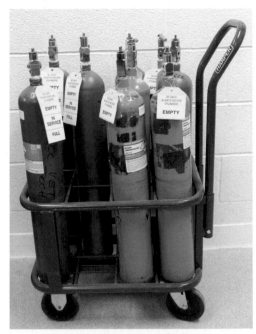

FIG. 5.11 Cart for size E compressed gas cylinder storage. A cart such as this one is used to store E tanks in an upright position and prevent them from being dropped, kicked, or otherwise damaged.

or animals in its path. Likewise, since cylinders are tall and narrow, they are inherently unstable when standing free and are prone to falling over if not secured. Even an empty tank can cause severe injury if it falls on one's feet or legs.

To prevent damage, cylinders must be handled with care and approved storage methods must be used. Chain or belt large cylinders to a wall and always store them in an upright position (see Chapter 4, Fig. 4.19). Small tanks should always be attached to an anesthetic machine, chained or belted to the wall, or stored in an approved cart (Fig. 5.11). Tanks should not be stored in a horizontal position on the floor as they may present a tripping hazard and can be kicked or bumped while moving other equipment such as anesthetic machines and mop buckets, risking damage to the valve. Valve caps should be used on all large cylinders that are not connected to gas lines to protect the valves from damage (Fig. 5.12).

Gas cylinders should be stored away from emergency exits or areas with heavy traffic. If a large cylinder must be moved to another location, a handcart should be used; do not drag or roll the cylinder.

Full tanks should be kept separate from empty tanks and also should be clearly labeled for quick identification. The use of tearoff labels helps eliminate confusion regarding the empty, in use, or full status of a given compressed air cylinder. The current status of the tank is indicated on the outermost section of the label (see Chapter 4, Fig. 4.30). Cylinders should be used in the order in which they are received (i.e., first in, first out).

ACCIDENTAL EXPOSURE TO INJECTABLE AGENTS

All anesthetic agents are potentially toxic to personnel handling them. Skin exposure, eye splash, or oral ingestion of injectable drugs or inhalation agents may be hazardous (or even fatal).

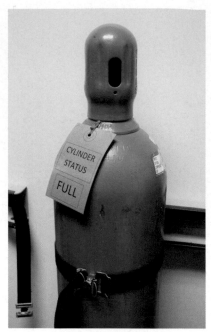

FIG. 5.12 Size H compressed gas cylinder valve cap. A valve cap should be kept on an H-tank when the tank is not in use to prevent damage to the valve.

The injectable drugs of most concern are the ultrapotent opioids (UPOs), etorphine (Immobilon, M99) and thiafentanil (Thianil, A3080), which are used for the restraint and capture of wildlife, particularly large ungulates. Although not available since 2016, carfentanil (Wildnil) is another UPO that was used for many years for this purpose. These drugs are classified as ultrapotent because they are thousands of times more potent than morphine (approximately 6000 times in the case of both etorphine and thiafentanil, and approximately 10,000 times more potent in the case of carfentanil). Even the reversal agent diprenorphine (although not commercially available at the time of writing) has some agonist effects in humans and can be dangerous. These agents are absorbed readily through mucous membranes or broken skin. Exposure may also occur through accidental injection, eye splash, or oral ingestion.

Accidental exposure can occur under a wide variety of circumstances and at any time during the process of handling these drugs. Reported accidents include situations in which the drug is sprayed into the face of the operator during loading or firing blow darts, accidental injections, exposure to a contaminated needle following administration or during recapping, contact with contaminated skin around the site of injection, and exposure during cleanup of the equipment.

Human exposure to even a minute amount of these agents by any route can cause rapid onset of unconsciousness, respiratory failure, and death. All personnel must therefore be trained in safe use; strict principles of safe handling must be observed at all times to prevent exposure; and adequate volumes of reversal agents such as naloxone or naltrexone must be drawn up and ready to use if human exposure occurs. A minimum of two people should be present when using UPOs in case of an emergency arising due to accidental exposure. See Procedure 5.2 for precautions that must be taken when handling these agents.

PROCEDURE 5.2   **Principles of Handling Ultrapotent Opioids Used for the Restraint and Capture of Wildlife (Etorphine and Thiafentanil)**

General Principles
- These agents should be stored in a locked safe (Fig. 1).

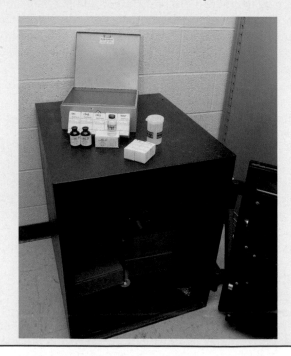

- Never handle these agents unless you have been adequately trained in their safe use, potential adverse effects, and treatment in case of exposure.
- Never work with these agents alone.
- Be sure that an oxygen source with an appropriate mask is available for immediate use.
- Have a written emergency response plan for on-site treatment of exposed personnel, including provision for cardiovascular and respiratory support, notification of emergency personnel, and transport to the emergency room.
- Have a stocked emergency exposure kit immediately available at all times. This kit should contain emergency procedures and protocols, syringes and needles, and adequate amounts of reversal agent (Fig. 2).

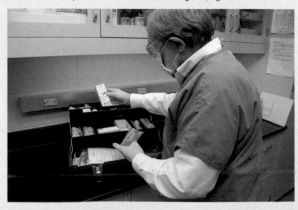

PROCEDURE 5.2 Principles of Handling Ultrapotent Opioids Used for the Restraint and Capture of Wildlife (Etorphine and Thiafentanil)—cont'd

When Handling These Agents

- Never handle these agents unless a trained person certified in cardiopulmonary resuscitation is present and in the immediate vicinity.
- Inform all personnel of the potential danger. Be sure that only personnel directly involved in the procedure are present.
- Wear personal protective equipment, including gloves (double gloves are preferred), mask and goggles or preferably a face shield, and long pants and sleeves when handling these agents (Fig. 3).

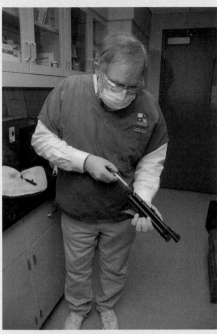

- Naloxone must be drawn up and ready for use. Note that up to three 10-mL bottles (concentration 0.4 mg/mL for a total of 12 mg) may be necessary to antagonize a single drop of these opioids. So a total of at least 30–40 mg (three to four 10-mL bottles of naloxone at a concentration of 1 mg/mL) may be needed to reverse the effects of an accidental injection effectively. Some cases may require upward of three times that volume. Note that some experts recommend naltrexone as an alternative reversal agent in the event that naloxone is ineffective or unavailable.

- Prepare the drug in an area that can easily be cleaned in the event that it is spilled. Have a source of running water or, if none is available, a bucket of fresh water in the immediate vicinity.
- Avoid distractions and have all uninvolved personnel out of the room when preparing these agents.
- Do NOT inject air into the drug vial (overpressurize the vial) before drawing the drug up. This will minimize the possibility of the drug leaking out of the rubber stopper when the needle is withdrawn.
- Use a device designed to prevent needle sticks when removing or replacing a needle cap (Fig. 4).

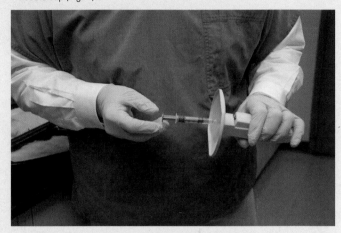

- Transport loaded darts in a labeled, impenetrable, unbreakable, leakproof container.
- Clearly mark the injection site on the skin of the animal so all personnel can visually identify it. Do not touch this area.
- Dispose of used needles and syringes in a closed container immediately after use.
- All reusable equipment used to inject the patient should be washed thoroughly with copious amounts of water.
- If exposure occurs, immediately wash skin and clothing with copious amounts of cold water and make those around you aware so that emergency procedures may be instituted.

Other injectable agents that may be hazardous include the dissociatives (ketamine, tiletamine), which have been reported to cause disorientation, excitement and other behavioral changes, dizziness, and unconsciousness after an accidental eye splash. Human exposure to alpha$_2$-agonists (e.g., xylazine, dexmedetomidine, detomidine, or romifidine) by injection or skin contact may cause profound sedation, hypotension, bradycardia, respiratory depression, and coma.

Safety precautions for prevention of exposure to any injectable agent include the use of personal protective equipment if there is a risk of spillage or eye splash, careful loading of syringes, avoidance of needle sticks, and proper disposal of used needles and syringes in an approved sharps container. If accidental exposure occurs, the exposed person should

BOX 5.2 Principles of Avoiding Exposure to Injectable Agents

- When loading a syringe, use a Luer lock syringe when available.
- Be sure needles are tightly attached to the syringe.
- Wear appropriate eye protection.
- Use gloves when using potentially dangerous agents.
- Avoid recapping of needles—instead, dispose of the syringe and needle immediately after use in an approved sharps container.
- When a needle is recapped, use the one-handed technique (Fig. 5.13).

receive prompt first aid (eye wash, flushing of exposed skin with large amounts of water, respiratory support) and subsequent transport to a medical center. See Box 5.2 for principles of avoiding exposure to injectable agents.

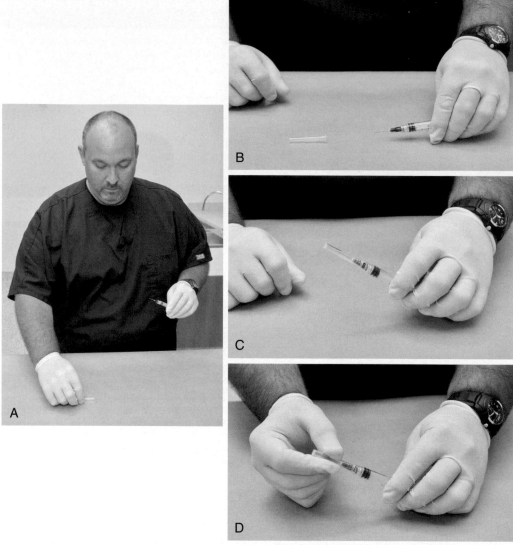

FIG. 5.13 One-handed technique for recapping needles. **(A)** Remove the needle cap with the nondominant hand and place it on a countertop or other flat surface. After injecting the medication, the needle should be immediately recapped. **(B)** and **(C)**, While keeping the nondominant hand away from the cap, "scoop up" the cap with the needle, using the dominant hand. **(D)** Hold the cap near the opening with the nondominant forefinger and thumb and snap it into place.

KEY POINTS

1. Anesthesia presents several potential health risks to hospital personnel, including exposure to waste anesthetic gas and hazardous injectable agents and accidents associated with handling of compressed gas cylinders.

2. Waste anesthetic gases and vapors are breathed by all personnel working in areas in which animals are anesthetized or are recovering from inhalation anesthesia. Filling or emptying vaporizers and the cleanup of accidental spills also may result in significant exposure.

3. Exposure to waste anesthetic gas is associated with short-term problems such as fatigue, headache, drowsiness, nausea, depression, and irritability.

4. Long-term exposure to high levels of waste anesthetic gases, as may occur in environments without scavenging, may be associated with reproductive disorders, liver and kidney damage, and nervous system dysfunction, although the evidence of epidemiologic studies is sometimes contradictory and difficult to interpret. Nevertheless, most authorities recommend that exposure to high levels of waste anesthetic gas be avoided, particularly by pregnant women.

5. Anesthetics such as isoflurane and sevoflurane, which undergo very little hepatic metabolism and renal excretion, are considered to be a lower hazard than anesthetics that are significantly eliminated by these routes (e.g., the older halogenated agents methoxyflurane and halothane).

6. The National Institute for Occupational Safety and Health (NIOSH) recommended exposure limit is 2 parts per million (ppm) for halogenated anesthetics when used alone. Surveys of veterinary clinics show wide variations in waste gas levels, depending on the sampling site, scavenging system, and anesthetic techniques used.

7. Installation and use of an effective gas scavenging system greatly reduces waste gas exposure. Caution should be used to prevent the scavenger from applying negative pressure to the breathing circuit.

8. Equipment leak testing should be done on a daily basis to detect and allow correction of leakage from the anesthetic machine and compressed gas cylinders. Tests should be done on both the high-pressure and low-pressure components of the machine.

9. Certain anesthetic techniques are associated with excessive release of waste gas. These include the use of anesthetic chambers, masks, and uncuffed endotracheal tubes. Procedures such as turning off the vaporizer before disconnecting the animal from the machine are helpful in reducing waste gas contamination of hospital air.

10. Vaporizers should be filled and emptied with care, using appropriate equipment and protective clothing.

11. Waste gas levels should be monitored regularly by professional occupational hygienists or by the use of detector badges.

12. Compressed air cylinders should be transported, used, and stored with care. Special hazards include a risk of fire in areas in which cylinders are stored and the risk of sudden release of pressurized gas from damaged cylinders.

13. Potent injectable opioids such as etorphine and thiafentanil have considerable potential to cause serious, even fatal, reactions. Special training is necessary to handle these agents safely, and sufficient quantities of an appropriate reversal agent must be readily available in case of human exposure.

ANSWERS TO CASE PRESENTATION

Case Presentation 5.1

Question #1: Parts of the machine that are frequently removed or disassembled for cleaning or maintenance, such as the Y-piece, breathing hoses, and CO_2 absorber canister, are common areas of leakage. Parts made of rubber and other materials that degrade over time, such as the reservoir bag and connecting hoses, are also commonly affected.

Question #2: Other possible sources of the leak include the APL valve, the unidirectional valves, and the air intake valve. Any part of the breathing circuit can be involved, as well as tubes connecting machine parts downstream from the flowmeter, such as the tube connecting the flowmeter and the vaporizer inlet port and the tube connecting the vaporizer outlet port and the fresh gas inlet or the common gas outlet. Each of these parts must be checked.

Question #3: First, always check that the machine is correctly assembled, and that detachable parts such as breathing hoses and the breathing bag are securely connected. Visually inspect each part for holes, tears, or other damage. Sometimes the leak is obvious and other times it is not. For instance, you may hear an obvious hissing noise coming from a part such as the neck of the reservoir bag that allows you to locate the leak quickly and easily. When the source of the leak is not obvious, you may have to put your ear close to various parts and listen carefully for the leak, or you may have to replace suspect parts such as the breathing hoses to see if the leak stops.

Outcome of This Case

By checking each part very carefully, Jennifer detected a very quiet hiss coming from the area of the unidirectional valves. Because this machine had an air intake valve on top of the inhalation valve (like the machine in Chapter 4, Fig. 4.50) this part became suspect. By temporarily taping over the air holes on the valve, she was able to stop the leak, confirming this as the source. Under normal circumstances, an air intake valve should only admit air in the event that a vacuum develops in the breathing circuit. In this case, the broken valve was allowing air to exit the breathing circuit when pressurized. This not only allows waste gas to leak from the system but also would prevent the anesthetist from being able to ventilate the patient manually when needed. So the machine could not be safely used until it was repaired.

This case illustrates the importance of performing a low-pressure system leak test on each anesthetic machine at the beginning of the day.

REVIEW QUESTIONS

1. The governmental agency that may issue citations for a failure to keep exposure to waste anesthetic gases under a recommended maximum allowable level is:
   a. FDA
   b. EPA
   c. NIOSH
   d. OSHA

2. Short-term problems associated with waste anesthetic gas exposure include all but one of the following. Which one is not considered to be a short-term effect?
   a. Miscarriage
   b. Fatigue or drowsiness
   c. Nausea
   d. Headache

3. Long-term toxicity of inhalation anesthetics is thought to be caused by
   a. Inhalation of the gas.
   b. Inherent sensitivity of the exposed individual.
   c. The release of toxic metabolites.
   d. Chronic use of a high vaporizer dial setting.

4. The volatile inhalant general anesthetic thought to be least toxic, because very little is retained and metabolized, is:
   a. Isoflurane
   b. Halothane
   c. Methoxyflurane
   d. Nitrous oxide

5. In the United States, the National Institute for Occupational Safety and Health (NIOSH) recommends that the levels of waste anesthetic gases for anesthetics such as isoflurane and sevoflurane should not exceed ___ ppm.
   a. 0.2
   b. 2
   c. 20
   d. 200

6. As long as you cannot smell any waste anesthetic gas, you can be reasonably sure that the levels are below recommended exposure limits.
   True
   False

7. When using oxygen as the only carrier gas and isoflurane anesthetic, which of the following machine leak tests must be performed regularly to detect leaks of WAGs?
   a. Low-pressure leak test
   b. High-pressure leak test
   c. Both the low-pressure and a high-pressure leak test
   d. Neither leak test need be performed

8. Rooms in which animals are recovering from anesthesia may be highly contaminated with waste gas.
   True
   False

9. Which of the following can be used effectively to monitor waste anesthetic gas levels?
   a. Odor of waste gas
   b. Radiation monitor
   c. Regular preventive maintenance by qualified personnel
   d. Passive dosimeter badge

10. Long-term exposure to more than 50 ppm of waste isoflurane, sevoflurane, or desflurane is known to be harmful.
    True
    False

11. How often should a test for low-pressure leaks be conducted?
    a. Each day that the machine is used
    b. At least once per week
    c. At least once per month
    d. When the anesthetist smells anesthetic gases

12. Activated charcoal canisters
    a. Are designed to scavenge isoflurane, sevoflurane, and nitrous oxide
    b. May be less efficient at high carrier gas flow rates
    c. Can remove waste anesthetic gases for at least 1 month
    d. Are more efficient than an active scavenger

13. The ventilation system in a room in which waste anesthetic gases are present should be capable of providing a minimum of _____ air changes per hour.
    a. 5
    b. 10
    c. 15
    d. 30

14. Which of the following drugs is not classified as an ultrapotent opioid?
    a. Carfentanil
    b. Etorphine
    c. Thiafentanil
    d. Fentanyl

15. OSHA expects anesthetic machines including breathing circuits to be serviced by a qualified technician every:
    a. 3 to 4 months
    b. 4 to 12 months
    c. 1 to 2 years
    d. 5 to 10 years

16. The safest way to transport a large compressed-gas cylinder, such as an oxygen tank, is by:
    a. Carrying it
    b. Rolling it along the floor
    c. Using a handcart
    d. Dragging it by the neck

For the following questions, more than one answer may be correct.

17. The interface of a scavenging system is designed to:
    a. Prevent excessive vacuum in the breathing circuit.
    b. Hold the waste gas until it is removed by the evacuation system.
    c. Prevent the excessive pressure in the breathing circuit.
    d. Accept waste gas from the transfer tubing.

18. Unless a scavenging system is used, waste anesthetic gases may originate from:
    a. The APL valve
    b. A main stream capnograph
    c. The negative pressure relief valve
    d. A cryosurgery unit

19. A technician may reduce the amount of waste gases by:
    a. Using cuffed endotracheal tubes.
    b. Ensuring that the anesthetic machine has been tested for leaks.
    c. Using an injectable agent rather than a mask or chamber.
    d. Using high fresh gas flows.

20. To conduct a low-pressure test on an anesthetic machine (with a rebreathing circuit), you must:
    a. Close the APL valve and occlude the patient end of the breathing circuit.
    b. Pressurize the circuit with a volume of gas.
    c. Turn off the oxygen tank.
    d. Compress the reservoir bag.

SELECTED READINGS

American Association of Nurse Anesthetists (AANA): *Management of waste anesthetic gases.* https://www.aana.com/docs/default-source/practice-aana-com-web-documents-(all)/professional-practice-manual/management-of-waste-anesthetic-gas.pdf?sfvrsn=600049b1_4. Accessed August, 2020.

American College of Veterinary Anesthesia and Analgesia: *Commentary and recommendations on control of waste anesthetic gases in the workplace*, Revised November 18, 2013. www.acvaa.org. Accessed August, 2021.

Aragonés JMM, Ayora AA, Ribalta AB, et al: Occupational exposure to volatile anaesthetics: a systematic review, *Occup Med (Lond)* 66(3):202–207, 2016. doi:10.1093/occmed/kqv193.

Boivin JF: Risk of spontaneous abortion in women occupationally exposed to anaesthetic gases: a meta-analysis, *J Environ Med* 54:541–548, 1997.

Burkhart JE, Stobbe TJ: Real-time measurement and control of waste anesthetic gases during veterinary surgeries, *Am Ind Hyg Assoc J* 51(12):640–645, 1990.

Byhahn C, Wilke HJ, Westpphal K: Occupational exposure to volatile anaesthetics: epidemiology and approaches to reducing the problem, *CNS Drug* 15(3):197–215, 2001.

California Department of Public Health: *Workplace hazard update.* 2019. https://www.cdph.ca.gov/Programs/CCDPHP/DEODC/OHB/HESIS/CDPH%20Document%20Library/IsofluraneGas.pdf. Accessed August, 2021.

Canadian Centre for Occupational Health and Safety. *OSH answer fact sheet: waste anesthetic gases, hazards of.* Updated June 1, 2017. https://www.ccohs.ca/oshanswers/chemicals/waste_anesthetic.html#Air. Accessed August, 2021.

Coleman D: *Anesthesia machines: finding leaks*, 2016, Clinician's Brief. https://www.cliniciansbrief.com/article/anesthesia-machines-finding-leaks. Accessed August, 2021.

da Costa MG, Kalmar AF, Struys MRF: Inhaled anesthetics: environmental role, occupational risk, and clinical use, *J Clin Med* 10(6):1306, 2021.

Hoerauf K, Lierz M, Wiesner G, et al. Genetic damage in operating room personnel exposed to isoflurane and nitrous oxide, *Occup Environ Med* 56(7):433–437, 1999.

Korczynski RE: Anesthetic gas exposure in veterinary clinics, *Appl Occup Environ Hyg* 14:384–390, 1999.

McKelvey D: *Safety handbook for veterinary hospital staff*, Lakewood, CO, 1999, American Animal Hospital Association Press.

Meyer RE: Anesthesia hazards to animal workers. In Lanley RL, editor: *Occupational medicine state of the art reviews*, Philadelphia, PA, 1999, Hanley and Belfus.

National Institutes of Health (NIH), Division of Occupational Health and Safety (DOHS), Office of Research Services Waste Anesthetic Gas: *Waste anesthetic gas*, 2023. https://ors.od.nih.gov/sr/dohs/Documents/WAG-Program.pdf. Accessed May 9, 2023.

National Institute for Occupational Safety and Health (NIOSH): *Waste anesthetic gases: occupational hazards and hospitals*, September 2007. https://www.cdc.gov/niosh/docs/2007-151/pdfs/2007-151.pdf?id=10.26616/NIOSHPUB2007151. Accessed May 9, 2023.

Occupational Safety and Health Administration (OSHA): *Anesthetic gases: guidelines for workplace exposures*, May 18, 2000. Revised May 18, 2000. https://www.osha.gov/waste-anesthetic-gases/workplace-exposures-guidelines. Accessed May 9, 2023.

Petrini KR, Keyler DE, Lind L, et al: Immobilization agents—developing an urgent response protocol for human exposure, *Proc Am Assoc Zoo Vet* 15:146–155, 1993.

Schenker MB, Samuels SJ, Green RS, et al: Adverse reproductive outcomes among female veterinarians, *Epidemiol* 132:96–106, 1990.

Seibert PJ Jr: *Safety issues for the veterinary hospital staff*, ed 6, Calhoun, TN, 2014, SafetyVet. www.safetyvet.com.

Shirangi A, Fritschi L, Holman CD: Maternal occupational exposures and risk of spontaneous abortion in veterinary practice, *Occup Environ Med* 65(11):719–725, 2008.

Shuhaiber S, Einarson A, Radde IC, et al: A prospective-controlled study of pregnant veterinary staff exposed to inhaled anesthetics and x-rays, *Int J Occup Med Environ Health* 15(4):363–373, 2002.

Anesthetic Monitoring

LEARNING OBJECTIVES

When you have completed this chapter, you will be able to:
- Explain the principles of anesthetic monitoring, including the reasons for and goals of monitoring.
- List the physical monitoring parameters and classify each in one of the following categories: (1) vital signs, (2) reflexes, (3) other indicators of anesthetic depth.
- List and describe each of the stages and planes of anesthesia.
- List the monitoring parameters used primarily to determine whether or not the patient is safe and group them according to whether they primarily assess circulation, oxygenation, or ventilation.
- Explain and demonstrate assessment of each of the vital signs, reflexes, and other indicators of anesthetic depth.
- List normal values for each physical monitoring parameter and identify values that should be reported to the attending veterinarian.
- Explain setup, operation, care, maintenance, and trouble-shooting of an esophageal stethoscope, electrocardiograph, Doppler monitor, oscillometric blood pressure monitor, pulse oximeter, and capnograph.
- Describe the information derived from anesthetic gas monitoring, oxygen monitoring, and anesthetic depth monitoring.

- Interpret output and data from an esophageal stethoscope, electrocardiograph, Doppler monitor, oscillometric blood pressure monitor, pulse oximeter, and capnograph.
- Describe how to determine the blood pressure using a Doppler monitor, oscillometric blood pressure monitor, or arterial catheter and transducer.
- Identify the following rhythms on an electrocardiograph tracing: normal sinus rhythm (NSR); sinus arrhythmia (SA); sinus bradycardia and tachycardia; first-, second-, and third-degree atrioventricular (AV) heart block; supraventricular premature complexes (SPCs) and ventricular premature complexes (VPCs); supraventricular tachycardia (SVT) and ventricular tachycardia (VT); atrial and ventricular fibrillation; and QRS and T-wave configuration changes.
- Identify machine-generated data that should be reported to the VIC.
- Identify abnormal monitoring parameters and list common causes of abnormal monitoring parameters.
- Use monitoring parameters to determine anesthetic depth.
- Explain adverse consequences of hypothermia and identify strategies to prevent hypothermia.

KEY TERMS

Anesthetic gas analyzer	Doppler blood flow detector	Partial pressure of oxygen
Atelectasis	Esophageal stethoscope	Percent oxygen saturation
Blood gas analysis	External active rewarming	Pressure transducer
Blood pressure	External passive warming	Pulmonary thromboembolism
Calculated oxygen content	Flaccid	Pulse oximeter
Capnogram	Icterus	Respiration
Capnograph	Mean arterial pressure	Respirometer
Cardiac arrhythmias	Monitor	Sphygmomanometer
Central venous pressure	Multiparameter monitor	Systolic blood pressure
Circulation	Oscillometer	Tachypnea
Core rewarming	Oxygen analyzer	Ventilation
Diastolic blood pressure	Oxygenation	

INTRODUCTION TO MONITORING

The word monitor comes from the Latin word *monere,* which means "to warn." It is a fitting definition for this aspect of anesthesia because the main purpose of monitoring is to warn the anesthetist of changes in anesthetic depth and patient condition in enough time to permit intervention before they become dangerous.

Throughout any anesthetic event, a delicate balance must be maintained. There must be sufficient central nervous system (CNS) depression, analgesia, muscle relaxation, and immobility for the procedure to be performed, yet cardiopulmonary function must not be dangerously compromised. Monitoring is therefore necessary for two reasons. First, it is necessary to keep the patient safe and second, it is necessary to regulate anesthetic depth. To keep the patient safe, the anesthetist must monitor the patient at many points in time to ensure that vital signs remain within acceptable limits. Failure to monitor and maintain vital signs within acceptable limits may lead to devastating consequences such as permanent brain damage or even death. The anesthetist also must maintain the animal at an appropriate anesthetic depth (i.e., one that is neither too light nor too deep) by monitoring reflexes and other indicators. Failure to maintain an adequate depth of anesthesia may result in perception of pain and premature arousal from anesthesia. On the other hand, maintaining an animal at an excessive depth of anesthesia may lead to anesthetic overdose or slow recovery.

> **TECHNICIAN NOTE** Monitoring is necessary for two reasons. First, it is necessary to keep the patient safe, and second, it is necessary to regulate anesthetic depth.

When monitoring, the anesthetist must observe various parameters that can be separated into three classifications: (1) vital signs, (2) reflexes, and (3) other indicators of anesthetic depth. Although information from all these monitoring parameters is used to determine the depth of anesthesia and patient well-being, some are more helpful in determining anesthetic depth and others are more helpful in determining whether the patient is safe.

The term *vital signs* refers to those variables that indicate the response of the animal's homeostatic mechanisms to anesthesia, including heart rate (HR), heart rhythm, respiratory rate (RR) and depth, mucous membrane color, capillary refill time (CRT), pulse strength, blood pressure (BP), and temperature. The patient's vital signs indicate how well the patient is maintaining basic circulatory and respiratory function during anesthesia and therefore are the best indicators of patient well-being. Although vital signs also generally reflect the anesthetic stage and plane, they are not reliable indicators of anesthetic depth.

The term *reflex* refers to an involuntary response to a stimulus (such as an eye blink in response to touching the skin at the corner of the eye or a kick in response to a tap on the patellar tendon). Reflexes used in veterinary anesthesia include the palpebral, corneal, pedal, swallowing, and laryngeal reflexes as well as the pupillary light reflex (PLR). *Other indicators of anesthetic depth* include spontaneous movement, eye position, pupil size, muscle tone, nystagmus, salivary and lacrimal secretions, and response to surgical stimulation. Both reflexes and other indicators are useful for determining anesthetic depth but are not useful for assessing cardiopulmonary function or homeostasis.

The 2020 AAHA Anesthesia and Monitoring Guidelines for Dogs and Cats recommend the use of hands-on assessment as well as a multiparameter monitor to track cardiovascular function, respiratory function, body temperature, and anesthetic depth for all anesthetized patients. Specific parameters that should be monitored include those listed in Box 6.1.

The 2009 Recommendations for Monitoring Anesthetized Patients published by the American College of Veterinary Anesthesia and Analgesia (ACVAA) offer somewhat more detailed guidelines for monitoring small animals that address each of the following topics:

- Assessment of circulation, oxygenation, ventilation, and body temperature
- Monitoring of patients under, and recovering from, neuromuscular blockade
- Record-keeping
- Monitoring during the recovery period

BOX 6.1   Recommended Monitoring for General Anesthesia

- Heart rate and rhythm (by electrocardiography)
- Capillary refill time and mucous membrane color
- Blood pressure (by Doppler or oscillometer monitor)
- Respiratory rate
- Ventilation (ETCO$_2$) (by capnography)
- Oxygen saturation of hemoglobin (SpO$_2$) (by pulse oximetry)
- Body temperature
- Anesthetic depth (by monitoring physical parameters)

(Adapted from the 2020 AAHA Anesthesia and Monitoring Guidelines for Dogs and Cats)

TECHNICIAN NOTE Anesthetic monitoring is based on the principle that in the average patient, each monitoring parameter is expected to show a predictable response at any given anesthetic depth.

- Recommendations regarding personnel
- Monitoring sedated patients

The focus of these recommendations is an assessment of vital signs and therefore primarily address the problem of keeping the patient safe.

AAHA and ACVAA monitoring guidelines recommend using mechanical means to monitor heart rate and rhythm, oxygen saturation, carbon dioxide levels, arterial blood pressure, and core body temperature. In practice, this means that each patient should ideally have ECG electrodes, a pulse oximeter probe, a capnograph sensor, a Doppler probe and cuff or oscillometric cuff, and a temperature probe, as shown in Fig. 6.1. For monitoring to be effective, the patient must be evaluated frequently during any anesthetic procedure. Although continuous monitoring of any anesthetized patient by a veterinary technician is ideal, it is not practical in many veterinary clinics. Therefore in lieu of continuous monitoring of all patients, the ACVAA recommends that class P1 and P2 patients should be monitored at least once every 5 minutes. In contrast, class P3, P4, and P5 patients, as well as horses receiving inhalant anesthetics or those that have been anesthetized for more than 45 minutes, should be monitored continuously.

Anesthetic monitoring is based on the principle that in the average patient, each monitoring parameter is expected to show a predictable response at any given anesthetic depth. For instance, swallowing and pedal reflexes are expected to be present when the patient's anesthesia level is too light but are absent during surgical anesthesia. Muscle tone, HR, and RR are expected to be high during light anesthesia and to decrease gradually as anesthetic depth increases. The eyes are in a central position during light anesthesia, generally rotate into a ventromedial position during surgical anesthesia, and return to a central position as anesthetic depth increases.

Interpretation of these indicators is quite challenging in practice, however, because a number of factors, including drugs, disease, and individual variation, may alter expected responses, producing contradictory evidence. In other words, a patient may show some signs that indicate one stage of anesthesia and other signs that indicate another. For instance, a dog that received an opioid agonist may have a smaller than expected pupil size while in surgical anesthesia. A patient with preexisting heart failure may have a higher HR than expected at a given depth. A patient given an alpha$_2$-agonist such as dexmedetomidine may have significant hypotension and bradycardia, whereas another given atropine may have tachycardia, even though both are in the same plane. Therefore is it important to observe multiple parameters and make decisions based on the predominant evidence. This requires careful observation, rapid decision making, and safe and appropriate action.

Stages and Planes of Anesthesia

During World War I, Arthur Guedel, MD, a U.S. Army doctor, developed a classification system of stages and planes of general anesthesia based on observation of patient responses to the

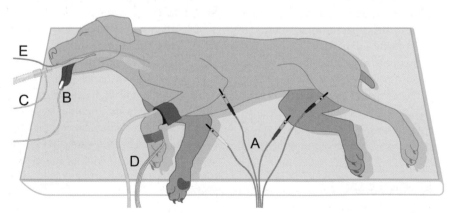

FIG. 6.1 Illustration showing the monitoring probes and devices recommended by both the AAHA Anesthesia and Monitoring Guidelines and the American College of Veterinary Anesthesia and Analgesia (ACVAA) 2009 Recommendations for Monitoring Anesthetized Patients. **(A)** ECG electrodes to monitor heart rate and rhythm; **(B)** pulse oximeter probe to measure oxygen saturation; **(C)** capnograph sensor to monitor carbon dioxide levels; **(D)** Doppler probe and cuff (or oscillometer cuff) to measure arterial blood pressure; **(E)** temperature probe for continuous monitoring of body temperature.

inhalant anesthetic diethyl ether. Under this system, general anesthesia was divided into four stages (I to IV) and stage III was subdivided into four planes (1 to 4) based on eye movement, pupil size, and later, eyelid movement. Development of this system gave anesthetists a basis to accurately assess the depth of anesthesia using detailed observation. Although responses to modern general anesthetics differ somewhat from responses to ether, this system is still used today in an altered form.

Overview of Anesthetic Stages and Planes

As an agent is given to induce general anesthesia, the patient passes through stage I and, as it loses consciousness, it enters stage II. The loss of consciousness marks the border between these stages. As the anesthetic depth increases, the patient then enters stage III, the period of surgical anesthesia. The loss of spontaneous muscle movement marks the border between stages II and III. If the depth continues to increase, the patient will enter stage IV. The loss of all reflexes, widely dilated and unresponsive pupils, flaccid muscle tone, and cardiopulmonary collapse mark this stage which, if not aggressively managed, is closely followed by cardiopulmonary arrest and death of the patient. As the animal passes through each stage, there is a progressive decrease in pain perception, motor coordination, consciousness, reflex responses, muscle tone, and eventually cardiopulmonary function (Fig. 6.2). Expected responses of selected monitoring parameters during each stage and plane are summarized in Table 6.1.

> **TECHNICIAN NOTE**
> - Loss of consciousness marks the border between stages I and II
> - Loss of spontaneous muscle movement marks the border between stages II and III
> - Loss of all reflexes, widely dilated pupils, flaccid muscle tone, and cardiopulmonary collapse mark stage IV

Stage I—Period of Voluntary Movement

During stage I, the patient begins to lose consciousness. This stage is usually characterized by fear, disorientation, and struggling. The HR and RR increase, and the patient may pant, urinate, or defecate. A patient in stage I is typically difficult to handle. Near the end of stage I, the patient loses the ability to stand and becomes recumbent.

Stage II—Period of Involuntary Movement

During stage II, also known as the *excitement stage*, the patient loses voluntary control and breathing becomes irregular. This stage is usually characterized by involuntary reactions in the form of vocalizing, struggling, chewing, or paddling. The HR and RR are often elevated, pupils are dilated, muscle tone is marked, and reflexes are present and in fact, may appear exaggerated. Although animals in stage II may appear to be "fighting" the anesthesia, the actions are not under conscious control. Rather, they are thought to occur because the anesthetic selectively depresses neurons in the brain and spinal cord that normally inhibit and control the function of motor neurons. Stage II ends when the animal shows signs of muscle relaxation, slower RR, and decreased reflex activity.

This stage is unpleasant and potentially hazardous for both the animal and hospital personnel. There is a risk of epinephrine release and the possibility of cardiac arrhythmias or arrest. The struggling patient may injure itself, the restrainer, or the anesthetist. Therefore it is desirable to plan the procedure such that the patient passes through this stage as quickly as possible by administration of additional anesthetic until stage III is reached.

Premedicated animals in which anesthesia is rapidly induced with an injectable anesthetic often appear to pass from consciousness directly to stage III. Although these patients pass through stages I and II, they are not clinically evident. In contrast, stages I and II are often very pronounced in animals in which anesthesia is mask or chamber induced without premedication (a practice that is potentially dangerous and recommended only as a last resort), sometimes creating a challenging and unpleasant situation for the anesthetist and patient.

Stage III—Period of Surgical Anesthesia

During stage III, the patient is unconscious and progresses gradually from light to deep anesthesia. This stage is characterized by progressive muscle relaxation, decreasing HR and RR, and loss of reflexes. The pupils gradually dilate, tear production decreases, and the PLR is lost. The increase in HR, BP, and RR seen in response to surgical stimulation during light anesthesia is also gradually lost.

Although Dr. Guedel originally divided stage III into four planes numbered 1 through 4, many anesthetists now use a system that divides stage III into three planes most often referred to as light, moderate, and deep surgical anesthesia or, stated more simply, light, moderate, and deep anesthesia. There is no universal agreement as to the precise meaning of these terms, however, so in this text, the terms "light stage III anesthesia," "surgical anesthesia," and "deep stage III anesthesia" will be used to denote inadequate depth, optimum depth, and excessive depth, respectively.

When a patient transitions from stage II to light stage III anesthesia, the respiratory pattern becomes regular and involuntary limb movements cease. The respiratory rate may be normal, increased, or decreased, depending on the circumstances. The eyeballs may start out in a central position but will gradually start to rotate ventromedially. The pupils often become somewhat constricted and the pupillary response to bright light is diminished. The gagging, laryngeal, and swallowing reflexes are depressed such that an endotracheal tube may be successfully passed, allowing the patient to be connected to a gas anesthetic machine. Other reflexes (such as the pedal and palpebral reflexes) are present; however, responses are less brisk than in stage II. Although unconscious, the patient will not tolerate surgical procedures at this light plane of anesthesia, and will move and exhibit increased HR, RR and respiratory depth, and BP in response to painful stimuli. This plane is inadequate for surgery although this is somewhat dependent on the nature of the procedure. For instance, it may be adequate for some minor procedures such as a skin biopsy but is not typically adequate for a major surgery such as a fracture repair.

Surgical anesthesia is the optimum depth for surgical and other invasive procedures. The respirations are usually regular but may be somewhat shallow, and the RR, HR, pulse strength, and BP are often mildly decreased. Surgical stimulation may evoke a mildly increased HR or RR, but the patient remains unconscious and immobile. Pupil size is moderate, the PLR is sluggish, lacrimation is decreased, and ventromedial eye rotation also

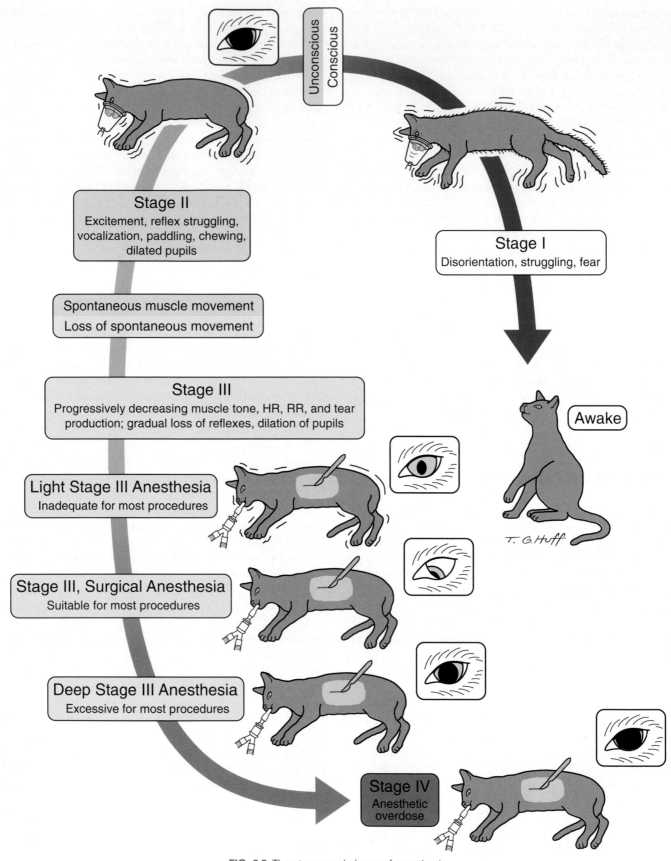

FIG. 6.2 The stages and planes of anesthesia.

TABLE 6.1 Expected Responses of Selected Monitoring Parameters

Stage of Anesthesia	Behavior	Respiration	Cardiovascular Function
I	Disorientation, struggling, fear	Respiratory rate increased; dogs may pant	Heart rate increased
II Excitement stage	Excitement: reflex struggling, vocalization, paddling, chewing	Irregular; may hold breath or hyperventilate	Heart rate often increased
III/Light stage III anesthesia	Unconscious; possible movement in response to surgical stimulation	Regular; rate high, normal, or low	Heart rate often high normal; pulse strong
III/Surgical anesthesia	Unconscious; immobile	Regular and shallow; rate often normal or mildly decreased	Heart rate often normal or mildly decreased, capillary refill time (CRT) normal; pulse strength decreased
III/Deep stage III anesthesia	Unconscious; immobile	Shallow; rate often below normal; may see abdominal breathing	Heart rate low normal to well below normal; pale mucous membranes; CRT normal or prolonged; pulse strength significantly decreased
IV	Unconscious; immobile	Apnea	Cardiovascular collapse

generally occurs at this time. The skeletal muscle tone is more relaxed, pedal and swallowing reflexes are absent, and laryngeal and palpebral reflexes are diminished or lost. So loss of the pedal and swallowing reflexes marks entry into this plane.

In deep stage III anesthesia, significant depression of circulation and respiration is often present and for this reason, this plane is considered to be excessively deep. In the dog or cat, the HR and RR are low and the tidal volume (V_T) is significantly decreased. HR, RR, V_T, and BP are nonresponsive to surgical stimulation. As depth continues to increase, abdominal breathing may be observed, which occurs as the intercostal muscles progressively become less active and the diaphragm is increasingly responsible for ventilation. Abdominal breathing is recognized by a "rocking" motion in which the abdomen expands and contracts in an attempt to move air into and out of the lungs. Manual or mechanical ventilation may be necessary in some small-animal patients and most large-animal patients. Pulse strength is often significantly reduced because of a fall in BP. The mucous membrane color is increasingly pale and CRT may be prolonged. The PLR is poor throughout this plane and may be absent. The eyeballs are central, the pupils are moderately to widely dilated, and the corneas gradually become dry because of an absence of lacrimal secretions. Reflex activity is totally absent. Skeletal muscle tone may be so relaxed that no resistance occurs when the mouth is opened (i.e., jaw tone is flaccid or slack).

> **TECHNICIAN NOTE** Stage III is most often divided into three planes:
> - Light stage III anesthesia (inadequate depth)
> - Surgical anesthesia (optimal depth)
> - Deep stage III anesthesia (excessive depth)

Stage IV—Period of Anesthetic Overdose

If anesthetic depth continues to increase, the animal enters stage IV anesthesia. At this stage, there is cessation of respiration and the cardiovascular system is markedly depressed, with a dramatic drop in HR and BP, accompanied by pale mucous membranes and a prolonged CRT. If not recognized and managed, circulatory collapse and death will quickly follow. Immediate resuscitation is necessary to save the patient's life.

ASSESSMENT OF ANESTHETIC DEPTH

Reflexes and Other Indicators of Anesthetic Depth

At all times during an anesthetic procedure, the anesthetist must accurately assess the patient's anesthetic depth. Like many things, this is more complex than it first seems and requires detailed observation and interpretation of subtle changes in physical signs. In practice, the subtleties of anesthetic monitoring are all too often neglected for a variety of reasons, including a lack of adequate skill, a sense of complacency born of past experience with many successful anesthetic procedures (and a subsequent attitude that can be summarized by the statement "it's not a big deal—my patients never have any problems"), or more job demands than the technician can reasonably handle. When not given due attention, monitoring is turned into a crude and alarmingly simplified system consisting of the following three stages of anesthesia: "awake," "asleep," and "dead."

Obviously, the anesthetist needs considerably more detail than that. The goal of monitoring is to ensure throughout the entire procedure that the patient is at a depth that provides immobility, unconsciousness, and lack of awareness of pain while avoiding conditions that endanger the patient such as hypoventilation, hypoxemia, hypotension, and hypothermia. Achieving this balance is not always easy and requires a timely and effective response to changes in monitoring parameters. Although vital signs provide some help, reflexes, muscle tone, pupil size, eye position, and response to surgical stimulation are the best indicators of anesthetic depth (Table 6.2).

> **TECHNICIAN NOTE** In practice, the subtleties of anesthetic monitoring are all too often neglected for a variety of reasons. When not given due attention, monitoring is turned into a crude and alarmingly simplified system consisting of the following three stages of anesthesia: "awake," "asleep," and "dead."

Reflexes

A reflex is an unconscious response to a stimulus. All healthy, conscious animals demonstrate predictable reflex responses. One example is the cough reflex, which is a response to the presence of foreign material in the airways. Reflex responses help protect the animal from injury (in the case of the cough reflex by clearing

TABLE 6.2 Indicators of Anesthetic Depth

| | INDICATORS OF ANESTHETIC DEPTH | | |
Parameter	Light Stage III	Surgical	Deep Stage III
Swallowing	Maybe	No	No
Vaporizer setting	Low (approximately 1 × MAC)	Medium (approximately 1.5 × MAC)	High (approximately 2 × MAC)
Palpebral reflex	Present	Decreased or absent	Absent
Pedal reflex	Present	Absent	Absent
Corneal reflex[a]	Present	Present	Absent
Pupillary light reflex	Present	May be present	Absent
Spontaneous movement	Maybe	No	No
Muscle tone[b]	Marked	Moderate	Flaccid
Eyeball position	Usually central	Usually ventromedial	Central
Pupil size[b]	Midrange to constricted	Usually midrange	Dilated
Heart rate	Often high or high normal	Often moderate	Often decreased
Respiratory rate	Often high or high normal	Often moderate	Often decreased
Nystagmus (horses)	Fast	Slow	Absent
Salivation, lacrimation	Normal	Decreased	Absent
Response to surgical stimulation	Marked	Moderate	None

[a]The corneal reflex is not reliable in small animals.
[b]Strongly influenced by anesthetic protocol and signalment.
MAC, Minimum alveolar concentration.
Modified from Haskins SC: General guidelines for judging anesthetic depth, *Vet Clin North Am Small Anim Pract* 22:432–434, 1992.

upper airway obstructions and preventing aspiration of harmful material). These protective reflexes gradually decrease in response to an increasing depth of anesthesia such that by deep stage III anesthesia, few to no reflex responses remain. The reflexes most commonly monitored in veterinary anesthesia include the swallowing, laryngeal, pedal, palpebral, and corneal reflexes as well as the PLR. When describing the status of these reflexes verbally to other surgical team members or in written records, the terms "present," "decreased" or "depressed," and "absent" are often used.

> **TECHNICIAN NOTE** When describing the status of reflexes verbally to other surgical team members or in written records, the terms "present," "decreased" or "depressed," and "absent" are often used.

Swallowing reflex. The swallowing reflex is a response to the presence of saliva or food in the pharynx. This reflex is monitored by watching for swallowing motions in the ventral neck region. The swallowing reflex is present in light stage III anesthesia, is lost in surgical anesthesia, and returns during recovery just before the patient regains consciousness. The return of the swallowing reflex during recovery is the main indicator used to determine when it is safe to remove the endotracheal tube. Animals that vomit after this point usually will swallow rather than aspirate the vomited material, and the endotracheal tube is therefore no longer needed to protect the airway. In fact, if the endotracheal tube is not removed at this point, the patient will begin to chew on it.

> **TECHNICIAN NOTE** The return of the swallowing reflex during recovery is the main indicator used to determine when it is safe to remove the endotracheal tube.

Laryngeal Reflex. The laryngeal reflex is an immediate closure of the epiglottis and vocal cords when the larynx is touched by any object. This reflex protects the animal from tracheal aspiration. The laryngeal reflex may be observed during intubation, is present if the animal is in a lighter plane of anesthesia, and can make it difficult to pass the endotracheal tube. It is strong in cats, pigs, and small ruminants. A sustained or exaggerated laryngeal reflex, referred to as *laryngospasm*, is most commonly seen in these species and is a complication of endotracheal intubation.

> **TECHNICIAN NOTE** The palpebral reflex should be absent during surgical anesthesia in small animals maintained with isoflurane or sevoflurane. In most horses, a very slight response indicates a surgical plane of anesthesia. Ruminants tend to have a slightly stronger reflex than horses, although spontaneous blinking is almost always associated with a plane of anesthesia that is too light.

Palpebral reflex. The palpebral reflex (blink reflex) is a blink in response to a light tap on the medial or lateral canthus of the eye (Fig. 6.3). In the conscious animal, this reflex helps protect the eye from injury. When eliciting this reflex, it is important to use a light touch because vigorous tapping may artificially cause the eyelid to move, giving the anesthetist a false-positive response. Some anesthetists prefer to test this reflex by lightly stroking the hairs of the upper eyelid. As with most reflexes, the palpebral reflex is gradually lost as anesthetic depth increases. Most animals retain the palpebral reflex in light stage III anesthesia and lose it during surgical anesthesia, although the exact point at which it is lost varies among individuals, species, and agents. In small animals maintained with isoflurane or sevoflurane, this reflex should be absent during surgical and deep levels

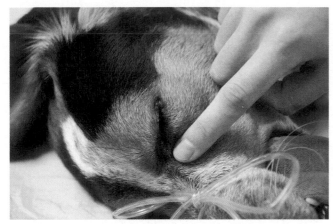

FIG. 6.3 Assessing the palpebral reflex by lightly tapping the medial or lateral canthus.

of anesthesia. Therefore when gas anesthetics are used in small-animal patients, the presence of this reflex indicates that the anesthetic depth is inadequate, although the absence of the reflex cannot be used to determine whether the anesthetic depth is excessive. In most horses, a very slight palpebral response (very slow closure of the eyelid) indicates a surgical plane of anesthesia. Ruminants tend to have a slightly stronger eyelid reflex than horses, although spontaneous blinking is almost always associated with a plane of anesthesia that is too light. During recovery, return of the reflex usually indicates impending arousal.

> **TECHNICIAN NOTE** The pedal reflex is present during light stage III anesthesia and is lost during surgical anesthesia. It is particularly important in animals undergoing mask induction, in which the presence of a mask makes assessment of other reflexes or jaw tone somewhat difficult.

Pedal reflex. The pedal reflex is flexion or withdrawal of the limb in response to vigorous squeezing and twisting or pinching of a digit or pad (Fig. 6.4). This reflex is useful only in small-animal patients. The pedal reflex varies depending on the anesthetic depth from a very subtle contraction of muscles to a full withdrawal of the limb. Because false-negative responses are

common, accurate assessment of this reflex requires a stimulus of a surprisingly high intensity (a really hard squeeze and twist) although obviously, it must not be so forceful as to injure the patient. This is an important point when learning to elicit this reflex because many novices are often surprised at how much force is required to obtain an accurate response.

This reflex is present during light stage III anesthesia, is lost during surgical anesthesia, and is particularly important in animals undergoing mask induction, in which the presence of a mask makes assessment of other reflexes or jaw tone somewhat difficult. Once the patient reaches surgical anesthesia, this reflex is not useful in detecting the onset of excessive anesthetic depth because the reflex is absent in both surgical and deep stage III anesthesia.

> **TECHNICIAN NOTE** The corneal reflex should be present in light and surgical planes of anesthesia and is lost when the anesthetic depth is excessive, but it is unreliable in small animals. It is therefore used primarily to tell the anesthetist when a large-animal patient is anesthetized too deeply.

Corneal reflex. The corneal reflex involves retraction of the eyeball within the orbit and/or a blink in response to stimulation of the cornea. It is tested by touching the cornea with a sterile object (a drop of saline or artificial tear solution is commonly used). As an alternative, the cornea can be stimulated with indirect digital pressure through the upper eyelid (Fig. 6.5). This

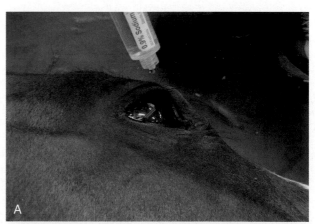

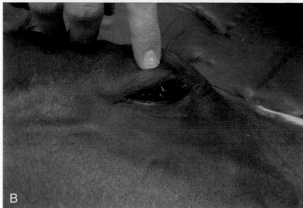

FIG. 6.5 **(A)** Assessing the corneal reflex in the horse with a drop of sterile saline. **(B)** Assessing the corneal reflex by applying digital pressure through the upper eyelid.

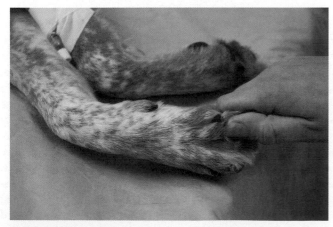

FIG. 6.4 Assessing the pedal reflex by vigorously squeezing and twisting or pinching a digit or pad.

reflex is most useful in large animals but is very difficult to elicit in small animals except when the patient is under very light anesthesia. Retraction of the eye is often subtle and best seen by positioning oneself so that the line of sight is near the same horizontal plane as the cornea.

This reflex should be present in light stage III and surgical planes of anesthesia and is lost when the anesthetic depth is excessive, but this is unreliable in small animals. It is therefore used primarily to tell the anesthetist when a large animal patient is too deeply anesthetized and should be reserved for this purpose only so that damage to the cornea is avoided.

Pupillary light reflex. The PLR is a constriction of the pupils in response to shining a bright light onto one of the retinas. It is elicited by following the steps described in Chapter 2. This reflex gradually diminishes with increasing anesthetic depth and should be present in light stage III and surgical anesthesia, but is lost during deep stage III anesthesia.

Dazzle reflex. The dazzle reflex is a blink in response to shining a bright light on the retinas. It has the same significance as the PLR but is generally lost very early.

Other Indicators of Anesthetic Depth

Spontaneous movement. Spontaneous movement in an unconscious patient demonstrates a very light plane of anesthesia and often indicates imminent arousal. This may manifest as shivering, alternating flexion and extension of the limbs, muscle twitching, or tremors. However, some drugs, including etomidate, propofol, and opioids, may be associated with focal muscle twitching, even in animals under a surgical plane of anesthesia.

> **TECHNICIAN NOTE** When assessing jaw tone, it is important to avoid opening the patient's mouth too wide because when the mouth is open to the maximum extent, the anesthetist will feel resistance, regardless of the muscle tone, and will thus falsely interpret the muscle tone as being greater than it actually is.

Muscle tone. Assessment of muscle tone gives the anesthetist an indication of the degree of skeletal muscle relaxation. Muscle tone is usually assessed by attempting to open the jaws from a closed position and estimating the amount of passive resistance (referred to as *jaw tone*) (Fig. 6.6). When assessing jaw tone, it is important to avoid opening the patient's mouth too wide because when the mouth is open to the maximum extent, the anesthetist will feel resistance, regardless of the muscle tone, and will thus falsely interpret the muscle tone as being greater than it actually is. If the anesthetist does not have access to the mouth, muscle tone can also be assessed by noting the size of the anal orifice (referred to as *anal tone*).

With increasing depth of anesthesia, the resistance to movement of the jaw will progressively decrease and the anal orifice will progressively increase in size. Tone generally is "marked" in light stage III anesthesia, "moderate" in surgical anesthesia, and "flaccid" in deep stage III anesthesia.

The degree of muscle relaxation observed in the patient depends not only on anesthetic depth but also on the patient's signalment and the agents used. For example, dogs with very

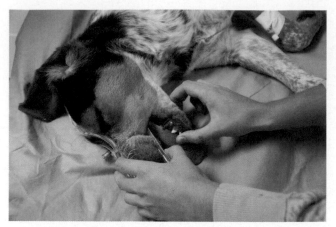

FIG. 6.6 Assessing jaw tone by attempting to open the jaws from a closed position and estimating the amount of passive resistance.

strong muscles of mastication (such as Rottweilers) will have a higher tone than dogs with smaller jaw muscles. This reflex is unreliable in pediatric patients (which normally have little tone regardless of the plane). Tone is generally decreased in patients receiving benzodiazepines, alpha$_2$-agonists, and other muscle relaxants, absent in patients receiving neuromuscular blockers, and increased in patients receiving dissociative anesthetics, such as ketamine.

Jaw tone is not useful in large animal patients because their large masseter muscles (for chewing and grinding plant material) and relatively small mouth openings make it impossible to detect changes in muscle tone.

> **TECHNICIAN NOTE** In small animals and ruminants, the eye is generally central during light stage III anesthesia, ventromedial during surgical anesthesia, and central during deep stage III anesthesia. In horses, the eye can rotate in any direction and sometimes the eyes will rotate in opposite directions. Generally, rotation of one or both eyes indicates adequate anesthetic depth for surgery.

Eye position. Eye position refers to the orientation of the cornea in relation to the palpebral fissure. Eye position changes from central to ventromedial (the patient appears to be looking toward its chin) and back to central with increasing anesthetic depth, although there is considerable variation among individuals in exactly when these changes occur (Fig. 6.7). When the eye is ventromedial, only the sclera and conjunctiva are visible, which precludes assessment of the pupil size and the PLR. In small animals, the eye is generally central during light stage III anesthesia, ventromedial during surgical anesthesia, and central during deep stage III anesthesia. Some anesthetics (e.g., ketamine) do not cause eye rotation, even at moderate anesthetic depth. Eye position in ruminants is often similar to that in dogs, and the eyes rotate ventromedially during surgical anesthesia. In horses, the eye can rotate in any direction, and sometimes the eyes will rotate in opposite directions. Generally, rotation of one or both eyes indicates adequate anesthetic depth for surgery. The eyes of swine are quite sunken and are often unhelpful when trying to determine the depth of anesthesia in pigs.

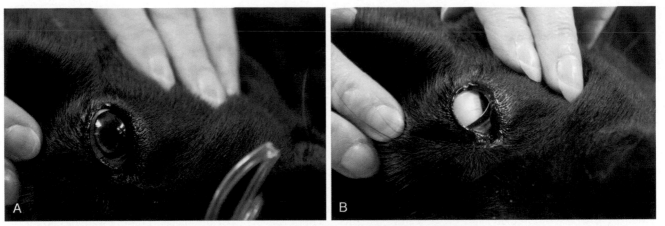

FIG. 6.7 Eye position. **(A)** Central position. **(B)** Ventromedial position.

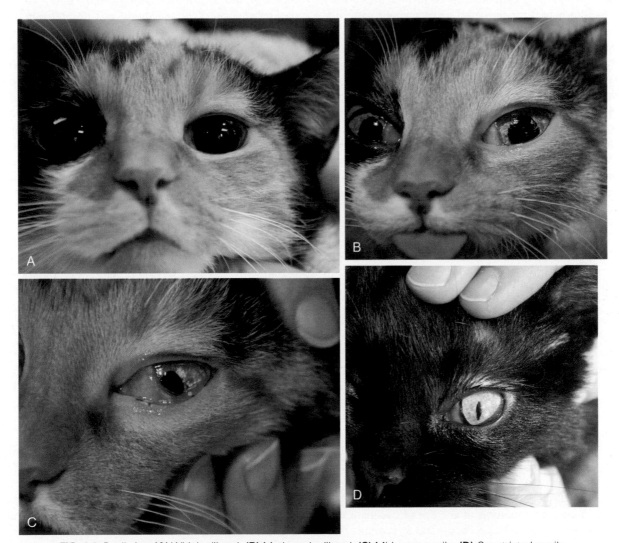

FIG. 6.8 Pupil size. **(A)** Widely dilated. **(B)** Moderately dilated. **(C)** Midrange pupils. **(D)** Constricted pupils.

Pupil size. The size of the pupil also varies with anesthetic depth; pupils are dilated (mydriatic) during stage II anesthesia, normal or constricted (miotic) during light stage III anesthesia, progressively dilate as anesthetic depth increases, and are widely dilated during deep stage III anesthesia (Fig. 6.8). This indicator is influenced by drugs, however, including opioids, cyclohexylamines, and parasympatholytics. Atropine ophthalmic ointment should not be used to lubricate the eyes during an anesthetic event because it causes significant pupil dilation.

> **TECHNICIAN NOTE** Nystagmus is commonly seen in horses during certain planes of anesthesia. Fast nystagmus occurs in very light anesthesia and gradually slows as the anesthetic depth increases. Very slow nystagmus may still be present as a "roving eye" during surgical anesthesia.

Nystagmus. Nystagmus is an oscillation of the eyeballs that is commonly seen in horses during certain planes of anesthesia. Fast nystagmus occurs in very light anesthesia (including recovery) and gradually slows as the anesthetic depth increases (or once anesthesia wears off at the end of the procedure). Very slow nystagmus may still be present as a "roving eye" during surgical anesthesia. In horses in which this occurs, one eye is rotated either rostrally or caudally, and the other eye remains central or rotated in the opposite direction ("divergent eye signs"). After a period of time, the eyes will then very slowly rotate to the alternate position. This eye movement pattern is typically associated with an adequate plane of anesthesia for surgery.

Ruminants and small animals rarely show nystagmus under anesthesia.

Salivary and lacrimal secretions. The presence or absence of salivary and lacrimal secretions may give clues about anesthetic depth, particularly in an animal that has not received anticholinergics. Normal production of tears and saliva diminishes with increasing anesthetic depth and is totally absent in deep stage III anesthesia. A lack of production is recognized as a dry appearance to the cornea, which loses its glistening appearance, and tacky mucous membranes. Because of the relative absence of tears, the use of ophthalmic artificial tear drops or ointment every 2 to 3 hours is advised for all animals undergoing general anesthesia. Note that application of ointment may decrease the ability to test the corneal reflex. In horses, increased lacrimation and salivation indicate light anesthesia.

Heart and respiratory rates. Although not reliable indicators of anesthetic depth, HR and RR can be used to supplement other data. Both values tend to decrease as anesthetic depth increases, and increase as anesthetic depth decreases. Caution should be used in interpreting both HR and RR because each is subject to many influences in addition to anesthetic depth. For example, HR increases in response to a fall in BP. The HR and RR may also increase in response to surgical stimulation or to a painful stimulus.

Some anesthetic drugs and adjuncts (e.g., cyclohexylamines and parasympatholytics) increase HR, whereas many other agents decrease HR. Bradycardia may be induced by endotracheal intubation or manipulation of the eye as occurs during ocular surgery. Hypercarbia (high $Paco_2$) and hypoxemia (low Pao_2) can also increase RR.

> **TECHNICIAN NOTE** An increase in HR, RR, V_T, or BP in response to surgical stimulation does not usually reflect a conscious perception of pain. The anesthetist should not necessarily interpret these signs as an indication that the animal's anesthetic depth is inadequate unless other evidence supports this conclusion.

Response to surgical stimulation. Surgical stimulation (e.g., incising the tissue, manipulating viscera, manipulating bones during fracture repair, or pulling on the suspensory ligament of the ovary) may cause an increase in HR, RR, V_T, or BP. These responses do not usually reflect a conscious perception of pain. The anesthetist should not necessarily interpret these signs as an indication that the animal's anesthetic depth is inadequate unless this conclusion is supported by other evidence. Minor changes in HR during surgery are considered normal and in fact, are absent when anesthetic depth is excessive.

Finding the Optimum Depth

So how does the anesthetist determine when a patient is at an optimum depth of anesthesia? This question has no easy answer because what is "optimum" differs for every patient, depending on the procedure it is undergoing and the interaction of a complex set of factors. The anesthetist may be guided in discovering an optimum depth for each patient, however, by seeing that the objectives of surgical anesthesia are fulfilled.

The objectives of surgical anesthesia are that the patient does not move, is not aware, does not feel pain, and has no memory of the procedure afterward. At the same time, the anesthetist must avoid excessive anesthetic depth, which will result in a dangerous depression of the cardiovascular and respiratory systems.

Studies in human patients suggest that with increasing depth of anesthesia, most patients lose the memory of the procedure first; awareness during the procedure second; unconscious movement in response to a painful stimulus third; and an increase in BP, HR, V_T, or RR in response to a painful stimulus fourth. So although a patient that moves in response to a painful stimulus such as a surgical incision may or may not feel pain depending on the anesthetic depth, these studies support the assumption that a patient that does not move in response to a painful stimulus is not aware, does not perceive pain, and will have no memory of the procedure afterward. Therefore a lack of unconscious movement may be considered evidence of sufficient depth to fulfill the objectives of surgical anesthesia. Although a lack of increase in the HR, RR, V_T, or BP in response to a painful stimulus is further evidence that these objectives are fulfilled, some patients will have adverse cardiopulmonary effects that prevent this depth from being maintained. Thus some reflex increase in these vital signs is not uncommon and is even expected when the patient is at optimum depth.

Maintaining the delicate balance required to fulfill the objectives of surgical anesthesia can be challenging. There are times in any procedure when even the experienced anesthetist will feel unsure. When in doubt, it is usually safer to err on the side of caution and to maintain the patient at the least depth required to fulfill the objectives. In any case, gauging anesthetic depth is a dynamic process that requires frequent reassessment with subsequent adjustments in the rate of anesthetic administration throughout the procedure.

> **TECHNICIAN NOTE** The objectives of surgical anesthesia are that the patient does not move, is not aware, does not feel pain, has no memory of the procedure afterward, and does not have dangerous depression of the cardiovascular and respiratory systems.

DETERMINING WHETHER OR NOT THE PATIENT IS SAFE

Determining whether or not the patient is safe during any anesthetic procedure is accomplished primarily by assessing vital signs. Vital signs may be assessed either by physical means (i.e., touch, hearing, and vision) or through the use of various instruments and machines such as an electrocardiograph, BP monitor, capnograph, Doppler blood flow detector, or pulse oximeter. The vital signs can be grouped according to whether they reflect circulation (HR and heart rhythm, pulse strength, CRT, mucous membrane color, and BP), oxygenation (mucous membrane color, hemoglobin saturation, measurement of inspired oxygen, and measurement of arterial blood oxygen [Pao_2]), or ventilation (RR and respiratory depth, breath sounds, end-expired CO_2 [$ETco_2$] levels, arterial carbon dioxide [$Paco_2$], and blood pH).

Although a competent technician can safely monitor most patients without the use of specialized instruments, the use of monitoring devices may be of significant benefit. Instruments offer continuous monitoring, whereas the technician in a busy veterinary practice is seldom able to sit with the patient constantly. Instruments also allow precise measurement of variables that are impossible to determine by observation alone, such as BP and the percent oxygen saturation of the hemoglobin.

On the other hand, monitoring instruments are subject to malfunction, failure, and artifacts, and are not able to capture completely the full range of information that is required for safe and effective monitoring. In addition, these instruments may divert the anesthetist's attention by requiring frequent adjustment of probes, cuffs, catheters, electrodes, or other equipment used to gather data. Consequently, the anesthetist may become frustrated, question the accuracy of abnormal data, and inadvertently may miss important information that requires action. Therefore no matter how sophisticated, expensive, convenient, or complex, instruments must never be used as a replacement for a skilled and conscientious anesthetist but must be used only as a supplement to careful physical monitoring.

This section describes indicators of circulation, oxygenation, and ventilation, including physical means as well as mechanical means that can be used to monitor the following variables:

* HR (esophageal stethoscope)
* heart rhythm (electrocardiograph)
* BP (Doppler blood flow detector, oscillometer, and transducer with direct arterial line)
* central venous pressure (CVP) (manometer)
* Pao_2 and $Paco_2$ (blood gases)
* oxygen saturation (pulse oximeter)
* RR and tidal volume (respirometer)
* expired carbon dioxide (capnograph)
* body temperature (esophageal or rectal temperature probes).

Note that electrocardiographs, BP monitors, and pulse oximeters also measure HR, and the capnograph also measures RR (Table 6.3).

> **TECHNICIAN NOTE** No matter how sophisticated, expensive, convenient, or complex, instruments must never be used as a replacement for a skilled and conscientious anesthetist but must be used only as a supplement to careful physical monitoring.

Indicators of Circulation

The objective of the ACVAA monitoring guidelines for circulation is "to ensure adequate circulatory function." To meet this objective, the ACVAA makes the following recommendations:

Continuous awareness of heart rate and rhythm during anesthesia, along with gross assessment of peripheral perfusion (pulse quality, mucous membrane color and CRT) are mandatory. Arterial blood pressure and ECG should also be monitored. There may be some situations where these may be temporarily impractical, e.g., movement of an anesthetized patient to a different area of the hospital.

TABLE 6.3 Monitoring Instruments and the Parameters They Measure

Equipment	HR	Rhythm	P_{SYS}	MAP	P_{DIA}	Blood Gases	PaO_2/SpO_2	RR	V_T	$ETCO_2$
ECG Unit	Y	Y								
Esophageal stethoscope	Y (relative value only[a])	Y[b] (normal vs. abnormal)						Y (if the room is quiet)		
Doppler blood flow detector	Y (relative value only[a])	Y[b] (normal vs. abnormal)	Y							
Oscillometric BP monitor	Y		Y	Y	Y					
Direct arterial line	Y		Y	Y	Y	Y	Y (Pao_2)			
Pulse oximeter	Y						Y (Spo_2)			
Respirometer								Y	Y	
End-tidal CO_2 Monitor								Y		Y

[a]"*relative value only*" means that an audible indicator of cardiac contraction is produced, so that the anesthetist can hear relative changes in rate, but the HR is not visually displayed.

[b]"*normal vs. abnormal*" means that an abnormal cardiac rhythm that produces a change in the audible pattern may be detected by the anesthetist, but the exact rhythm will not be known unless an ECG tracing is available. Note that some abnormal rhythms such as first-degree atrioventricular (AV) block do not produce an audible change.

BP, Blood-pressure; *CO_2*, carbon dioxide; *ECG*, electrocardiograph; *$ETCO_2$*, end-tidal carbon dioxide; *HR*, heart rate; *MAP*, mean arterial pressure; *P_{DIA}*, diastolic arterial pressure; *P_{SYS}*, systolic arterial pressure; *RR*, respiratory rate; *V_T*, tidal volume.

Heart Rate

The HR may be physically assessed by palpation of the apical pulse through the thoracic wall, palpation of a peripheral pulse, or auscultation with a stethoscope or with the assistance of an esophageal stethoscope, which is a device that amplifies the heart sounds. It may be measured mechanically with an electrocardiograph, a BP monitor (Doppler blood flow detector or oscillometric monitor), or an intra-arterial line attached to a transducer. Most mechanical monitors generate an audible beep, flashing light, or other visual indicator to make each heartbeat detectable from a distance. Many also show a digital readout of the HR in beats per minute (bpm). Some monitors can be adjusted to sound an alarm when the HR moves above or below limits set by the anesthetist.

When assessing the HR with a stethoscope during anesthesia, be aware that the heartbeat can be harder to hear than when the patient is awake for two reasons: first, because of a decreased strength of contraction often associated with anesthesia and, second, because the heart will gravitate to the lowest aspect of the thoracic cavity, making the heartbeat hard to hear if the stethoscope is placed in the customary locations. For instance, if the patient is in dorsal recumbency, as are many anesthetized patients, the heartbeat is often difficult to hear at all through the chest wall, especially in cats or obese patients. If the patient is lying in lateral recumbency, the heartbeat can generally be heard but is often audible only on the dependent side because of the effect of gravity on the position of the heart.

TECHNICIAN NOTE If the patient is lying in lateral recumbency, the heartbeat can generally be heard but is often audible only on the dependent side because of the effect of gravity on the position of the heart.

The HR is typically decreased in anesthetized animals owing to the depressant effect of many anesthetics. Alpha$_2$-agonists and opioids are particularly likely to cause bradycardia. Some drugs (e.g., anticholinergics and cyclohexylamines) have the opposite effect and can elevate HR. The minimum acceptable, maximum acceptable, and typical HRs for anesthetized patients are listed in Table 6.4. Bradycardia is commonly caused by excessive anesthetic depth or adverse effects of drugs, and common causes of tachycardia are inadequate anesthetic depth, pain during surgical anesthesia, hypotension, blood loss, shock, hypoxemia, and hypercapnia.

Heart Rhythm

The heart rhythm is assessed along with the HR. During anesthesia, normal sinus rhythm (NSR) is the most common rhythm in normal dogs, cats, and other small animals. Some normal dogs, however, especially if young and fit, have a sinus arrhythmia (SA) that can at times be quite pronounced and that can easily be mistaken for a cardiac arrhythmia (see page 205 for a discussion of SA). The anesthetist can usually differentiate SA from an abnormal rhythm by listening for the cyclic decrease in rate during expiration and increase in rate during inspiration characteristic of SA. Large animals typically have an NSR but may also have an SA. First- or second-degree block is also considered to be normal in the athletic horse, provided that when the patient is conscious, the rhythm returns to SA or NSR after gentle exercise or stimulation.

TECHNICIAN NOTE The anesthetist can usually differentiate SA from an abnormal rhythm by listening for the cyclic decrease in rate during expiration and increase in rate during inspiration that is characteristic of SA.

TABLE 6.4 Normal Vital Signs During Anesthesia

Species	Heart Rate (bpm)	Heart Rhythm	Respiratory Rate (Breaths/Minute), V_T, and Effort[a]	Body Temperature
Dog	60–150[b]	NSR or SA	8–20	97°F–100°F (36.1°C–37.8°C)
Report to veterinarian if:	<60 or >140 (lg) <70 or >160 (sm)	Any other rhythm is present	<6 or >20	>103.5°F (39.7°C) or <97°F (36.1°C)
Cat	120–180	NSR	8–20	97°F–100°F (36.1°C–37.8°C)
Report to veterinarian if:	<100 or >200	Any other rhythm is present	<6 or >20	>103.5°F (39.7°C) or <97°F (36.1°C)
Horse	28–40	NSR, SA, or first- or second-degree AV heart block	6–12	97°F–100°F (36.1°C–37.8°C)
Report to veterinarian if:	<25 or >60	Any other rhythm is present	<6 or >20	>101.5°F (38.6°C) or <97°F (36.1°C)
Cattle	50–80	NSR or SA	6–12, although rapid, shallow breathing is very common	97°F–100°F (36.1°C–37.8°C)
Report to veterinarian if:	<40 or >100	Any other rhythm is present	<6 or >20	>103.5°F (39.7°C) or <97°F (36.1°C)

[a]Respiratory effort should be normal, and V_T is typically decreased by approximately 25%. Any increase in effort or >25% decrease in V_T should be reported to the attending veterinarian.
[b]Owing to the extreme variability of size, large dogs tend to have lower rates, whereas small dogs and puppies have higher rates.
AV, Atrioventricular; lg, large; NSR, normal sinus rhythm; SA, sinus arrhythmia; sm, small; V_T, tidal volume.

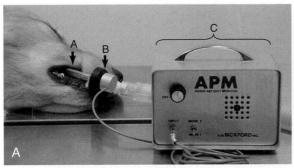

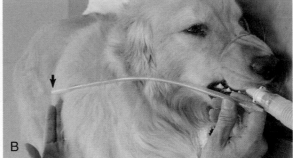

FIG. 6.9 **(A)** Esophageal stethoscope: *A,* catheter; *B,* sensor; *C,* base unit. **(B)** Measurement of the catheter to the level of the fifth rib or the caudal border of the scapula *(arrow).*

The anesthetist can generally develop a high degree of suspicion of a cardiac arrhythmia by its irregular sound but some, such as first-degree heart block, defy detection this way. The only certain way to identify this and other abnormal rhythms is by using an electrocardiograph monitor, which reveals the electrical activity of the heart. Cardiac arrhythmias are not uncommon during anesthesia and are commonly caused by anticholinergics, alpha₂-agonists, cyclohexylamines, and barbiturates, but they are also caused by a number of states and disease conditions including hypoxia, hypercarbia, heart disease, trauma, and gastric dilatation–volvulus. Disturbances in cardiac rhythm should always be brought to the attention of the veterinarian for assessment because benign arrhythmias can quickly degenerate into dangerous rhythms if not recognized and managed.

> **TECHNICIAN NOTE** Disturbances in cardiac rhythm should always be brought to the attention of the veterinarian for assessment because benign arrhythmias can quickly degenerate into dangerous rhythms if not recognized and managed.

Instruments used to monitor heart rate and rhythm

Esophageal stethoscope. An esophageal stethoscope (Fig. 6.9) permits auscultation of the heart from a distance even when the patient's chest is covered with surgical drapes and conventional auscultation is difficult. The esophageal stethoscope consists of a thin, flexible catheter attached to an audio monitor that electronically amplifies the heart sounds. Some catheters are combined with a temperature probe that enables core body temperature to be monitored continuously. The catheters come in various sizes (small, medium, and large) to fit small-animal patients of varying sizes. There are multiple holes near the patient end, which is covered with a plastic sheath. The opposite end has a hole that fits into a sensor, which in turn transfers the heart sounds to an amplifier. The distal end of a conventional stethoscope tube, with the diaphragm/bell detached, can also be attached to the catheter as an alternative.

To allow an esophageal stethoscope to be used, the catheter tube is lubricated with a small amount of water or lubricating jelly and the patient end is inserted through the oral cavity into the patient's esophagus to about the level of the fifth rib. The position of the catheter is adjusted a little at a time and the

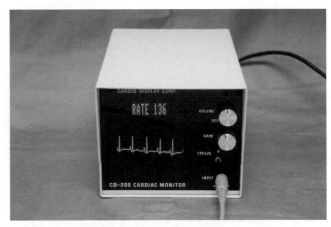

FIG. 6.10 An electrocardiograph (ECG) monitor. A device such as this, which displays a real-time ECG tracing on a screen, is most often used to monitor anesthetized patients.

volume on the monitor is adjusted until the heartbeat is audible. Although it does not give quantitative information (i.e., HR), this relatively simple, reliable, and inexpensive instrument allows the anesthetist or surgeon to hear the heart sounds easily anywhere in the surgical suite.

Esophageal stethoscopes require relatively little maintenance. Some catheters are designed for single use, whereas others are designed for multiple use. Catheters are considered to be semicritical items (because they contact mucous membranes and if reused, should be cleaned and treated with a high-level disinfectant (see Chapter 4 for a discussion of equipment cleaning and disinfection). When cleaning them, do not immerse the catheter or allow water to enter the hole in the end of the catheter. Some audio amplifiers use nonrechargeable batteries, which must be changed periodically.

Electrocardiography

Electrocardiograph monitor. The electrocardiograph (ECG) monitor is a device used to display electrical impulses generated by the cardiac conduction system that initiate each heartbeat. The pattern of electrical impulses, referred to as the heart rhythm, may be either displayed on a screen or permanently recorded on ECG paper.

When monitoring the heart rhythm of an anesthetized patient, a device called an ECG monitor generates a continuous real-time tracing of the heart rhythm on a screen and often produces an audible beep with each heartbeat (Fig. 6.10). Some

ECG monitors may allow the tracing to be "frozen" temporarily on the screen for a more detailed analysis, and may also allow small sections of interest to be printed out. An ECG monitor may be self-standing or may be part of a multiparameter monitor (Fig. 6.11), which concurrently tracks and displays other data such as blood pressure, oxygen saturation, and body temperature.

Electrocardiography is used not only to monitor anesthetized animals but also to guide the treatment of cardiac arrest and to assess the cardiac conduction system of both well and ill patients. When used for these purposes, most often, a machine is used that prints out the tracing on ECG paper (referred to herein as a "standard ECG machine") (Fig. 6.12).

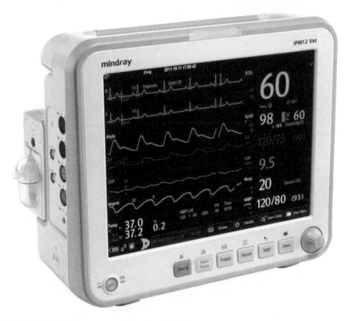

FIG. 6.11 Multiparameter monitor. iPM12 Vet Veterinary Monitor. (Courtesy Mindray.)

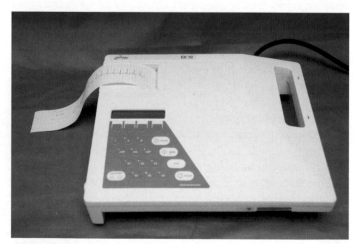

FIG. 6.12 A standard electrocardiograph (ECG) machine. This device prints out the ECG tracing on paper and is most often used to perform complete ECG examinations on well and ill patients.

> **TECHNICIAN NOTE** Cardiac arrhythmias occur commonly in anesthetized animals and vary in significance from innocuous to life-threatening. Therefore the anesthetist must assess the patient's heart rhythm at many points during any anesthetic procedure to keep the patient safe.

Cardiac arrhythmias occur commonly in anesthetized animals and often appear and disappear suddenly and without warning. The term *cardiac arrhythmia* (also known as *cardiac dysrhythmia*) may be defined as any pattern of cardiac electrical activity that differs from that of the healthy awake animal. Arrhythmias vary in significance from innocuous to life-threatening depending on the cause and the patient's general condition. Therefore the anesthetist must assess the patient's heart rhythm at many points during any anesthetic procedure to keep the patient safe.

Only a veterinarian can make an electrocardiographic diagnosis but when acting as anesthetist, the technician or nurse must be able to differentiate normal from abnormal, and dangerous from nondangerous rhythms. Although an alert anesthetist may strongly suspect an arrhythmia based on careful auscultation and palpation of the pulse, electrocardiography is the only monitoring tool that allows definitive identification of the heart rhythm.

> **TECHNICIAN NOTE** Only a veterinarian can make an electrocardiographic diagnosis but when acting as anesthetist, the technician or nurse must be able to differentiate normal from abnormal and dangerous from nondangerous rhythms.

Electrocardiograph machine electrodes and controls. All ECG machines and monitors have a set of three to five electrodes (usually alligator clips, atraumatic clips, flat contact plates with straps, or adhesive electrodes) (Fig. 6.13) that are attached to the patient's skin. These electrodes detect the electrical impulses which are then conveyed to the machine, where they are graphed out on paper or on a screen. The electrodes are color-coded according to the location on the body where they are to be placed. When using standard positioning, with a small-animal patient in right lateral recumbency, the white electrode (labeled "RA," corresponding to "right arm" in people) is placed on the right forelimb, the black electrode (labeled "LA") is placed on the left forelimb, the green electrode (labeled "RL," corresponding to the right leg in people) is placed on the right hindlimb, and the red electrode (labeled "LL") is placed on the left hindlimb. Some machines also have one or more brown electrodes (labeled "V") that are not routinely used in veterinary species. Note that patient positioning and electrode placement are different for large-animal patients when using the base apex lead (see Box 6.2 for standard patient position and electrode placement for electrocardiography for both SA and LA patients and well as an alternate position for small-animal patients undergoing abdominal or hindlimb surgery).

A standard ECG machine records the electrical impulses using six different leads (I, II, III, aVR, aVL, and aVF). Each

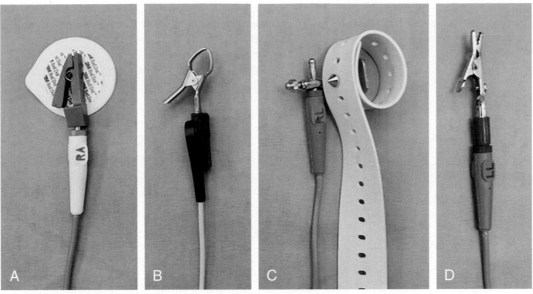

FIG. 6.13 Electrocardiograph (ECG) electrodes. **(A)** Adhesive electrode, which is applied to clipped, clean area of skin after removing the backing. **(B)** Atraumatic clip, which is applied on a folded area of loose skin but as the name implies, causes less trauma than conventional alligator clips. **(C)** Flat contact plate, which is held against distal limb skin by encircling the limb firmly with the strap. **(D)** Alligator clip, which is applied on a folded area of loose skin.

BOX 6.2   Standard Patient Position and Electrode Placement for Electrocardiography

General Principles
- The patient should be on a nonconductive surface
- Make sure the electrodes are clean and firmly attached to the skin
- Wet the skin–electrode contact points with a small amount of electrode gel or ultrasound gel, normal saline, or alcohol

Small Animals
Standard Patient Position: (Fig. 1)

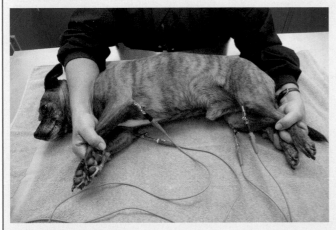

- Place the patient in right lateral recumbency if obtaining a full diagnostic electrocardiogram (ECG); both the forelimbs and hindlimbs should be held perpendicular to the body.
- If monitoring patients undergoing anesthetic procedures, position does not matter

- Sternal position is an alternative for a conscious cat or ferret that resists restraint or for small-animal patients with heart or lung disease or any other problem that would result in undue stress if put in the standard position

Standard Electrode Placement: (Fig. 2)

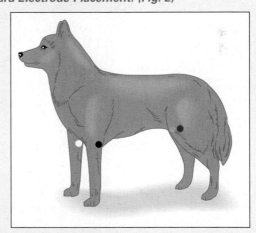

- White electrode on right forelimb
- Black electrode on left forelimb
  - Ideally, forelimb electrodes should be placed slightly proximal to the elbows, although any location on the limb distal to that point is acceptable
- Green electrode on right hindlimb
- Red electrode on left hindlimb
  - Rear limb electrodes should be placed slightly proximal to the stifle joints, although any location on the limb distal to that point is acceptable

Continued

BOX 6.2   Standard Patient Position and Electrode Placement for Electrocardiography—cont'd

Alternative Electrode Placement for Small Animals (Base Apex Lead)[a] (Fig. 3)

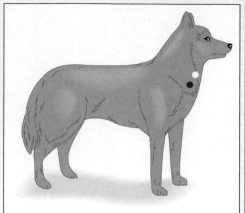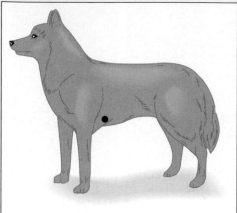

Note that this option may be preferable for patients undergoing abdominal or hindlimb surgery to minimize motion artifact
- Position white and red electrodes over the right or left jugular furrow (right is preferred)

- Position black electrode over the opposite thoracic wall caudal to the heart
- Recording on lead I setting will result in a negative R wave, whereas recording on lead III setting will result in a positive R wave

Large Animals
Electrode Placement for Large Animals (Base apex lead): (Fig. 4)

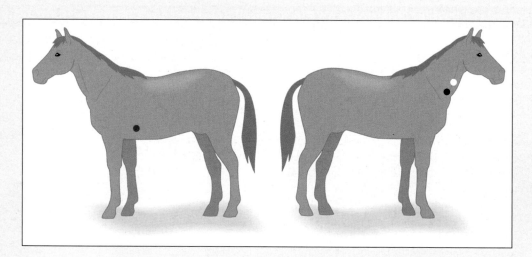

- Obtain ECG before anesthesia with the patient in a standing position as long as the patient is cooperative
- If monitoring for patients undergoing procedures, position does not matter
- Place the electrodes on the following locations:
  - White electrode on the right jugular furrow

- Black electrode on the right jugular furrow a few centimeters away from the white electrode
- Red electrode at the apex of the heart (left lateral thorax)
- Record the ECG tracing using lead II setting

[a]Anesthetic Monitoring: Devices to Use & What the Results Mean by Jeff Ko and Rebecca Krimins. Today's Veterinary Practice, March/April 2012.

lead "views" the electrical impulse from a slightly different angle and when analyzed together, these six leads allow a multidimensional assessment of the heart muscle. In small animals, lead II with standard electrode placement is most commonly used by itself to evaluate heart rhythm because when recorded using this lead, the waveforms are large and easy to evaluate. In horses, the base apex lead (which is an alternative way to position the limb electrodes) is typically used (see Fig. 6.14 for diagrams of lead II tracings in dogs and cats, and base apex lead tracing in horses).

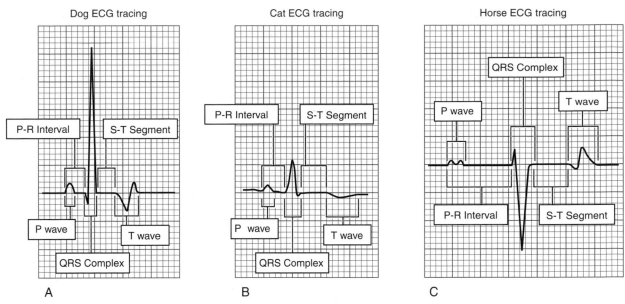

FIG. 6.14 Appearance of the normal electrocardiograph (ECG) waveforms, intervals, and segments in **(A)** the dog (lead II); **(B)** the cat (lead II); **(C)** the horse (base apex lead placement).

> **TECHNICIAN NOTE** In small animals, lead II with standard electrode placement is most commonly used by itself to evaluate heart rhythm because when recorded using this lead, the waveforms are large and easy to evaluate. In horses, base apex lead placement (which is an alternative way to position the limb electrodes) is typically used.

Most standard ECG machines have a set of common controls, including an on/off switch, a lead selector (I, II, III, aVR, aVL, aVF, or V), paper speed setting measured in millimeters per second (mm/s), and a sensitivity setting measured in centimeters per millivolt (cm/mV). The lead selector allows the operator to select and change the lead used to record the tracing (usually lead II for the purpose of monitoring heart rhythm). The paper speed controls the speed at which the paper exits the machine as the tracing is recorded (25 mm/s or 50 mm/s) and consequently, the width of the waveforms, intervals, and segments. The sensitivity setting controls the amplification of the impulses (0.5 cm/mV, 1 cm/mV, or 2 cm/mV) and consequently, the height of the waveforms.

An ECG monitor generally records a continuous tracing using a single lead (often lead I or II), and many have only two or three electrodes as opposed to four or five as with a traditional ECG machine. The equipment manual will indicate which lead is generated and will include instructions regarding how to change the lead if desired.

Acquiring a diagnostic electrocardiograph tracing. When acquiring a diagnostic ECG tracing, the patient should be placed on a nonconductive surface such as a towel or blanket, or a foam, fleece, or rubber mat. Proper patient positioning is important when performing a complete electrocardiographic evaluation with an ECG machine because patient and electrode position affects the shape and size of the waveforms. Patient positioning is not as critical, however, when evaluating heart rhythm only (as is done with an ECG monitor during an anesthetic event).

Consequently, the patient may be placed in any position requested by the surgeon. However, when a nonstandard position is used, the waveforms will change shape and may be too small to observe easily or to generate an audible signal. In these situations, the position of the electrodes can be changed to increase the size of the waveforms. The owner's manual of the equipment you are using will have instructions regarding how to do this.

> **TECHNICIAN NOTE** Patient positioning is not critical when evaluating heart rhythm only (as is done with an ECG monitor during an anesthetic event). Consequently, the patient may be placed in any position requested by the surgeon.

When performing a complete six-lead ECG examination with a standard ECG machine (with the patient in standard position and standard electrode placement), five to six complexes of each of the six standard leads should be recorded with a 1- to 2-minute tracing of lead II (see Box 6.3 for instructions regarding how to record a standard ECG tracing). When monitoring a patient continuously during an anesthetic event, a single lead is used (often lead I or II). When using an ECG monitor for this purpose, adjust the sensitivity so that the "R"

> ## BOX 6.3 **Recording a Standard Electrocardiograph Tracing**
>
> 1. Turn the machine on.
> 2. Set the paper speed at 50 mm/s for small animals (dog, cat, and ferret) or 25 mm/s for large animals (horse and cow).
> 3. Adjust the sensitivity setting to 1 cm/mV. If the complexes are very small (e.g., in cats), use 2 cm/mV. If the complexes exceed the width of the paper, use 0.5 cm/mV.
> 4. Record five or six complexes for each lead (I, II, III, aVR, aVL, aVF).
> 5. Record 1–2 min of lead II at 25 mm/s to assess rhythm.

wave can be adequately visualized on the screen and make sure the "R" wave is large enough to trigger the audible beep.

The generation of the electrocardiograph tracing. The normal electrocardiograph tracing (aka: electrocardiogram or ECG) is a graphic representation of the electrical activity of the heart as it travels through the cardiac conduction system (Fig. 6.15) and heart muscle. The wave of electrical activity starts in the sinoatrial node and travels through the internodal tracts, causing atrial contraction. Next, it is conducted to the atrioventricular (AV) node, where it briefly slows down to allow the ventricles to fill with blood. It then travels to the ventricles via the bundle of His, bundle branches, and Purkinje fibers, causing ventricular contraction. Although the precise appearance of the tracing varies according to the lead, the patient position, the species, and other factors, it always has the same general pattern of waveforms, intervals, and segments (see Fig. 6.14).

The "baseline" is the horizontal part of the tracing between the waveforms. As the electrical impulse moves through the heart, the heart muscle cells depolarize (change electrical polarity). If the wave of electrical depolarization is primarily traveling toward a positive electrode, the waveform will go up (above the baseline); if the wave is primarily traveling toward the negative electrode, the waveform will go down (below the baseline); and if the wave is traveling perpendicular to a line drawn between the positive and negative electrodes, there will be no deflection. So the shape of the waveforms is determined by the general direction that the electrical impulses travel in relation to the electrodes.

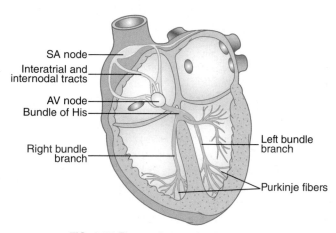

FIG. 6.15 The cardiac conduction system.

The appearance of normal waveforms, intervals, and segments. In order to differentiate normal ECG tracings from abnormal ECG tracings, it is necessary for the technician to have a detailed knowledge of the appearance of the normal waveforms, intervals, and segments (see Fig. 6.14).

The P wave, the first waveform, precedes contraction of the atria. It is normally small, rounded, and positive in lead II and is often "double humped" (also known as *bifid*) in adult large animals. It is separated from the QRS complex by the P-R interval. The P wave is measured from the point that it leaves the baseline to the point that it returns to the baseline. It is considered abnormal if it is abnormal in shape, if its duration or amplitude exceeds a maximum value, or if its relationship with the QRS complex is altered.

The P-R interval represents the time required for the impulse to move from the sinoatrial node to the Purkinje fibers. It is measured from the beginning of the P wave to the beginning of the QRS complex. In normal patients, the P-R interval must be within a range of 0.06 to 0.13 seconds in a dog, 0.05 to 0.09 seconds in a cat, and 0.22 to 0.56 seconds in a horse (see Table 6.5 for normal amplitudes and durations of waveforms, intervals, and segments in common domestic species).

The QRS complex represents contraction of the ventricles and follows the P-R interval. The shape of the QRS complex is variable depending on the species and the lead. It is the largest waveform, is pointed (peaked), and is primarily positive in small animals on lead II and negative in large animals when the base apex lead is used. The QRS is made up of three components: (1) the Q wave, which is the first negative deflection after the P-R interval; (2) the R wave, which is the first positive deflection after the P-R interval; and (3) the S wave, which is the first negative deflection after the R wave. A normal QRS complex may consist of any of these three components in any combination (R, QR, RS, QRS, and so on) depending on the species and the lead as well as other factors; however, they are typically referred to as the QRS complex when discussing cardiac rhythm.

The QRS complex is measured from the point that it leaves the baseline to the point that it returns to the baseline. It is considered abnormal if it is abnormal in shape, if its duration or amplitude exceeds a maximum value, or if its relationship with the P wave is altered.

The S-T segment is located between the QRS complex and the T wave. It should deviate very little from the baseline.

TABLE 6.5	**Normal Electrocardiographic Values in Common Domestic Species**				
Species	P-Wave Duration (Maximum in Seconds)	P Wave Amplitude (Maximum in mV)	P-R Interval (Seconds)	QRS Duration (Maximum in Seconds)	QRS Amplitude (Maximum in mV)
Dog	0.04	0.4	0.06–0.13	0.05 (small breed)	2.5 (small breed)
	0.05 (giant breed)			0.06 (large breed)	3.0 (large breed)
Cat	0.04	0.2	0.05–0.09	0.04	0.9
Horse	0.20		0.22–0.56	0.08–0.17 (range)	
Cow	0.10		0.16–0.30	0.08–0.14 (range)	
Ferret	0.04	0.1	0.04–0.06	0.04	2.5

From Edwards NJ: *ECG manual for the veterinary technician*, Philadelphia, 1993, Saunders.

The T wave, which follows the QRS complex, represents repolarization of the ventricles in preparation for the next contraction. It is variable in appearance but is normally no more than one-quarter the amplitude of the QRS complex. It is measured from the end of the S-T segment to the point at which the T wave returns to the baseline.

Using standard electrocardiograph paper. Note that the boxes created by the dots and/or lines on standard ECG paper are used to measure waveforms, intervals, and segments (Fig. 6.16). The small boxes (delineated by the dots or thin lines) are 1 mm on a side. The large boxes (delineated by the thicker lines) are 5 mm on a side. This means that at a paper speed of 50 mm/s, a horizontal distance of 50 1-mm boxes (10 large boxes) is equal to 1 second, and one 1-mm box is equal to 0.02 seconds (because 1 second/50 = 0.02 seconds). At a speed of 25 mm/s, a horizontal distance of 25 1-mm boxes (five large boxes) is equal to 1 second, and one 1-mm box is equal to 0.04 seconds (because 1 second/25 = 0.04 seconds).

To measure the P-R interval, multiply the number of small (1-mm) boxes between the beginning of the P wave and the beginning of the QRS by 0.02 seconds (when evaluating a tracing recorded at 50 mm/s) or by 0.04 seconds (when evaluating a tracing recorded at 25 mm/s). Fig. 6.16 shows how to measure the P-R interval.

Recognition and elimination of artifacts. ECG artifacts are movements, irregularities, or undulations of the baseline that are not due to a disease condition. They occur primarily as a result of patient body movement, electrode movement, and electrical interference. Artifacts are a frequent source of frustration for the operator because they make ECG interpretation difficult.

Motion artifacts are less common with anesthetized patients than patients that are awake but occur nonetheless if the anesthetist moves the patient or adjusts the patient's position during the procedure, or if the patient has exaggerated breathing movements, muscle tremors, or spontaneous body movements during light anesthesia (see Figs. 6.17–6.19 for examples of motion artifacts that might be seen during anesthetic events). These artifacts are avoided by keeping the patient and electrodes as still as possible.

A 60-cycle electrical interference artifact appears as uniform sawtooth, up-and-down movements of the baseline caused by contact of the patient or electrodes with a metal object, poor electrode–skin contact, electrode overwetting, or a variety of

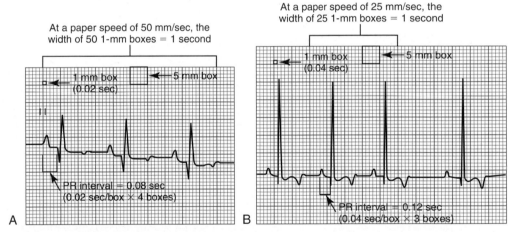

FIG. 6.16 Standard electrocardiograph (ECG) paper. On each tracing, the small boxes delineated by the dots or thin lines (e.g., the *small red box*) are 1 mm on a side. The large boxes delineated by the thicker lines (e.g., the *large red box*) are 5 mm on a side. **(A)** At a paper speed of 50 mm/s, a horizontal distance of 50 1-mm boxes is equal to 1 second and one 1-mm box is equal to 0.02 seconds. So the P-R interval on this tracing is approximately 0.08 seconds (0.02 seconds/box × 4 boxes). **(B)** At a speed of 25 mm/s, a horizontal distance of 25 1-mm boxes is equal to 1 second and one 1-mm box is equal to 0.04 seconds. The P-R interval in this tracing is approximately 0.12 seconds (0.04 seconds/box × 3 small boxes).

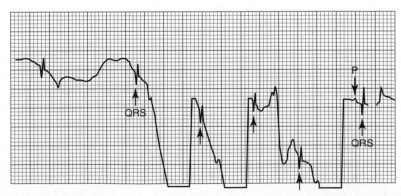

FIG. 6.17 Patient or electrode motion artifact. Dog, lead aVR; 25 mm/s, 1 cm/mV. The large deviations of the baseline in this tracing are characteristic of artifacts that might occur if the patient is moved or shifted.

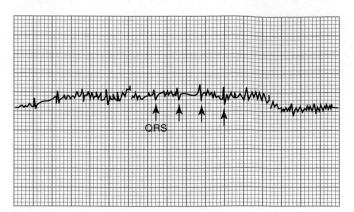

FIG. 6.18 Muscle tremor artifact. Feline, lead III; 25 mm/s, 1 cm/mV. The small irregular deviations of the baseline in this tracing are characteristic of muscle tremor artifact that might be seen in a patient that is in a light plane of anesthesia.

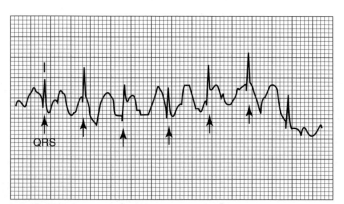

FIG. 6.19 Respiratory motion artifact. Dog, lead II; 25 mm/s, 1 cm/mV. The repetitive upward deviations of the baseline are characteristic of respiratory motion artifact that might be seen if a patient is experiencing forceful exhalations when lightly anesthetized or panting when awake.

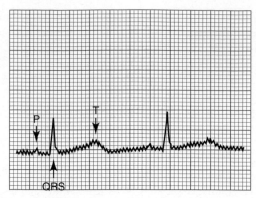

FIG. 6.20 Sixty-cycle electrical interference artifact. Cat, lead II; 50 mm/s, 1 cm/mV. The uniform sawtooth, up-and-down movements of the baseline are characteristic of 60-cycle electrical interference artifact.

BOX 6.4 Strategies for Preventing 60-Cycle Electrical Interference Artifact

1. Use a nonconductive surface and make sure the patient is not in contact with a metal table.
2. Make sure that the electrodes are clean and firmly attached to the skin.
3. Use a wetting agent on the electrodes but do not overwet them.
4. Make sure the electrodes do not touch each other.
5. Make sure the holder is not touching any electrodes.
6. Make sure no electrical cords are touching the table.
7. Turn off other electrical equipment that may be on the same circuit.
8. If the problem persists, have the equipment serviced.

---

other factors (Fig. 6.20). It is avoided by following the principles in Box 6.4.

Evaluating the electrocardiograph tracing. A complete evaluation of the ECG tracing requires the anesthetist to determine the HR, and then to analyze each waveform, interval and segment for: (1) location (where is it?), (2) shape (what does it look like?), (3) duration (how wide is it?), and (4) amplitude (how tall is it?). As with any skill, this takes some time to learn, but with experience, the anesthetist can learn to quickly recognize deviations from normal that must be reported to the attending veterinarian.

Most electrocardiograph monitors display the heart rate on the screen, so calculation of the HR is not necessary. When analyzing a paper tracing, however, the heart rate must be calculated as indicated in Box 6.5.

After determining the HR, a systematic approach is used to evaluate the waveforms, intervals, and segments. This can be done by performing a visual inspection and answering the five questions of ECG interpretation listed in Table 6.6. Determining the answers to these questions should be approached as follows:

Question #1: *Is there a P wave preceding every QRS complex?* This question is aimed at determining whether there are missing P waves. To answer this question, identify the QRS complexes on the tracing and check that there is a P wave immediately preceding each one.

Question #2: *Is there a QRS complex following every P wave?* This question is aimed at determining whether there are missing QRS complexes. To answer this question, identify the P waves on the tracing and check that there is a QRS after each one.

Question #3: *Are all of the Ps and all of the QRSs the same and do they appear normal?* This question has two parts. This first part is to look at all of the P waves on the tracing to be sure that they are normal in shape, size, and appearance, and that they are all the same. The second part is to repeat the process for all of the QRS complexes on the tracing.

Question #4: *Are the P-R intervals normal in duration and are they the same?* This question is used to determine whether the distance between each P wave and its corresponding QRS complex is normal and whether this distance is consistent over the entire tracing.

Question #5: *Are the R-R intervals the same?* This question is used to determine whether the distance between R waves is approximately the same. Realize that the distance between R waves may shorten or lengthen slightly on a normal tracing as the heart rate changes.

The answers to these five questions and the HR are then used to determine whether the electrocardiographic rhythm is normal or abnormal.

Although comprehensive interpretation of ECGs is complex and beyond the scope of this text, the anesthetist should be familiar with the following rhythms, which are commonly

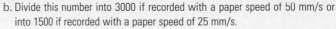

BOX 6.5   **Determining the Heart Rate (bpm) Using Standard Electrocardiograph Paper**

Method #1 to Determine the HR
a. Locate a 3- or 6-s segment of the tracing.
b. Count the number of QRS complexes in that time.
Multiply the number by 20 or 10, respectively, to calculate the HR in bpm.

Method #2 to Determine the HR (to be Used Only if the R-R Intervals Are Uniform)
a. Determine the number of 1-mm boxes between two R waves.

b. Divide this number into 3000 if recorded with a paper speed of 50 mm/s or into 1500 if recorded with a paper speed of 25 mm/s.
   Fig. 1 In this tracing, there are 7 complexes in 3 sec, so using method #1, the calculated HR is 140 bpm (7 × 20). Although the R-R intervals are not completely uniform, there are about 22 1-mm boxes between the two R waves marked. Using method #2, the calculated HR is 136 bpm (3000/22 = 136).

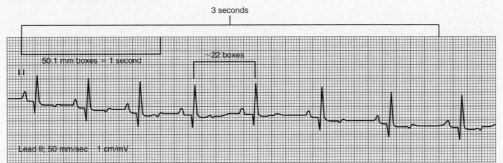

---

encountered in anesthetized patients. Table 6.7 summarizes findings including answers to the five questions of ECG interpretation for each rhythm.

- *Normal sinus rhythm.* NSR is a regular rhythm in which the HR is normal and the distance between successive heartbeats (each QRS complex) is approximately equal (Figs. 6.21 and 6.22). When an NSR is present, the answer to each of the five questions of ECG interpretation is "Yes." NSR is normal in anesthetized dogs, cats, horses, and cattle.
- *Sinus arrhythmia.* SA is a cyclic change in the HR coordinated with respiration in which the HR decreases (recognized by an increased distance between QRS complexes) during expiration and increases (recognized by a decreased distance between QRS complexes) during inspiration (Fig. 6.23). In other words, the R-R intervals vary in a cyclic manner. SA is normal in dogs, especially if young and healthy, and normal in horses and cattle but is not normal in cats.
- *Sinus bradycardia.* Sinus bradycardia (an abnormally slow HR; Fig. 6.24) is common during anesthesia and has a variety of causes, including excessive anesthetic depth and drug reactions (see Chapter 13). Treatment, if necessary, may include administration of appropriate reversal agents or anticholinergics.
- *Sinus tachycardia.* Sinus tachycardia (an abnormally fast HR) is less common than bradycardia during anesthesia. It has a variety of causes, including inadequate anesthetic depth, drug reactions, and surgical stimulation (see Chapter 13). Treatment depends on the underlying cause.
- *AV heart block.* AV heart block involves a delay or interruption in conduction of the electrical impulse through the AV node. There are three types (first-degree, second-degree, and third-degree), which vary in appearance but all involve a change in the relationship between the P wave and QRS complex.
  - *First-degree AV block* is recognized by a prolonged P-R interval (Fig. 6.25). It is often abnormal but is seen in normal resting or anesthetized horses.

- *Second-degree AV block* appears as occasional missing QRS complexes. In other words, not all P waves are followed by a QRS complex (Fig. 6.26). The P-R intervals may also be prolonged and may vary. Like first-degree AV block, it is often abnormal but is also seen in normal resting or anesthetized horses as long as no more than one QRS is skipped in a row, and it resolves with exercise or stimulation. It decreases cardiac output but may or may not require treatment, depending on how severe it is. Both first- and second-degree AV heart block are commonly seen after the administration of alpha$_2$-agonists such as dexmedetomidine. Other causes include high vagal tone, hyperkalemia, and cardiac disease.
  - *Third-degree AV block* is an abnormal rhythm in which the atrial and ventricular waveforms occur independently. It is recognized by a complete loss of the normal relationship between the P waves and QRS complexes and is characterized by randomly irregular P-R intervals (Fig. 6.27). This rhythm indicates cardiac disease and is infrequently seen in anesthetized patients but, when present, decreases cardiac output and requires treatment.
- *Premature complexes.* A premature complex is one that occurs too early. If the premature complex is associated with a heartbeat or pulse, it may be referred to as a *premature contraction.*
  - *Supraventricular premature complexes* (SPCs) appear as one or more normal QRS complexes that closely follow the previous QRS, interrupting an otherwise regular rhythm (Fig. 6.28). P waves may or may not be present but if present, are almost always different from normal P waves. *Atrial premature complexes* (APCs) are a specific type of SPC.
  - *Supraventricular tachycardia* (Fig. 6.29) is a series of three or more SPCs in a row. SPCs are abnormal but may or may not require treatment, depending on the frequency.
  - *Ventricular premature complexes* (VPCs) appear as one or more wide and bizarre QRS complexes that closely

TABLE 6.6   The Five Questions of Electrocardiograph Tracing Analysis

QUESTIONS	ANSWERS	
	Yes	No
1. Is there a P wave preceding every QRS complex?	Normal tracing	Missing P waves. There are no P waves preceding any of the QRSs in this tracing.
2. Is there a QRS complex following every P wave?	Normal tracing	Missing QRS complex following the second P wave.
3. Are all of the Ps and all of the QRSs the same and do they appear normal?	Normal tracing	QRS complexes of variable shape and size. Some are wide and bizarre in appearance.
4. Are the P-R intervals normal in duration and are they the same?	Normal tracing	P-R intervals of variable duration. The P-R interval on the far right is prolonged.
5. Are the R-R intervals the same?	Normal tracing	R-R intervals of variable duration.

TABLE 6.7 Summary of Electrocardiograph Analysis: Characteristics of Common Normal and Abnormal Rhythms

ANSWERS TO THE FIVE QUESTIONS OF ECG TRACING ANALYSIS (SEE TABLE 6.5)

Name of Rhythm	Normal or Abnormal?	HR	#1 (Is there a P wave before every QRS?)	#2 (Is there a QRS after every P wave?)	#3 (Are the waveforms normal and the same?)	#4 (Are the P-R Intervals normal and the same?)	#5 (Are the R-R intervals the same?)
Sinus Rhythms							
Normal sinus rhythm (NSR)	Normal for all species	Normal	Yes	Yes	Yes	Yes	Yes
Sinus arrhythmia	Normal (dog and horse at rest only)	Normal	Yes	Yes	Yes	Yes	No (R-R intervals vary cyclically with breathing)
Sinus bradycardia	Abnormal	Low	Yes	Yes	Yes	Yes	Yes
Sinus tachycardia	Abnormal	High	Yes	Yes	Yes	Yes	Yes
Heart block							
First-degree AV heart block	Abnormal (except in horses at rest/anesthetized)	Usually normal or low	Yes	Yes	Yes	No (P-R intervals are prolonged)	Yes
Second-degree AV heart block	Abnormal (except in horses at rest/anesthetized)	Usually normal or low	Yes	No (some QRS complexes are missing)	Yes	Variable (some or all P-R intervals may be prolonged)	No
3rd-Degree AV Heart Block	Abnormal	Low (ventricular rate)	P waves and QRS complexes are not related	P waves and QRS complexes are not related	P waves normal; QRS complexes may be normal or abnormal	No (no relationship between P waves and QRS complexes)	Y (usually)
Premature Impulse Formation							
Supraventricular premature complexes (SPC)/ supraventricular tachycardia	Abnormal	Often normal (SPC) or high (supraventricular tachycardia)	Variable	Yes	(P waves usually abnormal; QRS complexes normal)	No (P-R interval may be abnormals before SPCs)	No (the abnormal QRS complexes are early)
Ventricular premature complexes (VPC)/ ventricular tachycardia	Abnormal/ V-tachycardia is dangerous	Often normal (VPC) or high (ventricular tachycardia)	Variable	Yes	No (QRS complexes are wide and bizarre)	No (the P-R intervals are often abnormal before VPCs)	No (the abnormal complexes are early)
Fibrillation							
Atrial fibrillation	Abnormal	High	No P waves	N/A	Yes (QRS complexes normal)	N/A	No (R-R intervals are irregular)
Ventricular Fibrillation	Abnormal/dangerous	No measurable HR	No P waves	No QRS complexes	N/A	N/A	N/A

N/A, Not applicable.

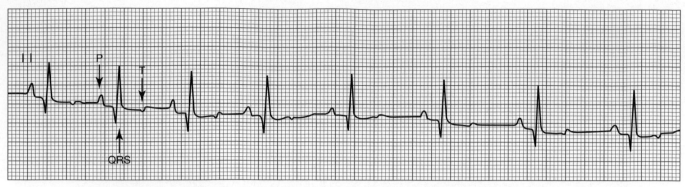

FIG. 6.21 Normal sinus rhythm (dog, lead II; 50 mm/s, 1 cm/mV).

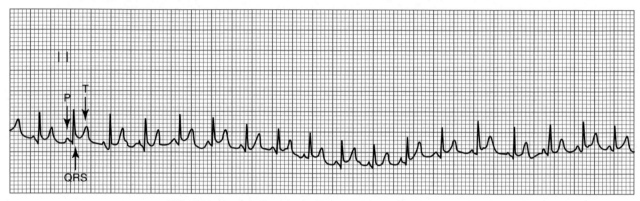

FIG. 6.22 Normal sinus rhythm (cat, lead II; 25 mm/s; 1 cm/mV).

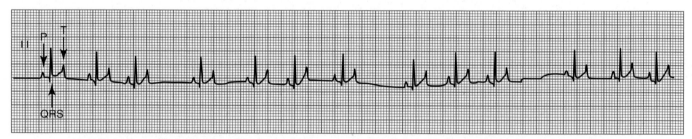

FIG. 6.23 Sinus arrhythmia (dog, lead II; 25 mm/s, 1 cm/mV). Note the regular acceleration and slowing of the heart rate as evidenced by the cyclic lengthening and shortening of the R-R intervals. This waxing and waning correlates with breathing.

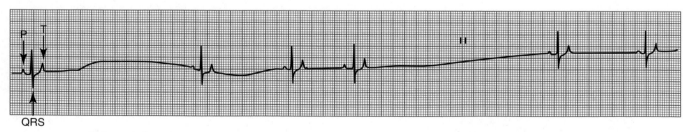

FIG. 6.24 Sinus bradycardia (dog, lead II; 25 mm/s, 1 cm/mV). Note that this tracing also exhibits sinus arrhythmia.

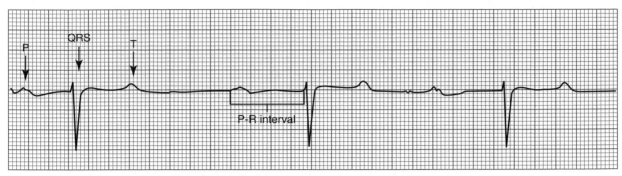

FIG. 6.25 First-degree atrioventricular heart block (horse, base apex lead; 25 mm/s, 1 cm/mV). This tracing was recorded at 25 mm/s. Therefore each box = 0.04 seconds. Note the wide P-R interval before the second QRS complex of approximately 0.72 seconds (0.04 seconds/box × 18 boxes) (normal 0.22 to 0.56 seconds).

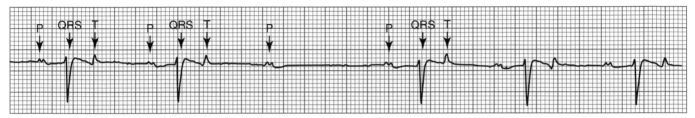

FIG. 6.26 Second-degree atrioventricular (AV) heart block (horse, base apex lead; 25 mm/s, 1 cm/mV). Note that there is a missing QRS complex after the third P wave from the left.

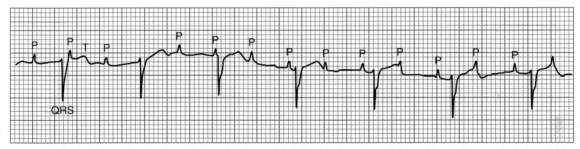

FIG. 6.27 Third-degree atrioventricular (AV) heart block (cat; 25 mm/s, 1 cm/mV). Note that the P waves are regular and are occurring independently of the QRS complexes. (From Bonagura JD, Twedt DC: *Kirk's current veterinary therapy XIV,* St Louis, MO, 2009, Elsevier.)

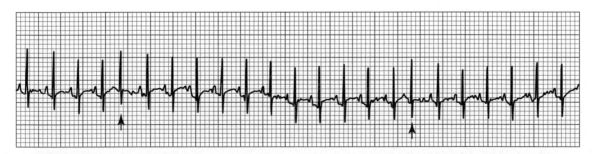

FIG. 6.28 Supraventricular premature complexes (cat; 25 mm/s, 1 cm/mV). Note the early complexes with normal QRS morphology *(arrows)*. (From Bonagura JD, Twedt DC: *Kirk's current veterinary therapy XIV,* St Louis, MO, 2009, Elsevier.)

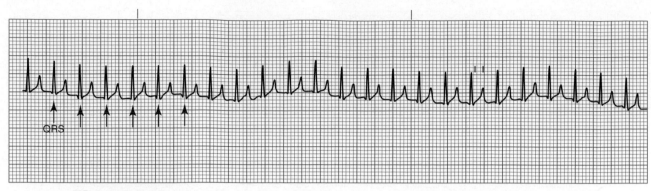

FIG. 6.29 Supraventricular tachycardia (dog, lead II; 25 mm/s, 1 cm/mV). Note the very rapid heart rate with normal QRS complexes. The P waves are superimposed over the T waves and so are not easily visualized.

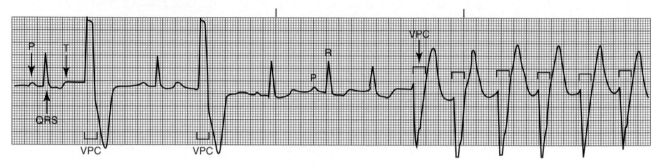

FIG. 6.30 Ventricular premature complexes (dog, lead II; 50 mm/s, 1 cm/mV). Note the early wide, bizarre QRS complexes, second and fourth from the left (ventricular premature complexes [VPCs]) and the last six complexes (which represent an episode of ventricular tachycardia). (From Birchard SJ, Sherding RG: *Saunders manual of small animal practice*, ed 3, St Louis, MO, 2006, Elsevier.)

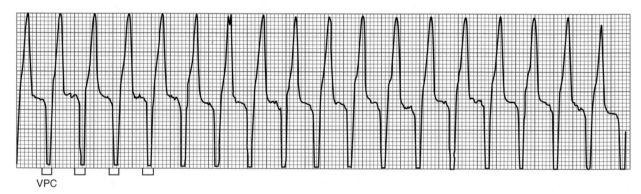

FIG. 6.31 Ventricular tachycardia (dog, lead II; 25 mm/s, 1.6 cm/mV). This is a series of wide, bizarre QRS complexes followed by T waves.

follow the previous QRS, interrupting an otherwise regular rhythm (Fig. 6.30). Like SPCs, they are early, but unlike SPCs, they appear different from normal QRS complexes. Isolated VPCs are commonly seen in anesthetized animals. They have a variety of causes, including heart disease, drug effects, hypoxia, and acid–base or electrolyte disorders. Epinephrine release in fearful patients is also a potent stimulus of VPCs. This is one reason why it is unwise to restrain a struggling animal forcibly during induction because release of epinephrine may potentiate severe and even fatal arrhythmias (particularly in patients given arrhythmogenic agents). VPCs may or may not require treatment, depending on the frequency.

- *Ventricular tachycardia* (Fig. 6.31) is a series of three or more VPCs in a row. It is a dangerous rhythm that significantly compromises cardiac output and requires intervention. Intravenous (IV) lidocaine is the most common treatment for severe VPCs.

- *Fibrillation.* Fibrillation is the chaotic, uncoordinated contraction of small muscle bundles within the atria or ventricles that appears as an undulating baseline with or without QRS complexes.

  - *Atrial fibrillation* appears as fine undulations of the baseline (often referred to as *f waves*), an absence of P waves, a high HR, and normal QRS complexes with irregular intervals between them (Fig. 6.32). This rhythm, which is usually caused by heart disease, decreases cardiac output and requires treatment.

  - *Ventricular fibrillation* appears as an irregular, undulating baseline, with complete absence of recognizable

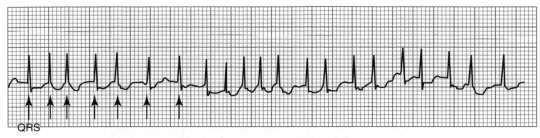

FIG. 6.32 Atrial fibrillation (cat; 25 mm/s, 1 cm/mV). Note the absence of P waves, the undulating baseline (f waves), and the irregular ventricular rate. (From Bonagura JD, Twedt DC: *Kirk's current veterinary therapy XIV*, St Louis, MO, 2009, Elsevier.)

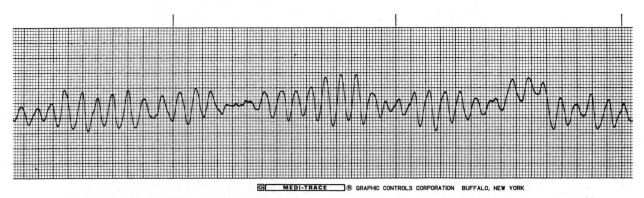

FIG. 6.33 Ventricular fibrillation (dog, lead II; 50 mm/s, 1 cm/mV). This is chaotic electrical activity unassociated with organized contraction of the heart muscle. (From Birchard SJ, Sherding RG: *Saunders manual of small animal practice*, ed 3, St Louis, MO, 2006, Elsevier.)

QRS complexes (Fig. 6.33). Ventricular fibrillation is associated with cardiac arrest and requires emergency treatment.

A change in the configuration of the QRS complex or T wave over time indicates hypoxia of the cardiac muscle, is dangerous, and requires immediate intervention.

Pulseless electrical activity (PEA) is the cessation of heart contractions and/or palpable pulses in the presence of a normal or nearly normal ECG and is associated with cardiac arrest. Because the ECG is not a sure indicator of mechanical activity of the heart, electrocardiographic monitoring must always be accompanied by physical monitoring of the heartbeat, apical pulse, and arterial pulses.

Capillary Refill Time

The CRT is the rate of return of color to oral mucous membranes after the application of gentle digital pressure (Fig. 6.34) and is indicative of the perfusion of the peripheral tissues with blood. The pressure applied to the mucous membranes compresses the small capillaries and temporarily blocks blood flow to that area. When the pressure is released, the capillaries rapidly refill with blood and the color returns, provided perfusion is adequate. Normal capillary refill is not always a reliable indicator of adequate circulation, however (e.g., CRT may appear normal shortly after euthanasia in some animals).

A prolonged CRT (>2 seconds) indicates that tissues in the area tested have reduced blood perfusion. This may be a result of vasoconstriction caused by epinephrine release. Poor perfusion may also be a result of low BP caused by anesthetic drugs

(including acepromazine, alpha$_2$-agonists, propofol, and inhalation agents), hypothermia, cardiac failure, excessive anesthetic depth, blood loss, or shock. Poor perfusion will also result in reduced temperature of the affected part.

Blood Pressure

BP is the force exerted by flowing blood on arterial walls. This monitoring parameter is used during anesthesia to evaluate tissue perfusion. BP is determined by complex interactions among HR, stroke volume (the volume of blood ejected by the heart on each beat), peripheral vascular resistance (the diameter of the vessels), arterial compliance (elasticity), and blood volume. Therefore it is altered by anything that affects these factors, including drugs, disease, surgical stimulation, and hydration status.

Normal BP varies throughout the cardiac cycle as the ventricles contract and relax. Systolic blood pressure (P_{SYS}) is produced by the contraction of the left ventricle as it propels blood through the systemic arteries. Diastolic blood pressure (P_{DIA}) is the pressure that remains in the arteries when the heart is in its resting phase between contractions. Mean arterial pressure (MAP) is the average pressure through the cardiac cycle and is the most important value from the anesthetist's standpoint because it is the best indicator of blood perfusion of the internal organs. MAP is automatically calculated by some instruments or can be mathematically calculated as follows:

$$MAP = P_{DIA} + \frac{1}{3}(P_{SYS} - P_{DIA})$$

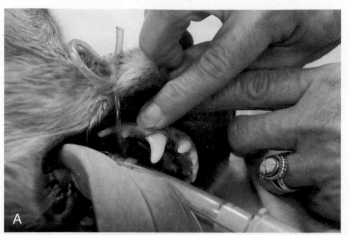

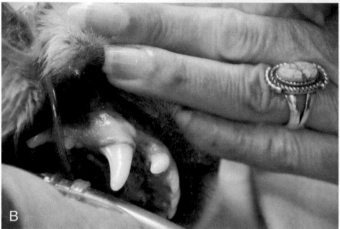
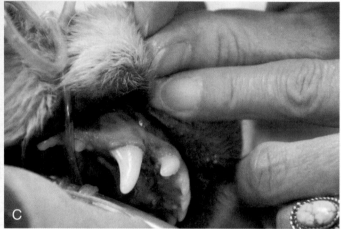

FIG. 6.34 Capillary refill time. **(A)** Application of digital pressure. **(B)** Blanching of the mucous membranes. **(C)** Return of color, which in a normal patient should occur in 2 seconds or less.

TECHNICIAN NOTE MAP is the average pressure through the cardiac cycle and is the most important value from the anesthetist's standpoint because it is the best indicator of blood perfusion of the internal organs.

All BP monitoring instruments can measure P_{SYS}, and some are able to measure P_{DIA} and MAP as well (transducers and oscillometric BP monitors). Because BP can be difficult to measure accurately, changes rapidly, and is subject to many influences, it is best to monitor trends rather than a single value. BP that is below normal limits is called *hypotension,* and BP that is above normal limits is called *hypertension.* BP may be decreased by anything that decreases HR, stroke volume, vascular resistance, or blood volume, and increased by anything that increases these parameters. Box 6.6 lists common causes of hypotension in anesthetized patients. Because of the complexity of the interactions among these parameters, interpretation of the significance of BP changes is not always straightforward. For example, under normal circumstances, the body compensates for MAP values between 60 and 150 mmHg by changing vascular resistance to maintain blood flow, and therefore the MAP can fall to as low as 60 mmHg without a significant change in tissue perfusion. In contrast, in situations when vascular resistance is high and cardiac output is

BOX 6.6 Common Causes of Hypotension

- Anesthetic agents (especially acepromazine, alpha$_2$-agonists, inhalant agents, propofol, and barbiturates)
- Excessive anesthetic depth
- Vasodilatation secondary to allergic reactions or endotoxic shock
- Blood loss
- Dehydration
- Cardiac arrhythmias
- Preexisting heart disease
- Positive-pressure ventilation
- Gastric distention

low, BP may remain normal even though perfusion is poor. So under normal circumstances in an awake animal, BP does not always reflect tissue perfusion.

During anesthesia, however, BP is a good indicator of tissue perfusion. This is because when inhalant anesthetics are used, the body's ability to compensate decreases as anesthetic depth increases, so that tissue perfusion is essentially directly determined by MAP. If MAP falls below 60 to 70 mmHg, blood flow to internal organs is reduced and tissues may become hypoxic. The kidneys are particularly sensitive to reduced perfusion and can fail postoperatively if the MAP is inadequate during anesthesia. This risk is increased by preexisting disease

TABLE 6.8 Normal Arterial Blood Pressure during Anesthesia

Species	Normal Systolic Arterial Blood Pressure (mmHg) (Anesthetized)	Normal Mean Arterial Blood Pressure (mmHg) (Anesthetized)	Normal Diastolic Arterial Blood Pressure (mmHg) (Anesthetized)	Report to the Veterinarian if:
Dog and cat	110–160	60–90	50–70	MAP <60–70; systolic <80–90
Horse	>80	60–90	>50	MAP <70; systolic <80
Cattle	>80	60–90	>50	MAP <60–70 systolic <80

and by some drugs, including nonsteroidal antiinflammatory drugs (NSAIDs). In horses, a MAP below 70 mmHg decreases blood flow to the muscle, predisposing the patient to postanesthetic myopathy.

When using a Doppler blood flow monitor, only the P_{SYS} can be measured. In these cases, P_{SYS} must be monitored in lieu of MAP and should not fall below 80 to 90 mmHg. (See Table 6.8 for normal blood pressure values during anesthesia.)

> **TECHNICIAN NOTE** During anesthesia, MAP is a good indicator of tissue perfusion. If MAP falls below 60–70 mmHg, blood flow to internal organs is reduced and tissues may become hypoxic. Every effort should be made to maintain a MAP of 60–70 mmHg or greater in small animals and ruminants, and 70 mmHg or greater in horses.

> **TECHNICIAN NOTE** When using a Doppler blood flow detector and sphygmomanometer, every effort should be made to maintain a P_{SYS} at 80–90 mmHg or greater in small animals.

Hypotension is common during anesthesia because most anesthetic drugs, with the exception of dissociatives, decrease BP, and because many common complications of anesthesia and surgery, including blood loss, also decrease it. Although a modest drop in BP is acceptable during anesthesia, every effort should be made to maintain a MAP of 60 to 70 mmHg or greater (70 mmHg or greater in horses). Changes in BP over the course of an anesthetic procedure give the anesthetist valuable information that can be used to warn of situations that may endanger the patient, including excessive blood loss, excessive anesthetic depth, decreased heart function, or changes in blood vessel tone. BP lower than minimum safe levels signals the need for intervention to support perfusion of vital tissues. Box 6.7 lists strategies to prevent hypotension.

Pulse strength. Pulse strength is a physical parameter that can be used as a rough indicator of BP. It is assessed by palpating a peripheral artery in one of several locations. Peripheral arteries appropriate to assess pulse strength include the lingual (dogs only) (Fig. 6.35 A), femoral (small animals and small ruminants only) (see Fig. 6.35 B), dorsal pedal (see Fig. 6.35 C), facial (horses only) (see Fig. 6.35 D), auricular (large animals only) (see Fig. 6.35 E and F), and carotid. A normal pulse should be strong and should occur shortly after each apical beat or S1 heart sound. During anesthesia, in most cases, the pulse strength naturally decreases, but the pulse should still be palpable during all stages.

BOX 6.7 Strategies to Prevent Hypotension

- Avoid excessive anesthetic depth
- Provide adequate analgesia
- Use preanesthetic medications to decrease the amount of general anesthetic required
- Minimize vaporizer dial settings by selecting balanced protocols designed to maintain the patient with a combination of injectable and inhalant agents
- Use caution when administering drugs that decrease cardiac output, induce bradycardia, or cause vasodilatation
- Administer intravenous (IV) fluids at a rate sufficient to maintain blood pressure.
- Some patients may require medication to maintain blood pressure (such as ephedrine, dobutamine, or dopamine)

Caution must be used when interpreting pulse strength because interpretation is subjective and normal pulse strength among healthy animals varies widely. Also, pulse strength does not always correlate well with BP because pulse strength is determined by the difference between P_{SYS} and P_{DIA}, vessel diameter, and other factors that do not always correlate with MAP or with tissue perfusion.

For example, the pressure difference between a P_{SYS} of 100 mmHg and a P_{DIA} of 30 mmHg is 70 mmHg. This relatively large difference will produce a strong pulse that will be subjectively interpreted as normal, even though the MAP in this patient is approximately 55 mmHg, which is inadequate. In contrast, the pressure difference between a P_{SYS} of 100 mmHg and a P_{DIA} of 70 mmHg is 30 mmHg, which will feel weak and will be interpreted as indicative of hypotension, even though the MAP is about 80 mmHg, which is within the normal range.

Despite these inaccuracies, by comparing pulse strength during the preanesthetic period with the pulse strength throughout the anesthetic period, many relative changes in BP can be detected that may indicate a problem and require further assessment by instrumentation.

Instruments used to monitor blood pressure. There are two general types of BP monitor: direct and indirect. When BP is monitored directly, the reading is obtained by means of a catheter inserted into an artery and attached to a pressure transducer (pressure sensor) and monitor. In the case of indirect BP monitoring, the reading is obtained by using an external sensor and cuff.

Direct BP monitoring is infrequently performed in small animal veterinary practice but is used commonly in equine practice and in research and referral institutions. An indwelling catheter is placed in the femoral or dorsal pedal artery (small animals) or the facial or auricular artery (large animals) by means of a surgical cutdown or percutaneous insertion technique. The catheter is

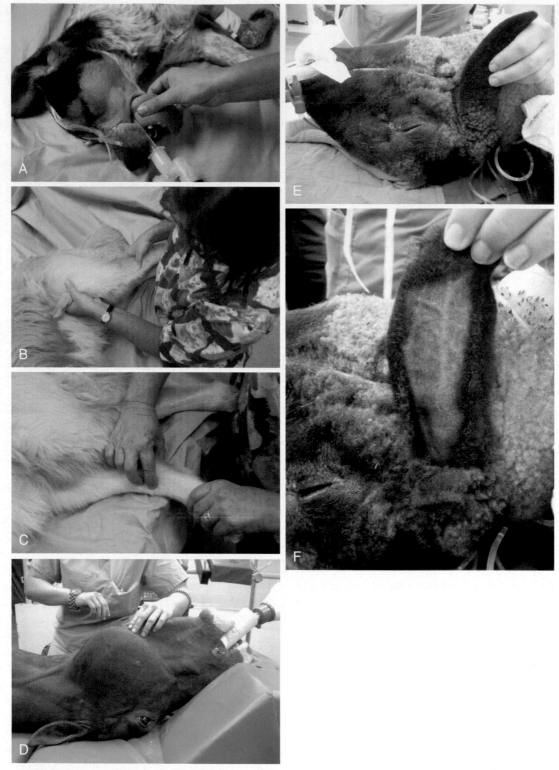

FIG. 6.35 Assessment of pulse strength. **(A)** Lingual artery (dog). Place the forefinger firmly but gently over the ventral aspect of the midline of the tongue. **(B)** Femoral artery (dog). Cup the hand under the thigh from a cranial approach. Place the forefinger or second finger firmly but gently over the caudomedial aspect of the proximal femur. **(C)** Dorsal pedal artery (dog). Place the forefinger over the dorsomedial aspect of the tarsus. **(D)** Facial artery (horse). Place the forefinger firmly but gently over the ventrolateral aspect of the ramus of the mandible. **(E)** and **(F)** Auricular artery (sheep). Firmly but gently pinch the pinna of the ear over the artery (located near the line visible down the center of the ear in Fig. 6.35 F) between the thumb and forefinger or second finger.

connected by a length of fluid-filled tubing to a manometer or pressure transducer, which displays the pressure as directly measured from within the artery. Direct BP monitoring gives the anesthetist a continuous reading of the BP throughout the cardiac cycle and is more accurate than indirect methods. More detail concerning direct BP monitoring may be found in Chapter 10. In general practice, BP is more commonly determined by indirect methods, which are noninvasive and technically less demanding than direct monitoring. There are two basic types of indirect method, Doppler and oscillometric, both of which use a cuff to occlude and release blood flow sequentially in a major artery of a limb or the tail. These systems differ in the way the pressure is measured.

> **TECHNICIAN NOTE** In general practice, indirect monitors are most commonly used to measure BP. There are two basic types of indirect monitors, Doppler and oscillometric, both of which use a cuff to occlude and release blood flow sequentially in a major artery of a limb or the tail. These systems differ in the way the pressure is measured.

The photoplethysmograph is another method used to provide indirect BP measurements. This method uses infrared light to measure changes in volume caused by pulse pressure. This instrument, designed for humans, is not in common use in veterinary patients but may be especially useful for dogs and cats weighing less than 10 kg. It creates a continuous waveform tracing in real time and so is able to display systolic, diastolic, and mean pressures.

In human patients, BP is routinely determined by using a stethoscope to listen for blood flow in a peripheral artery as a cuff is sequentially inflated until the flow stops and deflated until the flow resumes. As the cuff is slowly deflated, the point at which flow is first audible (because of turbulent blood flow through a partially occluded artery) represents the P_{SYS} and the point at which it is no longer audible (because of restoration of normal flow) represents the P_{DIA}. This method is not practical in domestic animals because arterial flow is not audible with a stethoscope.

Doppler blood flow detector. The Doppler blood flow detector is a monitoring device that consists of an ultrasonic probe and an electronic monitor. The Doppler probe contains a crystal that emits ultrasound frequency waves and another crystal that receives the returning echoes. Outgoing waves bounce off red blood cells (RBCs) traveling inside a pulsating artery and return to the probe, where they are sent to an electronic monitor for processing. The monitor converts the returning echoes into a "whooshing" sound audible to the attendant via a speaker or earphones. The frequency (or pitch) of the sound changes in proportion to the velocity of the RBCs, and the intensity changes in proportion to the number of RBCs detected. This device can be used to monitor HR and heart rhythm continuously or can be used with a conventional cuff and sphygmomanometer to determine the P_{SYS}. P_{DIA} and MAP cannot be measured by most Doppler systems.

Use and operation. Choose a location to place the probe over a peripheral artery. In small-animal patients, the ventral surface of a paw just proximal to the metacarpal or metatarsal pad (over the median palmar or median plantar artery), the dorsomedial surface of the tarsus (over the dorsal pedal artery), the ventral surface of the tail base (over the coccygeal artery), or over the medial surface of the thigh in patients weighing under 5 kg (over the femoral artery) are all possible locations. In large-animal patients, the ventral tail is the most frequently used site. Fig. 6.36 shows common locations for placement of the probe.

After choosing the location, clip a 1- to 2-cm square patch of hair over the artery, gently cleanse the skin, and apply a generous amount of ultrasonic gel. Avoid lubricating jelly and gels

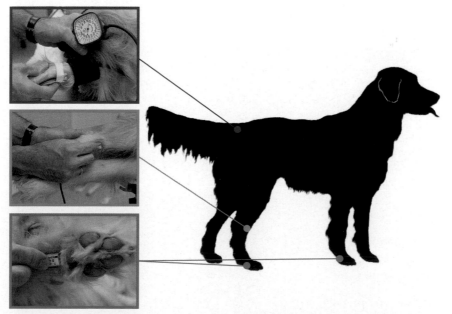

FIG. 6.36 Locations for Doppler probe placement. *Red,* Determination of P_{SYS} by use of a sphygmomanometer with the cuff placed around the tail base and the probe placed on the ventral surface of the tail distal to the cuff. *Green,* Probe over the dorsomedial surface of the hock. *Blue,* Probe proximal to the metatarsal pad or metacarpal pad.

containing electrolytic substances such as those used for electro-cardiographic leads. The concave surface of the probe must be oriented parallel to and precisely over the artery and must make firm but not excessive contact. Acquiring a good signal requires very fine changes in position of the probe, sometimes of only a millimeter or two. This can be a challenge, so the technician must be prepared to persevere until an audible signal is found. Once a signal has been found, the probe can be held in place manually by the technician if it is going to be used for only a short time (Fig. 6.37), but if it is to be used as a heart monitor for the duration of an entire procedure, it may be carefully taped in place.

Doppler probes are expensive and can easily be damaged. They must therefore be handled carefully. After use, clean the probe by wiping it gently with a gauze sponge. Gentle cleaning with mild detergent and warm water and wipe down with a manufacturer-recommended disinfectant is acceptable, but the probe must not be immersed, scrubbed, or autoclaved. It should be stored in a protective case.

Determining the blood pressure. When used with a cuff and sphygmomanometer, the Doppler monitor can be used to determine BP (see Fig. 6.36). A sphygmomanometer is an instrument, much like the pressure manometer on an anesthetic machine, which measures pressure within a cuff. The principle by which this system operates is as follows: when the cuff is inflated with a rubber bulb, an artery lying beneath the cuff is compressed. When the cuff pressure exceeds the P_{SYS}, blood flow through the artery stops and the sound is no longer audible. When the cuff pressure is slowly released, blood flow resumes and is again audible when the cuff pressure equals the P_{SYS}.

> **TECHNICIAN NOTE** When the BP is measured, the width of the cuff should be 30%–50% of the circumference of the extremity (ideally 40%), and the cuff should be placed firmly but not too tightly over a peripheral artery. The cuff should be wrapped slightly more tightly in large animals than in small animals and should ideally be at the same horizontal plane as the heart.

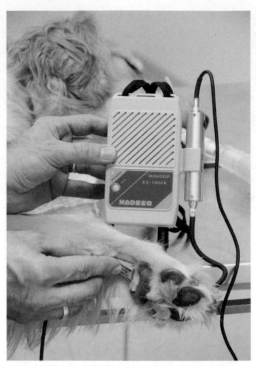

FIG. 6.37 Doppler monitor base unit with the probe positioned over the ventral surface of the metacarpus proximal to the metacarpal pad.

To determine the P_{SYS}, fit a cuff to the extremity. The width of the cuff should be 30% to 50% of the circumference of the extremity (ideally 40%) (Fig. 6.38, *inset*). Place the cuff firmly but not too tightly, proximal to the site where the probe is positioned. The cuff should be wrapped slightly more tightly on large animals than on small animals and should ideally be at the same horizontal plane as the heart (the level of the sternum when in lateral recumbency or the shoulder when in dorsal recumbency). All cuffs contain a balloon inside that inflates as

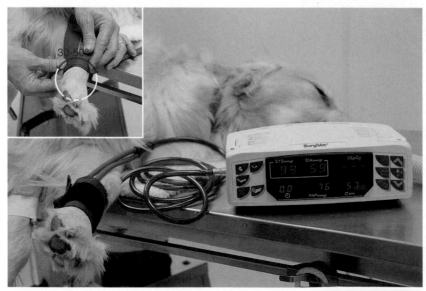

FIG. 6.38 Oscillometric blood pressure (BP) monitor with a cuff placed on the metacarpus. The following measurements are indicated: systolic BP (P_{SYS}), 99 mmHg; diastolic BP (P_{DIA}), 59 mmHg; mean arterial pressure (MAP), 76 mmHg; heart rate 57 bpm. *Inset,* Selecting an appropriately sized blood pressure cuff, the width of which should be 30% to 50% of the circumference of the extremity (ideally 40%).

PROCEDURE 6.1 Measuring Blood Pressure With a Doppler Device

1. Clip any hair from the area where the probe will be placed.
2. Apply ultrasound gel to the concave portion of the probe.
3. Select a cuff that has a width 30%–50% of the circumference of the extremity used for the reading (wrap intravenous [IV] tubing around the limb to measure it). Place the cuff snugly over the limb or tail, proximal to where the probe will be placed.
4. Place the probe over the appropriate artery distal to the cuff (coccygeal, median palmar, median plantar, or dorsal pedal artery).
5. Turn on the amplifier. Adjust the position of the probe until a signal is acquired.
6. Attach the manometer and bulb to the cuff tubing.
7. You may tape the probe in place, but do not apply the tape tightly or the artery will be occluded and no readings will be possible.
8. Inflate the cuff until the sound stops.
9. Slowly release pressure from the cuff until the first "whooshing" sound is heard. This represents the P_{SYS}.
10. Take five readings. Discard the highest and lowest values and average the remaining values to determine the P_{SYS}.

the cuff is pressurized. Some cuffs require the balloon to be centered over the artery but others do not, as specified in the manufacturer's equipment manual. After establishing a good Doppler signal, use the bulb to inflate the cuff until the signal can no longer be heard. While reading the manometer, gradually decrease the pressure until the pulsing signal first returns. This represents the P_{SYS}. P_{DIA} is the pressure indicated just before the sound becomes continuous but is difficult to determine reliably with this instrument. Procedure 6.1 describes the technique for measuring BP with a Doppler device.

Specific locations in which adequate superficial arteries are located include the medial aspect of the proximal forelimb (radial artery), over the palmar aspect of the metacarpus (median palmar artery—Fig. 6.39, *blue*), proximal to the tarsus over the dorsomedial aspect of the limb (cranial tibial artery), distal to the tarsus over the dorsomedial aspect of the limb (dorsal pedal artery—Fig. 6.39, *green*), and over the ventral aspect of the tail base (coccygeal artery—Fig. 6.39, *red*).

Doppler systems are accurate over a wide range of pressures and are the preferred instruments for cats and small dogs. They are labor intensive, however, because there is no automatic readout, and like most instruments, they are subject to various unique technical problems and artifacts, including the following:

- Doppler monitors underestimate the P_{SYS} in cats by about 15 mmHg but are fairly accurate in dogs and large animals. Therefore when taking a cat's BP, add 15 mmHg to the pressure indicated on the manometer.
- Values are affected by patient position in relationship to the probe and blood flow to the extremity and can be altered by ropes used to tie the patient to the table as well as many other factors. Therefore several readings should be taken and averaged.
- The signal is difficult to maintain over time and is commonly lost if the patient is moved or is shivering, the probe shifts, or the contact pressure is not exactly right.
- Finding the right location and tightness for the cuff can be challenging and requires experience. The use of a cuff that is too loose will give falsely high readings and a cuff that is too tight can cause discomfort and venous distention.
- The use of a cuff that is too narrow will give falsely high readings and a cuff that is too wide will give falsely low readings.

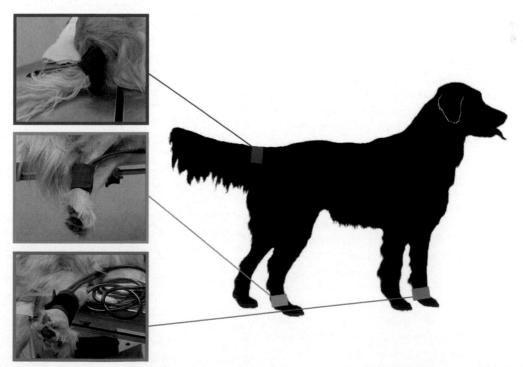

FIG. 6.39 Locations for placement of a blood pressure cuff. *Red*—base of the tail. *Green*—metatarsus. *Blue*—metacarpus. Note that the cuff may also be placed over the proximal forelimb above the carpus (not pictured) or proximal to the tarsus (not pictured).

Oscillometric blood pressure monitors. An oscillometric BP monitor (oscillometer) consists of a cuff with an internal pressure-sensing bladder connected to a computerized monitor (see Fig. 6.38). The machine inflates and deflates the cuff, and the computer measures the oscillations in intracuff pressure caused by the subtle volume changes of the extremity resulting from pulsations of the artery beneath the cuff. It then calculates the systolic, mean, and diastolic pressures, and the HR from the pressure changes.

Oscillometers are more expensive than Doppler devices but offer two significant advantages: they work automatically, and they determine the P_{DIA} and MAP in addition to P_{SYS}.

Use and operation. The cuff is selected in the same way and placed in the same locations as a Doppler cuff. Currently available machines are technologically sophisticated and will automatically inflate the cuff at preprogrammed intervals (such as every 5 minutes) or on demand (when a button is pushed). Alarm limits can be programmed for any of the parameters and the computer may be able to store or print patient data. These machines contain rechargeable batteries and require very little maintenance other than cleaning and periodic recharging.

As with Doppler detectors, oscillometers are subject to artifacts and technical problems, as follows:

- These instruments are relatively accurate in animals weighing over 7 kg but may have difficulty detecting pulsations in cats and other animals with small superficial arteries.
- They tend to underestimate high pressures and overestimate low pressures.
- They are also inaccurate in animals with significant hypotension, arrhythmias, or fast HRs.
- P_{SYS} measured by these instruments is generally 10 to 15 mmHg lower than that obtained by direct BP monitoring in dogs.
- The instrument may not work if the patient moves or is shivering, or if the cuff slips.
- If the cuff is too loose, the machine may be unable to measure the pressure. If too tight, the values will be inaccurate.

Central venous pressure. CVP is the BP in a large central vein such as the anterior vena cava. This value allows the veterinarian to assess blood return to the heart and heart function. This value is especially helpful in monitoring animals for right-sided heart failure because it can detect the increased pressure in the vena cava that results from this condition. It is also useful in preventing overhydration in animals receiving IV fluids because CVP values rise when blood volume is excessive.

CVP can be directly measured by inserting a long catheter percutaneously into the jugular vein or by cutting down into the jugular vein. The catheter is advanced into the anterior vena cava and toward the heart so that the tip of the catheter lies close to the right atrium. The catheter is connected to a water manometer to obtain a measurement. The manometer should be positioned so that "0" on the manometer is at the same horizontal plane as the right atrium (halfway between the shoulder and sternum in sternally recumbent patients, level with the sternum in laterally recumbent patients, and level with the shoulder in dorsally recumbent patients; Fig. 6.40). If the catheter is correctly positioned, the meniscus of the fluid in the manometer should rise and fall with each breath. Normal CVP

in dogs and cats is less than 8 cm H_2O. Pressures over 12 to 15 cm H_2O (taken during exhalation) are considered elevated. As with arterial BP, it is usually more valuable to monitor trends over time rather than base an assessment on a single reading.

Indicators of Oxygenation

The objective of the ACVAA monitoring guidelines for oxygenation is "to ensure adequate oxygenation of the patient's arterial blood." To meet this objective, the ACVAA makes the following recommendation:

Assessment of oxygenation should be done whenever possible by pulse oximetry, with blood gas analysis being employed when necessary for more critically ill patients.

Mucous Membrane Color

Mucous membrane color is most commonly assessed by observing the gingiva (see Fig. 6.34 C). Normal mucous membrane color is pink, although the color varies somewhat among patients. For this reason, mucous membrane color should be assessed before each procedure so that the anesthetist knows what is normal for the patient and can use this as a point of comparison. This parameter gives the anesthetist a crude assessment of both oxygenation and tissue perfusion. In patients with pigmented gums, alternative sites may be used to assess mucous membrane color, including the tongue, the conjunctiva of the lower eyelid, or the mucous membrane lining the prepuce or vulva.

Pale mucous membranes indicate intraoperative blood loss, anemia from any cause, or poor capillary perfusion (as may occur with vasoconstriction, excessive anesthetic depth, or prolonged anesthesia). Cyanosis (purple or blue discoloration of the mucous membranes or skin) indicates very low blood oxygen concentration (a partial pressure [Pao_2] of approximately 35 to 45 mmHg) in patients with a normal packed cell volume (PCV). Some common causes of cyanosis are respiratory arrest, oxygen deprivation (such as when the oxygen tank is empty or the flowmeters are inadvertently turned off), and severe pulmonary disease.

Mucous membrane color is not a reliable indicator of perfusion because many other factors affect it, including body temperature, vascular resistance, and gum disease. It is a crude indicator of oxygenation for two reasons. First, in animals with a normal PCV, the blood oxygen concentration is so low by the time cyanosis occurs that the situation is already a medical emergency. Second, there must be a minimum concentration of deoxygenated hemoglobin for cyanosis to occur. Consequently, animals with severe anemia may not have enough hemoglobin to reach this threshold and may not become cyanotic, even though tissues are hypoxic.

Before examination of the ways in which oxygen is measured, it is important to understand how oxygen is carried in the bloodstream.

TECHNICIAN NOTE Pale mucous membranes indicate intraoperative blood loss, anemia from any cause, or poor capillary perfusion. Cyanosis indicates very low blood oxygen concentration.

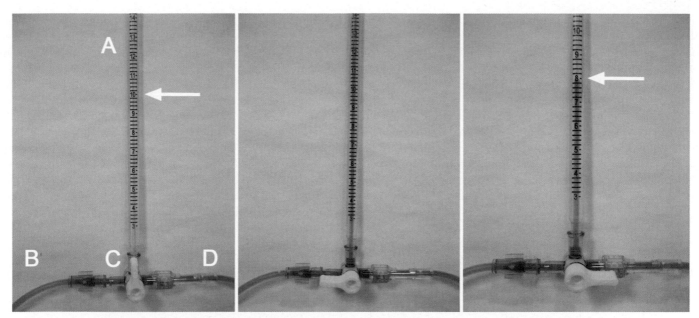

FIG. 6.40 Central venous pressure (CVP) manometer. *Left:* Setup for measuring CVP. A manometer calibrated in centimeters **(A)** is connected to a three-way stopcock **(C)** that is inserted between the extension tubing leading to the central venous catheter in the patient **(B)** and the intravenous (IV) fluid bag **(D)**. Note that the fluid has been colored red for clarity in this image. As CVP can range from slightly positive to slightly negative, a convenient reference point should be chosen as the zero, in this case 10 cm *(arrow)*. This zero point should be placed level with the right atrium of the patient by attaching the apparatus to a sliding IV stand. With the three-way stopcock off to the manometer, IV fluids flow from the bag to the patient. *Middle:* Obtaining a CVP measurement requires two steps. First, the three-way stopcock is turned so that the IV fluid bag and the manometer are connected. Fluid should be allowed to flow up the manometer to a point above the zero mark. *Right:* Second, the three-way stopcock is turned so that the manometer is now connected to the extension tubing leading to the patient. The fluid column in the manometer will then equilibrate. Once the fluid in the manometer stops falling or rising, this can be read as the CVP. In this case, the fluid fell to 8 (arrow), which is 2 less than 10 (used as the zero point). The CVP is therefore −2 cm H_2O. Note that at the point of equilibration, there will be small movements of the fluid column due to changes in pressure in the chest during breathing. These changes will be more apparent with larger animals and patients being ventilated. Once the CVP reading has been recorded, the stopcock is returned to the position on the left.

Physiology of Oxygen Transport

As discussed previously, tissues must have adequate oxygen at all times to perform metabolic processes. This need is paramount in the brain and heart, which use the highest proportion of oxygen and which will be damaged within seconds or minutes when oxygen levels are decreased. Consequently, assessment of blood oxygen levels is a critical component of patient monitoring.

The total oxygen content of the blood is carried in two forms: as free, unbound O_2 molecules dissolved in plasma; and as oxygen that is chemically bound to the hemoglobin contained in RBCs. Each hemoglobin molecule has four oxygen binding sites, each of which can bind one molecule of O_2. Thus each hemoglobin molecule can carry four oxygen molecules if all the binding sites are full. When all available binding sites are occupied with oxygen, the hemoglobin is said to be 100% saturated.

In healthy patients, dissolved oxygen in plasma represents a small amount of the total blood oxygen content, whereas bound oxygen represents the majority. For example, in a healthy animal breathing room air (with approximately 21% oxygen), the amount of oxygen dissolved in arterial blood is approximately

1.5% of the total content and the remaining 98.5% is bound to hemoglobin. Thus the majority of oxygen necessary for normal cell function is carried by hemoglobin. That is why PCV is such an important determinant of oxygen available to the tissues.

> **TECHNICIAN NOTE** In nonanemic animals (with normal hemoglobin concentration), saturation alone gives the anesthetist a good estimate of oxygen available to the tissues. In contrast, a patient with anemia may have severely decreased oxygen availability even though saturation is normal.

Blood Oxygen is Measured in One of Three Ways:

1. Calculated oxygen content measures the total volume of oxygen in the blood, including both dissolved and bound forms, expressed in milliliters per deciliter (mL/dL). This system of measurement accurately measures total oxygen available to the tissues. Arterial oxygen content is calculated by using the following formula: $Cao_2 = (Hb \times 1.39 \times Sao_2/100) + (Pao_2 \times 0.003)$, where Cao_2 = calculated arterial oxygen content, Hb = hemoglobin in grams per deciliter

(g/dL), Sao_2 = arterial oxygen saturation (expressed as a percent), and Pao_2 = partial pressure of oxygen in arterial blood (mmHg). In a healthy animal breathing room air (with ~21% oxygen) with 15 g/dL of hemoglobin that is 100% saturated, each deciliter of arterial blood contains about 21.15 mL of oxygen (0.3 mL dissolved in plasma and 20.85 mL bound to hemoglobin). In this situation, oxygen availability is largely dependent on hemoglobin concentration and saturation. Therefore in nonanemic animals (with normal hemoglobin concentration), saturation alone gives the anesthetist a good estimate of oxygen available to the tissues. In contrast, a patient with an anemia may have severely decreased oxygen availability, even though saturation is normal.

2. **Partial pressure of oxygen** (Po_2) measures the unbound O_2 molecules dissolved in the plasma and is expressed in millimeters of mercury (mmHg). Partial pressure differs depending on whether arterial, capillary, or venous blood is measured. Oxygen content is highest after oxygen is picked up by blood in the lungs, decreases as it is consumed by the tissues, and is lowest as the blood travels back to the heart before reoxygenation in the lungs. Normal partial pressure of oxygen in arterial blood (Pao_2) in an animal breathing room air is about 90 to 110 mmHg (100 mmHg for practical purposes). In contrast, the partial pressure of oxygen in venous blood (Pvo_2) is about 40 mmHg owing to extraction of the difference (60 mmHg) by the tissues. Partial pressure represents only a small portion of the total amount of oxygen available to tissues (1.5%) because it does not measure bound oxygen at all.

3. **Percent oxygen saturation** (So_2) measures the percentage of the total number of hemoglobin binding sites occupied by oxygen molecules. Like partial pressure, oxygen saturation varies depending on whether it is sampled in the arterial blood, capillary blood, or venous blood. Normal arterial oxygen saturation (Sao_2) is 97% or above. Normal venous saturation (Svo_2) is about 75%. Unlike partial pressure, percent oxygen saturation measures the majority of oxygen available to tissues (98.5%).

The relationship between partial pressure and oxygen saturation. The partial pressure of oxygen in the plasma is dependent almost exclusively on the amount of oxygen in the alveoli and the health of the lungs. Decreased inspired oxygen or lung disease will decrease partial pressure. Partial pressure in turn influences saturation of the hemoglobin because there must be an adequate level of dissolved oxygen in the blood for binding to occur. Thus partial pressure and oxygen saturation are directly related (when one goes up, the other does also). This relationship is relatively predictable in healthy patients; knowing one allows the anesthetist to estimate the other.

However, this direct relationship between the two is not linear but looks rather more like the first big hill on a roller coaster. This means that as the partial pressure decreases, the saturation decreases very slowly at first, but the decrease gradually accelerates. For example, when a patient is breathing 100% oxygen, the Pao_2 is about 500 mmHg and hemoglobin is nearly 100% saturated (Box 6.8, Fig. 1). When the Pao_2 decreases from 500 mmHg to 100 mmHg (a drop of 400 mmHg), as for a patient breathing room air, saturation drops only from 100% to about 98% (see Box 6.8, Fig. 2). As Pao_2 drops from 100 to 80 mmHg (a drop of 20 mmHg), the saturation decreases from 98% to 95% (see Box 6.8, Fig. 3). Below this point, the saturation drops more quickly. As Pao_2 drops from 80 to 60 mmHg (also a drop of 20 mmHg), the saturation drops from 95% to 90% (see Box 6.8, Fig. 4). When Pao_2 drops from 60 to 40 mmHg (again, a drop of 20 mmHg), the saturation drops much more quickly, from 90% to 75% (see Box 6.8, Fig. 5). Therefore in animals with normal hemoglobin, the total oxygen available to the tissue decreases very little at partial pressures above 80 mmHg (saturation above 95%), whereas the total oxygen available to the tissues decreases much more rapidly below this level.

In contrast, when hemoglobin is low (the patient is anemic), neither of these parameters gives an accurate measure of oxygen availability. This is because even if the partial pressure and/or saturation is normal, the carrying capacity of the blood is severely decreased because of the decrease in the number of hemoglobin binding sites. For example, a patient with a hemoglobin of 5 g/dL (equivalent to a very anemic patient with a PCV of about 15%) breathing room air or 100% oxygen will have a total blood oxygen content of only slightly more than one-third of the normal level, even though percent saturation and partial pressure are both normal. Therefore with anemic patients, the value of these parameters in predicting patient tissue oxygenation is limited.

> **TECHNICIAN NOTE** When a patient is anemic, neither Pao_2 nor Spo_2 gives an accurate measure of oxygen availability. This is because even if the Pao_2 and/or Spo_2 is normal, the carrying capacity of the blood is severely decreased because of the decrease in the number of hemoglobin binding sites.

Once hemoglobin is 100% saturated, as occurs when the partial pressure is near 120 mmHg, any further increase in inspired oxygen will have almost no effect on the oxygen-carrying capacity of the blood and thus will be of little benefit to the patient. When the partial pressure of oxygen decreases to values lower than about 80 mmHg, as could occur with lung disease, lack of oxygen, inadequate ventilation, or shunting, the saturation begins to decrease more quickly. Saturation is therefore an early warning sign that can alert the anesthetist to a potentially devastating decrease in the oxygen content of the blood.

When patients are breathing pure oxygen from an anesthetic machine, the amount of dissolved oxygen (Pao_2) can increase markedly (up to about 500 mmHg). But as dissolved oxygen represents only a very small proportion of the total oxygen content and because hemoglobin is already nearly 100% saturated when the patient is breathing room air, this extra oxygen contributes only about a 10% increase in the total oxygen content of the blood.

Both Po_2 and So_2 can be measured, although by different instruments. Blood gas analyzers measure Pao_2; pulse oximeters measure Spo_2. Both values reflect inspired oxygen and how well the lungs deliver oxygen to the blood. Most anesthetized

BOX 6.8 How to Read Oxygen Dissociation Curves

At the top of each figure is the oxygen dissociation curve, which illustrates the relationship between partial pressure of oxygen and oxygen saturation (with Po_2 on the x-axis and So_2 on the y-axis).

When the amount of dissolved oxygen (Po_2) is above 100 mmHg (after oxygenation in the lungs), nearly all (at least 98%) of the binding sites on the hemoglobin molecules are occupied. However, as the blood reaches the systemic capillaries, oxygen diffuses into the tissues causing the Po_2 to decrease. As the Po_2 decreases, oxygen separates or "dissociates" from the hemoglobin to meet tissue needs.

The bar below the dissociation curve labeled "Hemoglobin Saturation" compares the proportion of the binding sites on the hemoglobin molecules that are occupied (in green) with the proportion of the binding sites that are unoccupied (in purple). The bar to in the lower right represents the relative color of the blood at the indicated saturation. Note that as the number of sites occupied decreases, the color of the hemoglobin and the blood gradually changes (representing the change in light absorption associated with decreased saturation). Although exaggerated in these illustrations, a change in color actually occurs in live, nonanemic patients, leading to visible cyanosis in patients with dangerously decreased saturation.

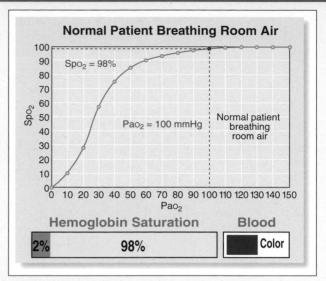

FIG. 2 When breathing 21% oxygen, a patient will have a Pao_2 of approximately 100 mmHg and a Spo_2 of approximately 98%. In this scenario, approximately 2% of the available binding sites are unoccupied and the color is subtly changed.

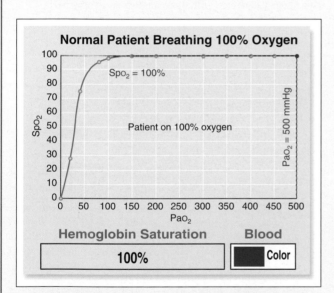

FIG. 1 When breathing 100% oxygen, a patient will have a Pao_2 of approximately 500 mmHg and a Spo_2 of nearly 100%. In this scenario, all binding sites on the hemoglobin molecules are occupied and the blood is bright red.

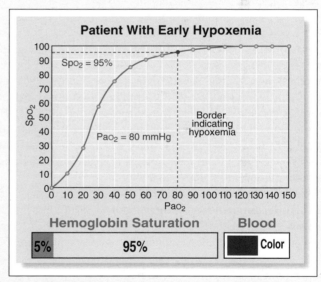

FIG. 3 A patient with a Pao_2 less than 80 mmHg or a Spo_2 less than 95% is considered to be hypoxemic. In this scenario, approximately 5% of the available binding sites are unoccupied and the color is changed to a slightly greater degree.

Continued

BOX 6.8 How to Read Oxygen Dissociation Curves—cont'd

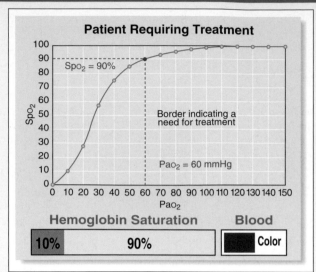

FIG. 4 A patient with a Pao_2 less than 60 mmHg or a Spo_2 less than 90% requires treatment. In this scenario, approximately 10% of the available binding sites are unoccupied and the color is noticeably changed.

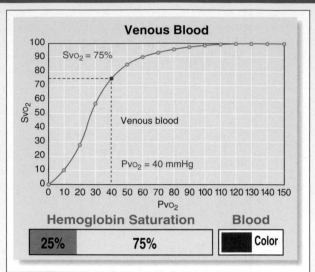

FIG. 5 The Pvo_2 of venous blood is approximately 40 mmHg and the Svo_2 is approximately 75%. In this scenario, approximately 25% of the available binding sites are unoccupied and the color is significantly changed. If the oxygen content of arterial blood decreases approximately to this level in a patient with a normal packed cell volume (PCV), cyanosis will occur, indicating a critically low oxygen level, which will rapidly lead to death if not immediately corrected.

animals show a greatly elevated Pao_2 (up to 500 mmHg compared with the normal 90 to 110 mmHg for an awake patient breathing room air) because they are breathing almost 100% oxygen from the anesthetic machine, whereas the conscious animal breathes approximately 21% oxygen in room air. Similarly, Spo_2 readings from anesthetized animals breathing pure oxygen are usually high (97% to 99%).

Low Pao_2 and Spo_2 values are sometimes observed during anesthesia. A Pao_2 value below 80 mmHg (Spo_2 95%) indicates hypoxemia and a value below 60 mmHg (Spo_2 90%) indicates the need for oxygen supplementation and possibly assisted ventilation.

Pulse Oximeter

A pulse oximeter estimates the saturation of hemoglobin (So_2) expressed as a percentage of the total binding sites. Pulse oximeters are readily available, relatively inexpensive, noninvasive, portable, and relatively easy to use. A pulse oximeter is equipped with a probe, which is sensitive to both the absorption of light by hemoglobin and to blood pulsations in the small arterioles (Fig. 6.41).

Red- and infrared-wavelength light emitted by the probe is passed through or reflected off the tissue bed, and the frequency of the emergent light is read by a sensor and analyzed. The machine determines the oxygen saturation (Spo_2) by calculating the difference between levels of oxygenated and deoxygenated hemoglobin based on subtle differences in absorption of light. The HR is determined by detecting pulsations in the small arterioles. Both the HR and the oxygen saturation are digitally displayed.

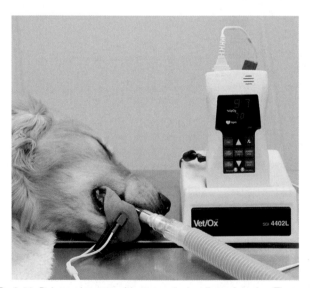

FIG. 6.41 Pulse oximeter with transmission lingual probe. The upper number (97) represents the percent oxygen saturation (Spo_2). The lower number (70) represents the heart rate in beats per minute.

Some pulse oximeters also display a plethysmogram, which is a graphic representation of the blood pressure pulse wave in the small arterioles. This waveform helps the anesthetist determine if tissue perfusion is adequate to produce a reliable signal, in which case, the plethysmogram should closely resemble the waveform produced by a direct intraarterial blood pressure monitor (Fig. 6.42). This suggests that the displayed

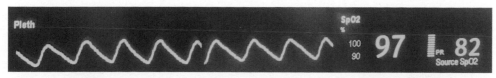

FIG. 6.42 Normal plethysmograph wave form on a pulse oximeter, showing an SpO_2 of 97% and a pulse rate of 82 bpm. A normal waveform and $SpO_2 > 95\%$ suggests perfusion of the tissue is adequate.

SpO_2 is accurate. A weak signal (waveform that is smaller than normal) may indicate that the displayed SpO_2 is not accurate because perfusion of the tissue is poor or the probe needs to be repositioned or cleaned. Checking to see if the probe functions correctly on a person will eliminate the possibility that the probe has stopped functioning and needs to be replaced. Thus use of a machine with a plethysmograph display helps the anesthetist determine whether or not abnormal SpO_2 values are real or artifactual and respond in an appropriate and timely manner.

Normally, when pure oxygen is breathed, the hemoglobin in the lungs is at least 98% saturated with oxygen. For practical purposes, during oxygen administration, the oxygen saturation should be equal to or greater than 95%. A pulse oximeter reading of 90% to 94% must be investigated because it indicates that the patient's hemoglobin is not adequately saturated and the patient is hypoxemic. Saturation of less than 90% indicates serious hypoxemia and a need for therapy. Saturation of less than 85% for longer than 30 seconds is a medical emergency. (See Table 6.9 for interpretation of oxygen saturation values during anesthesia.)

TECHNICIAN NOTE
- When breathing 100% oxygen, the oxygen saturation should be equal to or greater than 95% (>97% in most cases)
- A pulse oximeter reading of 90%–94% must be investigated because it indicates that the patient is hypoxemic
- Saturation of less than 90% indicates serious hypoxemia and a need for therapy
- Saturation of less than 85% for longer than 30 sec is a medical emergency

---

Use and operation. Pulse oximeters usually come with a variety of probes, each of which analyzes light either passed through or reflected off a tissue bed. The probes are classified as transmission or reflective. Transmission probes are constructed in a "clothespin-" type configuration. One of the jaws houses a light source and the other houses a sensor that detects the transmitted light. Transmission probes must be applied over a nonpigmented tissue bed that is thin enough to allow light transmission through the tissue. In anesthetized animals, the tongue is commonly used, but the probe may also be applied to the pinna, toe web, vulvar fold, prepuce, Achilles tendon, lip, or any other area that is thin, relatively hairless, and nonpigmented. Although these probes are able to function through a thin hair coat, excessive hair will prevent operation. Fig. 6.43 shows examples of probe types and placement.

Reflective probes reflect light off a tissue bed. The light source and sensor are located next to each other on one side of the probe. These probes are placed inside a hollow organ such as the esophagus or rectum, or against the ventral surface of the tail, with the light source and sensor in contact with a tissue bed. During placement of a reflective probe in the rectum, care must be taken to displace the feces from the wall of the rectum using a finger and place the side of the probe that houses the light source and sensor against the tissue.

Pulse oximeter probes can be frustrating to work with because the probes may be temperamental and often give inaccurate readings or lose the signal altogether. When this happens, values will no longer appear on the display, the numbers will be incorrect, or an alarm may sound. Tissue pigmentation, motion, excessive pressure, drying of mucous membranes, and patient conditions such as anemia, icterus, vasoconstriction, hypotension, hypothermia, or edema will all decrease accuracy or result in signal loss. Other factors such as interference from ambient light, use of electrosurgery, or use of a probe made from a different manufacturer from the specific monitor you are using may also interfere with the signal. Box 6.9 contains suggestions for troubleshooting signal loss.

Even when a good signal is obtained, it is important to keep in mind that an adequate SpO_2 does not always mean that tissue oxygenation is adequate. Circumstances in which SpO_2 does not accurately represent tissue oxygenation include the presence of carboxyhemoglobin (hemoglobin bound to carbon monoxide in an animal with carbon monoxide poisoning), which will cause falsely high SpO_2 levels; the presence of methemoglobin (hemoglobin that is unable to carry oxygen due to exposure to certain drugs or toxins), which may cause either falsely high or falsely low SpO_2 levels; and severe anemia (low red blood cell mass), which will register as adequate saturation in the face of inadequate oxygen delivery the tissues. So as with any other piece of monitoring equipment, information provided by a pulse oximeter should never be relied upon solely as an indicator of patient well-being.

Pulse oximeters require little maintenance but must be handled with care. Transmission probes should be cleaned with

---

TABLE 6.9 Interpretation of Oxygen Saturation Values During Anesthesia

SpO_2 Value	Significance	Action
95%–100%	Normal	None
90%–94%	Early hypoxemia	Explore possible causes
85%–89%	Severe hypoxemia—therapy required	Take steps to increase oxygenation
<85%	Medical emergency	Aggressive treatment required

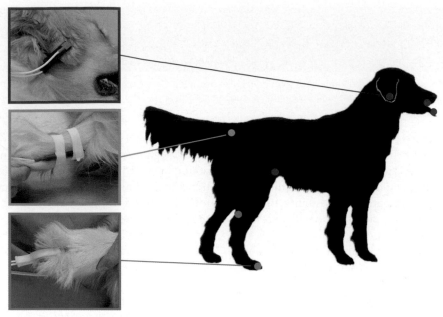

FIG. 6.43 Examples of pulse oximeter probes and locations for placement. *Red*—transmission probe on the ear flap. Additional red dots show alternate placement locations for this probe (tongue, lip, and flank fold). *Green*—reflective probe taped to the ventral surface of the tail base. *Blue*—"C-probe" (a transmission probe) on the toe web. The other blue dot shows an alternate placement location for this probe (the skin fold between the Achilles tendon and the tibia).

BOX 6.9 Suggestions for Troubleshooting Pulse Oximeter Signal Loss

Transmission Probes
- Make sure the patient is stable by assessing vital signs
- Remove the probe and place it in a slightly different location
- When using a lingual probe, if the tongue is dry, rewet it
- Be sure there is not excessive or inadequate pressure on the tissue
- When possible, the jaw with the sensor should be oriented toward the ceiling to avoid interference from ambient light
- Choose a different area that is not pigmented, covered with excessive hair, icteric, or edematous
- If the area is heavily haired, clip and gently cleanse the area

Reflective Probes
- Make sure the patient is stable by assessing vital signs
- Be sure the side with the light source and sensor is oriented toward the tissue
- Check for adequate tissue contact
- When the probe is placed in the rectum, be sure that feces are not between the probe and the tissue

---

70% isopropyl alcohol or manufacturer-recommended high-level disinfectant after use. Reflective probes should be covered with a plastic sleeve supplied by the manufacturer before insertion into the rectum or esophagus. None of the probes can be immersed, scrubbed, or autoclaved.

If pulse oximeter readings are abnormally low during anesthesia, the anesthetist should consider the following questions:
- Is the instrument working correctly? Readings may be affected by factors such as probe placement, external light sources, and motion.
- Do any of the drugs used cause vasoconstriction? Some anesthetic agents (especially alpha$_2$-agonists such as dexmedetomidine) cause vasoconstriction and decreased peripheral perfusion, which may significantly lower Spo$_2$ values.
- Is the tissue under the probe adequately perfused? Regardless of the anesthetic agents used, perfusion of an extremity such as the tongue may decrease gradually with time and give artificially reduced Spo$_2$ readings. If this is the case, readings may improve if the probe is moved to a different location. If higher readings cannot be obtained, the patient should be evaluated for hypothermia, hypotension, blood loss, and other causes of reduced perfusion.
- Is adequate oxygen being delivered to the patient? Inadequate oxygen delivery may result from esophageal intubation, an oxygen flow rate that is too low, an empty oxygen tank, endotracheal tube blockage or disconnection, or respiratory failure.
- Is oxygen being transferred from the alveoli to the blood? This process may be impeded by inadequate ventilation or preexisting lung disease.
- Is circulation adequate? Heart disease, bradycardia, severe arrhythmias, or pulmonary embolism may decrease oxygenation.

Regardless of the cause, patients with subnormal Pao$_2$ or Spo$_2$ readings may require supplemental oxygen delivery, or ventilation through bagging or use of a ventilator.

Pulse oximeters can be used not only on anesthetized patients but also on animals that are in intensive care because of trauma, heart failure, respiratory difficulty, or unconsciousness. Their chief limitation is the difficulty of finding a suitable probe site in alert and mobile patients.

Blood Gas Analysis

Blood gas analysis is an alternative method used to evaluate oxygenation. This monitoring tool is discussed in detail in the next section (indicators of ventilation).

Indicators of Ventilation

The objective of the ACVAA monitoring guidelines for ventilation is "to ensure that the patient's ventilation is adequately maintained." To meet this objective, the ACVAA makes the following recommendations:

> *Qualitative assessment of ventilation is essential by either (1) Observation of thoracic wall movement or observation of breathing bag movement when thoracic wall movement cannot be assessed, or (2) Auscultation of breath sounds with an external stethoscope, an esophageal stethoscope, or an audible respiratory monitor; and capnography is recommended, with blood gas analysis as necessary.*

The term *ventilation* refers to the movement of gases in and out of the alveoli, whereas respiration is a more general term that means the processes by which oxygen is supplied to and used by the tissues and carbon dioxide is eliminated from the tissues. The following monitoring parameters and indicators give the anesthetist information about ventilation.

Respiratory Rate

The RR is the number of breaths per minute (breaths/min). It is most often monitored by watching the chest wall. In situations in which the chest excursions are not visible, such as when the patient is covered by a surgical drape, it may also be monitored by observing movements of the reservoir bag. Auscultation of breath sounds is not a particularly good way to determine the RR because the low V_T typically seen during anesthesia renders respiratory sounds inaudible or nearly so in many anesthetized patients. RR may also be monitored mechanically with a capnograph, which displays a digital readout of the RR in breaths per minute. The minimum acceptable, maximum acceptable, and typical RR for anesthetized patients are listed in Table 6.4. During anesthesia, there is normally a decrease in the RR. Inhalant anesthetics, opioids, and alpha$_2$-agonists are particularly likely to cause respiratory depression. Propofol, alfaxalone, and thiopental sodium typically cause bradypnea or apnea during induction, especially if given quickly or at high doses.

An increase in RR is called tachypnea. Tachypnea must be differentiated from panting, in which breaths are rapid but shallow and air is taken in through an open mouth. Panting (only seen in conscious, nonintubated patients) is a common side effect of neuroleptanalgesia. True tachypnea has many possible causes, including hypercapnia, pulmonary disease, or a response to a mild surgical stimulus. For example, tachypnea is often apparent when the surgeon pulls on the suspensory ligament of the ovary during an ovariohysterectomy. An elevated RR may also indicate progression from surgical to light stage III anesthesia and is one of the first signs of arousal from anesthesia. Some patients (particularly obese dogs) breathe rapidly, even at a moderate depth of anesthesia.

Tidal Volume

The V_T is the amount of air inhaled during a breath. As with RR, V_T is monitored by watching the chest wall or movement of the reservoir bag. Normal V_T is generally considered to be 10 to 15 mL/kg, but it decreases by at least 25% to 30% in most anesthetized animals, largely because most preanesthetic and general anesthetic drugs decrease the contraction of the intercostal muscles on inspiration. As the animal's breaths become more shallow (i.e., as V_T decreases), some alveoli in the lungs may not receive amounts of air adequate for normal gas exchange. As a result, the alveoli will partially collapse (a condition called atelectasis). This is most pronounced in the "down" lung (also called the dependent lung) of a patient that is lying on its side and in the dorsal lung fields of a patient lying on its back. In its early stages, atelectasis can be reversed by gentle inflation of the lungs by the anesthetist. In this procedure, called *bagging* or *sighing* the patient, the reservoir bag of the anesthetic machine is carefully squeezed, forcing air into the patient's breathing passages. When bagging a patient, the anesthetist should closely observe the animal's chest to ensure that it rises only slightly, as with a normal breath, to prevent overinflation of the lungs. Some anesthetists routinely bag every patient under inhalation anesthesia once every 5 to 10 minutes. Alternatively, hypoventilation and atelectasis may be prevented by use of a mechanical ventilator (see Chapter 7).

Anesthetized patients may occasionally have increased V_T (hyperventilation). As with tachypnea, hyperventilation may result from hypercapnia or surgical stimulation.

The V_T can be measured using a respirometer (Fig. 6.44), which is placed between the expiratory hose of a rebreathing circuit and the exhalation unidirectional valve. When the patient breathes out, vanes within the respirometer turn small dials on the front of the device. All dials are cumulative and therefore can be used to monitor the patient's minute volume (breaths/min × V_T). The respirometer dials are easily reset to zero by depressing the buttons at the top, much like a stopwatch.

TECHNICIAN NOTE In its early stages, atelectasis can be reversed by gentle inflation of the lungs. In this procedure, called *bagging* or *sighing* the patient, the reservoir bag of the anesthetic machine is carefully squeezed, forcing air into the patient's breathing passages until the animal's chest rises as with a normal breath. Some anesthetists routinely bag every patient under inhalation anesthesia once every 5–10 min.

Respiratory Character

Respiratory character refers to the effort required to breathe, the relative length of inhalation and exhalation, and regularity. Respiratory character is monitored by watching the chest wall.

The anesthetized animal's breathing should be smooth and regular, with both thoracic and diaphragmatic components (i.e., both the chest wall and the diaphragm should move). Gasping, difficult, or labored breathing (dyspnea) indicates a problem requiring intervention, including airway blockage, respiratory disease, pressure buildup in the breathing circuit, or hypoxemia, and must be brought to the veterinarian's attention.

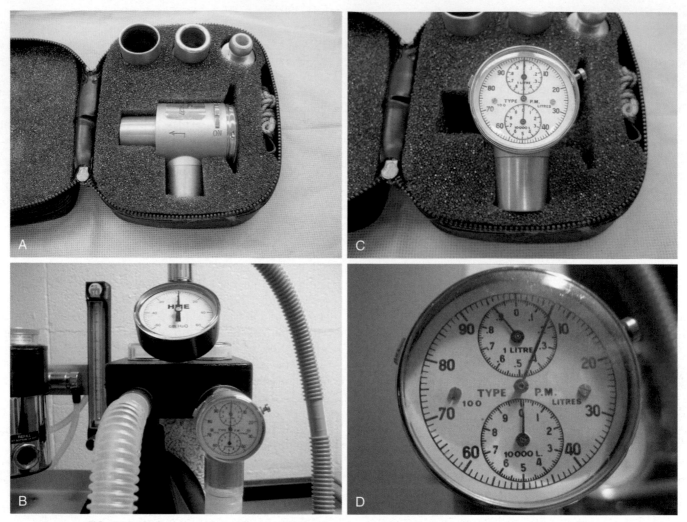

FIG. 6.44 (A) Side view of respirometer. (B) Respirometer positioned between expiratory breathing tube and exhalation unidirectional valve. (C and D) Face of the respirometer. The upper small dial is cumulative and displays volumes between 0 and 1 L. The large dial is cumulative and displays volumes between 1 and 100 L. The lower small dial is cumulative and displays volumes between 100 and 10,000 L.

The time relationship between inspiration and expiration may vary also. Normal inspiration lasts 1 to 1.5 seconds, and expiration lasts at least 2 to 3 seconds. Expiration is usually followed by a pause before the next inspiration begins. Animals anesthetized with ketamine may exhibit an apneustic respiratory pattern in which there is a prolonged pause between inspiration and expiration.

Auscultation of the chest is useful to assess respiratory function. Normal respiratory sounds are almost inaudible in the dog and cat. Harsh noises, crackles, gurgling, whistles, or squeaks may indicate narrow or obstructed airways or the presence of fluid in the airways or alveoli, and should be brought to the veterinarian's attention.

Capnograph (End-Tidal CO$_2$ Monitor)

A capnograph measures the amount of CO$_2$ in the air that is breathed in and out by the patient. Capnography is a noninvasive, continuous, and practical method of monitoring CO$_2$ levels in anesthetized patients without the need to catheterize an artery, as is necessary with blood gas analysis. Although

this monitoring device does not measure blood CO$_2$ directly, expired CO$_2$ closely mirrors arterial CO$_2$ (Paco$_2$). Specifically, end-tidal CO$_2$ (ETco$_2$) is approximately 2 to 5 mmHg less than Paco$_2$.

A capnograph consists of a sensor and a computerized monitor with a digital readout (Fig. 6.45). The sensor measures infrared light absorption, which is directly proportional to the CO$_2$ level. Sensors are of two general types. A mainstream capnograph is an instrument in which the sensor chamber is placed directly between the endotracheal tube and the breathing circuit. A sidestream capnograph is one in which the sensor chamber is located in the computerized monitor and air is pulled into it through a tube attached to a sampling spacer placed between the endotracheal tube and breathing circuit. Both systems measure the CO$_2$ in the air that passes into and out of the endotracheal tube on both inspiration and expiration, and display this information as a waveform (called the capnogram) and as a numeric display of the ETco$_2$.

On sidestream capnographs, the sampling spacer (placed between the endotracheal tube and breathing circuit) is very

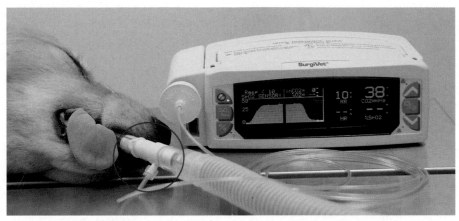

FIG. 6.45 A sidestream capnograph registering an end-tidal CO_2 level of 38 mmHg and a respiratory rate of 10 *(upper right)*. The sampling spacer *(circled)* is located between the breathing circuit and the endotracheal tube connector. The graph indicates the carbon dioxide levels throughout the respiratory cycle, which in normal patients is 35 to 55 mmHg during expiration and 0 mmHg during inspiration.

light in weight but does add additional mechanical dead space (typically ~5 mL) to the circuit (see Box 4.1 in Chapter 4 for a detailed discussion of dead space). For small patients, these units often come with special endotracheal tube connectors with a port for the sampling tube which, when used in place of the regular endotracheal tube connector, decreases dead space often to between 0.5 mL and 2 mL depending on its design.

There is a 2- to 3-second delay in the display of CO_2 levels with these units. Also, these units typically sample between 50 and 200 mL of air per minute from the circuit, which may cause a significant loss of gas and false readings when very low oxygen flow rates are used.

Mainstream samplers produce an immediate reading with no delay. However, the sensor chamber, which is placed between the endotracheal tube and the breathing circuit, is relatively large and heavy in some units and is heated to prevent condensation. This results in increased dead space, a greater risk that the endotracheal tube will kink, and a risk that the patient may be burned.

In recent years, very small, lightweight mainstream units have become available, such as the EMMA Mainstream Capnometer, Masimo, Irvine, CA These units come with adult and pediatric sampling chambers that are not heated (Fig. 6.46).

TECHNICIAN NOTE Blood CO_2 levels are determined by the following three factors:
1. The rate of production by the cells
2. The rate of transport to the lungs
3. The rate of elimination from the lungs

Generation of the capnogram. Carbon dioxide is produced in cells as a byproduct of cellular metabolism. After diffusing into venous blood, CO_2 is transported from the cells to the lungs, where it is eliminated on expiration (Fig. 6.47). Blood CO_2 levels are determined by the following three factors:
1. The rate of production by the cells (determined by cellular metabolism)
2. The rate of transport to the lungs (determined by cardiovascular output and pulmonary perfusion)

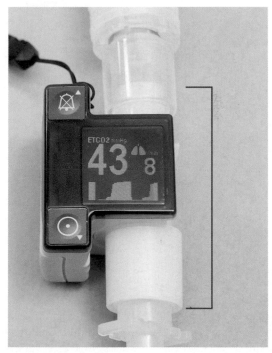

FIG. 6.46 EMMA Mainstream Capnometer (Masimo, Irvine, CA) registering an end-tidal CO_2 level of 43 mmHg and a respiratory rate of 8. The sampling chamber (within the *red bracket*) is located between the breathing circuit *(top)* and the endotracheal tube connector *(bottom)*. An adult chamber may be exchanged with a pediatric chamber in small patients to reduce dead space.

3. The rate of elimination from the lungs (determined by respiratory system health, RR, and V_T)

The $ETco_2$ level, as well as the configuration of the waveform, is thus influenced by the interactions among all three factors (metabolism, perfusion, and ventilation), as well as equipment function. Interpretation of a capnogram requires knowledge of normal and abnormal $ETco_2$ values, common abnormal waveform configurations, and causes of each abnormality. Therefore interpretation is somewhat complex and may

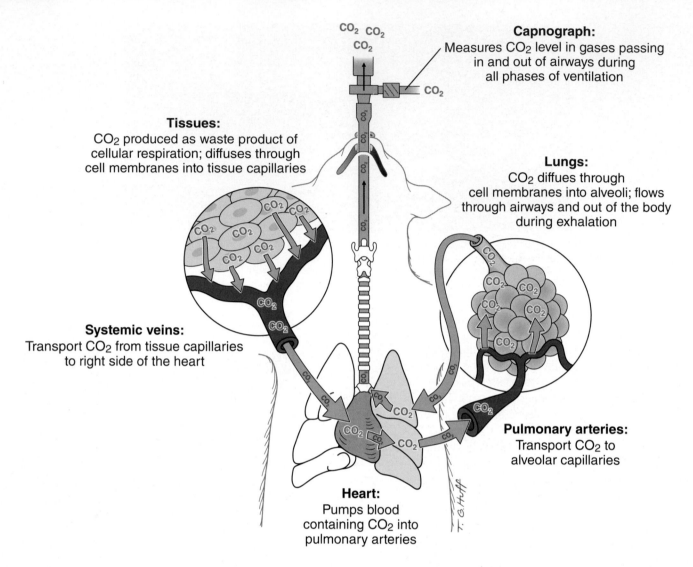

CO₂ CO₂
CO₂

Capnograph:
Measures CO₂ level in gases passing
in and out of airways during
all phases of ventilation

CO₂

Tissues:
CO₂ produced as waste product of
cellular respiration; diffuses through
cell membranes into tissue capillaries

Lungs:
CO₂ diffues through
cell membranes into alveoli; flows
through airways and out of the body
during exhalation

Systemic veins:
Transport CO₂ from tissue capillaries
to right side of the heart

Pulmonary arteries:
Transport CO₂ to
alveolar capillaries

Heart:
Pumps blood
containing CO₂ into
pulmonary arteries

FIG. 6.47 Generation of the capnogram.

be confusing until the anesthetist acquires some experience. Once mastered, however, the capnogram is an extremely valuable tool that can alert the anesthetist to a wide variety of anesthetic problems.

Appearance of a normal capnogram. On the capnogram, the x-axis displays time and the y-axis displays the CO₂ level (Fig. 6.48). The configuration of the waveform is determined by the levels of CO₂ passing through the machine end of the endotracheal tube and is divided into four phases (0, I, II, and III). During the respiratory cycle, the composition of the air measured by the capnograph changes from fresh gas to alveolar gas, with two brief periods during inhalation and exhalation when the amount of CO₂ in the sampled air rapidly decreases or increases, respectively.

Provided the anesthetic machine is working correctly and appropriate oxygen flow rates are used, inspired fresh gas contains oxygen and gas anesthetic but no CO₂, whereas expired alveolar gas (gas originating from the alveoli) is high in CO₂. Therefore as the patient inspires, the CO₂ level abruptly drops to 0 mmHg as pure exhaled alveolar gas is rapidly replaced by inspired fresh gas at the level of the sampling

port. This phase is referred to as phase 0 or the *inspiratory downstroke*.

Phase I (the *inspiratory baseline*) constitutes a transition between the end of inhalation and the beginning of exhalation, during which the CO₂ level remains at 0 mmHg. This is because the inhaled fresh gas contains no CO₂, nor does the first part of exhaled dead space gas, which comes from the ETT, bronchi, and other tubes that were filled with fresh gas during the previous inhalation.

During phase II (the *expiratory upstroke*), the CO₂ level abruptly increases to about 40 mmHg as exhaled dead space gas is rapidly replaced with CO₂-rich alveolar gas. Phase III (the *expiratory plateau*) consists of the end of exhalation and the expiratory pause that follows. During this time, CO₂ levels are relatively constant but increase slightly until right before the next breath. This is followed by a rapid drop back to 0 mmHg during the next inhalation (phase 0).

The shape of the resulting waveform can be described as a modified rectangle. It is called an "end-tidal" monitor because the CO₂ value at the end of the expiration (which is displayed as a number on the video monitor) is most reflective of arterial CO₂ levels.

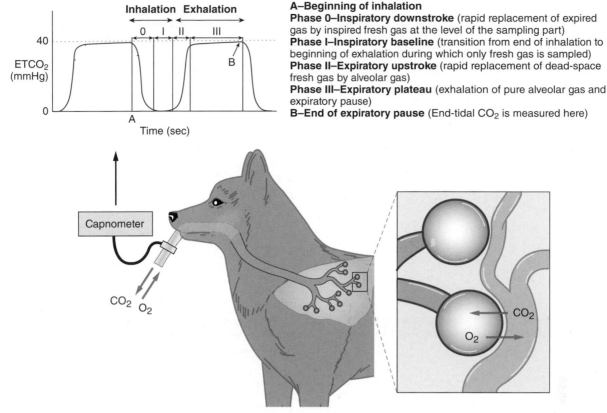

A–Beginning of inhalation
Phase 0–Inspiratory downstroke (rapid replacement of expired gas by inspired fresh gas at the level of the sampling part)
Phase I–Inspiratory baseline (transition from end of inhalation to beginning of exhalation during which only fresh gas is sampled)
Phase II–Expiratory upstroke (rapid replacement of dead-space fresh gas by alveolar gas)
Phase III–Expiratory plateau (exhalation of pure alveolar gas and expiratory pause)
B–End of expiratory pause (End-tidal CO_2 is measured here)

FIG. 6.48 Normal capnogram. The capnograph measures the partial pressure of CO_2 in the air moving between the endotracheal tube and the breathing circuit. As long as the patient is not rebreathing expired gases and the CO_2 absorbent is not exhausted, CO_2 is 0 mmHg during peak inspiration (phase I). As the patient exhales, (phase II or the expiratory upstroke), CO_2 rapidly increases to about 40 mmHg (phase III or the expiratory plateau), then continues to increase slightly until immediately before the next inhalation. This represents the $ETco_2$. Immediately after the beginning of the next inhalation, the CO_2 again rapidly decreases to 0 mmHg (phase 0 or the inspiratory downstroke).

> **TECHNICIAN NOTE** In a nonanesthetized patient, an $ETco_2$ of 35 to 45 mmHg is considered normal. In contrast, when a patient is anesthetized, up to 60 mmHg (typically 40 to 55 mm Hg) is considered acceptable because the respiratory depression produced by most anesthetics causes the body to retain CO_2.

In a nonanesthetized patient, an $ETco_2$ of 35 to 45 mmHg is considered normal. In contrast, when a patient is anesthetized, up to 60 mmHg (typically 40 to 55 mm Hg) is considered acceptable because the respiratory depression produced by most anesthetics causes the body to retain CO_2.

Effective interpretation requires evaluation of four distinct aspects of the capnogram:
1. The baseline value
2. The $ETco_2$ value
3. The waveform shape
4. The rate at which changes occur (suddenly, rapidly, or gradually)

> **TECHNICIAN NOTE** Effective interpretation of the capnogram requires evaluation of four distinct aspects:
> 1. The baseline value
> 2. The $ETco_2$ value
> 3. The waveform shape
> 4. The rate at which changes occur (suddenly, rapidly, or gradually)

Appearance of an abnormal capnogram. A change in metabolism, perfusion, or ventilation, as well as equipment malfunction, will affect $ETco_2$ levels and/or the waveform configuration. In most normal patients, provided metabolism and perfusion are normal, abnormal CO_2 levels are most commonly a result of changes in ventilation (hyperventilation, hypoventilation, apnea) or equipment problems. What follows are some common abnormalities:

- Hyperventilation caused by increased RR or V_T or overzealous mechanical or manual ventilation will cause CO_2 to be exhaled more quickly than it is produced and will consequently cause a gradual decrease in the $ETco_2$ (a shorter rectangle).
- Hypoventilation (decreased RR or V_T or inadequate mechanical or manual ventilation) will cause a gradual increase in $ETco_2$ (a taller rectangle).
- Detachment of the endotracheal tube from the sensor fitting, esophageal intubation, a blocked endotracheal tube, or apnea will cause a sudden loss of the waveform (a flat line) because in each of these circumstances, no CO_2 will reach the sensor.
- A malfunctioning exhalation unidirectional valve or exhausted CO_2 absorbent will cause the baseline to rise above 0, reflecting rebreathing of CO_2 in the inspired air (a failure of the baseline to return to 0 during inspiration) and increased $ETco_2$.

- A leaky cuff or partially kinked endotracheal tube will cause a sloppy upstroke and downstroke (rounding of the edges of the rectangle).

Many other conditions not related to ventilation or equipment can also cause abnormal $ETco_2$ values or waveforms, including pulmonary or heart disease, shock, changes in BP and body temperature, cardiac arrest, blood loss, and pulmonary thromboembolism.

The following are examples of these abnormalities:

- Cardiac arrest will cause a rapid loss of the waveform because CO_2 is no longer circulated to the lungs, and the waveform will rapidly reappear with the return of spontaneous circulation (ROSC) if cardiopulmonary resuscitation (CPR) is successful.
- Hypotension or a sudden decrease in cardiac output will cause a rapid decrease in the $ETco_2$ (a shorter rectangle).
- Hypothermia will cause a gradual decrease in the $ETco_2$ because of a decrease in the metabolic rate and therefore CO_2

production (a shorter rectangle). Hyperthermia will cause a gradual increase (a taller rectangle).

Other, more subtle changes in the configuration of the waveform may occur as a result of high or low gas flow, the type of breathing circuit used, the amount of dead space, and other factors. Also, capnograph malfunctions will affect the waveform, including excess moisture in the sampling line, blockage of the line, or a leak in the system. Table 6.10 shows common changes in the capnogram and associated causes. See Case Presentation 6.1 for an example of the value of capnography as a monitoring tool.

Blood Gas Analysis

Blood gas analysis refers to the measurement of blood pH and of dissolved oxygen and carbon dioxide gas in arterial (Pao_2 and $Paco_2$) or venous (Pvo_2 and $Pvco_2$) blood. It is therefore an indicator of both oxygenation and ventilation, as well as acid–base status. Each of these variables is influenced by respiratory function, which can be roughly evaluated by observation of the

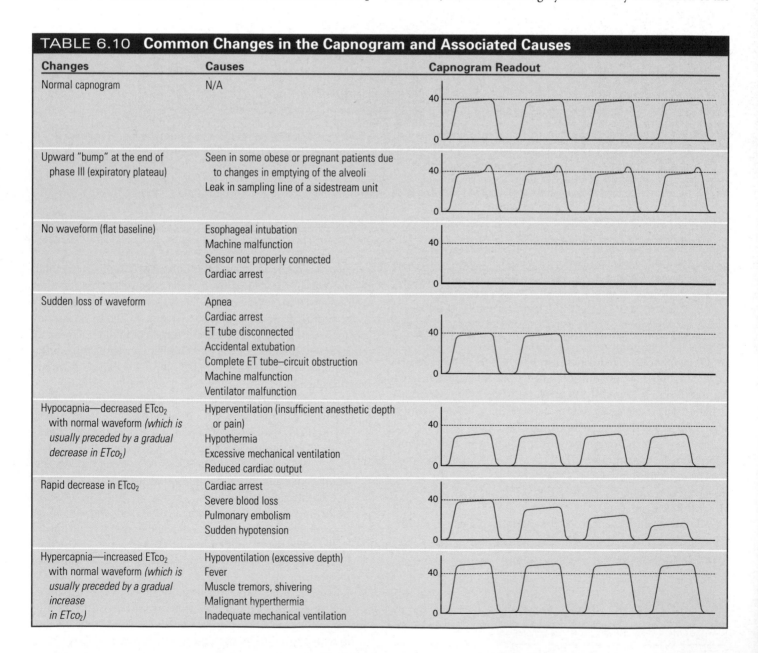

TABLE 6.10   Common Changes in the Capnogram and Associated Causes

Changes	Causes	Capnogram Readout
Normal capnogram	N/A	
Upward "bump" at the end of phase III (expiratory plateau)	Seen in some obese or pregnant patients due to changes in emptying of the alveoli Leak in sampling line of a sidestream unit	
No waveform (flat baseline)	Esophageal intubation Machine malfunction Sensor not properly connected Cardiac arrest	
Sudden loss of waveform	Apnea Cardiac arrest ET tube disconnected Accidental extubation Complete ET tube–circuit obstruction Machine malfunction Ventilator malfunction	
Hypocapnia—decreased $ETco_2$ with normal waveform *(which is usually preceded by a gradual decrease in $ETco_2$)*	Hyperventilation (insufficient anesthetic depth or pain) Hypothermia Excessive mechanical ventilation Reduced cardiac output	
Rapid decrease in $ETco_2$	Cardiac arrest Severe blood loss Pulmonary embolism Sudden hypotension	
Hypercapnia—increased $ETco_2$ with normal waveform *(which is usually preceded by a gradual increase in $ETco_2$)*	Hypoventilation (excessive depth) Fever Muscle tremors, shivering Malignant hyperthermia Inadequate mechanical ventilation	

TABLE 6.10 Common Changes in the Capnogram and Associated Causes—cont'd

Changes	Causes	Capnogram Readout
Rapid increase in ETco₂	Return of spontaneous circulation after successful CPR Malignant hypothermia	
Increase in baseline CO₂ (usually with gradual increase in ETco₂)	Usually due to rebreathing of CO₂ due to: • Malfunction of expiratory unidirectional valve • Saturation of CO₂ absorbent • Inadequate fresh gas flow with NRS • Excessive dead space • Leak in the inner tube of a Bain coaxial system May be due to contamination of sensor with secretions	
Sudden, temporary increase in ETco₂	Release of a tourniquet Administration of sodium bicarbonate	
Slow upward stroke ("shark-fin" appearance to waveform)/increased angle of the plateau	Slow expiration due to asthma or other obstructive lung disease Partially obstructed endotracheal tube or breathing circuit	
Plateau irregular or terminal "dip" in plateau	Dilution of expired CO₂ by fresh gas or ambient air due to: • Leak in sampling line of sidestream unit • Excessive fresh gas flow rate	
Sloppy upstroke and downstroke	Leaky ET tube cuff Partially kinked ET tube	
Cleft in the expiratory plateau (sometimes referred to as "curare cleft")	Pushing on the chest wall during exhalation Spontaneous breaths in a patient that is on a ventilator Spontaneous breaths in a patient recovering from neuromuscular blockade	
Oscillations during end expiration and phase 0	Caused by cardiac contractions (more common with low RR and V_T)	

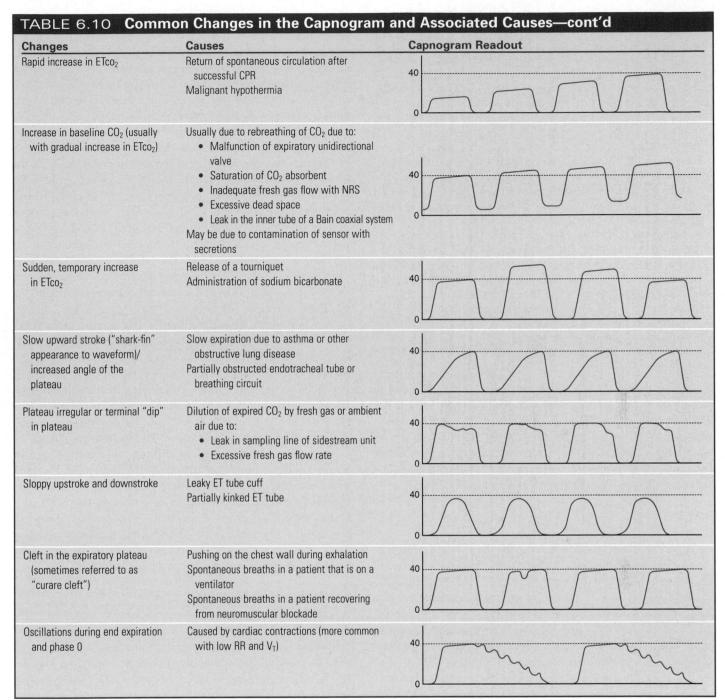

CO₂, Carbon dioxide; CPR, cardiopulmonary resuscitation; ET, endotracheal; ETco₂, end-tidal CO₂; NRS, nonrebreathing system.

rate, depth, and character of the patient's respiration. However, physical monitoring may give an inaccurate impression of the patient's status because although breathing may appear normal, oxygenation and ventilation may in fact be abnormal.

Blood gas monitoring is most commonly used for large-animal patients and is seldom used in small-animal practice, outside of specialty practices, for several reasons. First, sample collection may be difficult because blood intended for blood gas analysis is most often obtained from an artery (as opposed to routine blood samples, which are taken from a vein). In certain situations, a venous sample may be used. For example, the lingual vein has extensive anastomoses with arteries in the tongue, the blood gas values obtained from lingual vein samples are close to arterial values, and the head is often easily accessed by the anesthetist during surgery. Second, sample handling is labor intensive. Once obtained, the blood sample must be stored on ice and values should be measured within 2 hours. Many veterinary reference laboratories and some veterinary hospitals are equipped to perform these tests, and some human hospital laboratories may be willing to accept samples from nonhuman patients. Portable analyzers have recently been introduced to the veterinary market.

CASE PRESENTATION 6.1   The Value of Capnography

Cooper, a 1-year-old, 17-kg male Beagle mix, was anesthetized in preparation for a routine castration. Based on preanesthetic assessment, he was classified as a physical status class P1 patient. Cooper was premedicated with 0.1 mg/kg acepromazine by intramuscular (IM) injection 15 minutes before anesthetic induction and was induced with a mixture of 5.5 mg/kg ketamine and 0.28 mg/kg diazepam intravenously. He was intubated and placed on a semiclosed rebreathing system. After reaching surgical anesthesia, he was maintained with isoflurane at a rate of 1.5% to 2.0% and oxygen at a rate of 0.5 L/min. Pulse oximetry was used to monitor Cooper via a transmission probe placed on the tongue.

During surgical preparation, the anesthetist determined that Cooper was in surgical anesthesia, but he had a slightly increased respiratory rate (22 breaths/min) and tidal volume. An investigation ensued to determine the cause of the hyperventilation, but an immediate cause was not identified. Oxygen saturation (Spo$_2$) was in the range of 97%–98% and all other vital signs were normal.

A decision was made to use a capnograph to assess carbon dioxide levels. It was immediately noted that the ETco$_2$ was 62 mmHg (normal 35–55) and the carbon dioxide level on inspiration was about 25 mmHg (normal 0 mmHg).

1. What machine problems or patient conditions might cause these changes on the capnograph?
2. What steps would you take to manage this case?

Carbon dioxide (CO_2) is transported through the blood in three ways. About 20% to 30% is bound to hemoglobin in the RBCs. About 5% to 10% is dissolved in plasma and is measurable as Pco_2 (the CO_2 partial pressure in the vessels). The remainder (about 60% to 70%) reacts with water to form carbonic acid, which is quickly converted into bicarbonate and hydrogen ions according to the following reaction:

$$CO_2 + H_2O = H_2CO_3 = HCO_3^- + H+$$

The anesthetist can evaluate how well the patient is eliminating CO_2 by measuring $Paco_2$ through blood gas determination. $Paco_2$ is often elevated during anesthesia (45 to 60 mmHg compared with less than 45 mmHg in the awake patient) because the respiratory depression produced by most anesthetics causes the body to retain CO_2 (i.e., the patient is hypoventilating). In other words, the patient does not breathe often enough and/or deeply enough to eliminate the normal amount of CO_2. A $Paco_2$ greater than 60 mmHg indicates that the hypoventilation is significant and requires intervention. If this happens, the anesthetist needs to determine whether the patient is in trouble by assessing the oxygenation, cardiac rhythm, BP, and anesthetic depth. It may be necessary to assist ventilation by compressing the reservoir bag or using a ventilator (see Chapter 7).

TECHNICIAN NOTE $Paco_2$ is often 45–60 mmHg during anesthesia because the respiratory depression produced by most anesthetics causes the body to retain CO_2. A $Paco_2$ greater than 60 mmHg indicates that hypoventilation is significant and requires intervention.

Because of high CO_2 levels, anesthetized patients may also become mildly acidotic (i.e., excess hydrogen ions are produced from CO_2 according to the previous equation). The blood pH in anesthetized animals usually reflects this mild respiratory acidosis and is commonly 7.2 to 7.3 compared with the normal animal's blood pH of 7.35 to 7.45. Cellular enzymes do not work well outside certain pH ranges, so when acid–base disturbances are suspected or present, maintaining a pH between 7.2 and 7.5 is advisable. The correction of the underlying cause often results in improvement of acid–base status; thus treatment should be discussed with the attending veterinarian. Blood pH measurement can be performed at the same time as blood gas determinations are made to help the anesthetist determine the acid–base status of the body and the adequacy of the patient's respiration. In the absence of elevated $Paco_2$, a decreased pH is evidence of metabolic acidosis, which should be brought to the attention of the attending veterinarian. Blood pH that is elevated (>7.45) when $Paco_2$ is decreased (<35 mmHg) indicates hyperventilation, which may be caused by light anesthetic depth, overzealous ventilation, pain, or hypoxemia. Blood pH that is elevated with a normal $Paco_2$ indicates metabolic alkalosis, which may be caused by obstruction of outflow from the pylorus of the stomach or by excessive administration of $NaHCO_3$.

Pao_2 is the partial pressure of dissolved oxygen in arterial blood. This should be approximately five times the inspired concentration of oxygen. Therefore when a patient is breathing room air, which is approximately 21% O_2, Pao_2 is approximately 100 mmHg, and when it is breathing 100% O_2 under general anesthesia, Pao_2 is approximately 500 mmHg. Clinically significant hypoxemia is present if Pao_2 is below 80 mmHg, and Pao_2 below 60 mmHg requires intervention such as mechanical ventilation (see Chapter 7). Causes of hypoxemia are hypoventilation, a decreased fraction of inspired oxygen, shunting of blood flow (blood bypasses the lungs and is returned, unoxygenated, to the systemic arteries), and decreased ability of oxygen to diffuse from the lung into the bloodstream (in diseases such as pneumonia or pulmonary edema). In the absence of disease, small animals and ruminants are rarely hypoxemic during anesthesia. Anesthetized horses are commonly hypoxemic regardless of health status (see Chapter 10).

Miscellaneous Monitors
Anesthetic Gas Analyzers

Anesthetic gas analyzers are machines that measure the concentration of inhalant anesthetic (isoflurane, sevoflurane, or desflurane) in the breathing circuit. Gas is sampled via a spacer placed between the endotracheal tube connector and the breathing circuit in a similar way to a capnograph, and gas concentration is measured by a technology called infrared absorption spectrometry. End-tidal concentration (concentration of the inhalant agent in the expired gases) is displayed. This monitor provides a way to compare the concentration in the exhaled gases to the dial setting and can enable the anesthetist to identify and respond to situations in which the patient is receiving less than the amount of inhalant anesthetic indicated on the dial and therefore may be in danger of awaking prematurely. This may happen in a number of situations including (1) when the vaporizer is first turned on but before the agent reaches a state of equilibrium, (2) in larger dogs and large-animal patients, or (3) when using low fresh gas flows (under 250 to 500 mL/min). The Riken FI-8000P Anesthetic Gas Analyzer (Fig. 6.49) is an example of this type of analyzer.

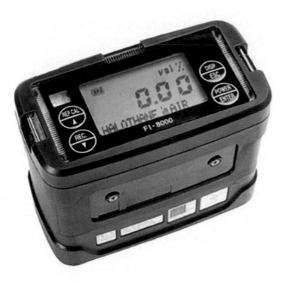

FIG. 6.49 Riken FI-8000P anesthetic gas analyzer.

Oxygen Analyzers

Oxygen analyzers measure the percentage of oxygen in inspired gases (fraction of inspired oxygen or FiO_2) by sampling gas from a spacer that can be placed between the inspiratory tube and the y-piece. These monitors enable the anesthetist to monitor the % oxygen in the breathing circuit and detect problems such as loss of oxygen flow due to a tank being empty or an oxygen flow meter that is not turned on. Use of an FiO_2 monitor is recommended when multiple carrier gases are used, such as medical air or nitrous oxide mixed with oxygen, to prevent inadvertent delivery of a hypoxic mixture of gas.

Monitors for Depth of Anesthesia

For many years, measurement of electrical activity in the brain (electroencephalography or EEG analysis) has been used in human patients to monitor anesthetic depth and to ensure that a patient is not aware during a general anesthesia procedure. One of the most common methods used to do this is the bispectral index (BIS) monitor, which evaluates brain activity and generates a number between "0" (no brain activity) and "100" (wakefulness). This technology has not been found to reliably correlate with anesthetic depth as evaluated by conventional means in anesthetized animals. Consequently, EEG monitoring has not found acceptance for monitoring of patient depth in clinical practice.

Multiparameter Monitors

As implied by the name, multiparameter monitors (see Fig. 6.11) are capable of measuring and displaying multiple machine parameters previously discussed (such as HR, ECG tracing, P_{SYS}, P_{DIA}, and MAP, SpO_2, FiO_2, RR, $ETco_2$, Pao_2, $Paco_2$, blood pH, and body temperature). The number of parameters that can be monitoring simultaneously depends on the specific model. Some enable monitoring of more than one patient at a time and offer features such as touch screen capability, depending on their sophistication. Use of such a monitor overcomes the necessity of setting up, operating, and maintaining multiple separate monitors on one patient.

BODY TEMPERATURE

The objective of the ACVAA monitoring guidelines for body temperature is "to ensure that patients do not encounter serious deviations from normal body temperature." To meet this objective, the ACVAA makes the following recommendations:

Temperature should be measured periodically during anesthesia and recovery and if possible checked within a few hours after return to the wards.

Core body temperature is another vital sign that although not an indicator of circulation, oxygenation, or ventilation, is nonetheless vital to patient well-being for reasons indicated later in this section. Core body temperature should be monitored at least every 15 to 30 minutes during anesthesia using a digital rectal thermometer or an esophageal or rectal probe attached to a continuous display monitor.

Core body temperature, which may be defined as the temperature of deep tissues, internal organs, and the brain, is tightly regulated in homeotherms (animals that maintain a constant body temperature independent of environmental temperature). This is accomplished through a complex physiologic process called thermoregulation, which employs a variety of metabolic and physical means that include panting, sweating, shivering, release of hormones, peripheral vasoconstriction and vasodilatation, and changes in metabolism to keep the internal temperature within a range of approximately 0.2°C in most mammals. The hypothalamus of the brain is the "control center" for thermoregulation.

The gold standard for measuring core body temperature involves insertion of a catheter into a pulmonary artery, which is not a safe or practical option in a clinical setting. Therefore temperatures must be measured in other locations that are easily accessible during an anesthetic procedure by use of a thermometer or probe, and that correlate most closely with the true core temperature. The rectum and esophagus are two such sites that are commonly used for this purpose.

Most electronic rectal thermometers and esophageal or rectal temperature probes use either a thermistor or a thermocouple, which are devices capable of measuring and displaying temperature rapidly, accurately, and continuously. In order to accurately measure core temperature, rectal thermometers and probes must be inserted to an adequate distance (which may be as much as 5 to 8 cm in a large dog), and ideally must be next to the mucosa, as feces may decrease the accuracy of the measurement. Esophageal probes should be inserted to the caudal third of the esophagus, between the heart base and descending aorta, as measurements taken cranial or caudal to this location will be artificially low or high, respectively.

Measurement of temperature in peripheral locations, such as the skin, axilla, or the ear canal, with an infrared monitoring device show significant variability and poor correlation with core body temperature, and so should not be used for anesthetized animals.

Hypothermia

With few exceptions, anesthetics decrease the body temperature by depressing the hypothalamus, reducing muscular activity, and slowing the metabolic rate. For this reason, hypothermia is a frequent and even an expected response to general anesthesia that, if not prevented, recognized, and controlled, will cause a variety of adverse effects, including prolonged recovery. In severe cases of hypothermia, depressed CNS and heart function will endanger the patient. Temperature loss is greatest in the first 20 minutes and can be 3°C or more during the course of a prolonged procedure. (See Table 6.4 for typical body temperatures during anesthetic procedures.) Several factors contribute to this effect:

- Animals are routinely shaved before surgery and the skin is often prepared with antiseptic and alcohol solutions that cool the skin by evaporation
- An anesthetized animal is incapable of generating heat by shivering or muscular activity
- The metabolic rate of an anesthetized animal is less than that of a conscious animal, resulting in less heat generation
- During the course of surgery, a body cavity may be opened and the viscera exposed to air at room temperature
- Some preanesthetic and general anesthetic agents cause peripheral vasodilation, resulting in an increased rate of heat loss
- Pediatric and geriatric animals are less able to maintain thermoregulation and are therefore even more predisposed to hypothermia than adult animals
- Small patients lose heat faster because the body surface area is proportionately greater than the surface area of larger patients
- Administration of room temperature IV fluids will further decrease body temperature
- Patients placed on nonrebreathing systems constantly breathe fresh gas, which is cold and dry; they therefore expend energy warming and humidifying this gas.

TECHNICIAN NOTE During anesthesia, body temperature loss is greatest in the first 20 min. Body temperatures in the range of 32°C–34° C (89.6°F–93.2°F) prolong anesthetic recovery and significantly decrease the dose of anesthetic agents required. Temperatures below 32°C (89.6°F) cause dangerous CNS depression and changes in heart function.

The magnitude of hypothermia determines the effects, but temperatures as low as 36°C (96.8°F) do not cause significant harm.

There are several potential problems associated with hypothermia during the maintenance and recovery periods. Body temperatures in the range of 32°C to 34°C (89.6°F to 93.2°F) delay anesthetic recovery and significantly decrease the dose of anesthetic agents required to maintain surgical anesthesia by slowing the rate at which liver enzymes metabolize the drugs. This predisposes the patient to anesthetic overdose if the rate of administration is not reduced. Shivering during recovery will increase the patient's oxygen demands by as much as six times. This can cause significant complications when the patient is unable to respond to this increase in demand (as may be the case in a patient not receiving adequate oxygen or with cardiopulmonary disease). Temperatures below 32°C (89.6°F) cause dangerous CNS depression and changes in heart function. To avoid these problems, the anesthetist should endeavor to monitor the patient's temperature and maintain it within the normal range as much as possible.

Used to Minimize Heat Loss and Manage Hypothermia

A variety of techniques to minimize heat loss and manage hypothermic patients can be used, and fall into one of three categories: (1) external passive warming; (2) external active rewarming; and (3) core rewarming. External passive warming helps to minimize hypothermia by using various methods (such as the use of towels, blankets, or bubble wrap) to conserve body heat. These methods do not involve production of additional heat. External active rewarming raises body temperature by using external heat-producing devices (such as circulating warm water blankets or warm air blankets) to manage hypothermic patients. Core rewarming involves the use of various devices (such as IV fluid warmers—see Fig. 6.50) and practices (such as using rebreathing circuits when possible and avoiding high oxygen flow) to either warm the patient internally or to prevent excessive heat loss from the respiratory tract (see Box 6.10 for a summary of these techniques).

Potential Complications of Rewarming

Never use electric heating pads unless specifically designed for anesthetized patients because consumer-grade heating pads are not usually temperature regulated and often exceed the maximum safe operating temperature of 42°C (107.6°F). Thus severe burns can result from their use.

Active rewarming the patient by placing homemade devices such as microwave-heated water bottles or bags of solid materials such as rice or lentils should be used with great caution or not at all, because it is impossible to closely regulate the temperature

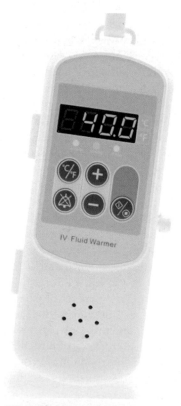

FIG. 6.50 Intravenous fluid warmer.

BOX 6.10 Strategies to Minimize Heat Loss and Manage Hypothermia in Anesthetized Patients

External Passive Warming Techniques

- Avoid excessively cold temperatures in the surgery suite or treatment room
- Always place an insulating barrier such as a towel or blanket between the patient and tabletops, especially those made of stainless steel
- Dry the patient's haircoat
- Wrap the patient's extremities in bubble wrap

External Active Rewarming Techniques

- Place a circulating warm water blanket between the patient and the table. These quilted vinyl blankets are attached to a unit that circulates warm water through the blanket
- Place the patient on a forced warm air blanket. These devices consist of a quilted plastic blanket (similar to a pool floater) that is placed under and sometimes over the patient. A device is attached that circulates warm air through the blanket.

Core Rewarming Techniques Include the Following

- Use a rebreathing circuit whenever possible and appropriate
- Avoid excessive oxygen flow rates
- Consider use of a coaxial breathing circuit, such as an F-circuit or a Bain circuit (although the benefit derived from using these circuits for this purpose is dependent on many factors)
- Use a heat and moisture exchanger in the breathing circuit to warm and humidify inspired gas (see Chapter 4 for a discussion of heat and moisture exchangers)
- Use an in-line intravenous (IV) fluid warmer such as the IV Fluid Warmer (Midmark Corporation, Dayton, OH [see Fig. 6.50]) to raise the temperature of the IV fluids prior to administration
- Flush the abdominal cavity with warmed fluids.

of these devices, which may dangerously overheat the patient. Aggressive external rewarming can also cause afterdrop, a complication caused by dilatation of peripheral vessels and shunting of cool blood from the extremities to the core. This results in a further drop in core temperature and so worsens hypothermia instead of helping to restore it. In addition, dilation of the peripheral vasculature may decrease BP and release substances toxic to the heart that may accumulate in hypoxic tissues.

Core rewarming should never be attempted by warming a fluid bag in a microwave oven, which can heat the fluids unevenly and because it is impossible to determine the temperature of the fluids by feeling the outside of the bag. Fluid temperatures over 42°C (107.6°F) cause hemolysis and damage to the vascular endothelium and organs.

Hyperthermia

Hyperthermia (increased body temperature) is occasionally seen in anesthetized animals. Hyperthermia may occur for several reasons, including excessive administration of external heat, drug-induced reactions (e.g., opioid administration in some cats, excessive muscular activity after drugs such as ketamine), inability to dissipate heat (e.g., large dogs with thick coats under surgical drapes and/or placed on low-flow or closed system anesthesia in which the rebreathed gases are warmer). Hyperthermia in these cases is often noted during or just before recovery. Cooling methods should be applied, such as administering cold fluids

intravenously, intraperitoneally, or rectally, and performing surface cooling with fans and ice or alcohol. When opioids have been given to cats, administration of acepromazine (0.03 to 0.05 mg/kg) or reversal using naloxone should be considered. If the patient is still anesthetized, increasing the flow rate of oxygen to nonrebreathing levels will also help.

One particular type of hyperthermia, malignant hyperthermia (MH), is most commonly seen in pigs, although there are reports of susceptible individuals in other species. In pigs, this is caused by a genetic defect that results in excess muscle metabolism in the presence of some anesthetic drugs such as the halogenated inhalant agents and the muscle relaxant succinylcholine. Restraint can also precipitate this syndrome, so stress should be minimized during handling of susceptible swine. Clinically, the anesthetized pig will become hot and stiff to the touch, pink pigs will turn red, large amounts of CO_2 are produced, and tachyarrhythmias occur. Anesthesia should be halted immediately, 100% oxygen administered, and cooling methods applied. The only medical treatment for MH is dantrolene, which is typically available only in large veterinary or human hospitals.

JUDGING ANESTHETIC DEPTH

During the course of anesthesia, the anesthetist should monitor as many variables as possible and weigh all available evidence before judging the anesthetic depth of the patient. No one piece of information is unfailingly reliable, and it is unwise to determine the anesthetic plane by monitoring only one or two reflexes or vital signs. In addition, each animal is unique and has an individual response to increasing anesthetic depth. For example, many animals develop bradypnea and hypoventilation shortly after induction with injectable general anesthetics while still in a light plane of anesthesia. If RR is used as the sole criterion for judging anesthetic depth, the animal that develops respiratory depression may be incorrectly judged to be too deeply anesthetized. Decreasing the concentration of anesthetic delivered to such a patient might easily result in the patient becoming inadequately anesthetized. Observation of the other indicators of anesthetic depth will give the anesthetist a more balanced view of the situation and a more accurate assessment of true anesthetic depth. Examples of the use of judgment in interpreting anesthetic depth are given in Case Presentations 6.2–6.4.

Similarly, observation of the amount of anesthetic being delivered to the patient (e.g., the vaporizer setting) does not in itself indicate the patient's anesthetic depth. Although high vaporizer settings result in increased delivery of anesthetic to

CASE PRESENTATION 6.2 Assessment of Readiness for Intubation

Mia, a 3-year-old intact female domestic shorthair (DSH) cat is being prepared for a routine spay. She is induced with intravenous (IV) propofol. The anesthetist notes that the cat appears unconscious and relaxed. The pulse is strong and the heart rate is 144 bpm. The respirations are regular and the respiratory rate is 20 breaths/min. The pupils are centrally positioned. The palpebral reflex is brisk, but no pedal or swallowing reflex is present. The anesthetist wishes to intubate the animal.

1. Is Mia at a sufficient depth to allow intubation?
2. What other steps could the anesthetist take to determine anesthetic depth?

the patient and subsequently, an increase in anesthetic depth, there is tremendous variation in patient response. This variation results in part from the patient's response to the anesthetic and in part from the influence of other drugs given to the animal. One animal may be maintained at stable surgical anesthesia with a vaporizer setting of 3% isoflurane, whereas another animal may require 2%, and still another may be satisfactorily maintained at 1% or even 0.5%. The concentration of anesthetic gas received by the animal also is not necessarily the concentration indicated by the vaporizer setting; it may vary with the oxygen flow rate, the quality of respiration, and other factors (see Chapter 4). Nevertheless, the vaporizer setting and the length of time for which the animal has been anesthetized are additional evidence that must be considered. The basic rule is that if there is doubt about the level of anesthesia in a particular patient possibly being excessive, one should decrease the vaporizer setting and continue to monitor the animal closely.

RECORDING INFORMATION DURING ANESTHESIA

The objectives of the ACVAA monitoring guidelines for record-keeping are as follows:

1. To maintain a legal record of significant events related to the anesthetic period.
2. To enhance recognition of significant trends or unusual values for physiologic parameters and allow assessment of the response to intervention.

To meet these objectives, the ACVAA makes the following recommendations:

1. Record all drugs administered to each patient in the peri-anesthetic period and in early recovery, noting the dose, time, and route of administration, as well as any adverse reaction to a drug or drug combination.
2. Record monitored variables on a regular basis (minimum every 5 to 10 minutes) during anesthesia. The minimum variables that should be recorded are heart rate and respiratory rate, as well as oxygenation status and blood pressure if these were monitored.
3. Record heart rate, respiratory rate, and temperature in the early recovery phase.
4. Any untoward events or unusual circumstances should be recorded for legal reasons, and for reference should the patient require anesthesia in the future.

Complete and accurate medical records are a legal requirement in veterinary practice. Most jurisdictions require that some form of anesthetic record be maintained during anesthesia. In many cases, this record can be in the form of a logbook in which information is listed, such as the date, client and patient identification, preoperative physical status, nature of the procedure performed with the patient under anesthesia, and the anesthetic protocol. A brief description of the animal's response to anesthesia should also be given. Records of this type allow the veterinarian to review the total number of anesthetic procedures that have been carried out in a given period and determine the frequency and nature of complications. This information may be helpful in assessing the anesthetic protocols. Controlled substance logs must be meticulously maintained to document use of benzodiazepines, opioids, cyclohexylamines, barbiturates, and other controlled drugs.

In addition, medical information regarding the anesthetic procedure must be written in the patient's record. This allows the veterinarian to review the animal's anesthetic history quickly and may be helpful in determining the best anesthetic protocol to use for future procedures. For example, if the record indicates that the animal was induced with propofol and maintained on isoflurane and experienced significant hypotension or hypoventilation, the veterinarian may choose to use a different protocol in the future. On the other hand, if a patient with a preexisting disease was recently anesthetized without incident with a particular agent, the veterinarian would be justified in using the same agent for the next anesthesia.

In some practices, an anesthesia form such as shown in Fig. 6.51 is used to record a detailed description of an anesthetic procedure. This type of record contains information on the patient's preoperative status (e.g., vital signs and the results of diagnostic tests), the anesthetic protocol used (including fluids administered and the amounts of drugs given), the patient's vital signs throughout anesthesia (e.g., pulse, respiration, BP, and temperature), laboratory results, the times at which anesthesia commenced and was terminated, the beginning and end of surgery, and the time required for recovery. Typically, the information is recorded chronologically to allow an overview of the patient's responses at every point throughout the procedure. Fig. 6.52 is an example of a completed record. Detailed records of this type are not always used in general veterinary practice; however, they are common in teaching, referral, or research institutions.

ANESTHESIA RECORD

Date: _____   Monitor:_____

Patient Name:_____ Wt:_____ Species:_____ Breed:_____ Sex:_____ Age:_____

Premedications:	Amount Given:	Route:	Time:	NOTES:
				Physical Status Class:
				Procedure:
				Anesthetist/Surgeon:

Induction Agents:	Amount Given:	Route:	Time:	Pre-op/Post-op data:

Maintenance Agents:	% Range/Total:	Route:

Reversal Agents:	Amount Given:	Route:	Time:

SpO₂ (%)
ETCO₂ (mm Hg)

TIME   00   15   30   45   00   15   30   45   00   15   30   45   Comments

Oxygen Flow (L/min)   6 4 2 1 0

Inhalant Agent:

Vaporizer Setting (%)   6 5 4 3 2 1 0

CODE:

● HR (monitor q5 min)

○ RR (monitor q5 min)

v Systolic BP (mm Hg)
X Mean BP (mm Hg)
∧ Diastolic BP (mm Hg)

S -Ⓢ (begin-end surgery)
P -Ⓟ (begin-end procedure)
Ⓘ-Ⓔ (intubate-extubate)

Monitoring:
❑ Esophageal stethoscope
❑ ECG monitor
❑ Doppler monitor
❑ Oscillometric BP
❑ Direct BP monitoring
❑ Pulse oximeter
❑ Capnograph
❑ Apnea monitor
❑ Temperature probe

Anesthetic System:
Machine: SA❑; LA❑; Ventilator ❑
Checked/leak tested/APL valve set ❑
Non-rebreathing ❑; Rebreathing ❑
ET tube size _____ Bag size _____

(graph vertical axis values: 220, 200, 180, 160, 140, 120, 100, 80, 60, 40, 35, 30, 25, 20, 15, 10, 8, 6, 4, 2)

Temperature (monitor q 15 min)

Line #	
Meds/Fluids:	1
	2
	3
	4
	5

FIG. 6.51 An example of an anesthesia record used to document the anesthetic procedure.

ANESTHESIA RECORD

Date: 3/25/19   Monitor: LINDA D.

Patient Name: JEAN _____ Wt: 21.4 kg Species: CANINE Breed: SHEP X Sex: F Age: 2 YOA.

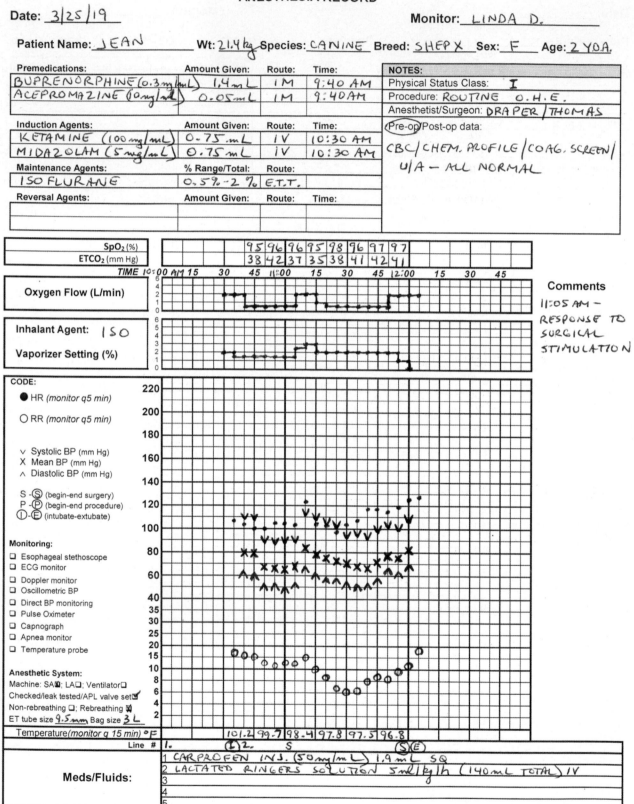

Premedications:	Amount Given:	Route:	Time:
BUPRENORPHINE (0.3 mg/mL)	1.4 mL	IM	9:40 AM
ACEPROMAZINE (10 mg/mL)	0.05 mL	IM	9:40 AM

Induction Agents:	Amount Given:	Route:	Time:
KETAMINE (100 mg/mL)	0.75 mL	IV	10:30 AM
MIDAZOLAM (5 mg/mL)	0.75 mL	IV	10:30 AM

Maintenance Agents:	% Range/Total:	Route:
ISOFLURANE	0.5% - 2%	E.T.T.

Reversal Agents:	Amount Given:	Route:	Time:

NOTES:
Physical Status Class: I
Procedure: ROUTINE O.H.E.
Anesthetist/Surgeon: DRAPER / THOMAS
(Pre-op)/Post-op data:
CBC / CHEM. PROFILE / COAG. SCREEN /
U/A — ALL NORMAL

SpO₂ (%)	95	96	96	95	98	96	97	97	
ETCO₂ (mm Hg)	38	42	37	35	38	41	42	41	

TIME 10:00 AM 15   30   45   11:00   15   30   45   12:00   15   30   45

Oxygen Flow (L/min)

Inhalant Agent: ISO
Vaporizer Setting (%)

Comments
11:05 AM —
RESPONSE TO
SURGICAL
STIMULATION

CODE:
● HR (monitor q5 min)
○ RR (monitor q5 min)
∨ Systolic BP (mm Hg)
X Mean BP (mm Hg)
∧ Diastolic BP (mm Hg)
S - Ⓢ (begin-end surgery)
P - Ⓟ (begin-end procedure)
Ⓘ - Ⓔ (intubate-extubate)

Monitoring:
☐ Esophageal stethoscope
☐ ECG monitor
☐ Doppler monitor
☐ Oscillometric BP
☐ Direct BP monitoring
☐ Pulse Oximeter
☐ Capnograph
☐ Apnea monitor
☐ Temperature probe

Anesthetic System:
Machine: SA☒; LA☐; Ventilator☐
Checked/leak tested/APL valve set☑
Non-rebreathing ☐; Rebreathing ☒
ET tube size 9.5 mm Bag size 3 L

Temperature (monitor q 15 min) °F	101.2	99.7	98.4	97.8	97.5	96.8

Line #	I.	Ⓘ	2.	S	Ⓢ Ⓔ

Meds/Fluids:
1 CARPROFEN INJ. (50 mg/mL) 1.9 mL SQ
2 LACTATED RINGERS SOLUTION 5 mL/kg/h (140 mL TOTAL) IV
3
4
5

FIG. 6.52 Completed anesthesia record. Looking at this finished record permits all details of this procedure to be easily reviewed, including patient data; doses, times, and routes of administration of all agents, adjuncts, and fluids; physical and machine-generated monitoring parameters; and detailed observations about the procedure.

KEY POINTS

1. The American College of Veterinary Anesthesia and Analgesia (ACVAA) has published guidelines for anesthetic monitoring intended to help veterinary anesthetists make sound monitoring decisions.

2. During any anesthetic procedure, the anesthetist must monitor the animal closely to ensure that the patient is safe and that the degree of central nervous system (CNS) depression or anesthetic depth is appropriate.

3. Effective monitoring is based on the principle that at any given anesthetic depth, monitoring parameters show predictable responses. Much discernment is required on the part of the anesthetist to interpret the significance of these parameters, however.

4. Knowledge of the anesthetic stages and planes gives the anesthetist a framework for meaningful interpretation of monitoring parameters.

5. The objectives of surgical anesthesia are that the patient does not move, is not aware, does not feel pain, has no memory of the procedure afterwards, and has stable cardiopulmonary function.

6. Physical monitoring parameters can be grouped into one of the following three classifications: (1) vital signs, (2) reflexes, and (3) other indicators of anesthetic depth.

7. Vital signs (including heart rate and rhythm, pulse strength, capillary refill time, mucous membrane color, respiration rate and depth, and temperature) are most helpful to determine whether the patient is safe.

8. Reflexes (including the laryngeal, swallowing, pedal, palpebral, corneal, and pupillary light reflex) and other indicators (including spontaneous movement, muscle tone, eye position, pupil size, response to surgical stimulation, lacrimation, salivation, and nystagmus) are most helpful to determine whether the anesthetic depth is appropriate.

9. Physical and machine monitoring parameters can be grouped according to whether they assess circulation, oxygenation, ventilation, or anesthetic depth.

10. Monitoring equipment, although not mandatory for effective patient monitoring, is necessary to meet the current standard of care, and in any case, generates data (including oxygen saturation, arterial blood pressure, cardiac electrical activity, inspired and expired CO_2 levels, blood gases, heart rate [HR], respiratory rate [RR], and tidal volume [V_T]) that help the anesthetist accurately assess patient status. This equipment often warns of impending problems early, so that the anesthetist can take action before they reach crisis level.

11. Effective monitoring requires the anesthetist to memorize normal monitoring parameters and to know what levels signal a need to inform the attending veterinarian.

12. The anesthetist must keep accurate and complete records of anesthetic procedures, the nature of which will vary depending on the clinical situation.

REVIEW QUESTIONS

1. When using commonly accepted doses, which of the following IV induction agents or combinations would be expected to depress respiratory function the least?
   a. Propofol
   b. Dexmedetomidine/fentanyl
   c. Alfaxalone
   d. Ketamine/midazolam

2. The plane of anesthesia most suitable for surgical procedures occurs during:
   a. Stage I
   b. Stage II
   c. Stage III
   d. Stage IV

3. Breath holding, vocalization, and involuntary movement of the limbs are most likely an indication that the animal is in what stage or plane of anesthesia?
   a. Stage I
   b. Stage II
   c. Stage III, light
   d. Stage III, deep

4. Anatomic dead space is considered to include:
   a. Air within the breathing tubes and the endotracheal tube
   b. Air within the digestive tract
   c. Air within the trachea, pharynx, larynx, bronchi, and nasal passages
   d. Air within the alveoli

5. The minimum acceptable heart rate for an anesthetized large-breed dog is _____ bpm.
   a. 60
   b. 70
   c. 80
   d. 100

6. Which of the following rhythms seen on an ECG tracing of a canine patient is generally most dangerous and requires immediate intervention?
   a. Supraventricular premature complexes
   b. Sinus arrhythmia
   c. Second-degree heart block
   d. Ventricular tachycardia

7. In general, a respiratory rate of less than _____ breaths/min in an anesthetized dog should be reported to the veterinarian.
   a. 4
   b. 6
   c. 10
   d. 15

8. A plethysmograph is a monitoring parameter that is displayed on some pulse oximeters. The plethysmograph is displayed as a waveform that helps the anesthetist determine if:
   a. The probe should be checked and readjusted
   b. Mean arterial pressure is acceptable
   c. Oxygen saturation is within a safe level
   d. The machine should be serviced

9. Tachypnea is:
   a. An increase in respiratory depth (tidal volume)
   b. An increase in respiratory rate
   c. A decrease in respiratory depth (tidal volume)
   d. A decrease in respiratory rate

10. A patient that has been anesthetized will often have a:
    a. Mild metabolic acidosis
    b. Mild metabolic alkalosis
    c. Mild respiratory acidosis
    d. Mild respiratory alkalosis

11. A 20-kg dog has been anesthetized by mask induction with isoflurane and after intubation, is maintained on 2% isoflurane with a flow rate of 2 L/min of oxygen. The heart rate is 80 bpm, respiratory rate is 4 breaths/min and shallow, the jaw tone is fully relaxed, pupils are dilated, and all reflexes are absent. This animal is most likely in what stage of anesthesia?
    a. Stage II
    b. Stage III, light
    c. Stage III, surgical
    d. Stage III, deep

12. An end-tidal CO_2 monitor can be used to detect each of the following except one. Which one cannot be determined with this monitoring device?
    a. Carbon monoxide poisoning
    b. Esophageal intubation
    c. Excessive dead space
    d. Cardiac arrest

13. Pulse oximetry allows accurate estimation of:
    a. Arterial blood pressure
    b. Pulse pressure
    c. Pao_2
    d. Percent saturation of hemoglobin with oxygen

14. During anesthesia, a mean arterial blood pressure of less than 60 mmHg in a dog or cat indicates:
    a. Inadequate tissue perfusion
    b. Imminent cardiac arrest
    c. A normal expected value during anesthesia
    d. Uncontrolled pain

15. The most accurate way to determine core body temperature in a German Shepherd is by:
    a. Directing an infrared monitoring device into the ear canal
    b. Placing a temperature probe in the caudal third of the esophagus
    c. Directing an infrared monitoring device toward axillary skin
    d. Placing a temperature probe at least 2 to 3 cm into the rectum

16. A pulse oximeter reading of 89% indicates:
    a. A normal value
    b. A state of hypoxemia but no need for therapy
    c. Significant hypoxemia and a need for supportive therapy
    d. A medical emergency

17. An $ETco_2$ level of 65 would commonly be caused by:
    a. Hyperventilation
    b. Decreased tidal volume
    c. Detachment of the endotracheal tube from the connector
    d. Hypothermia

18. Regarding oxygen transport:
    a. Most oxygen travels in the blood dissolved in plasma
    b. Spo_2 is an accurate indicator of oxygen available to the tissues even in anemic animals
    c. Pao_2 is closely related to Spo_2 (as one goes up, the other does also)
    d. When a patient is breathing 100% oxygen, the Pao_2 is expected to be in the range of 100 to 120 mmHg

For the following questions, more than one answer may be correct.

19. Which of the following statements about body temperature is/are correct?
    a. Body temperatures of 32°C to 34°C (89.6°F to 93.2°F) cause prolonged anesthetic recovery
    b. Dangerous CNS depression and changes in cardiac function may be seen at body temperatures less than 32°C (89.6°F)
    c. Ideally, IV fluids should be warmed to about 37.5°C (approximately 100°F) before administration to surgical patients
    d. Circulating warm water blankets should be set at 45°C (approximately 111°F)

20. For a patient that is in light stage III anesthesia, which of the following monitoring parameters may change in response to surgical stimulation (e.g., making a surgical incision or pulling on viscera)?
    a. Heart rate
    b. Respiratory rate
    c. Blood pressure
    d. Respiratory depth

21. When maintaining a patient with a halogenated inhalant anesthetic, which of the following changes in monitoring parameters are expected to occur as anesthetic depth increases?
    a. Blood pressure progressively decreases
    b. Respiratory minute volume progressively decreases
    c. Saliva and tear production progressively decreases
    d. Capillary refill time progressively decreases

22. Which of the following statements about nystagmus as a monitoring tool is/are accurate?
    a. Nystagmus is commonly seen in horses under very light anesthesia
    b. Nystagmus is not a useful indicator of anesthetic depth in small animals
    c. In a horse, a "divergent eye sign" is typically associated with an adequate plane of anesthesia for surgery
    d. Ruminants rarely show nystagmus under anesthesia

23. The AAHA and ACVAA monitoring guidelines recommend that heart rate, respiratory rate, mucous membrane color, capillary refill, and body temperature should be monitored on all patients. They also recommend monitoring of additional parameters that can only be measured by mechanical means. Which of the following parameters are on this list?
    a. Oxygen saturation
    b. Carbon dioxide levels
    c. Blood gases
    d. Arterial blood pressure

24. Pale mucous membranes commonly indicate:
    a. Blood loss
    b. Anemia
    c. Decreased perfusion
    d. Hypertension

25. An animal under surgical stage III anesthesia would exhibit which of the following signs?
    a. Brisk palpebral reflex
    b. Regular respiration
    c. Moderate skeletal muscle tone
    d. Dilated pupils

ANSWERS TO CASE PRESENTATIONS

Case Presentation 6.1

Question #1: Machine problems that can cause an increase in $ETco_2$ include saturation of the CO_2 absorbent and malfunction of the expiratory unidirectional valve. A variety of patient conditions that affect production of CO_2 at the cellular level or elimination of CO_2 from the lungs will also cause increased $ETco_2$, including hypoventilation, malignant hyperthermia, fever, and muscle tremors. In this case, the baseline CO_2 level was also increased. This happens only when CO_2 is being rebreathed, a situation that is generally caused by a machine malfunction or inadequate oxygen flow when using a nonrebreathing system.

Question #2: Management of a case such as this requires a rapid and efficient response because rebreathing CO_2 can cause the patient to decompensate very quickly. The best thing to do would be to remove the patient from the breathing circuit immediately and change to a spare machine if one was available. As long as the exhalation unidirectional valve was functional, a very high oxygen flow (200 to 300 mL/kg/min) could be used to flush CO_2 out of the system until the absorbent could be replaced, but if the unidirectional valve was at fault, either the patient would have to be changed to a different machine or, if one was not available, a nonrebreathing circuit designed for animals over 7 kg used. If no other option was available, the patient could be allowed to breathe room air until a suitable alternative was available. In the last scenario it may also be necessary to maintain anesthesia using injectable agents.

Outcome of This Case

Knowing that these levels suggested rebreathing of CO_2, the anesthetist immediately examined the carbon dioxide absorber canister and the unidirectional valves. The absorbent granules had not changed in color or appearance and had been recently changed. The unidirectional valves were difficult to evaluate because of the presence of a large amount of condensation inside the domes. Careful examination revealed that the expiratory valve leaflet had temporarily become stuck to the top of the dome because of the presence of the moisture within the valve. The patient was immediately disconnected from the breathing circuit and another machine was used for the duration of the procedure. Within a short time of placement on the new machine, Cooper's breathing and capnogram returned to normal and the procedure was completed without further incident.

Later, the valve was disassembled, cleaned, and reassembled. Although there was nothing wrong with the valve, it appeared that a combination of factors had caused the valve to malfunction. Apparently, during a particularly forceful exhalation, the valve leaflet had been momentarily forced to the top of the dome, where it adhered to the inner surface of the dome because of the presence of the excess moisture, preventing proper closure.

This case illustrates the importance of vigilant monitoring, shows how monitoring equipment can provide vital information not available from physical monitoring parameters, and underscores the importance of monitoring multiple parameters whenever possible. Although the anesthetist initially identified the problem by observation of physical signs, the capnograph allowed her to identify, isolate, and correct the problem rapidly and efficiently before the patient was seriously affected.

Case Presentation 6.2

Question #1: Without more information, the question cannot be answered. Mia appears to be in light stage III anesthesia and may be deeply anesthetized enough to intubate, but this cannot be definitively determined.

Question #2: The anesthetist should assess the jaw tone and observe (1) whether there is any resistance when the tongue is gently pulled, and (2) whether or not the mouth can be held open without patient movement before assuming that intubation is possible.

This case highlights the importance of assessing multiple parameters before making a decision regarding anesthetic depth.

Case Presentation 6.3

Question #1: Chester is indeed adequately anesthetized and in fact, may be at an excessive anesthetic depth. The respiratory rate and tidal volume are low. The absence of the reflexes, the central pupils, and the flaccid jaw tone all indicate that the animal may be in deep stage III anesthesia. At this point, the anesthetist should consider reducing the isoflurane setting to 1% to 1.5% and monitor the animal for signs of decreased depth. After doing this, the anesthetist should carefully monitor the animal for signs that may be indicative of pain perception (e.g., increased respiratory rate, increased blood pressure, or voluntary movement) to ensure that the vaporizer setting is high enough for adequate analgesia. Even in animals at adequate anesthetic depth, the heart rate and respiratory rate will commonly increase slightly in response to surgical stimulation.

This case illustrates the importance of frequent assessment of monitoring parameters with special attention to subtle changes that signal a change in anesthetic depth.

Case Presentation 6.4

Question #1: The anesthetist cannot be sure whether the anesthetic depth is appropriate or excessive because some parameters indicate stage III surgical anesthesia (heart rate, jaw tone), but others indicate deep stage III anesthesia (respiratory rate, reflexes, eye position, and PLR). The patient has been given glycopyrrolate and ketamine, which may have stabilized or even elevated the heart rate. Jaw tone is often not a completely reliable indicator of anesthetic depth because it is influenced by so many factors. At this point, the anesthetist should assume the patient is excessively deeply anesthetized and should reduce the concentration of sevoflurane. At the same time, the anesthetist should monitor the patient for signs of arousal.

This case highlights the importance of critical thinking and careful consideration in accurate determination of anesthetic depth.

SELECTED READINGS

American College of Veterinary Anesthesia and Analgesia: *Recommendations for monitoring anesthetized veterinary patients*. Available from: www.acvaa.org. Accessed September, 2021.

Clark-Price S: ECG and blood pressure monitoring in anesthetized patients, DVM360.com, CVC in Washington, DC, Proceedings. May 1, 2011.

Cooley KG, Johnson RA: *Veterinary anesthetic and monitoring equipment*, ed 1, Ames, IA, 2018, John Wiley & Sons, Inc.

Doherty T, Valverde A: *Manual of equine anesthesia and analgesia*, Ames, IA, 2022, Blackwell Publishing, Ltd.

Grimm KA: Arterial blood gas analysis and interpretation in anesthetized patients. DVM360.com. Vet Med. Accessed November 1, 2010.

Grubb T, Sager J, Gaynor JS, et al: 2020 AAHA Anesthesia and Monitoring Guidelines for dogs and cats, *J Am Anim Hosp Assoc* 56(2):59–82, 2020.

Haskins SC: Monitoring. In Grimm KA, Tranquilli WJ, Lamont LA, editors: *Essentials of small animal anesthesia and analgesia*, ed 2, Ames, IA, 2011, Wiley-Blackwell, pp 197–239.

Haskins SC: Monitoring anesthetized patients. In Grimm KA, Lamont LA, Tranquilli SA, editors: *Lumb & Jones' veterinary anesthesia and analgesia*, ed 5, Ames, IA, 2015, John Wiley & Sons, Inc., pp 86–113.

Ko J, Krimins R: *Anesthetic monitoring your questions answered*, 2012, Today's Veterinary Practice.

Ko J, Krimins R: *Anesthetic monitoring devices to use & what the results mean*, 2012, Today's Veterinary Practice.

Ko J, Krimins R: *Anesthetic monitoring therapeutic actions*, 2012, Today's Veterinary Practice.

McNurney T: Measuring blood pressure and managing hypotension in the surgical patient, *Firstline* 18(2), 2021.

Muir WM, Hubbell JA: *Equine anesthesia*, ed 2, St. Louis, MO, 2008, Saunders Elsevier.

Muir WW, Hubbell JA, Bednarski RM, et al: *Handbook of veterinary anesthesia*, ed 5, St. Louis, 2013, Elsevier.

Murrell JC: Monitoring the anesthetized horse. In Doherty T, Valverde A, editors: *Manual of equine anesthesia and analgesia*, Ames, IA, 2022, Blackwell, pp 187–205.

Pablo LS: Monitoring the anesthetized patients, DVM360.com, CVC in Kansas City Proceedings. August 1, 2011.

Quandt J: *Hypothermia in the operating room*, 2018, Today's Veterinary Practice.

Reed R: *Image gallery: capnography*, Clinician's Brief. Available from: https://www.cliniciansbrief.com/article/image-gallery-capnography. 2017 Web exclusive.

Robertson SA, Gogolski SM, Pascoe P, et al: AAFP Feline Anesthesia Guidelines, *J Feline Med Surg* 20:602–634, 2018.

Rowland S. Blood pressure management in equine anesthesia, *Vet Tech* 34(7), 2013.

Schauvliege S: Patient monitoring and monitoring equipment. In Duke-Novakovski T, DeVries M, Seymour C, editors: *BSAVA manual of canine and feline anaesthesia and analgesia*, ed 3, Glouchester, UK, 2016, British Small Animal Veterinary Association, pp 77–96.

Scislowicz O: *Blood pressure measurement*, 2018, Veterinary Team Brief.

Sidari H: *The veterinary nurse's role in reading blood gases*, 2021, Today's Veterinary Nurse, Summer.

Special Techniques

OUTLINE

LEARNING OBJECTIVES

When you have completed this chapter, you will be able to:
- Define or explain the terms local anesthesia, sensory neuron, motor neuron, infiltration, line block, nerve block, ring block, splash block, epidural anesthesia, cauda equina, and sympathetic blockade.
- List the advantages and disadvantages associated with the use of local anesthetic agents.
- Describe the ways in which local anesthetic agents may be used, including topical, infiltration, regional, intraarticular, epidural, intravenous administration, and intraperitoneal lavage.
- Outline the methods for performing a nerve block and a line block, and list clinical situations in veterinary practice in which these blocks are used.
- Describe the technique for performing an epidural block and give examples of clinical situations in which this block could be used.

- Explain the risks involved and the adverse effects that may be seen with the use of local anesthetic agents.
- Define or explain the terms tidal volume, respiratory minute volume, atelectasis, controlled ventilation, assisted ventilation, manual ventilation, and mechanical ventilation.
- Explain the difference between assisted and controlled ventilation.
- Describe the techniques of manual, mechanical, periodic, and intermittent mandatory ventilation and their application to anesthesia.
- List the indications for the use of neuromuscular blocking agents and the hazards associated with their use.
- Describe the differences between the two classes of neuromuscular blocking agents, including mode of action and reversibility.

KEY TERMS

Assisted ventilation
Atelectasis
Bagging
Cauda equina
Controlled ventilation
Dependent
Epidural anesthesia
Eutectic mixture
Hypercarbia
Infiltration

Intermittent mandatory ventilation
Intraperitoneal splash block
Line block
Local anesthesia
Manual ventilation
Mechanical ventilation
Motor neurons
Nerve block
Neuromuscular blocking agents
Paralysis

Paresis
Paresthesia
Positive pressure ventilation
Respiratory minute volume
Ring block
Scoliosis
Sensory neurons
Splash block
Sympathetic blockade
Tidal volume

The anesthetic agents and techniques used for routine procedures on most veterinary patients are described in Chapters 9, 10, and 11. In addition, one or more specialized techniques such as local anesthesia, mechanical ventilation, and/or the use of neuromuscular blocking agents may be indicated for a patient. This chapter describes these techniques and indicates the circumstances in which they may be useful.

LOCAL ANESTHESIA

The term *local anesthesia* (also referred to as *local analgesia* because local anesthesia blocks pain transmission) can be defined as the use of a chemical agent on sensory neurons to produce a disruption of nerve impulse transmission, leading to a temporary loss of sensation.

Local anesthesia is an effective, practical, and inexpensive means of producing anesthesia when the patient is tractable, when general anesthesia is undesirable or of high risk, or when the means to deliver general anesthesia safely are unavailable. The advantages of local anesthesia include low cardiovascular toxicity, low cost, excellent pain control in the immediate postoperative period, and minimal patient recovery time. Local anesthetics are therefore commonly used in ruminants for obstetric and abdominal procedures, often without sedation. Local anesthesia is frequently used to complement standing sedation in horses. Although local anesthesia is less commonly used instead of general anesthesia for canine and feline patients, it may be a viable alternative in some patients. The choice between local anesthesia and general anesthesia is made by the attending veterinarian on the basis of such factors as the temperament, age, species, and physical status of the patient; cost; the nature of the operation to be performed; and the anesthetist's skill in performing the local anesthesia procedure.

Local anesthetics are also first-tier agents used in conjunction with general anesthesia to enhance pain control during and after many surgical procedures including ovariohysterectomies, castrations, dental extractions, surgery involving the mandible, limb amputations and other orthopedic surgeries, thoracic surgery, and abdominal surgery. The dose of the general anesthetic required may be significantly reduced because of the analgesia provided by the local anesthetic. The practice of providing preemptive analgesia by performing nerve blocks and regional blocks using local anesthetics has become increasingly common over the past several years and will likely continue to do so.

> **TECHNICIAN NOTE** Local anesthetics are first-tier agents used in conjunction with general anesthesia to enhance pain control during and after surgery. The dose of the general anesthetic required may be significantly reduced because of the analgesia provided by the local anesthetic.

Local Anesthetic Agents

Many local anesthetic agents are available. These agents vary in strength, duration of effect, and method of use (Table 7.1). Lidocaine, bupivacaine, mepivacaine, and procaine are the agents most commonly used for skin infiltration and application to mucous membranes. Tetracaine and proparacaine are reserved chiefly for ophthalmic use.

Of the various local anesthetic agents available, lidocaine and bupivacaine are most commonly used in veterinary medicine. Lidocaine is available at a concentration of 0.5% to 2% and bupivacaine as a 0.25% or 0.5% solution. Both agents can be diluted with sterile saline (not water) if a lower concentration is desired. Bupivacaine has a slower onset of action (20 minutes) and a longer duration (6 hours) than lidocaine (almost immediate onset, duration 1 to 2 hours).

TABLE 7.1 Local Analgesics

Agent (Generic Name)	Agent (Trade Name)	Potency (Procaine = 1)	Dose	Onset and Duration of Action
Lidocaine[a]	Xylocaine	2	0.5%–2% for injection 2%–4% for topical use Do not exceed 10 mg/kg SC or 4 mg/kg IV in dogs; do not exceed 10 mg/kg SC and 2 mg/kg IV in large animals; do not exceed 4 mg/kg SC or 0.5 mg/kg IV in cats	Immediate onset; duration 1–2 hrs with epinephrine, 1 hr without; IV administration should be done slowly over 15–20 min
Mepivacaine	Carbocaine	2.5	1%–2% for injection Do not exceed 5 mg/kg in dogs or 2.5 mg/kg in cats	Immediate onset; duration 90–180 min
Tetracaine	Pontocaine	12	0.1% for injection 0.2% for topical use	Onset 5–10 min; duration 2 hrs
Bupivacaine	Marcaine	8	0.25%–0.5% for injection Give SC only Do not exceed 2 mg/kg in dogs or 1 mg/kg in cats	Onset 20 min; duration 4–6 hrs
Procaine	Novocain	1	1%, 2%, 10%	Immediate onset, duration 1 hr

[a]Sodium bicarbonate (8.4%, 1 mEq/mL) is used as follows: add 1 mL sodium bicarbonate to 10 mL of 2% lidocaine.
IV, Intravenously; *SC*, subcutaneously.
From Skarda RT: Local and regional analgesia. In Short CE, ed.: *Principles and practices of veterinary anesthesia*, Baltimore, 1987, Williams & Wilkins.

Characteristics of Local Anesthetics

Local anesthetics differ from general anesthetics in several important respects:

- Local anesthetics are not general anesthetics. The term *general anesthetic* is reserved for those drugs such as inhalant anesthetics, propofol, ketamine, or alfaxalone that primarily affect neurons in the brain and produce unconsciousness. Like general anesthetics, local anesthetics exert their effect on neurons, with the target neurons being in the peripheral nervous system and spinal cord. Local anesthetics normally do not affect the brain and have no sedative effect. The patient remains fully conscious unless other agents such as tranquilizers, neuroleptanalgesics, or general anesthetics are used.
- If the appropriate dose and route of administration are used, local anesthetics have relatively few effects on the cardiovascular or respiratory systems. In contrast, preanesthetic medications and general anesthetics may have significant cardiovascular and respiratory effects. For this reason, local anesthesia may be preferable to general anesthesia for certain high-risk patients. However, local anesthetics are not without risk of toxicity and the anesthetist should use caution to avoid overdosage, especially in small patients.
- Whereas general anesthetics are widely distributed throughout the body, local anesthetics primarily exert their effects in the area closest to the site of injection. Effective use of local anesthetics requires precise placement of the drug immediately adjacent to the target nerve (avoiding injection into the nerve). The veterinarian or technician performing the procedure must be familiar with the technique involved for each type of nerve block. For example, it is possible to block the sensory nerve of a tooth in a dog to perform a dental procedure; however, accurate and detailed knowledge of the neuroanatomy of the oral cavity is necessary. Local anesthetics are relatively ineffective in areas where drug diffusion is impeded by fat, bone, cartilage, fascia, tendon, and other connective tissues, as well as the presence of inflammation and infection.
- Unlike general anesthetics, local anesthetics are not normally transferred across the placenta to the fetus. For this reason, local anesthesia is used for cesarean sections and obstetric manipulations, particularly in ruminants, and also in small-animal patients when general anesthesia is considered high risk.

> **TECHNICIAN NOTE** Local anesthetics do not cross the placenta to the fetus. They are therefore useful for cesarean section and obstetric manipulation, particularly in ruminants.

Mechanism of Action

The peripheral nervous system and spinal cord are made up of many types of neurons. The primary targets of local anesthetic drugs are the neurons that convey sensations (i.e., pain, heat, cold, and pressure) from the skin, muscles, and other peripheral tissues to the brain. These neurons (called *sensory neurons*) are affected by even small amounts of local anesthetic, provided the drug is deposited in proximity to the neuron. Local anesthetics result in antagonism, also referred to as blockade, of sodium channels. When the sodium channels of a neuron are blocked, the neuron cannot generate electrical impulses. A local anesthetic drug therefore acts as a membrane stabilizer, stopping the process of nerve depolarization. The result is a loss of nerve conduction. Reversal of this effect occurs as the drug is absorbed into the local circulation. Local anesthetics are then redistributed to the liver, where they are metabolized.

Another type of neuron (called a *motor neuron*) conveys impulses from the brain to muscle fibers and is responsible for initiating and controlling voluntary movements. Motor neurons are also sensitive to the effect of local anesthetics, and administration of a local anesthetic may cause temporary paresis (weakness) or paralysis (loss of voluntary movement) in the area served by the affected motor neurons.

> **TECHNICIAN NOTE** Because motor neurons are also sensitive to the effect of local anesthetics, administration of a local anesthetic may cause temporary paresis (weakness) or paralysis (loss of voluntary movement) in the area served by the affected motor neurons.

Loss of sensation and loss of motor ability can be seen concurrently. For example, use of a local anesthetic near the terminal end of the spinal cord (called an *epidural block*) will result in loss of sensation and voluntary movement to all areas in the caudal abdomen and pelvic limbs. The sensations that are lost are, in order of loss: pain, cold, warmth, touch, joint sensation, and deep pressure. After an epidural block, the patient will be unable to move the pelvic limbs, and the muscles, including the anal sphincter, will appear relaxed.

Local anesthetics also affect the neurons of the autonomic nervous system. These neurons convey impulses between the brain and the blood vessels and internal organs (including the heart). If these neurons are exposed to local anesthetics, there may be a temporary loss of function. This is most important in the sympathetic nervous system, and the loss of function of these neurons is called a sympathetic blockade. The main effect in the peripheral tissues is vasodilation, resulting in flushing and increased skin temperature of the affected area. If severe, vasodilation may cause blood pressure to fall, leading to clinically significant hypotension. Sympathetic blockade can also be seen after epidural blocks with lidocaine and other local anesthetics because sympathetic ganglia adjacent to the vertebrae are affected. If sympathetic blockade occurs within the thoracic spinal cord (as may occur if local anesthetic is allowed to diffuse into the thoracic spinal canal), sympathetic innervation to the heart may be blocked, resulting in bradycardia and impaired ventricular contractions, both of which are undesirable.

> **TECHNICIAN NOTE** Local anesthetics also affect the neurons of the autonomic nervous system, causing sympathetic blockade. Signs include flushing and increased skin temperature of the affected area and, if severe, hypotension. Treatment consists of intravenous crystalloid fluid administration at a rate of 20 mL/kg over a 15–20 min period.

Route of Administration of Local Anesthetics

Local anesthetic techniques are often used in conjunction with neuroleptanalgesics, tranquilizers, or other injectable medications. This helps to ensure adequate restraint, allowing accurate and safe injection of the local anesthetic and preventing movement of the patient during the surgical procedure.

Local anesthetics can be administered by a variety of routes, including topical application, infiltration (injection), or introduction into a joint (intraarticular), nerve plexus, vein, or the epidural space.

Topical Use

Local anesthetics such as lidocaine are usually ineffective when applied directly to intact skin because the drug molecules are unable to penetrate the epidermis and reach the dermis, where the peripheral nerves are located. However, local anesthetics can be used for topical analgesia in some clinical situations:

- A cream formulation containing a eutectic mixture of 2.5% lidocaine and 2.5% prilocaine (EMLA cream) can be used to desensitize intact skin for superficial minor procedures such as catheterization. A thick layer of cream is applied to intact shaved skin in the area to be anesthetized and covered with an occlusive dressing for 10 minutes. The duration of effect is 1 to 2 hours. EMLA cream is available in 5-g or 30-g tubes and in single-dose anesthetic discs. It should not be applied to the eyes or to inflamed or broken skin. The patient should be prevented from licking treated areas.
- Wounds or open surgical sites (e.g., lateral ear resection, dewclaw removal) can be treated with topical anesthetic sprays such as 10% lidocaine or by direct application of 0.25% bupivacaine. Sterile gauze sponges soaked with a mixture of local anesthetic and saline can also be placed on an open surgical site. The use of sprays or soaked gauze sponges is called a splash block. The efficacy of this technique has not been well established, but it appears to be most effective if the surgical field is relatively dry, with minimal bleeding. Care must be taken to avoid local anesthetic overdose, which is a particular concern with small patients. The dose of lidocaine given by this route should not exceed 4 mg/kg for the dog and 2 mg/kg for the cat. For bupivacaine, the dose should not exceed 2 mg/kg in dogs and 0.5 mg/kg in cats.

> **TECHNICIAN NOTE** When applying local anesthetics to wounds or open surgical sites, care must be taken to avoid local anesthetic overdose, which is a particular concern with small patients.

- Bupivacaine can be instilled through a chest tube placed during thoracic surgery. Local anesthetic administration should be delayed until the patient is awake because instillation of bupivacaine into the chest cavity of an anesthetized patient may cause cardiac arrhythmias.
- Local anesthetics can be absorbed by mucous membranes, including the conjunctiva, nose, mouth, larynx, and lining of the urethra. They can be administered as topical sprays, drops, or ointment applied to these areas. For example, lidocaine spray is used to desensitize the larynx and prevent laryngospasm in cats. Another example of topical use of local anesthetics is the application of 0.5% proparacaine or tetracaine to the surface of the eye. This procedure desensitizes the cornea and conjunctiva, allowing procedures such as conjunctival scraping or tonometry. Gel containing local anesthetic (lidocaine or tetracaine) can be applied to a urinary catheter to ease catheterization. In each case, analgesia of the mucous membrane results within 60 to 90 seconds and allows procedures to be performed with less discomfort to the patient. Analgesia lasts for 10 to 15 minutes.
- Lidocaine patches are available that are applied to the skin and are effective for management of superficial wounds or incisional pain.

Although topical anesthetics are useful in the situations previously mentioned, they generally offer less pain relief and a shorter duration of effect than local anesthetics given by infiltration.

Infiltration

Local anesthetics may be infiltrated (injected) into tissues, preferably in proximity to the target nerve. The local anesthetic can be given intradermally, subcutaneously, or between muscle planes. Infiltration techniques are used to provide analgesia for surgery involving superficial tissues, including skin biopsies, removal of small skin tumors, and repair of minor lacerations.

The procedure used for infiltration of local anesthetics is relatively simple. The area must be clipped and a skin antiseptic applied in a manner similar to surgical preparation. This prevents inadvertent contamination of the tissues with skin bacteria when the local anesthetic is injected. A small needle (23- or 25-gauge in small-animal and equine patients, 20- or 22-gauge in ruminants) is often used to prevent tissue damage and allow for more precise placement of the drug. The amount of the drug to be injected varies with the location and procedure used and may be as little as 0.1 mL or as much as several milliliters in a dog, or several to tens of milliliters in large-animal patients. The onset of analgesia is usually 3 to 5 minutes after the injection of lidocaine.

Before surgery commences, it is advisable to test the effectiveness of the block by gently pricking the skin with a 22-gauge needle. If sensation is still present, the anesthetist should wait several minutes longer and consider repeating the injection or using another anesthetic protocol if the block does not take effect.

The infiltration of local anesthetics is not universally effective. Deep tissues such as muscles are unlikely to be affected when only superficial neurons are blocked. In addition, obstacles such as scar tissue or fibrous tissue, fat, edema, and hemorrhage impede diffusion of local anesthetic. Local anesthetics are also relatively ineffective when injected into inflamed or infected areas. In areas of active inflammation, tissue pH is acidic, resulting in rapid inactivation of the drug. For this reason and also for the prevention of contamination of other tissue, local anesthetics should not be infiltrated into infected tissues.

Once the local anesthetic reaches the neuron, the duration of effect depends on the type of drug being used (see Table 7.1) and the rate of absorption by local blood vessels. This in turn will depend on whether epinephrine is used with the local anesthetic or not. Lidocaine, the drug most commonly used for local injection, may be purchased with or without epinephrine. In the combined solution, the concentration of epinephrine is 0.01 mg/mL.

Epinephrine is added to lidocaine for the two reasons:

1. Epinephrine causes constriction of blood vessels in the area of the injection. This decreases the rate of drug absorption and thereby prolongs the effect of the lidocaine by approximately 50%.
2. By causing vasoconstriction, epinephrine reduces the concentration of local anesthetic that enters the circulation at any given time, thereby reducing toxicity of the drug. This is most effective for short-acting drugs such as lidocaine and less helpful for long-acting drugs such as bupivacaine.

Lidocaine without epinephrine may be preferred to lidocaine with epinephrine in some situations. A solution containing epinephrine should not be used at an incision site because it may impair tissue perfusion and healing. Lidocaine with epinephrine should not be used on the ears, tail, or digits because circulation to these areas may be compromised. Epinephrine also increases the risk of ventricular arrhythmias and should be used with caution in animals with known cardiac disease. Lidocaine without epinephrine is used for intravenous (IV) techniques.

> **TECHNICIAN NOTE** Local anesthetics with epinephrine should not be administered intravenously and should be avoided when blocks of extremities are performed as circulation to these areas may become compromised.
>
> Local anesthetic injections may be painful in the awake patient, in part because they are acidic. Some anesthetists, when administering lidocaine, add sodium bicarbonate (at one-tenth the volume of local anesthetic) to buffer and raise the pH, which will decrease pain on injection.
>
> Two techniques are commonly used for infiltration of local anesthetics: nerve blocks and **line blocks**.

Nerve Blocks

A nerve block is achieved by injecting local anesthetic in proximity to a nerve to desensitize a particular anatomic site. One familiar example is the use of Novocain (procaine) in human dentistry. Nerve blocks are used commonly in anesthesia of large animals and also may be used in small animals, provided the location of the target nerve is known exactly. Some nerve blocks are performed using ultrasound to determine that the needle is in the correct location prior to local anesthetic injection. Reference texts contain illustrations that indicate the location of nerve blocks for different species and particular areas of the body. Before a nerve block is performed, the nerve is palpated to determine its location, although this may not always be possible if the nerve is small.

Once the location of the nerve supplying the surgical site is known, the procedure is straightforward. After the skin has been clipped and prepared for surgery, a small amount of local anesthetic is injected immediately adjacent to the nerve. Lidocaine or bupivacaine can be used. The drug diffuses through the tissues to reach the target nerve. Caution should be used to avoid injecting directly into the nerve because temporary or permanent loss of nerve function can occur. If resistance is encountered during injection, it may indicate intraneural injection. The needle should be withdrawn and repositioned if this occurs. Also, IV injection of the local anesthetic should be avoided because this may cause unwanted central nervous system and cardiovascular effects. To avoid IV injection, always aspirate before injecting a local anesthetic. If blood appears in the syringe, the needle should be withdrawn and the location of the injection changed.

> **TECHNICIAN NOTE** To avoid intravenous injection, always aspirate before injecting a local anesthetic. If blood appears in the syringe, the needle should be withdrawn and the location of the injection changed.

Clinical situations in which nerve blocks can be used include but are not limited to the following:

- Dental blocks in dogs and cats: rostral maxillary nerve (infraorbital) block, caudal mandibular nerve block, and rostral mandibular nerve (mental) block (Fig. 7.1)
- Intercostal nerve blocks in animals undergoing chest surgery
- Infiltration of nerves during amputation of a limb (0.5 mL of 0.5% bupivacaine, injected into and around the nerves during the operation)
- Nerve blocks to provide analgesia for declawing cats (Procedure 7.1)
- Paravertebral blocks for abdominal surgery or cesarean sections in cattle (Procedure 7.2)
- Cornual blocks for dehorning cattle
- Diagnostic nerve blocks in awake horses as part of a lameness examination

Specialty textbooks and journal articles provide complete descriptions of these and other nerve blocks. Specific nerve blocks of the head that are easy to perform and have few side effects include the rostral maxillary nerve (infraorbital) block, the caudal mandibular nerve block, and the rostral mandibular nerve (mental) block (see Fig. 7.1). Blocking the nerves in the forelimb of the cat before declaw surgery is also a straightforward procedure (see Procedure 7.1).

Regardless of the technique used, it is important to allow sufficient time for the tissues to absorb the drug (15 to 20 minutes) before the surgical or dental procedure is started. When properly performed, these blocks not only decrease the amount of general anesthetic required but also provide excellent short-term analgesia after the procedure.

Line Blocks

Often, the attending veterinarian will perform an operation on an area of tissue that is served by numerous small nerves. In this situation, a line block, consisting of a continuous line of local anesthetic, can be placed in the subcutaneous or subcuticular tissues immediately proximal to the target area (Fig. 7.2 A). If the line of local anesthetic completely encircles an anatomic part, such as a digit or teat, it is called a **ring block**.

A line block should be positioned between the target area and the spinal cord because this will block the sensory neurons

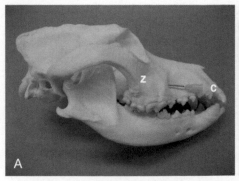
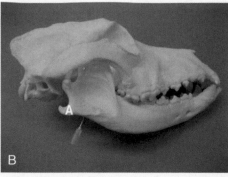
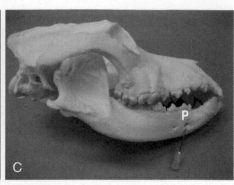

FIG. 7.1 **(A)** Rostral maxillary nerve (infraorbital) block. Blocking the infraorbital nerve desensitizes the upper lip, the nose, the roof of the nasal cavity, and the skin overlying these structures, up to the level of the infraorbital foramen. The nerve is blocked as it exits the infraorbital canal. The infraorbital canal is palpated on a line between the dorsal border of the zygomatic process *(Z)* and the gum line of the upper canine *(C)*. The needle is advanced parallel to the face into the canal to deposit local anesthetic. **(B)** Caudal mandibular nerve block. The mandibular nerve is blocked to anesthetize the teeth, skin, and mucosa of the lower jaw and lip. The needle is placed at the angle of the jaw, approximately 0.5 cm rostral to the angular process *(A)*, then advanced on the medial aspect of the ramus of the mandible for 1 to 2 cm before depositing local anesthetic. **(C)** Rostral mandibular nerve (mental) block. Analgesia of the lower lip alone can be achieved by blocking the mandibular nerve as it exits the mental foramen. The needle is positioned at the mental foramen directly below the second premolar tooth *(P)*.

PROCEDURE 7.1   Performing a Three-Point Nerve Block for Declawing a Cat

1. Diagrammatic view of needle placement for three-point nerve block for right forelimb declaw in a cat.

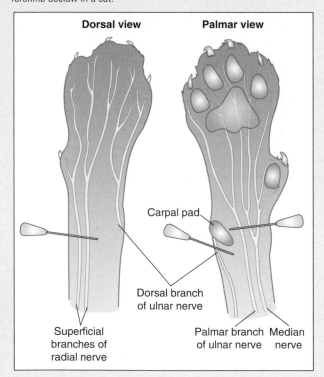

2. First, 0.2 mL of 2% lidocaine is deposited dorsally, proximal to the carpus, to target the branches of the radial nerve.

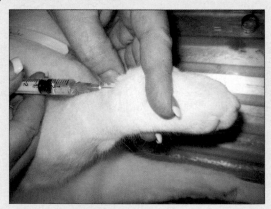

3. Second, 0.1 mL of 2% lidocaine is deposited on each side of the superficial digital flexor tendon to target the median nerve medially (left) and ulnar nerve laterally (right). Bupivacaine can be used in place of lidocaine, ensuring that a total dose of 1 mg/kg is not exceeded.

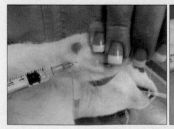
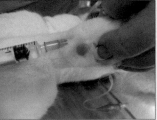

PROCEDURE 7.2 **Performing Paravertebral Anesthesia in a Cow**

1. The sites for paravertebral anesthesia of spinal nerves T13–L2 for flank laparotomy.

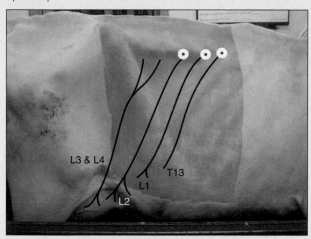

2. The space cranial to the transverse spinous process of L1 is palpated.

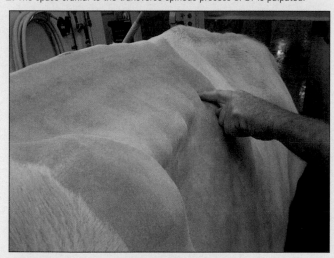

3. A 1.5-inch, large-gauge needle is inserted in the skin over the space, approximately 2.5–5 cm from the midline.

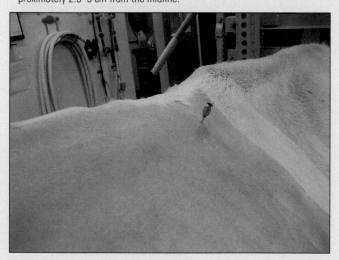

4. Then 2–3 mL of lidocaine is injected into the subcutaneous tissues.

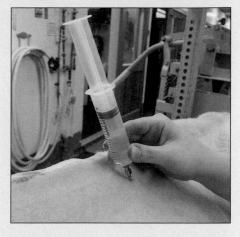

5. A 2.5–3.5-inch spinal needle is passed through the anesthetized tissue, in this case inside the short needle.

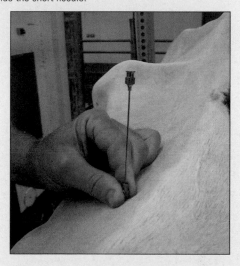

6. The remainder of the local anesthetic is deposited above and below the intertransverse fascia to anesthetize the dorsal and ventral branches of the spinal nerve.

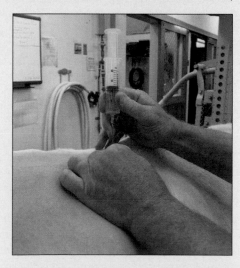

Continued

PROCEDURE 7.2 *Performing Paravertebral Anesthesia in a Cow—cont'd*

7. A correctly performed block will produce scoliosis toward the side of the block.

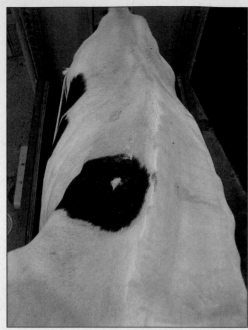

8. Skin sensitivity to a needle prick can be assessed before commencement of surgery.

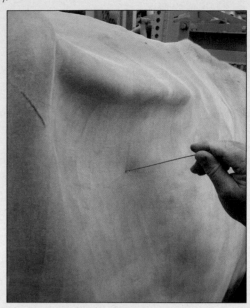

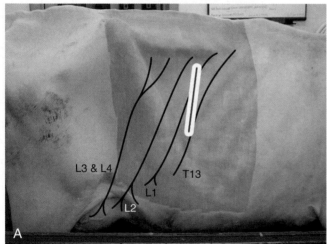

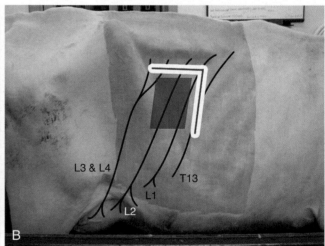

FIG. 7.2 Location for performing a line block or L-block in a cow for standing flank laparotomy. **(A)** Line for infiltrating local anesthetic. The surgical incision is made along the line where anesthesia has been infiltrated. **(B)** The line can be extended in an inverted L-shape to anesthetize the caudal part of the surgical field. The surgical incision is made anywhere in the box outlined to the left of the L.

most effectively. As with nerve blocks, the area is clipped and the skin prepared. A line block is performed by inserting the needle along the proposed line of infiltration, then gradually withdrawing the needle while simultaneously injecting a small amount of local anesthetic. If several injections are made, the needle should be inserted into a desensitized area of skin to avoid patient discomfort. Care should be taken to avoid inserting the needle into contaminated tissue (e.g., an infected wound).

> **TECHNICIAN NOTE** A line block is performed by inserting the needle along the proposed line of infiltration, then gradually withdrawing the needle while simultaneously injecting a small amount of local anesthetic.

Line blocks and ring blocks are used extensively in food animal and equine surgery, particularly in cattle. Examples include teat surgery and wound repair. A particular type of line block, called an *L-block*, is used for laparotomy in ruminants (see Fig. 7.2 B).

Specific Local Blocks

Incision block, testicular block, and intraperitoneal splash block or lavage are three specific types of local blocks used to provide analgesia for patients undergoing spays and castrations as well as other procedures (as indicated in the following paragraphs). They are relatively inexpensive, easy to perform, and effective as one part of a multimodal approach to perioperative pain control.

Incision block for spays and other abdominal surgeries. An incision block is a type of line block that can be used to provide preemptive analgesia for a variety of procedures including spays and other abdominal surgeries. To perform this block, bupivacaine (2 mg/kg in dogs or 1 mg/kg in cats) is injected subcutaneously along the planned site of the incision at least 20 minutes prior to surgery. For long incisions, it may be necessary to dilute the local anesthetic 1:1 with saline in order to have sufficient volume.

Testicular block. A testicular block is used specifically to provide preemptive analgesia for animals undergoing castration. Bupivacaine up to 0.5 mg/kg/testicle (dog or cat) is injected into the testicular tissue slowly until the testicle feels turgid. The block should be performed 20 minutes prior to surgical incision and can be completed after the initial surgical preparation to allow enough time for the local anesthetic to diffuse to the spermatic cord. As always, when injecting local anesthetic, it is important to aspirate prior to injecting to avoid IV injection.

Intraperitoneal splash block/lavage. An intraperitoneal splash block or lavage is a technique used to provide analgesia for patients undergoing a spay or other abdominal procedure, and it is performed by depositing local anesthetic in proximity to the affected tissues. Immediately prior to abdominal wall closure, bupivacaine (3 mg/kg in dogs and 2 mg/kg in cats) is administered into the abdominal cavity (lavage). In the case of ovariohysterectomy, the total volume can be divided in three, with a third of the injectate directed towards each of the ovarian pedicles and the uterine stump (splash block).

Intraarticular Administration

In certain circumstances, local anesthetics can be injected directly into a joint. For example, bupivacaine has been shown to provide significant analgesia when injected into the stifle joint at the conclusion of stifle arthroscopy and surgery. A dose of 0.4 mL/kg of 0.5% bupivacaine, diluted with sterile saline (not water) to a volume sufficient to fill the joint, has been recommended. The drug is injected immediately after closure of the joint capsule.

Liposome Encapsulated Bupivacaine (Nocita)

Liposome encapsulated bupivacaine (13.3 mg/mL) is available for placement between tissue layers at the end of surgery. This formulation allows for extended release of the local anesthetic and has a duration of action of up to 3 days. This gives the veterinary team an effective way to provide postoperative pain control for an extended time that does not require the owner to administer the medication at home. At the time of this writing, Nocita is licensed for use in dogs undergoing cranial cruciate stabilization surgery and in cats for 3-point nerve block for onychectomy. The dose is 5.3 mg/kg (0.4 mL/kg) that is infiltrated into all tissue layers during closure (cruciate surgery in dogs). In cats, the dose is 5.3 mg/kg (0.4 mL/kg) per forelimb. Detailed instructions regarding administration of this drug are provided by the manufacturer.

Regional Anesthesia

Regional anesthesia is a technique whereby a local anesthetic is injected into a major nerve plexus or in proximity to the spinal cord. This results in the blockade of nerve impulses to and from a relatively large area such as an entire limb or the caudal portion of the body. Examples of regional anesthesia in veterinary medicine include paravertebral, epidural, spinal (intrathecal), and brachial plexus blocks.

Paravertebral anesthesia (ruminants). This is an alternative to a line block for standing laparotomy in cattle. The dorsal and ventral branches of spinal nerves T13 to L2 are blocked, along with L3 to L4 if anesthesia of the paralumbar fossa is required (e.g., for flank cesarean section) (see Procedure 7.2).

Advantages include provision of a wide, uniform area of anesthesia and a shorter time required to perform the block. Disadvantages include the increase in technical difficulty, hindlimb weakness if L3 and L4 are blocked, and the development of scoliosis (lateral curvature of the spine) commonly seen with this technique, which may make closure of the incision more challenging.

Epidural anesthesia. Epidural anesthesia is a regional anesthesia technique that is commonly used in both large- and small-animal patients. The procedure is not difficult (Procedure 7.3) and, once mastered, allows the anesthetist to provide reliable sensory and motor blockade of the abdomen, pelvis, tail, pelvic limbs, and perineum. The technique is useful for tail amputation, anal sac removal, perianal surgery, urethrostomies, obstetric manipulations, cesarean sections, and some hindlimb operations. Epidural anesthesia is most commonly used in three classes of patients:
1. Ruminants, in which procedures such as replacement of a vaginal prolapse can be undertaken with epidural anesthesia alone or in combination with a sedative. Epidural procedures are also useful to prevent straining during obstetric procedures, including cesarean sections.
2. Debilitated small-animal patients in which general anesthesia is problematic but that may tolerate sedation and a lidocaine or bupivacaine epidural block. One example is a patient requiring a cesarean section.
3. Patients requiring profound pain control after surgical procedures involving the hindlimbs, pelvis, or caudal abdomen. For example, morphine or lidocaine epidural blocks are useful for animals undergoing surgical repair of a fractured femur.

> **TECHNICIAN NOTE** Epidural anesthesia is useful for tail amputation, anal sac removal, perianal and perineal surgery, urethrostomies, obstetric manipulations, cesarean sections, and some hindlimb operations.

The choice of drug used for epidural anesthesia is governed by the reason for the epidural: if immobility and anesthesia for surgery are required, a local anesthetic such as 2% lidocaine or 0.5% bupivacaine can be used at a dose of 1 mL per 3.5 to 4.5 kg of body weight. Duration of effect is 1.5 to 3 hours for lidocaine and 4 to 6 hours for bupivacaine. If the main objective is epidural analgesia to ensure postoperative pain control, an opioid such as morphine is used instead (see Chapter 8). Opioids and local anesthetics such as lidocaine can also be mixed together and delivered epidurally. Opioids administered epidurally are generally associated with fewer unwanted side effects than lidocaine or bupivacaine (less risk of sympathetic blockade and hypotension, unlikely to cause motor blockade, and therefore less ataxia), but they may cause pruritus (itching) and urinary retention in some patients. Opioids may also be combined with alpha$_2$-agonists for epidural analgesia in horses and cattle.

Anatomic considerations. To understand the technique used for epidural anesthesia, the anesthetist must be familiar with the anatomy of the terminal spinal cord region (see Procedure 7.3, Fig. 1). The spinal cord is made up of sensory, motor, and autonomic neurons and is surrounded by three membrane layers: the pia mater, arachnoid, and dura mater. The subarachnoid space, which is the area between the arachnoid and the pia mater, is filled with cerebrospinal fluid (CSF). This fluid surrounds the entire spinal cord and communicates with the CSF in the ventricles of the brain. The spinal cord and its membrane layers are encased within the spinal canal. This canal consists of bony vertebrae (cervical, thoracic, lumbar, sacral, and coccygeal) that protect the spinal cord from injury. Several ligaments also protect the vertebral canal, including the supraspinous ligament (which lies directly under the skin), the ligamentum flavum (also called the *ligamentum interarcuatum*), and the interspinous ligament (see Procedure 7.3, Fig. 1). The neurons that supply the tissues

---

PROCEDURE 7.3 Performing an Epidural Injection in a Dog

Steps

1. Gather the necessary equipment. This includes a short-beveled spinal needle with a stylet (18–22 gauge, 1.5 inches for small or thin dogs, and 2–3 inches for large or overweight dogs) and several sterile 3- or 5-mL syringes. If a catheter is to be placed, a thin-walled 18-gauge, 3-inch needle is required.
2. Sedate (or anesthetize) the patient to achieve adequate restraint and place them in sternal or lateral recumbency. The head is positioned higher than the spinal cord for at least the first 10 min of analgesia. This prevents forward migration of the drug into the region of the thoracic spinal cord, which could potentially affect the phrenic nerve (causing respiratory arrest) or cause a sympathetic blockade.
3. Identify the right and left cranial dorsal wings of the ilium, the spinous process of L7, and the sacral crest (Figs. 1 and 2). Shave and prepare the area (approximately 10 cm × 10 cm) surrounding the injection site between L7 and the sacral crest. Wear surgical gloves and mask for the procedure.

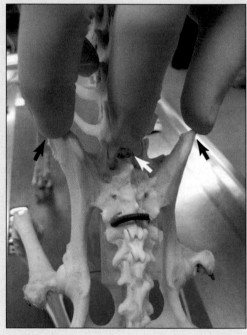

FIG. 2 Palpation of landmarks on a canine skeleton for a lumbosacral epidural. *Black arrows,* the most dorsal points of the wings of the ilia. *White arrow,* the lumbosacral space.

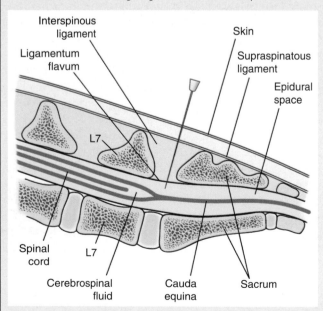

FIG. 1 Anatomy of the distal spinal canal, showing the placement of a needle for lumbosacral epidural analgesia. (From Fossum TW, editor: *Small animal surgery,* ed 4, St Louis, 2013, Elsevier.)

4. Palpate the lumbosacral space (between L7 and the sacrum), which is midway between the dorsal iliac wings (Fig. 3). The lumbosacral space is the depression just caudal to the L7 process and immediately cranial to the sacral crest, which feels like a series of small bumps under the skin. Place the spinal needle in the area of the greatest depression, perpendicular to the skin surface and exactly on the midline (Fig. 4). The bevel should be directed cranially and the stylet should be left in the needle to prevent introduction of skin or tissue into the epidural space. The needle is gently advanced perpendicular to the skin in the dog, passing through the skin, subcutaneous fat, supraspinous ligament, interspinous ligament, and ligamentum flavum (Fig. 5). Resistance may be encountered and a distinct "pop" often can be felt as the needle is advanced through

PROCEDURE 7.3 Performing an Epidural Injection in a Dog—cont'd

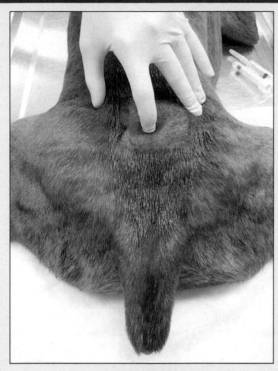

FIG. 3 Palpation of landmarks on a dog for a lumbosacral epidural. The anesthetist places their thumb and middle finger on the most prominent points of the wings of the ilia, and then places the index finger in the indentation at a midpoint between the thumb and middle finger, the lumbosacral junction.

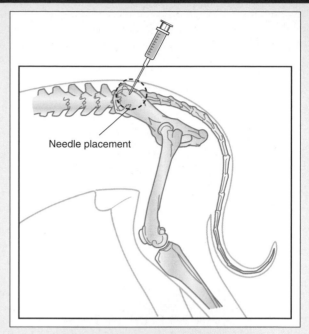

FIG. 5 Needle placement for a lumbosacral epidural in the dog.

Needle placement

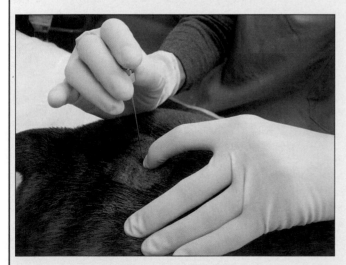

FIG. 4 The anesthetist then inserts the needle perpendicular to the spine.

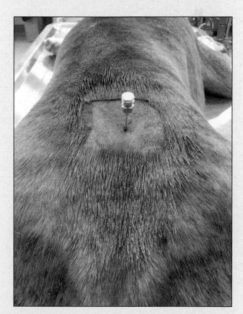

FIG. 6 Spinal needle after the epidural space has been entered.

the ligamentum flavum. Immediately after the ligamentum flavum is penetrated, the needle enters the epidural space. This usually occurs at a needle depth of 1–3 cm, depending on the size of the animal (Fig. 6). Occasionally, there is some difficulty in finding the intervertebral space, in which case the needle should be withdrawn, angled slightly caudally or cranially, and reinserted.

5. Remove the stylet and examine the needle hub for blood or cerebrospinal fluid (for 2 min). If cerebrospinal fluid is encountered, the needle is in the subarachnoid space. If this is the case, the procedure may be abandoned or the anesthetist may choose to administer 30%–50% of the original dose (provided the agent used has minimal spinal toxicity), which will induce spinal anesthesia. If blood is encountered, the needle has entered the venous sinus, and the procedure should be abandoned. If blood and cerebrospinal fluid are not observed, the needle should be aspirated to ensure that neither is present. To check further for proper needle placement, inject 0.5–1 mL of saline (drawn up so that 1–2 mL of air is above the fluid in the syringe); no resistance to injection should be felt, and the air should not compress more than 50% within the syringe. Alternatively, the stylet can be removed as it enters the skin. The hub can be filled with saline and as the needle penetrates the ligamentum flavum, the liquid will be drawn into the epidural space, indicating correct placement.

Continued

PROCEDURE 7.3 Performing an Epidural Injection in a Dog—cont'd

6. Inject the calculated dose of lidocaine or bupivacaine over 1 min (Fig. 7). More rapid injection may cause pressure damage to the spinal cord and nerves or result in local anesthetic infiltrating too far forward along the spinal canal. Injection will be resistance-free if the needle is positioned correctly. If continuous epidural anesthesia is required, a polyethylene catheter may be advanced through the needle and the needle subsequently withdrawn, leaving the catheter in place. Advance the catheter only 1 cm into the epidural space.

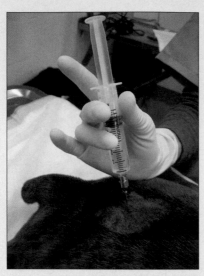

FIG. 7 Local anesthetic, opioid, or a combination of both is injected slowly. The anesthetist should feel no resistance to injection.

Onset of analgesia is approximately 5 min after lidocaine injection or 20 min after bupivacaine injection. The block normally affects the most distal body parts (toes and tail) first. If a bilateral effect is desired, position the patient in dorsal recumbency for 20 min after the injection. If unilateral analgesia is required, place the patient in lateral recumbency with the desired side positioned ventrally, allowing for gravitation of the local anesthetic within the epidural space to the targeted side of the spinal canal.

It has been reported that 12% of correctly performed epidural blocks are ineffective, perhaps because of individual variations in anatomy. Effectiveness of the block may be determined by a test with a needle prick or may become evident during preparation of the patient or application of towel clamps. The duration of analgesia is 4–6 hr for bupivacaine and 1.5–3 hr for lidocaine.

Drug Selection for an Epidural for Surgical Analgesia

If the epidural is performed for surgical analgesia and immobilization, lidocaine or bupivacaine is used. The dose of 2% lidocaine (without epinephrine) or 0.25%–0.5% bupivacaine will vary with the extent of analgesia required. The anesthetist often will choose to produce anesthesia as far cranially as L2 (which is sufficient for most caudal abdominal procedures and all pelvic and hindlimb procedures). The dose used in this case is 1 mL of local anesthetic for each 3.5–4.5 kg of body weight. The volume should be 0.25 mL/kg.

Drug Selection for an Epidural for Postoperative Pain Control

If the epidural is performed to provide postoperative analgesia, morphine or another opioid agent is used, either alone or combined with a local anesthetic. The procedure used is the same as just described. It is advisable that single-use vials of preservative-free morphine be used. See Chapter 8 for more information on the use of morphine epidurals for pain control.

---

exit from the spinal cord at regular intervals, emerging between the vertebrae and ultimately ending in the skin and other tissues. The spinal cord itself terminates in a group of neurons collectively called the cauda equina.

When epidural anesthesia is performed, local anesthetic is deposited in the epidural space, between the dura mater and the vertebrae. This is a potential space that is often filled with fat. Spinal nerves pass through the epidural space as they exit through the intervertebral foramina and are affected by local anesthetics and other drugs deposited in this space. In dogs, the location of the injection is between the last lumbar vertebra (L7) and the sacrum (see Procedure 7.3, Fig. 1). When properly performed, injection of local anesthetic into this area is unlikely to damage the spinal cord because the cord normally ends at the sixth or seventh lumbar vertebra (L6 or L7). In cats, the spinal cord extends farther caudally (as far as S1) and there is a chance of entering the subarachnoid space when performing epidural anesthesia.

Epidural anesthesia must be differentiated from spinal anesthesia, which is commonly performed in human patients. In spinal anesthesia, the local anesthetic is injected into the subarachnoid space, where it mixes with the CSF. Inadvertent injection of local anesthetic into the subarachnoid space when performing an epidural injection is more common in the cat than in the dog. If CSF is apparent in the needle, half the volume required for epidural injection should be delivered, as the injectate will travel further cranially and

the block produced will be more intense compared to epidural injection.

Because local anesthetics block not only sensory nerves (including those that transmit pain sensation) but also motor neurons, an animal that has undergone epidural anesthesia may be unable to walk until the block wears off. Opioids, however, have minimal effect on motor neurons, and movement of the limbs and tail is usually unimpaired after morphine epidural analgesia.

Intravenous regional anesthesia (Bier block). IV regional anesthesia is used to provide short-term (less than 1 hour) local anesthesia to an extremity. This technique is used most commonly for surgery of the lower extremity, including amputation of a digit. When a Bier block is performed, a calculated amount of lidocaine is injected into the distal segment of a superficial vein after a tourniquet has been applied proximally to the vein (Procedure 7.4). Bupivacaine is not used for this block because it is more cardiotoxic when given intravenously.

> **TECHNICIAN NOTE** Bupivacaine should not be used for intravenous regional anesthesia because cardiotoxicity is likely to occur after release of the tourniquet.

Systemic Administration

Lidocaine can also be administered intravenously (IV) by constant rate infusion to healthy anesthetized animals to reduce the

PROCEDURE 7.4   Performing a Bier Block in a Dog Undergoing Toe Amputation

A 22-gauge, 1.5-inch catheter is placed in a vein in the distal part of the limb (because the valves of the veins prevent the backward flow of local anesthetic if the drug is injected too far proximally). Once the catheter is in place, an elastic bandage is wrapped around the extremity, starting at the distal end and wrapping proximally to drive blood out of the veins (Fig. 1). A tourniquet is applied just proximal to the area requiring anesthesia (e.g., immediately above the elbow if the forelimb is to be anesthetized). The tourniquet must be tight or symptoms of local anesthetic toxicity may be evident after injection. The bandage is then removed and the drug injected into the vein via the catheter (Fig. 2). The typical dose used is 2–3 mL of 2% lidocaine without epinephrine, not to exceed 2 mg/kg. Within 3–5 min, there is total desensitization of the limb distal to the tourniquet, allowing 25–30 min of analgesia. An additional advantage of this technique is the relatively blood-free surgical site resulting from tourniquet application. As with other local anesthetic procedures, however, patient restraint may be a problem unless concurrent sedation or neuroleptanalgesia is provided. This technique can also be used in anesthetized patients.

Sensation returns to the affected area within a few minutes of release of the tourniquet. It is important to remove the tourniquet soon after the procedure has been completed. If the tourniquet is in place for more than 90 min, prolonged hypoxia of the tissues of the limb may result, leading to tissue damage and loss of function. In all patients, removal of the tourniquet should be gradual (i.e., over a 5-min period) because this helps prevent an excessive concentration of local anesthetic from reaching the heart and brain.

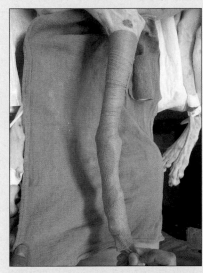

FIG. 1 The limb is tightly wrapped using, in this case, Vetrap (3M), or alternatively an Esmarch bandage, starting at and including the toes. A tourniquet is placed proximal to the bandage, and the bandage is then removed, starting at the toes and moving proximally.

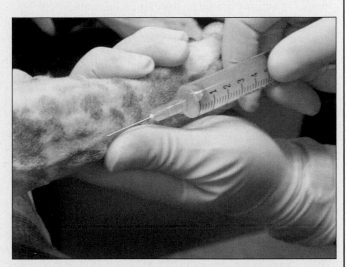

FIG. 2 Local anesthetic is injected into a vein distal to the tourniquet. Very little blood should be present in the vein if the bandage and tourniquet have been applied correctly. The tourniquet should be removed after 60 min of intravenous regional anesthesia.

dose of general anesthetic or analgesic required for painful operations and to prevent cardiac arrhythmias. The dose used is 2 to 3 mg/kg/h in dogs and horses. A constant rate infusion of lidocaine may also be used as part of a postoperative analgesic plan using these dosages.

Adverse Effects of Local Anesthetics

The use of local anesthetics is not without risk and several adverse effects have been reported, including the following:

1. **Motor neurons** may be affected by the local anesthetic and the patient may lose voluntary motor control of the body part innervated by the affected neurons. The loss of motor function to the limbs typically results in recumbency. This may be inconvenient (e.g., for a standing procedure in a cow) or undesirable and dangerous (e.g., a horse that falls and thrashes repeatedly as it tries unsuccessfully to stand).

2. If local anesthetic is injected into a nerve, temporary or permanent loss of function may result. Direct injection into a nerve should be avoided, except for animals undergoing an amputation.

> **TECHNICIAN NOTE** If local anesthetic is injected into a nerve, temporary or permanent loss of function may result.
> Direct injection into a nerve should be avoided, except for animals undergoing an amputation.

3. Tissue irritation may occur after injection of some local anesthetics. Some veterinarians prefer mepivacaine to other local anesthetics because it appears to cause less tissue irritation.

4. **Paresthesia,** an abnormal sensation of tingling, pain, or irritation, may be apparent during recovery from local anesthesia. (Human patients also experience this tingling sensation, for example, during recovery from "numbing" of the oral cavity with Novocain.) Animals should be monitored during recovery because they may chew or otherwise traumatize affected areas and may require chemical or physical restraint or the use of Elizabethan (E)-collars (for cats and dogs).

5. Human and animal patients may exhibit allergic reactions to local anesthetics, usually in the form of a skin rash or hives. Anaphylaxis is also occasionally seen. Local anesthetics should not be used in patients when an allergic reaction to these drugs has been previously observed.

6. Systemic toxicity may occur, particularly if a local anesthetic is inadvertently given intravenously without the use of a tourniquet. Systemic toxicity may be seen even with subcutaneous injections if a large amount of local anesthetic is injected. The most common signs of systemic toxicity originate in the central nervous system. The first sign of systemic toxicity is usually sedation, followed by nausea, restlessness, muscle twitching, hyperexcitability, seizures, respiratory depression, and eventually, coma. Treatment of central nervous system signs may include IV midazolam, lorazepam or diazepam, or intrarectal diazepam, and administration of oxygen. Cardiovascular effects may also be observed because of the direct effect of local anesthetics on the heart. IV injection of lidocaine may inhibit the conduction of electrical impulses within the heart muscle and decrease the force of cardiac contractions. This is undesirable when local anesthesia is performed but makes this drug useful in the treatment of some types of ventricular tachyarrhythmia. Bupivacaine is more cardiotoxic than lidocaine. The dose of lidocaine given subcutaneously to dogs, cows, and horses should not exceed 10 mg/kg and in cats, should not exceed 4 mg/kg to avoid systemic toxicity. The smallest possible dose should be used. If the drug is given intravenously, the dose of lidocaine should not exceed 4 mg/kg in dogs, 2 mg/kg in large animals, and 0.5 mg/kg in cats. The dose of bupivacaine given subcutaneously should not exceed 2 mg/kg in dogs and 1 mg/kg in cats. For the average (4-kg) cat, the maximum dose of 2% (20 mg/mL) lidocaine is 0.8 mL (16 mg) if given subcutaneously and 0.1 mL (2 mg) if given intravenously. For 0.5% (5 mg/mL) bupivacaine, the maximum subcutaneous dose for a 4-kg cat is 4 mg (0.8 mL). Bupivacaine should never be given by IV injection. Dilution of the calculated dose of lidocaine or bupivacaine with sterile saline is helpful in small patients because it increases the volume and decreases the concentration of the solution to be injected.

7. Epidural or spinal injection may rarely traumatize the spinal cord or cauda equina, particularly if the animal struggles during placement of the needle. Inflammation and fibrosis have been reported after epidural infiltration of local anesthetics containing preservatives. In addition, myelitis (spinal cord inflammation) and meningitis (inflammation of the pia mater, arachnoid, or dura mater) may occur if asepsis is not maintained.

8. If local anesthetics are permitted to infiltrate into the cranial portion of the spinal cord, serious toxicity and even death may occur. If the local anesthetic reaches the midthoracic

vertebrae, innervation of the intercostal muscles may be blocked, interfering with normal respiration. If local anesthetic diffuses as far forward as the cervical spinal cord, the phrenic nerve may be affected. This nerve innervates the diaphragm, and loss of function may result in respiratory paralysis. When epidural anesthesia is performed, care should be taken to keep the patient's head elevated to avoid gravitational flow of the anesthetic cranially to the level of the thoracic and cervical spinal cord. The anesthetist should be prepared to intubate and artificially ventilate any patient undergoing epidural anesthesia because this may be necessary if intercostal and phrenic nerve function is impaired.

9. Diffusion of local anesthetic into the cervical and thoracic spinal cord may also affect sympathetic nerves supplying the heart and blood vessels, resulting in a sympathetic blockade with symptoms of bradycardia, decreased cardiac output, and hypotension. If blood pressure measurement is unavailable, careful monitoring of the capillary refill time, heart rate, and pulse strength will alert the anesthetist to a fall in blood pressure. If this occurs before the entire dose has been administered, injection should be halted. Hypotension should be treated as discussed in Chapter 2, page 41. Once blood pressure has normalized, the attending veterinarian may decide to administer the rest of the injection or abandon the procedure (Case Presentation 7.1).

ASSISTED AND CONTROLLED VENTILATION

The anesthetist may be called on to assist or control patient ventilation during any period of general anesthesia. In assisted ventilation, the anesthetist ensures that an increased volume of air or, more commonly (when the patient is connected to an anesthetic machine and breathing circuit), oxygen and anesthetic gases, is delivered to the patient, although the patient initiates each inspiration. In controlled ventilation, the anesthetist delivers all of the air or anesthetic gases required by the patient and the patient usually does not make spontaneous

BOX 7.1 The Terminology of Assisted and Controlled Ventilation

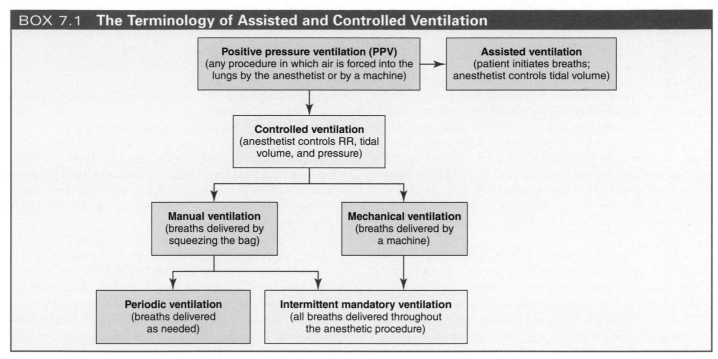

RR, Respiratory rate.

respiratory efforts. The anesthetist controls the respiratory rate and the volume and pressure of gas delivered to the animal.

Any procedure by which the anesthetist assists or controls the delivery of oxygen and anesthetic gas to the patient's lungs may be termed positive pressure ventilation (PPV). (See Box 7.1 for a summary of the terminology of ventilation.) Whether achieved by bagging the patient (applying pressure to the reservoir bag with the adjustable pressure limiting (APL) valve fully or partially closed) or by using a mechanical ventilator, PPV is intended to ensure that the animal receives adequate oxygen and is able to exhale adequate amounts of carbon dioxide. This is a concern in veterinary anesthesia because the patient's own respiratory effort may be inadequate to achieve these objectives.

Ventilation in the Awake Animal

To understand the use of PPV in anesthesia, it is necessary to review the mechanics of normal breathing and the reasons why they may be altered in the anesthetized animal. Ventilation is the physical movement of air (and anesthetic gases in an anesthetized patient) into and out of the lungs and upper respiratory passageways. Ventilation has two parts: an active phase (inhalation) and at rest, a passive phase (exhalation). Inhalation is initiated by the respiratory center in the brain and is normally triggered by an increased level of carbon dioxide in the arterial blood ($Paco_2$). As $Paco_2$ rises above a threshold level (approximately 40 mmHg), the respiratory center initiates the active inspiratory phase by stimulating the intercostal muscles to move the ribcage outwards and the diaphragm to flatten towards the abdomen, thus expanding the thorax. This creates a negative pressure within the chest, which causes the lungs to expand. As the lungs expand, air moves from the atmosphere via the mouth through the breathing passages and into the alveoli. When the lungs reach an adequate volume, nerve impulses send feedback to the respiratory center, signaling the brain to stop the active phase of respiration. The intercostal muscles and diaphragm then relax and exhalation takes place as the lungs deflate. Exhalation is passive, which means that no active muscle movement occurs (with the exception of exhalation during vigorous exercise, which has an active component). During exhalation, the carbon dioxide level in the blood begins to rise again, and after a short pause, the respiratory center responds by initiating another inspiration.

Normally, exhalation lasts approximately twice as long as inspiration. For example, in an animal breathing 20 times per minute, each inspiration will last approximately 1 second and each exhalation will last approximately 2 seconds.

The amount of air that passes into or out of the lungs in a single breath is the tidal volume (V_T). Animals that are breathing deeply have a relatively large V_T, whereas animals that have shallow breathing or that are panting have a relatively small V_T. Normal V_T in the awake animal is 10 to 15 mL/kg of body weight.

The respiratory rate or frequency is the number of breaths that occur in 1 minute. The respiratory minute volume is the total amount of air that moves into and out of the lungs in 1 minute. This value can be found by multiplying the average V_T by the respiratory rate.

> **TECHNICIAN NOTE** Respiratory minute volume is the total amount of air that moves into and out of the lungs in 1 min. This value can be found by multiplying the average V_T by the respiratory rate.

Ventilation in the Anesthetized Animal

Ventilation in the anesthetized animal differs significantly from normal ventilation described above. These differences include the following:

- Tranquilizers, opioids, and general anesthetics may decrease the responsiveness of the respiratory center in the brain to carbon dioxide. This means that inspiration does not occur as often in the anesthetized animal as in the healthy awake animal, despite the fact that the carbon dioxide level may be significantly elevated. This explains the observation that a respiratory rate of 8 to 20 breaths/min is expected in cats and dogs anesthetized with an inhalant, whereas the same animal would be expected to have a respiratory rate of approximately 15 to 30 breaths/min when awake.
- Tranquilizers and most general anesthetics relax the intercostal muscles and diaphragm, causing them to expand less than they normally do during the inspiratory phase. Because the chest does not expand fully, V_T is reduced. The anesthetist may become aware of the reduced V_T by noting that the reservoir bag does not collapse significantly during the inhalation phase (i.e., the volume of gas inhaled is relatively small). Because the V_T and respiratory rate are decreased, respiratory minute volume is also decreased.

As the amount of air entering and leaving the lungs in the anesthetized animal may be considerably reduced compared with the healthy awake animal, the anesthetist must be aware of the following potential problems that can arise:

- Hypercarbia. $Paco_2$ may rise in the anesthetized patient because carbon dioxide produced by the body is not eliminated as efficiently as in the awake animal. As the blood carbon dioxide level rises, carbon dioxide combines with water molecules in the bloodstream to form bicarbonate ions (HCO^{3-}) and hydrogen ions (H^+). The accumulation of hydrogen ions causes the pH of circulating blood to fall, leading to respiratory acidosis. Blood pH in the healthy awake animal is 7.38 to 7.42, whereas in the anesthetized animal the blood pH may be as low as 7.20.
- Hypoxemia. If the anesthetized animal is breathing room air, Pao_2 may fall below normal values as a result of the decreased respiratory minute volume. Less oxygen enters the lungs and therefore less is available to be absorbed into the blood.
- Atelectasis. Because V_T is reduced, the alveoli do not expand as fully as normal on inspiration. Under general anesthesia, some of the alveoli in dependent regions of the lungs (i.e., the parts of the lungs that are closer to the table or floor), may completely or partially collapse, a condition called atelectasis.

> **TECHNICIAN NOTE** In an anesthetized animal, V_T is reduced and consequently, the alveoli do not expand as fully as normal on inspiration. Some of the alveoli in dependent regions of the lungs may completely or partially collapse (a condition called atelectasis).

Some patients are at increased risk for having or developing these problems. Predisposing factors for hypercarbia, hypoxemia, and atelectasis include the following:

- Prolonged anesthesia (more than 90 minutes)
- Obesity
- Administration of neuromuscular blocking agents (NMBAs) (see following section)
- Preexisting lung disease such as pneumonia
- Recent head trauma
- Surgical procedures involving the chest or diaphragm. These animals may have preexisting cardiovascular or pulmonary disease and are at significant risk for cardiovascular collapse or respiratory arrest if conventional anesthesia with unassisted ventilation is attempted.
- Species differences. Horses in particular are prone to the problems listed previously, regardless of physical status. Adult ruminants also tend to hypoventilate and become hypercarbic.

The anesthetist has several ways of compensating for these effects. The Pao_2 can be elevated to normal levels (and, in fact, often above normal levels) if the patient is supplied with adequate oxygen. This is easily achieved because animals connected to anesthetic machines normally receive close to 100% oxygen. The healthy anesthetized patient connected to an anesthetic machine is unlikely to have a reduced Pao_2 unless a problem such as pulmonary edema or upper airway obstruction is present. Horses are the exception to this (see Chapter 10).

It is more difficult to prevent atelectasis or an increase in $Paco_2$ and resulting respiratory acidosis. In each of these situations, it may be advisable to take active steps to assist or control the patient's ventilation.

Types of Controlled Ventilation

The following are two ways to control the patient's ventilation in the anesthetized patient:

1. The patient's lungs are ventilated by the anesthetist using the anesthetic machine breathing circuit; this technique is referred to as manual ventilation (see Fig. 4.49). A common term that is also used to indicate manual ventilation is "bagging." In this type of PPV, the lungs are filled with oxygen by the pressure of gas entering the airways as the anesthetist squeezes the reservoir bag with the APL valve fully or partially closed. Exhalation is passive and occurs when the positive pressure is discontinued and the APL valve is opened fully, allowing the lungs to empty. For most patients, periodic bagging (one or two breaths every 2 to 10 minutes) is adequate to expand the lungs and reduce atelectasis. However, some patients require bagging throughout the anesthetic period, which is referred to as intermittent mandatory ventilation.
2. The patient's lungs are ventilated by a machine; this technique is called mechanical ventilation. In this type of PPV, the lungs are filled with oxygen by the pressure of gas from a special apparatus called a ventilator. As with manual ventilation, exhalation is passive and occurs when the positive pressure is discontinued. Ventilators used in anesthesia are not usually used to ventilate patients periodically but are most commonly used to provide intermittent mandatory ventilation.

Whether the patient's lungs are to be ventilated by manual or mechanical means, the patient must first be intubated and connected to an anesthetic machine. Ventilating the patient's lungs through an ordinary anesthesia mask does not deliver adequate amounts of oxygen to the lungs and may cause the stomach to fill with air, increasing the risk of regurgitation.

Periodic Manual Ventilation

Manual ventilation can be performed on a periodic basis (one or two breaths every 2 to 10 minutes) for any anesthetized patient. These periodic breaths, also called "sighs," help expand collapsed alveoli and reverse atelectasis. For the patient's lungs to be ventilated manually, the APL valve is closed and the reservoir bag is compressed until the lungs are inflated. When pressure on the reservoir bag is released, exhalation can occur. The anesthetist must use caution to ensure that the pressure used is not excessive: the patient's chest should rise only to the same extent as with normal awake respiration. When normal lungs are ventilated, the pressure manometer reading should not exceed 20 cm H_2O in small-animal patients and 40 cm H_2O in large-animal patients. The bag should be squeezed for 1 to 1.5 seconds. Excessive or prolonged pressure may damage lung tissue and impede venous return to the heart (see Box 7.2 for a summary of periodic manual ventilation).

> **TECHNICIAN NOTE** Manual ventilation can be performed on a periodic basis (one or two breaths every 2–10 min) for any anesthetized patient. These periodic breaths, also called "sighs," help expand collapsed alveoli and reverse atelectasis.

Intermittent Mandatory Ventilation

For some patients, respiratory depression is so severe that periodic bagging does not provide the necessary level of ventilation, placing increased demand on the anesthetist's time and attention. Animals with preexisting heart or lung disease or diaphragmatic hernias may go into respiratory arrest immediately after induction. Other patients continue to breathe under anesthesia, but their V_T is low (they have shallow breaths) and/or the respiratory rate is less than 6 breaths/min. These patients require intermittent mandatory manual or mechanical ventilation. (See Box 7.3 for a summary of the steps involved in providing intermittent mandatory ventilation.)

Intermittent mandatory manual ventilation can be performed using either a rebreathing or a nonrebreathing system. Nonrebreathing systems usually lack a manometer unless a universal control arm (Bain block) is used or the circuit is fitted with an in-circuit pressure manometer (see Chapter 4, Fig. 4.44). In this case, the anesthetist must use sight and touch to

BOX 7.2 Summary of Periodic Manual Ventilation

- Often performed routinely on anesthetized patients
- Provide one or two breaths every 2–10 min as needed
- Maximum pressure: (SA) – 20 cm H_2O; (LA) – 40 cm H_2O
- Squeeze bag for 1–1.5 sec

SA, small animal; *LA*, large animal

BOX 7.3 Providing Intermittent Mandatory Ventilation

Used for animals with preexisting heart or lung disease, diaphragmatic hernias, low V_T and/or respiratory rate (RR), 6 breaths/min.
1. Start immediately after intubation.
2. Give two to three larger than normal breaths manually, then connect the patient to a ventilator or initiate manual ventilation. Once connected to a ventilator or manually ventilated, the patient usually stops spontaneous breathing efforts within 1 min.
3. Provide assisted ventilation at a rate of 8–20 breaths/min, depending on the patient's size.
4. If after 5–10 min the patient still makes spontaneous breathing efforts, it may be necessary to use a neuromuscular blocking agent.
5. Once control has been established, a ventilation rate of 6–12 breaths/min is usually adequate.
6. A pressure of 15–20 cm H_2O is recommended for small animals (25–40 cm H_2O for large animals) unless the chest is open, in which case, higher pressures may be required.
7. The inspiratory time should be 1–1.5 sec. Expiratory time should be at least 2–3 sec.
8. When the surgical procedure is nearing completion, turn off the anesthetic vaporizer while continuing to ventilate the patient with oxygen. If a neuromuscular blocking agent has been used, it should be reversed if necessary.
9. Gradually reduce the rate of inspirations to approximately two to four per minute while observing the animal for evidence of spontaneous breathing. When this is seen, the patient's ventilation can then be assisted by squeezing a small amount of air from the reservoir bag with each inspiration. Eventually, the animal will regain the ability to maintain a normal respiratory rate and V_T, and ventilation assistance can be discontinued.

determine the optimal V_T or a capnograph (see Chapter 6, page 226) to assess the adequacy of ventilation.

To initiate intermittent mandatory manual ventilation, ventilation can be assisted starting immediately after intubation, at which point the anesthetist should use the reservoir bag to superimpose positive pressure breaths on the animal's own spontaneous breathing efforts. For many patients, it is adequate to give a few larger than normal breaths manually and then connect the patient to a ventilator or to initiate manual ventilation. The initial large V_T depresses the animal's urge to breathe by lowering blood carbon dioxide levels. Once the patient is connected to a ventilator or is undergoing appropriate manual ventilation, the patient usually stops spontaneous breathing efforts within 1 minutes. Initially, the assisted ventilation rate should be 8 to 20 breaths/minute, depending on patient size. If after 5 to 10 minutes, the patient still makes spontaneous breathing efforts, it may be necessary to use an NMBA, which paralyzes the muscles of respiration (see the following section).

Once control has been established, a ventilation rate of 6 to 12 breaths/min is usually adequate. A pressure of 15 to 20 cm H_2O is recommended in small animals (25 to 40 cm H_2O in large animals), unless the chest is open, in which case higher pressures may be required, depending on the degree to which the lungs are packed off by the surgeon to expose the surgical field. When the reservoir bag is squeezed, the inspiratory time should be 1 to 1.5 seconds. Expiratory time should be at least twice as long as inspiratory time. The APL valve must be closed or partially closed when the reservoir bag is squeezed; however, it should otherwise remain open to allow gas to escape from the circuit. This will allow the airway pressure to return to zero during expiration so that cardiopulmonary function can normalize (by improving venous return of blood to the heart and increasing stroke volume). Many small animal anesthetic machines are fitted with an APL occlusion valve (quick release button) below the APL valve that closes when depressed, allowing a positive pressure breath to be delivered. Releasing the button allows gas to exit the circuit via the APL valve.

> **TECHNICIAN NOTE** When providing manual ventilation, the patient's chest should rise only to the same extent as with normal awake respiration. When normal lungs are ventilated, the pressure manometer reading should not exceed 20 cm H_2O in small-animal patients and 40 cm H_2O in large-animal patients.

When assisting or controlling ventilation, the anesthetist may find it difficult to evaluate the adequacy of the ventilation efforts. Pulse oximetry and end-tidal capnography are valuable aids (see Chapter 6). For example, if the pulse oximeter reading is 95% or less or if end-tidal CO_2 is greater than 55 mmHg in a patient undergoing manual ventilation, the patient may need more frequent ventilation or ventilation at a greater pressure or volume to increase V_T.

When the surgical procedure is nearing completion, the anesthetist must transition the patient from the intermittent mandatory breaths given by the ventilator to spontaneous breathing. This is known as "weaning" the animal off mandatory manual ventilation and is accomplished by turning off the anesthetic vaporizer while continuing to ventilate the patient's lungs with oxygen. If an NMBA has been used, it should be reversed prior to turning the anesthetic agent off. The anesthetist should gradually reduce the rate of inspirations to approximately two to four per min while observing the animal for evidence of spontaneous breathing. When this is seen, the patient's ventilation can then be assisted by squeezing a small amount of air from the reservoir bag with each inspiration. Eventually, the animal will regain the ability to maintain a normal respiratory rate and V_T, and ventilation assistance can be discontinued. This may take several minutes to reestablish, particularly in older, hypothermic, or debilitated patients, and when ventilation has been controlled for a long time. Warming the patient or stimulating them by pinching the toe pads or gently rubbing the thorax and abdomen (small animals) or twisting an ear (large animals), may help the patient regain spontaneous respiratory movements.

Mechanical Ventilation

Mechanical ventilation is similar to intermittent mandatory manual ventilation in many respects. With mechanical ventilation, however, the patient's breathing is controlled by a ventilator, rather than by manual compression of the reservoir bag. When a ventilator is connected to the breathing circuit, it functionally replaces the reservoir bag and becomes a part of the breathing circuit. The ventilator automatically compresses a bellows or moves a piston, which forces oxygen and anesthetic gas into the patient's airways via an endotracheal tube.

Many types of ventilators can be used with a veterinary anesthesia machine, and they vary in the number and complexity of the controls (Fig. 7.3). The basic design is a bellows inside a housing, which is attached to the reservoir bag port of a rebreathing system. The bellows is compressed at a specified rate and a specified volume by a driving gas. Most ventilators have a double gas circuit pattern, with one circuit providing oxygen and anesthetic for the patient and the other circuit containing a separate gas (oxygen or air) to drive the bellows. The bellows can be "standing" if they move downwards, or "hanging" if they move upwards, when compressed by the driving gas during inspiration (Fig. 7.4). Ventilators are available for either large

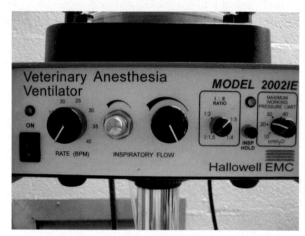

FIG. 7.3 Ventilator control panel of a Hallowell small animal anesthesia ventilator. From left to right, the controls are the on–off switch with indicator light; respiratory rate knob; inspiratory flow knobs (smaller silver knob for fine control, larger black knob for gross control); I:E ratio knob (controls ratio of inspiration to expiration); inspiratory hold button (allows the anesthetist to keep the patient's lungs expanded temporarily); and the pressure limit knob (allows the anesthetist to set the maximum pressure within the breathing system on inspiration—an alarm will sound if this pressure is reached).

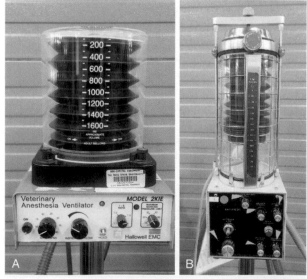

FIG. 7.4 **(A)** Hallowell small anesthesia ventilator with standing bellows; **(B)** Ohio ventilator with a hanging bellows. (A, Courtesy Hallowell EMC.)

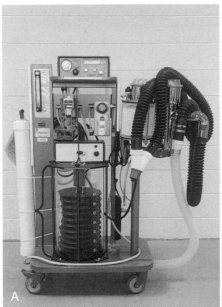
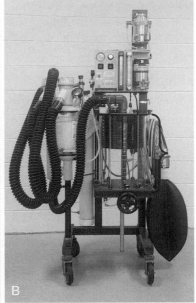

FIG. 7.5 (A) Mallard large-animal anesthetic machine. The ventilator on this machine uses a standing bellows. **(B)** Drager large-animal anesthetic machine. The ventilator on this machine has a hanging bellows. (In both photos, the red bracket delineates the bellows housing and the black corrugated object inside of the housing is the bellows.)

animal or small animal use, with ventilators typically being incorporated into the large animal anesthetic machine (Fig. 7.5). In both cases, the scavenger should be attached to the exhaust port of the ventilator.

Depending on the type of ventilator used, the anesthetist may choose to deliver gases on inspiration according to a pressure cycle, volume cycle, or time cycle. A pressure-cycled ventilator (such as the Bird Mark 7 Respirator) will deliver gases into the patient's lungs until the pressure reaches a preset level. A time-cycled ventilator (such as the Small Animal Ventilator by Drager) delivers gases according to a set inspiratory time. A volume-cycled type (such as the Ohio Metomatic) delivers a preset V_T regardless of the pressure required. In volume-cycled ventilators, the anesthetist must adjust the volume of gas to be delivered on inspiration (usually 10 to 15 mL/kg or less if respiration is to be assisted rather than controlled).

After connecting the ventilator to the breathing circuit, the anesthetist should closely observe the patient to ensure that the chest rises with each inspiration. Respiratory rate is usually 6 to 12 breaths/min. Duration of inspiration is set at 1 to 1.5 seconds and duration of expiration should be 2 to 6 seconds, with an inspiratory/expiratory ratio of 1:2 to 1:4. If a pressure-cycled ventilator is used, a pressure setting of 12 to 20 cm H_2O is normally selected for small-animal patients, or 25 to 40 cm H_2O for larger animals. These settings may be varied to adapt to the special needs of selected patients. For example, a dog with gastric dilatation–volvulus or a horse with colonic torsion may need higher airway pressures to deliver a minimal effective V_T. Obese cats and dogs often require normal rates but higher airway pressures to overcome the thoracic effects of obesity.

Like manual ventilation, mechanical ventilation is particularly indicated for patients with compromised respiration. It is not normally necessary for healthy anesthetized patients, where periodic manual bagging is usually sufficient. Mechanical ventilation is particularly helpful for animals undergoing a thoracotomy or other lengthy operation, when manually providing intermittent mandatory ventilation would be difficult for the anesthetist.

A large-animal ventilator that delivers V_T via an electronically controlled piston rather than by compressing bellows is available (Tafonius, manufactured by Hallowell) for animals weighing between 45 and 900 kg (Fig. 7.6). This ventilator has

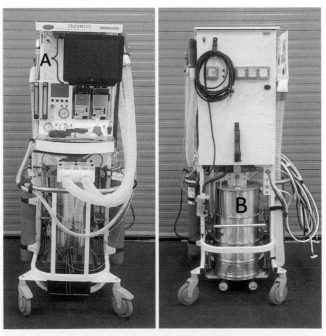

FIG. 7.6 Tafonius large-animal anesthetic machine (Hallowell). Note the touch screen control panel (A) and metal piston housing (B). (Courtesy Hallowell EMC.)

no bellows; therefore no driving gas is needed, which saves oxygen. The ventilator is controlled via an electronic touch screen interface which allows the anesthetist to precisely set V_T and other respiratory parameters.

Risks of Controlled Ventilation

Controlled ventilation, whether by manual ventilation with a reservoir bag or mechanical ventilation with a ventilator, has the potential to damage the animal's lungs if performed incorrectly.

- Excessive airway pressure may rupture alveoli, leading to pneumothorax and/or pneumomediastinum
- Cardiac output may be decreased if positive pressure is maintained throughout the respiratory cycle (during both expiration and inspiration)
- If the ventilation rate is too high, excessive amounts of carbon dioxide may be removed from the lungs, leading to respiratory alkalosis, which (if severe) can cause cerebral vasoconstriction and decreased cerebral blood flow. This can be alleviated by monitoring all ventilated patients with capnography.
- Controlled ventilation is generally more efficient at delivering anesthetic gas. A ventilator will thus deliver more inhalant anesthetic to the patient, which may lead to exacerbation of side effects such as hypotension and increased central nervous system depression. Consequently, it may be advisable to reduce the precision vaporizer setting slightly when PPV is initiated; otherwise, the patient's level of anesthesia may become too deep because of increased delivery of anesthetic. The anesthetist should monitor the patient closely and adjust the vaporizer setting according to the patient's anesthetic depth. Conversely, ventilators are often used as anesthetic delivery devices for large-animal patients to maintain a smoother plane of anesthesia than sometimes occurs with spontaneous breathing.
- Mechanical ventilation is not intended to relieve the anesthetist of the necessity for patient monitoring. The anesthetist must closely monitor all animals when ventilation is controlled or assisted to ensure that anesthetic depth and vital signs are maintained within acceptable limits. (See Case Presentation 7.2 for an example of the benefits and risks of providing ventilatory support.)

CASE PRESENTATION 7.2

Andrea is anesthetizing "Lottie," a Pomeranian weighing 4 kg, in preparation for bladder surgery. Anesthesia is being maintained with isoflurane. With the exception of end-tidal CO_2, which is 60 mmHg, Lottie's monitoring parameters are normal.

1. **What is the significance of the end-tidal CO_2 value?**
2. *How should Andrea approach this situation?*
3. *What possible complications should Andrea be aware of while she is managing this situation?*

NEUROMUSCULAR BLOCKING AGENTS

NMBAs are agents that paralyze skeletal muscles (including the muscles of respiration) by interrupting nerve transmission at the neuromuscular junction. They are often used in human anesthesia, but they have relatively limited use in veterinary practice. Paralysis of the muscles of respiration is undesirable in conventional veterinary anesthesia; however, it is useful in the following situations:

- Patients that require mechanical ventilation. The use of NMBAs prevents spontaneous inspiratory efforts by the patient and allows more rapid and complete control of ventilation. This is particularly useful for thoracic or diaphragmatic surgery.
- Orthopedic surgery. NMBAs provide excellent muscle relaxation, which may be helpful in orthopedic procedures.
- Ophthalmic surgery. NMBAs prevent movement of the eyeball and cause it to remain in a central rather than rotated position, which facilitates intraocular surgery.
- NMBAs may be useful in facilitating difficult intubation (e.g., intubating animals with laryngospasm) because they allow rapid control of the airway without coughing or gagging.

Occasionally, NMBAs are used in "balanced anesthesia" techniques. In balanced anesthesia, different drugs are used to provide the three components of general anesthesia (unconsciousness, muscle relaxation, and analgesia). Instead of using a high dose of a single agent such as propofol to induce general anesthesia, a balanced technique will include low doses of multiple agents (an analgesic, an NMBA, and an agent that induces unconsciousness). The aim is to induce general anesthesia with a minimum of cardiovascular and other side effects while gaining rapid control over the patient's airway.

TECHNICIAN NOTE Neuromuscular blocking agents prevent movement of the eyeball and cause it to remain in a central rather than a rotated position, which facilitates intraocular surgery but makes assessment of anesthetic depth more difficult. Also, animals given NMBAs cannot blink and are predisposed to corneal drying, necessitating application of an ophthalmic lubricant if the eye is not being operated on.

NMBAs should be administered only after the patient has become unconscious and respiration has been controlled by means of intermittent mandatory manual or mechanical ventilation. These agents should be considered to be an adjunct to rather than a replacement for anesthesia with other agents. Use of NMBAs in a conscious animal is inhumane because these agents have no tranquilizing, analgesic, or anesthetic properties. This means that a patient given only an NMBA will be fully conscious and have normal sensitivity to pain, but will be unable to move or otherwise resist the surgeon's efforts. Control of respiration is also essential after the administration of these drugs because the respiratory muscles will be paralyzed, making it impossible for the patient to breathe unaided.

NMBAs act by interrupting normal transmission of impulses from motor neurons to the muscle synapse. The site of action is the neuromuscular junction, where acetylcholine (ACh) is released by the neurons in proximity to the muscle endplate. There are two ways in which NMBAs may disrupt nerve transmission and they are classified as depolarizing or nondepolarizing, according to which of the two mechanisms applies.

Depolarizing agents, such as succinylcholine, act as agonists at the neuromuscular junction, causing a single, short surge of muscle activity. This is followed by a period in which the muscle is refractory to further stimulation. Animals given these agents may show spontaneous muscle twitching, followed by paralysis. Succinylcholine has a fast onset (20 seconds) but a short duration of effect and is useful for rapid intubation. Potential adverse effects of succinylcholine include hyperkalemia and cardiac arrhythmias.

Nondepolarizing agents, such as pancuronium, atracurium besylate, cisatracurium, rocuronium, and vecuronium, act by blocking the receptors at the endplates. As their classification suggests, they do not cause an initial surge of activity at the neuromuscular junction, and spontaneous muscle movements are not seen. Potential adverse effects of these agents include histamine release, hypotension or hypertension, tachycardia, and ventricular arrhythmias.

Concurrent use of inhalant anesthetics increases the potency of NMBAs. Animals that have undergone recent treatments with organophosphate insecticides also show an increased susceptibility to NMBAs. Other drugs, including corticosteroids, barbiturates, furosemide and other diuretics, antineoplastic drugs, epinephrine, tetracycline, and aminoglycoside antibiotics such as gentamicin, have been shown to affect the potency of NMBAs. Other factors that impact the duration of action include body temperature and blood pH.

NMBAs are normally given by slow IV injection. The dose required varies among patients and with the anesthetic protocol used. Most agents take effect within 2 minutes and the duration of paralysis is approximately 10 to 30 minutes (although this varies considerably, depending on the agent used). If more prolonged paralysis is required, repeated doses can be given. Alternatively, some agents may be given by constant IV infusion.

Regardless of the agent used, only voluntary (skeletal) muscles are affected. These agents do not affect the involuntary muscles, including cardiac muscle and the smooth muscle of the intestine and bladder. Skeletal muscles are affected in a predictable order: facial and neck paralysis is seen first, followed by paralysis of the tail, limbs, then abdominal and intercostal muscles, with the diaphragm being affected last.

Anesthetic depth may be difficult to assess in animals that have been given NMBAs because of the inhibition or absence of normal reflex responses and the absence of jaw tone. Heart rate and blood pressure may give some indication of anesthetic depth. If salivation, paradoxical tongue curling, or lacrimation is seen, the patient is likely not anesthetized deeply enough for surgery.

TECHNICIAN NOTE Anesthetic depth may be difficult to assess in animals that have been given neuromuscular blocking agents because of the inhibition or absence of normal reflex responses and the absence of jaw tone. Heart rate and blood pressure may give some indication of anesthetic depth.

Animals given NMBAs cannot blink and are predisposed to corneal drying. An ophthalmic lubricant must be used. The anesthetist must also monitor the patient for hypothermia, which is a common side effect resulting from the decreased muscle tone seen in patients given these agents. Hypothermia and acidosis can slow the metabolism of the agents and delay recovery from anesthesia.

Muscle paralysis following administration of depolarizing agents cannot be reversed—muscle function will return once adequate levels of ACh have built up. Nondepolarizing agents should be reversed with an anticholinesterase agent, even if the effects appear to be wearing off. The most commonly used reversal agents are edrophonium, neostigmine, and pyridostigmine. Another reversal drug, sugammadex, is a reversal drug that works by a different mechanism and is classified as a selective relaxant binding agent. It reverses neuromuscular blockade by binding to rocuronium and vecuronium, which rapidly decreases neuromuscular blockade. At the time of this writing, the cost of sugammadex is high (approximately $100/mL), making it cost prohibitive in veterinary anesthesia.

The patient should be maintained at a light anesthetic depth until the reversal agent has taken effect. After reversal of neuromuscular blockade, muscle function returns in the reverse order of onset of paralysis, with diaphragmatic movements resuming first. Sometimes the effect of the reversal agent wears off before the muscle-paralyzing agent is completely eliminated, in which case respiratory support and another dose of reversal drug may be required.

Reversal agents may have undesirable side effects such as bradycardia and increased bronchial and salivary secretions and should be given only after pretreatment with atropine or glycopyrrolate. Edrophonium and sugammadex have fewer side effects than neostigmine.

Neuromuscular blockade should be monitored using a peripheral nerve stimulator (Fig. 7.7). The most common method used to assess degree of blockade is train of four (TOF). Briefly, the nerve stimulator delivers four consecutive supramaximal impulses, and the presence or absence of twitches is observed visually or shown graphically on the monitor. The strength of the fourth twitch is compared to that of the first twitch. In the absence of blockade, all twitches will be equal, and the TOF ratio will be 1 (100%). As blockade develops, the twitches will become less strong starting with the fourth twitch, a concept referred to as "fade." All twitches will be absent with complete blockade and as muscle function returns, the twitches will return, starting with the first twitch. Neuromuscular function is considered to be adequate once TOF is 0.9 (90%).

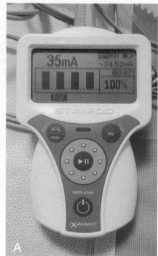
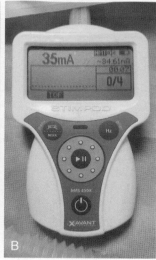
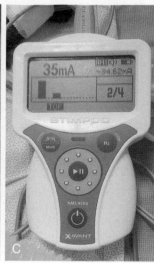
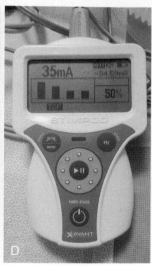

FIG. 7.7 Peripheral nerve stimulator used to monitor neuromuscular blockade (NMB) with train of four (TOF). **(A)** In the absence of NMBA, stimulation of a peripheral nerve (e.g., ulnar nerve in the forelimb, peroneus nerve in the hindlimb) with TOF will cause the limb to twitch four times. When these twitches (T1 through T4) are displayed graphically on the monitor, they will all be equal in height, and the T4/T1 ratio will be 1; that is, T4 is 100% of the height of T1; **(B)** All twitches are absent after administration of a neuromuscular blocking agent (NMBA) and the monitor will not display a ratio (0/4 indicates none of four twitches detected). **(C)** As the NMBA wears off, twitches will return, starting with T1. In this image, T1 and T2 have returned. **(D)** As the NMBA is further metabolized or reversed, all four twitches will return. In this case, the T4/T1 ratio is 50%. Reversal of NMB at the end of the procedure is considered to be adequate (i.e., the patient can breathe adequately unassisted and protective laryngeal function has returned) when the T4/T1 ratio is ³ 90% or greater. (Courtesy Xavant Technology.)

KEY POINTS

1. Local anesthesia is the use of a chemical agent on sensory and motor neurons to produce a temporary loss of pain sensation and movement. Because of low patient toxicity, low cost, and minimal recovery time, local anesthesia may be preferred to general anesthesia in some patients. Disadvantages include lack of patient restraint, risk of overdose in smaller patients, and technical difficulties.

2. If a sufficient quantity of local anesthetic reaches the sympathetic ganglia, sympathetic blockade may result. This causes flushing, increased skin temperature, and, occasionally, hypotension and bradycardia.

3. Local anesthetics have many topical uses, including application to the conjunctiva or the epithelium of the respiratory or urogenital tracts.

4. Local anesthetic techniques are recommended along with systemic agents (e.g., opioids) to optimize multimodal analgesia for many procedures, including orthopedic, dental, and soft tissue surgeries, including spays and castrations.

5. Local anesthetics may be injected in proximity to a peripheral nerve, blocking sensation from the tissues served by the nerve. Surgical preparation of the area is necessary before injection of a local anesthetic.

6. Epinephrine is commonly added to lidocaine to delay absorption of the local anesthetic agent from the site, but epinephrine must not be used at peripheral locations where blood supply may be compromised.

7. Epidural anesthesia is achieved by injecting local anesthetic into the epidural space between the dura mater and the vertebrae. In dogs and cats, the injection is performed between the last lumbar vertebra and the sacrum. This technique is useful for surgical procedures in patients that are debilitated and in patients that require profound analgesia of the caudal abdomen, limbs, or pelvis.

8. Intravenous injection of local anesthetics after tourniquet application may be useful for distal limb surgery, including amputation.

9. Local anesthetics may be harmful if injected into a nerve. They may also cause temporary paresthesia, which may result in self-mutilation.

10. Adverse systemic effects of local anesthesia include sedation, hyperexcitability, respiratory depression, and sympathetic blockade. Toxicity may be avoided by limiting the amount of lidocaine administered to the patient and avoiding intravenous injection of bupivacaine.

11. Controlled or assisted ventilation may be used to deliver oxygen and anesthetic to the patient. Either a mechanical ventilator or manual bagging may be used. These procedures are particularly useful for patients with poor respiratory function. Controlled or assisted ventilation helps prevent the development of hypercarbia, respiratory acidosis, and pulmonary atelectasis.

12. Intermittent mandatory manual ventilation can be achieved by gently squeezing the reservoir bag at a rate of 6 to 12 breaths/min and a pressure of 15 to 20 cm H_2O for small-animal patients. Inspiration time should be 1 to 1.5 seconds and expiratory time should be at least 2 to 3 seconds.

13. Mechanical ventilators may be incorporated into either a rebreathing or a Bain nonrebreathing system. Depending on the type of ventilator used, the anesthetist may control the pressure or volume of gas to be delivered, the respiratory rate, and the length of inspiration and expiration.

14. If controlled ventilation is used, the anesthetist must use caution to avoid excessive expansion of the alveoli, continuous positive pressure, and excessive ventilation rates.

15. Neuromuscular blocking agents may be useful in some anesthetic procedures to allow relaxation of voluntary muscles. They should never be used as the sole anesthetic agent.

16. Neuromuscular blocking agents may be depolarizing or nondepolarizing in their action. Nondepolarizing agents should be reversed, which is most commonly achieved by the administration of neostigmine or edrophonium. An anticholinergic should be administered prior to neostigmine.

17. Neuromuscular blocking agents necessitate the use of mechanical or manual ventilation because the muscles of respiration (diaphragm and intercostal muscles) will be paralyzed.

18. Many drugs, including isoflurane, aminoglycoside antibiotics, organophosphates, and diuretics, may alter the potency of neuromuscular blocking agents.

REVIEW QUESTIONS

1. In the healthy awake animal, the main stimulus to breathe is the result of:
   a. Excess oxygen concentration in the blood
   b. Excess carbon dioxide concentration in the blood
   c. Insufficient oxygen in the blood
   d. Insufficient carbon dioxide in the blood

2. In the healthy awake animal, exhalation lasts at least ___ times as long as inhalation.
   a. ½
   b. 2
   c. 3
   d. 4

3. The normal V_T in an awake animal is ___ mL/kg.
   a. 5 to 10
   b. 10 to 15
   c. 15 to 20
   d. 20 to 25

4. In the anesthetized animal that is breathing room air, the anesthetist may expect to see:
   a. An increase in the $Paco_2$ and a decrease in the Pao_2
   b. A decrease in the $Paco_2$ and an increase in the Pao_2
   c. A decrease in the $Paco_2$ and a decrease in the Pao_2
   d. An increase in the $Paco_2$ and an increase in the Pao_2

5. When used in a line block, a local anesthetic agent will have a direct effect on the:
   a. Peripheral nervous system
   b. Central nervous system
   c. Peripheral and central nervous systems
   d. Autonomic nervous system

6. Local anesthetics block transmission of nerve impulses from:
   a. Sensory neurons only
   b. Motor neurons only
   c. Sensory and motor neurons only
   d. Sensory, motor, and autonomic neurons

7. Local anesthetic agents work because:
   a. They mechanically block nerve impulse transmission
   b. They interfere with the movement of sodium ions
   c. They block all impulses at the spinal cord level
   d. They affect neurotransmission within the brain

8. When a local anesthetic is injected around a single major nerve, the procedure is referred to as a(n):
   a. Line block
   b. Epidural block
   c. Infiltration nerve block
   d. Intravenous anesthesia

9. Epinephrine may be mixed with a local anesthetic agent to prolong the effects of the drug.
   True
   False

10. When performing an epidural, one must be aware that the spinal cord in a cat may extend as far caudally as:
    a. T13
    b. L6
    c. L7
    d. S1
    e. The coccygeal vertebrae

11. The maximum subcutaneous dose of lidocaine for a dog is ___ mg/kg.
    a. 1
    b. 4
    c. 10
    d. 15

12. When performing intravenous regional anesthesia (Bier block), one should use lidocaine:
    a. With epinephrine
    b. Without epinephrine
    c. Either with or without epinephrine
    d. Lidocaine should not be used for this technique

13. The term *atelectasis* refers to:
    a. Excess fluid in the respiratory system
    b. The absence of breathing
    c. Collapse of the alveoli
    d. Bronchial constriction

14. What is the most common acid–base abnormality in anesthetized patients?
    a. Respiratory alkalosis
    b. Metabolic alkalosis
    c. Respiratory acidosis
    d. Metabolic acidosis

15. When intermittent mandatory manual ventilation is applied to a patient that is connected to a circle system with a precision vaporizer, it is customary to:
    a. Increase the vaporizer setting
    b. Decrease the vaporizer setting
    c. Disconnect the patient from the circle system before starting manual ventilation
    d. The lungs of patients that are connected to a circle system should not be manually ventilated

16. Which of the following can be used to monitor anesthetic depth in a patient that has been given a neuromuscular blocking agent?
    a. Heart rate
    b. Jaw tone
    c. Palpebral reflex
    d. Pedal reflex

17. A neuromuscular blocking agent will not only paralyze skeletal muscle, but also provide some analgesia.
    True
    False

18. When an animal is given a _____ neuromuscular blocking agent, an initial surge of muscle activity may be seen before there is paralysis of the muscles.
    a. Depolarizing
    b. Nondepolarizing

19. The muscle type that is most affected by neuromuscular blocking agents is:
    a. Cardiac
    b. Smooth muscle
    c. Skeletal muscle
    d. All types are equally affected.

20. Both depolarizing and nondepolarizing drugs can be reversed.
    True
    False

For the following questions, more than one answer may be correct.

21. Problems that may result from excessive controlled ventilation may include:
    a. A decreased cardiac output
    b. Muscle twitching
    c. A state of respiratory alkalosis
    d. Ruptured alveoli

22. Local anesthetic agents such as lidocaine or proparacaine work well when applied:
    a. Topically on the epidermis
    b. Topically on mucous membranes
    c. Topically on the cornea
    d. Through injection

23. Factors that may interfere with the action of local anesthetic agents include:
    a. Fat
    b. Scar tissue
    c. Rapid heart rate
    d. Hemorrhage

24. Clinical signs of systemic toxicity from a local anesthetic agent may include:
    a. Sedation
    b. Convulsions
    c. Muscle twitching
    d. Respiratory depression

25. The effects that could result from an epidural anesthetic if the drug reaches the thoracic and cervical spinal cord include:
    a. Sympathetic blockade
    b. Paralysis of intercostal muscles
    c. Paralysis of the diaphragm
    d. Hypertension

ANSWERS TO CASE PRESENTATIONS

Case Presentation 7.1

Question #1: There are multiple reasons for the heart rate to increase, including hypotension, decreased depth of anesthesia, hypoxemia, hypercarbia, and pain.

Question #2: The first step Sarah should take is to stop administration of the epidural injection. After informing the attending veterinarian of the problem, Sarah should assess Blanche's anesthetic depth briefly to make sure that it is not too light. Epidural injection with local anesthetic may cause hypotension, so Sarah's next step would be to measure Blanche's blood pressure. If Blanche's blood pressure is normal, then the other causes of the tachycardia should be ruled out. If Blanche is indeed hypotensive, steps should be taken to correct this, such as decreasing the depth of anesthesia if possible and administering fluids (colloids and/or crystalloids).

Question #3: The attending veterinarian should make the decision as to whether the epidural injection should be completed or whether the procedure should be aborted. If the increase in heart rate does not appear to be related to epidural administration, the injection will most likely be completed. If the injection is indeed the cause of the hypotension, the procedure may be aborted or the injection may be continued at a much slower rate while paying close attention to blood pressure and heart rate.

Case Presentation 7.2

Question #1: The end-tidal CO_2 is increased (acceptable during anesthesia: 40 mmHg to 55 mmHg). An end-tidal CO_2 of 60 mmHg indicates hypoventilation and respiratory acidosis, for which there are several possible causes in this situation.

Question #2: Andrea should support Lottie's ventilation, aiming to bring the end-tidal CO_2 down into the range of 40 to 55 mmHg. She has two options for doing so: she could provide manual ventilation or she could place Lottie on a mechanical ventilator. Various factors may influence her decision, including how much longer the procedure will last, the availability of a ventilator, and the number of other tasks she is currently performing. Decreasing the end-tidal CO_2 by manually bagging the patient is usually easy to achieve in a small dog, but will occupy a considerable portion of Andrea's time. If the procedure is likely to continue for some time, it may be better to begin mechanical ventilation in order to keep Andrea's hands free so that she can monitor Lottie more effectively. If a ventilator is not in the surgery room, someone will have to bring it and Andrea will have to set it up. She should set the ventilator to deliver approximately 40 mL per breath (i.e., 4 kg × 10 mL/kg) at a rate of 8 to 12 breaths/min. The end-tidal CO_2 values should decrease soon after initiating ventilation and stabilize within 15 to 20 minutes, after which further adjustments can be made as indicated.

Question #3: Manual or mechanical ventilation is achieved by forcing anesthetic gases into the patient's lungs (i.e., positive pressure ventilation). Positive pressure in the chest cavity decreases venous return of blood to the heart which decreases cardiac output, resulting in lower blood pressure. Furthermore, the increased respiratory minute volume that results from ventilation increases anesthetic gas delivery which, in turn, causes anesthetic depth to increase, which can result in vasodilation and contribute to hypotension. Andrea should therefore pay close attention to Lottie's depth of anesthesia and blood pressure after initiating ventilatory support.

SELECTED READINGS

Anderson DE, Miesner MD: Field surgery of cattle, *Vet Clin North Am Food Anim Pract* 24:211–226, 2008.

Campoy L, Read M, Peralta S: Canine and feline local anesthetic and analgesic techniques. In Grimm KA, Lamont LA, Tranquilli SA, editors: *Veterinary anesthesia and analgesia*, ed 5, Ames, IA, 2015, John Wiley & Sons, Inc., pp 827–856.

Epstein ME: *6 Practical loco-regional blocks you should be using*, March 1, 2011. https://www.dvm360.com/view/6-practical-loco-regional-blocks-you-should-be-using. Accessed November 3, 2022.

Gaynor JS, Muir WW: *Handbook of veterinary pain management*, ed 3, St. Louis, 2014, Elsevier.

Lerche P, Aarnes TK, Covey-Crump G, Taboada FM: *Handbook of small animal regional anesthesia and analgesia techniques*, Ames, IA, 2016, John Wiley & Sons, Inc.

Mosley CA: Anesthesia equipment. In Grimm KA, Lamont LA, Tranquilli SA, editors: *Veterinary anesthesia and analgesia*, ed 5, Ames, IA, 2015, John Wiley & Sons, Inc., pp 61–85.

Muir WW, Hubbell JAE: *Equine anesthesia*, ed 2, St. Louis, 2008, Elsevier.

Schock S, Shaver S: *Surgery STAT: The use of local anesthetic in spays and neuters*, DVM360.com, Volume 51, Number 1, January 2020. https://www.dvm360.com/view/surgery-stat-local-anesthetic-use-spays-and-neuters. Accessed November 3, 2022.

Tranquilli WJ, Grimm KA, Lamont LA: *Pain management for the small animal practitioner*, ed 3, Jackson, WY, 2022, Teton New Media.

Valverde A, Sinclair M: Ruminant and swine local anesthetic and analgesic techniques. In Grimm KA, Lamont LA, Tranquilli SA, Greene SA, Robertson SA, editors: *Veterinary anesthesia and analgesia*, ed 5, Ames, IA, 2015, John Wiley & Sons, Inc., pp 941–959.

8

Analgesia

OUTLINE

LEARNING OBJECTIVES

When you have completed this chapter, you will be able to:

- Define pain, nociception, physiologic pain, pathologic pain, inflammatory pain, neuropathic pain, idiopathic pain, visceral pain, somatic pain, preemptive analgesia, and pain scale.
- List the main steps of the pain pathway.
- List the benefits of multimodal analgesia.
- List the consequences of untreated pain.
- Explain how primary hyperalgesia (peripheral hypersensitivity) develops.
- Explain how secondary hyperalgesia (central hypersensitivity) develops.
- List common surgical and medical conditions that are considered to be painful.
- Describe how to recognize and assess pain-associated behaviors in animals.

- Compare and contrast major types of pain assessment tools and describe how to use each.
- List the routes by which analgesic drugs are commonly administered.
- List the uses for and adverse effects of opioid analgesics.
- Explain the mechanism of action of nonsteroidal antiinflammatory drugs.
- List the uses for and adverse effects of nonsteroidal antiinflammatory drugs.
- Describe the uses for and procedure for application of fentanyl transdermal patch.
- Define multimodal therapy and list two examples of multimodal therapy.
- Describe nursing care that relieves discomfort in hospitalized patients.

KEY TERMS

Acute pain
Adaptive pain
Allodynia
Analgesia
Catabolic state
Categorical numeric rating scale
Central nervous system hypersensitivity

Chronic pain
Distress
Emergence delirium
Idiopathic pain
Inflammatory mediators
Inflammatory pain
Locomotor

Maladaptive pain
Modulation
Morbidity
Mortality
Multimodal therapy
Neuropathic pain
Nociception

The veterinary team has the unique responsibility of assessing and treating animal pain. The role of the veterinary technician or nurse, either as anesthetist or patient caregiver, in the provision of analgesia cannot be overstated. The technician or nurse forms a vital part of the team through their understanding of pain physiology, pain-associated behaviors, pain assessment tools, analgesic drug pharmacology, and communication with the attending veterinarian regarding the welfare of patients. Pain assessment is considered to be an essential part of every patient evaluation, regardless of presenting complaint, and consequently many clinicians refer to pain as the fourth vital sign along with heart rate, respiratory rate, and temperature.

Under the currently accepted standard of practice, provision of analgesia is mandatory for patients that are deemed to be in pain or that undergo painful procedures, including surgery for any reason. Clients expect, request, or sometimes even demand pain control for their pets. Consequently, failure to provide effective pain control not only results in patient discomfort and suffering but may evoke anger, could damage the attending veterinarian's reputation, or, in extreme circumstances, could result in disciplinary action by a veterinary medical licensing board.

> **TECHNICIAN NOTE** Pain assessment is an essential part of every patient evaluation regardless of presenting complaint and consequently, many clinicians refer to pain as the fourth vital sign.

The science of pain control in veterinary patients is a relatively new field of study, and over the past several decades, interest in this discipline as a research topic has steadily increased. As a result, there is now a large body of clinical studies related to the science of pain and pain control. In 2007, the American Animal Hospital Association (AAHA) and the Association of Feline Practitioners (AAFP) jointly published an article addressing the principles of pain management for practitioners entitled "2007 AAHA/AAFP Pain Management Guidelines for Dogs and Cats." This publication was intended to "educate and inform members of the veterinary profession" regarding what was known about pain control at that time based on the results of scientific studies and expert opinion. These guidelines were updated in 2015 and again in 2022 to include knowledge gained from studies published in the intervening time. Collectively, these papers are a rich source of information regarding the current knowledge about the genesis, assessment, treatment, and prevention of pain. Much information about pain control is also available from a number of professional organizations, several of which are listed in Chapter 1, Box 1.1.

THE NATURE OF PAIN

Pain is a complex phenomenon that has been defined as an aversive sensory and emotional experience that elicits protective motor actions (such as a dog trying to bite when being given an injection), results in learned avoidance (the same dog exhibits fear the next time it is taken to the clinic for vaccine boosters), and may modify species-specific behavior traits, including social behavior. This experience is different for every individual animal, although within a given species, some physiologic and behavioral responses will be similar (e.g., dogs in pain will often seek attention from their owners, whereas cats are more likely to hide). If left untreated, pain can negatively affect a patient's behavior, physiology, metabolism, and immune system, causing a wide spectrum of consequences including poor performance, weight loss, and increased susceptibility to infection.

PHYSIOLOGY OF PAIN

Detection by the nervous system of the potential for or the actual occurrence of tissue injury is called nociception. This mechanism, by which noxious stimuli from potentially damaging factors such as chemicals, heat, cold, or trauma are processed by the nervous system, serves to protect the animal from harm. Pain is the unpleasant sensory and emotional experience that results.

There are many terms that are used to classify and describe pain that are related to its cause and duration. The protective sensation of pain that normally occurs when there is a possibility of or actual tissue injury is referred to as physiologic pain. This is the "ouch" pain (e.g., the pain you would feel that would warn you that you may be injured if you touched something sharp, hot, or chemically noxious, or that would make you avoid touching or moving an injured limb). Physiologic pain is adaptive pain because it promotes survival by preventing injury and by promoting healing of the injured body part. This type of pain is generally treatable and typically resolves when healing is complete. In contrast, pathologic pain is pain that is amplified and persistent. This type of pain is due to malfunction of or damage to the nervous system and is maladaptive pain because it serves no useful function and causes suffering. It is often difficult to treat. Inflammatory pain occurs at the site of tissue injury due to the release of inflammatory mediators such as prostaglandins and histamine, with the accompanying migration of white blood cells to the site. Neuropathic pain results from injury to the nervous system (e.g., due to nerve damage). The mechanism can also be classified as idiopathic pain if no identifiable cause can be determined. Acute pain refers to pain that has an immediate onset after a tissue injury and resolves when healing is complete. Examples include pain resulting from surgery, trauma, or medical conditions such as acute pancreatitis and gastrointestinal (GI) obstruction. It often has elements of physiologic pain and inflammatory pain and is usually treatable. Chronic pain lasts weeks, months, or years, and persists after the tissues have healed or when they will not heal, and it is more challenging to treat. Examples include patients with osteoarthritis, patients with long-standing medical conditions like cancer, and sometimes after surgery, as might be the case after a declaw where postoperative pain was inadequately treated.

Both physiologic and pathologic pain can also be classified based on the origin and the severity of pain. Pain can originate from organs, in which case it is visceral pain (e.g., pleuritis, pancreatitis, or colic due to intestinal distension), or from the musculoskeletal system, in which case it is somatic pain (e.g., bone fracture, skin incision). Somatic pain can be divided into superficial (i.e., skin) and deep (i.e., joints, muscles, bones) pain. Some diseases or surgeries may result in more than one of these types of pain—for example, abdominal surgery has components of somatic pain (skin and abdominal wall incisions)

and visceral pain (organ manipulation and surgery). Pain severity is often classified as none, mild, moderate, or severe, although more involved classifications exist (see the discussion of pain assessment tools later in this chapter).

Nociception

Nociception, or the pain pathway, is the process by which noxious stimuli are sensed by receptors in the peripheral nervous system and then communicated via peripheral nerves to the spinal cord and finally, the brain. Nociception consists of four main steps (Fig. 8.1). The first step is the transformation of noxious mechanical, thermal, or chemical stimuli into electrical signals, called *action potentials*, by nociceptors (pain receptors), and is called transduction. These sensory impulses are then conducted to the spinal cord via peripheral nerve fibers, a process known as transmission. In the spinal cord, where the fibers terminate, the impulses can be altered by other neurons, which can either amplify or suppress them. The general term to cover both possibilities is modulation. The final step is perception, in which the impulses are transmitted to the brain, where they are processed and recognized. At each level of the pain pathway, different receptors are involved in the nociceptive process, allowing the pain management team to choose drugs that target a specific receptor (e.g., nonsteroidal antiinflammatory drugs [NSAIDs], opioids, local anesthetics, or corticosteroids can all inhibit transduction via different mechanisms of action) (Table 8.1). A goal of pain management, particularly when dealing with severe pain, is to use multiple drugs to target different receptors in two or more of the steps of the pain pathway. This pain management strategy is called multimodal therapy and is preferable to using a single

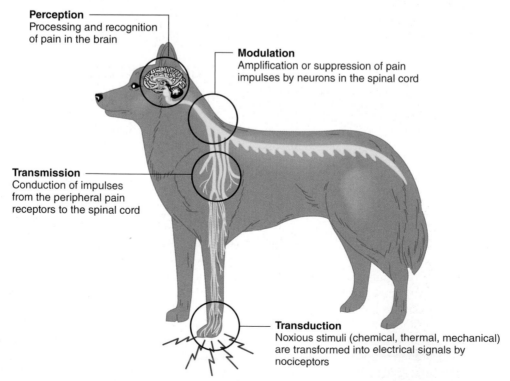

Perception
Processing and recognition of pain in the brain

Modulation
Amplification or suppression of pain impulses by neurons in the spinal cord

Transmission
Conduction of impulses from the peripheral pain receptors to the spinal cord

Transduction
Noxious stimuli (chemical, thermal, mechanical) are transformed into electrical signals by nociceptors

FIG. 8.1 Pain pathway and receptors. Steps of the nociceptive (pain) pathway.

TABLE 8.1   **Where Are Drugs Effective in the Nociceptive Pathway?**

Analgesic Agent Classes	NOCICEPTIVE PATHWAY			
	Transduction	Transmission	Modulation	Perception
Opioids	X		X	X
Nonsteroidal antiinflammatory drugs (NSAIDs)	X		X	
Local anesthetics	X	X	X	
Alpha$_2$-agonists		X	X	X
Ketamine			X	
Corticosteroids	X			
Sedatives/tranquilizers/general anesthetics				X
Tricyclic antidepressants			X	
Anticonvulsants			X	

analgesic because in addition to reducing pain signaling more effectively by inhibition of multiple receptors, lower dosages of each drug can be used, which lessens adverse effects and improves safety.

> **TECHNICIAN NOTE** Using several analgesic drugs, each with a different mechanism of action, is called *multimodal therapy*. This permits the use of lower doses of each drug, which lessens adverse effects and increases safety.

CONSEQUENCES OF UNTREATED PAIN

Pain that goes untreated has undesirable consequences for the patient.
- Pain produces a catabolic state, which may lead to wasting
- Pain suppresses the immune response, predisposing to infection and increasing hospitalization time and cost
- Pain promotes inflammation, which delays wound healing
- Anesthetic risk is increased because higher doses of anesthetic drugs are required to maintain a stable plane of anesthesia
- Pain causes patient suffering, which is also stressful for owners and caregivers (Fig. 8.2)

In the case of pathologic pain, tissue damage results in constant stimulation of the nerves involved in the nociceptive process. This constant noxious stimulation of the central nervous system (CNS) can alter the function of neurons and receptors involved in the pain pathway. The ability of the CNS to change in this way can result in hypersensitivity in both acute and chronic pain. Neurons in the periphery (limbs, organs) and central neurons (spinal cord) can be affected. Peripheral tissue trauma results in the release of substances called inflammatory mediators from damaged cells, and also attracts inflammatory cells (white blood cells), which release additional mediators. These inflammatory mediators combine to form what is called

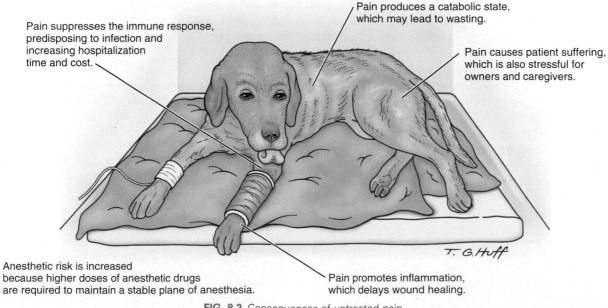

Pain suppresses the immune response, predisposing to infection and increasing hospitalization time and cost.

Pain produces a catabolic state, which may lead to wasting.

Pain causes patient suffering, which is also stressful for owners and caregivers.

Anesthetic risk is increased because higher doses of anesthetic drugs are required to maintain a stable plane of anesthesia.

Pain promotes inflammation, which delays wound healing.

FIG. 8.2 Consequences of untreated pain.

a "sensitizing soup" that lowers the threshold of the peripheral pain receptors, thus increasing their sensitivity. This peripheral hypersensitivity, referred to as primary hyperalgesia, manifests clinically as increased sensitivity to a painful stimulus. For example, if you fracture your wrist and someone touches the damaged area, you may feel an exaggerated sense of pain from that touch that is worse than can be accounted for by the extent of the injury. Centrally, in the spinal cord, neurons that are stimulated by constant nociceptive input from the periphery become hyperexcitable and sensitive to low-intensity stimuli that would not normally elicit a pain response. This central nervous system hypersensitivity, referred to as secondary hyperalgesia, is also referred to as "windup." Clinically, this may manifest as allodynia, a phenomenon in which an area close to the site of tissue injury is painful if stimulated with a normally nonnoxious stimulus. Using the previous example of a fractured wrist, if the fracture and pain remain untreated, it is likely that you will experience windup pain if someone touches your forearm, even though your forearm is not injured. A receptor in the CNS that is activated in windup pain but not in physiologic pain is the *N*-methyl-D-aspartate (NMDA) receptor. Drugs such as ketamine can be used to block this receptor.

Pain also causes physiologic changes. Neuroendocrine changes that occur in response to pain include release of adrenocorticotropic hormone (ACTH); elevation in cortisol, norepinephrine, and epinephrine; and a decrease in insulin. Over time, these changes result in a catabolic state, which, in addition to the fact that patients in pain may be reluctant or unable to eat, leads to wasting.

Sympathetic stimulation leads to vasoconstriction, increased myocardial work, and increased myocardial oxygen consumption, predisposing the patient to arrhythmias. Skeletal muscle blood flow tends to increase, whereas blood flow to the GI and urinary tract decreases.

The stress response caused by tissue injury (including the controlled tissue disruption that results from surgery) is important for immediate survival but if left unchecked, can lead to increased morbidity and mortality. An extreme form of stress, distress, occurs when stressors such as pain negatively affect the animal's physiology and behavior. An animal that is enduring pain is therefore suffering.

The quality of life of a patient in pain should be a concern of every veterinary professional and owner. Although not always easy to define, a high quality of life requires that several basic needs be met. Representing these basic needs, the "five freedoms" can help those caring for animals assess the quality of life (Box 8.1). As freedom from pain is a necessary element of a high quality of life, assessment of pain and provision of analgesia and comfort should be goals of treatment for all veterinary patients.

TECHNICIAN NOTE Freedom from pain is a necessary element of a high quality of life; thus assessment of pain and provision of analgesia and comfort should be goals of treatment of all veterinary patients.

BOX 8.1	**The Five Freedoms**

- Freedom from hunger and thirst
- Freedom from discomfort
- Freedom from disease
- Freedom from injury
- Freedom from pain

SIGNS OF PAIN IN ANIMALS

Animals cannot verbally express their pain. Pain recognition therefore relies on a sound understanding of normal animal physiology and behavior and stress-related or behavioral changes that may be indicative of painful conditions. A thorough, detailed history may also be helpful in assessing pain because the owner is more likely to be aware of behaviors that may be masked during a visit to the hospital or when the veterinarian is at a farm or stable. An understanding of the degree of pain that is expected and associated with specific diseases and surgeries is also helpful.

There is no single physiologic parameter that is a specific indicator of pain. Common pain-related physiologic changes are presented in Box 8.2; however, note that there are other causes for each change. It is important to avoid projecting complex human emotions onto animals (anthropomorphizing); however, the pain pathways and therefore pain perceptions in animals and people have much in common. Our personal experiences can therefore help us determine whether a disease or procedure is likely to be painful or not.

Many disease processes and surgical procedures are associated with moderate to severe pain (see Box 8.3 for some examples). Pain management can be initiated for these types of patients when they present to the clinic already in pain or before elective surgery. The administration of pain medication before pain occurs reduces the overall requirement for analgesics and the duration of analgesic administration postoperatively compared with waiting until after surgery to start analgesic therapy. Providing analgesia before tissue injury occurs is called preemptive analgesia. Preemptive analgesia is most commonly achieved by adding an

---

BOX 8.2	**Pain-Related Physiologic Changes**

Cardiovascular
Hypertension
Tachycardia, tachyarrhythmia
Peripheral vasoconstriction (pale mucosae)

Respiratory
Tachypnea
Shallow breathing (abdominal or thoracic guarding)
Exaggerated abdominal component
Panting (dogs)
Open-mouth breathing (cats)

Ophthalmic
Mydriasis

BOX 8.3 Examples of Diseases and Surgeries Associated With Moderate to Severe Pain

Disease Processes
Arthritis
Cancer
Cystitis
Pancreatitis
Peritonitis
Pleuritis

Surgical Procedures
Spinal surgery
Fracture repair
Total hip replacement
Joint surgery
Ear surgery
Dental extractions
Rhinotomy or sinus surgery
Surgical repair of traumatic injury
Eye surgery
Thoracotomy
Gastric dilatation–volvulus, colon torsion
Pyometra

analgesic to the premedication before anesthetizing a patient for surgery. Preemptive analgesia also helps to prevent windup which, through changes in the CNS from central sensitization, can lead to pain that lasts longer than anticipated and is more difficult to manage.

> **TECHNICIAN NOTE** Administering analgesics before surgery decreases analgesic requirements and minimizes CNS sensitization. This is called *preemptive analgesia.*

Behavioral responses to pain vary depending on the species, age, breed, and temperament of the patient and the nature, duration, and severity of pain. Younger patients are less likely to tolerate pain and more likely to vocalize, whereas older animals may be more stoic and are more likely to become aggressive. Cattle are generally much more stoic than other species. Within a species, certain breeds may have higher or lower pain thresholds (e.g., calm draft horses versus excitable Thoroughbreds; large breed versus toy breed dogs; Labradors versus Siberian Huskies and Greyhounds). Individuals within a breed will also respond differently to pain. It is important to recognize that nonspecific behaviors that indicate pain may also be observed in patients with nonpainful conditions.

Ideally, assessment of pain-associated behavior is performed using a multistep process. The value of this approach is that it avoids overlooking subtle changes. The downside is that it is time consuming and may require special facilities. Also, when an animal is obviously in pain, it is better to treat first.

Step #1: Prior to directly interacting with the patient, observe the patient at a distance.

It is useful to observe patient behavior when people are not present (e.g., via remote cameras or one-way windows), although this may not be possible in many clinics. This step is useful in assessing behavior because many animals change their behavior when the animal is aware that a human observer is watching, when a person interacts verbally, and finally, when undergoing physical examination. A thorough assessment of pain-related behavior can therefore be time consuming, although decreasing the time devoted to the assessment may result in subtle changes being overlooked. It is important to remember that animals may mask pain-related behavior in the presence of people, due either to a protective response to avoid looking like prey or to socialization instincts. Different species often respond differently when they are in pain; cats tend to hide, dogs tend to seek attention from their owners, and herd or flock animals tend to separate from the other animals.

Step #2: Remove clothing such as lab coats, which may be a source of anxiety or stress, then approach the patient's cage or stall and quietly observe the patient. Evaluate the patient's facial expressions, appearance, attitude, and posture. Note if vocalization is present or not. If the patient moves towards the observer, assess the gait and level of activity.

Facial expressions, appearance, and attitude may be altered in patients that are in pain (Fig. 8.3 and see Fig. 12.23). Common facial expressions encountered in dogs in pain include a glazed or fixed stare. Cats may squint, exhibit changes in the appearance of the muzzle and whiskers, and may have a furrowed brow. Horses and cattle will have an altered head carriage and may also curl their lips. Cattle will grind their teeth. Animals in pain do not typically groom themselves and may appear unkempt.

Vocalization is frequently associated with pain. Dogs tend to whine, growl, whimper, and groan. Cats are more likely to groan, growl, or purr. Large animals do not vocalize as commonly; however, groaning and grunting are associated with pain in these species. In small animals, particularly dogs, vocalization is common in the immediate postoperative period and may be caused by pain or emergence delirium. Emergence delirium can be differentiated from pain by the fact that it lasts for a short time (less than 5 minutes) and responds to sedation. Pain lasts longer and responds to analgesic administration.

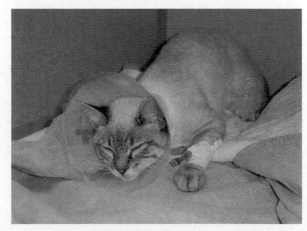

FIG. 8.3 This cat is experiencing abdominal pain. Note the squinted eyes and furrowed brow in addition to the head-down, sternal posture and arched back.

Changes in gait and level of activity such as lameness, limping, stiffness, and reluctance to move are all indicators of limb or joint pain. The development of exercise intolerance or a decrease in performance may also indicate the presence of limb pain. Arthritic dogs may not walk normally, whereas cats with arthritis show a reluctance to jump as high or as often as before. Horses will shift weight more frequently and point, rotate, or hang their limbs. Cows may arch their backs. A reluctance to lie down or a constant shifting of position is an indicator of thoracic or abdominal pain. Patients may stand, sit, or adopt a prayer position (head, chest, and thoracic limbs held lower than abdomen and hindquarters) rather than lie down, eventually becoming exhausted.

> **TECHNICIAN NOTE** Emergence delirium can be differentiated from pain by the fact that it lasts for a short time (less than 5 min) and responds to sedation. Pain lasts longer and responds to analgesic administration.

Step #3: Verbally interact with the patient by calling the animal by name or making encouraging sounds, while using a gentle tone of voice. Note if the patient moves towards the observer or not. Assess the change in behaviors listed above as well as gait and level of activity if the patient approaches. Hospitalized patients may sit staring at the back of the cage or stand at the back of the stall. Such patients may be unaware of their surroundings and not interested in interacting, often appearing stuporous or unwilling to move because of pain. Cats in pain will attempt to hide by moving as far from view as possible (a form of escape behavior) and will often become unresponsive to people. Remember that some hospitalized patients may be reluctant to come towards an observer even when not in pain. (See Fig. 8.4 for examples of pain-related behaviors.)

Step #4: Evaluate response to handling, palpation, or forced activity. Palpation or manipulation of a painful area may elicit pain. It is best to start a distance away from the area you think is the source of the pain and slowly and gently palpate closer to the source. For example, when assessing the pain associated with a surgical incision, start several centimeters away from the incision. Aggression is most commonly observed with severe acute pain that is elicited on palpation. Dogs may snarl or bite, cats may bite or hiss, and horses may bite or kick, or may try to flee. Pain may not consistently be present but can be elicited by an event such as forced activity (e.g., a horse that is not lame at the walk but is when it is encouraged to trot). This is often the

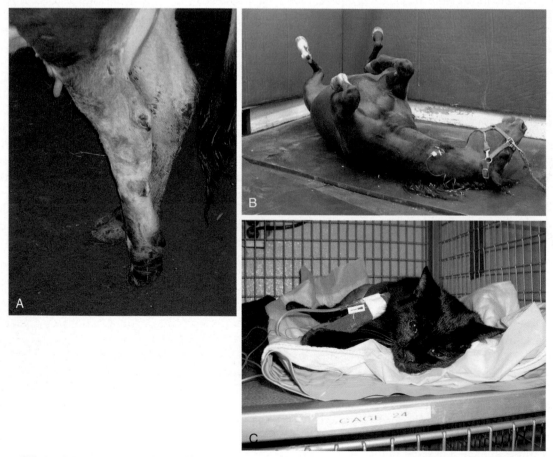

FIG. 8.4 Pain behaviors. **(A)** Signs of locomotor pain in a cow. This cow had a chronic wound of the hock joint and was three-legged lame. **(B)** Signs of abdominal pain in a horse. This horse, with severely painful colic, was violently thrashing in its stall and causing injury to itself. **(C)** General signs of pain in a cat. This cat suffered multiple trauma (fractured femur and ruptured bladder) from being hit by a car. Note the laterally recumbent posture, the vacant stare with dilated pupils, and the lack of interest in the photographer. (B, Courtesy OSU Equine Section.)

TABLE 8.2	Summary of Behavioral Signs of Pain in Domestic Animals				
Category	All Species	Dog	Cat	Horse	Cow
General behavior	Loss of grooming behavior; appear unkempt	Seek attention	Hide	Separate from herd	Isolate from herd
Facial expression	(Species dependent)	Glazed or fixed stare	Squinting, changes in muzzle and whiskers (see Feline Grimace Scale); furrowed brow	Altered head carriage; lip curl	Altered head carriage; lip curl; teeth grinding
Vocalization	(Species dependent)	Whine, growl, whimper, or groan	Groan, growl, or purr	Not as common; may groan or grunt	Not as common; may groan or grunt
Changes in gait	Lameness, limping, stiffness	(same)	(same)	(same)	(same)
Level of activity/response to forced activity	Reluctance to move; exercise intolerance; decreased performance	Trouble climbing stairs	Reluctance to jump as high or often	Shift weight more frequently; point, rotate, or hang limb; lame at trot (but not at walk)	May arch back
Body position	Reluctance to lie down; constant shifting of position (thoracic or abdominal pain);	May stand, sit, or adopt prayer position instead of lying down	May stand, sit, or adopt prayer position instead of lying down	May roll (sign of colic pain)	
Response to verbal interaction	Unresponsive; stuporous; stare at back of cage or stall		Attempt to hide; move from view	Remain at back of stall	Remain at back of stall
Response to handling/palpation	Aggression	Snarl; bite	Bite; hiss	Bite; kick; flee	Kick; flee

case with chronic pain (e.g., osteoarthritis). (See Table 8.2 for a summary of behavioral signs of pain in domestic animals.)

> **TECHNICIAN NOTE** While it is time consuming and may require specific facilities or equipment, a stepwise approach to assessing patient behaviors associated with pain will avoid missing subtle changes. A stepwise approach includes remote observation; quiet observation at the cage or stall; verbal interaction; and physical interaction. Note that if an animal is obviously in pain, then the priority should be treatment rather than assessment.

PAIN ASSESSMENT TOOLS

Pain assessment poses special challenges for veterinary patients because they are unable to verbally express their pain. This means that pain assessment in animals must involve evaluation of behaviors and physiologic parameters (as previously discussed) that change in response to pain. This process is, by its nature, subjective and requires the ability to detect subtle changes. In addition, because each patient responds differently to pain, it is important to find ways to help categorize and quantify these responses in a way that makes it easier to accurately compare pain levels among animals and in the same animal over time. Pain assessment tools (also called pain scales) are designed to meet this need. Use of such tools helps us to recognize and treat pain more effectively.

Most pain assessment tools used in human medicine rely on accurate self-reporting by the patient (e.g., answering the question, "On a scale of 0 to 10, how would you rate your pain?"). Consequently, these tools must be modified for use in animals in a way that allow us to more objectively evaluate the pain through careful observation, examination, and/or interaction with the patient.

In recent years, many pain assessment tools with varying degrees of complexity have been developed for veterinary patients. These assessment tools include verbal rating scales, simple descriptive scales, visual analog scales, numeric rating scales, categorical numeric rating scales, and comprehensive scales. Most of these tools require evaluator training for consistently meaningful results to be obtained. The more sophisticated scales are designed for specific types of pain (e.g., acute pain or chronic pain) caused by specific procedures or diseases (e.g., stifle surgery, colic) and are species specific (e.g., for use in dogs or in cats only).

A simple descriptive scale (Fig. 8.5) allows the assessor to rate the degree of pain (e.g., absent, mild, moderate, or severe). These scales are quick and easy to use, but they are subjective because they do not include a description of what to look for. It is therefore up to the assessor to decide when a patient is experiencing mild pain as opposed to moderate pain, severe pain, or no pain based on their impressions. In addition, these scales are not well suited to chronic or subtle changes, nor do they allow easy comparison of the progression of pain over time, as they are not very detailed in terms of design.

A visual analog scale consists of a "ruler." The left end of the line equates to no pain, and the right end of the line to the worst pain imaginable for the specific disease or surgical procedure (Fig. 8.6). The assessor places a mark (usually an X) on the line corresponding to the level of pain the assessor feels the animal is experiencing. The

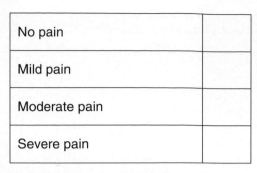

FIG. 8.5 Simple descriptive scale. The observer makes an overall assessment of the animal's pain and places an X in the box next to the descriptor.

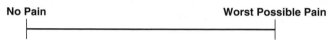

FIG. 8.6 Visual analog scale. The assessor places a mark (usually an X or a small vertical line) on the ruler corresponding to the level of pain the assessor feels the animal is experiencing.

assessor can rate the pain as being at any point along a continuum, which theoretically permits more discernment; however, like the simple descriptive scale, this scale is subjective.

Numeric Rating Scale

A numeric rating scale is similar to a simple descriptive scale in that pain is assigned to one of several levels but different in that each level is assigned a number (e.g., no pain = 0; mild pain = 1; moderate pain = 2; severe pain = 3).

The more sophisticated numeric rating scales include descriptions of behaviors or physiologic changes that correspond to each level (e.g., 0 = asleep, calm; 1 = agitated, vocalizing, looks at injury; 2 = severely agitated, vocalizing, thrashing), which makes assessment somewhat more objective.

The Colorado State University (CSU) Canine Acute Pain Scale, the CSU Feline Acute Pain Scale, and the CSU Equine Comfort Assessment Scale are numeric rating scales (Figs. 8.7–8.9). These scales have descriptors in each of three categories (psychological and behavioral, response to palpation, and body tension in the dog and cat; and behavior, clinical assessment, and postural features in the horse) that are used as a guide to classify the degree of pain on a scale of 0 to 4.

Categorical Numeric Rating Scale

A categorical numeric rating scale has a series of numeric rating scales with descriptions to rate each of several categories of behavior and/or physiologic changes, such as appearance, interaction, posture, and response to palpation of the wound, separately (Fig. 8.10). The points for each of the categories are totaled. A higher score indicates that the animal is in more pain. These scales are often species specific and may be designed for specific types of pain (e.g., acute or chronic) or for specific procedures (e.g., for horses undergoing castration).

A widely used scale that is of this type is the Short Form of the Composite Measure Pain Scale (CMPS-SF). This validated scale, which is available online from NewMetrica, University of Glasgow, at https://www.newmetrica.com/acute-pain-measurement/, is designed for evaluation of dogs with acute pain. It includes 30 descriptors in six categories (1) vocalization and (2) response to wound or painful area (assessed with the patient in the cage); (3) mobility (assessed by leading the dog out of the cage); (4) response to palpation of the wound or painful area; (5) overall demeanor; and (6) overall posture/comfort level. The maximum score is 24 points (or 20 if mobility cannot be assessed due to limb fracture, spinal disease, etc.). Administration of analgesics is recommended for patients with a score of 6 or more out of 24 points or 5 or more out of 20 points (if mobility is not assessed).

There is a similar scale designed for cats (Glasgow Composite Measure Pain Scale: CMPS-Feline), with 28 descriptors in 7 categories. These categories are similar to those used for the dog but include assessment of the cat's facial expression and response to stroking, and exclude assessment of mobility. Administration of analgesics is recommended for patients with a score of 5 or more out of 20 points.

The UNESP-Botucatu Multidimensional Composite Pain Scale from Universidade Estadual Paulista (UNESP) [aka: São Paulo State University], (available at: http://www.animalpain.com.br/en-us/escala-multidimensional.php) for cats with acute pain is another example of a validated categorical numeric rating scale that is available online. It includes 40 descriptors in 10 categories (including response to palpation of the wound, vocalization, posture, comfort, activity, attitude, appetite, and blood pressure). The maximum score of this scale is 30 points. Online, there are instructions for use of this scale along with a series of videos illustrating many of the behaviors described therein.

Feline Grimace Scale

The Feline Grimace Scale is a validated assessment tool developed in 2019 at Universite de Montreal for assessment of acute pain in cats (i.e., pain associated with medical, surgical, and oral conditions).

It is unique among pain scales in that it allows for rapid assessment by observing the patient at a distance and is based on changes in facial expression. Use of this scale involves assessment of five factors: (1) ear position; (2) orbital tightening; (3) muzzle tension; (4) position of the whiskers; and (5) head position. Each of these factors are given a score of 0, 1, or 2, and the scores are totaled. Analgesic administration is recommended when the total score is ≥4/10.

The website for this scale has a wide variety of information, including a training manual, practice cases, scientific publications related to the Grimace Scale, and a smart phone app is available that supports use of this scale at the point of care. More information about the Feline Grimace Scale may be found at: https://www.felinegrimacescale.com/.

Assessing Chronic Pain

Detecting the presence of chronic pain can be more challenging than detecting acute pain for a variety of reasons, especially when it is less severe and develops very gradually (e.g., pain associated with age-related arthritis or dental pain). Often, signs of chronic pain are very subtle and go unnoticed (e.g., changes

Your Clinic Name Here

Date _____

Time _____

Canine Acute Pain Scale

Rescore when awake	☐ **Animal is sleeping, but can be aroused - Not evaluated for pain** ☐ **Animal can't be aroused, check vital signs, assess therapy**

Pain Score	Example	Psychological & Behavioral	Response to Palpation	Body Tension
0	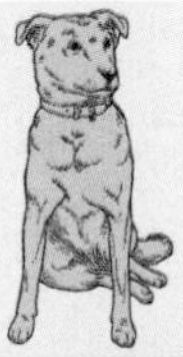	☐ **Comfortable** when resting ☐ **Happy, content** ☐ Not bothering wound or surgery site ☐ Interested in or curious about surroundings	☐ **Nontender** to palpation of wound or surgery site, or to palpation elsewhere	Minimal
1	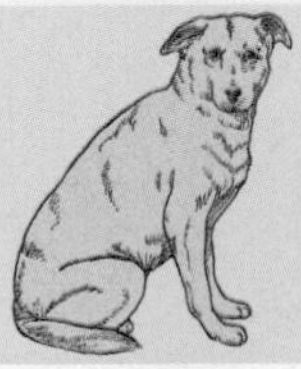	☐ **Content to slightly unsettled** or restless ☐ **Distracted easily** by surroundings	☐ **Reacts to palpation** of wound, surgery site, or other body part by **looking around, flinching,** or **whimpering**	Mild
2	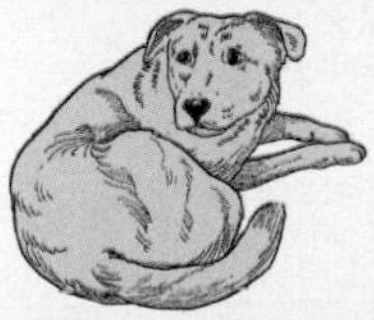	☐ Looks **uncomfortable** when resting ☐ May **whimper** or cry and may **lick or rub wound** or surgery site when unattended ☐ Droopy ears, **worried facial expression** (arched eye brows, darting eyes) ☐ **Reluctant to respond** when beckoned ☐ **Not eager to interact** with people or surroundings but will look around to see what is going on	☐ Flinches, whimpers cries, or guards/pulls away	Mild to Moderate **Reassess analgesic plan**
3	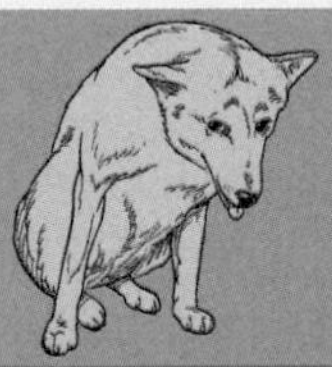	☐ **Unsettled, crying, groaning, biting or chewing** wound when unattended ☐ **Guards or protects** wound or surgery site by altering weight distribution (i.e., limping, shifting body position) ☐ **May be unwilling to move** all or part of body	☐ May be **subtle** (shifting eyes or increased respiratory rate) if dog is too painful to move or is stoic ☐ May be **dramatic**, such as a sharp cry, growl, bite or bite threat, and/or pulling away	Moderate **Reassess analgesic plan**
4	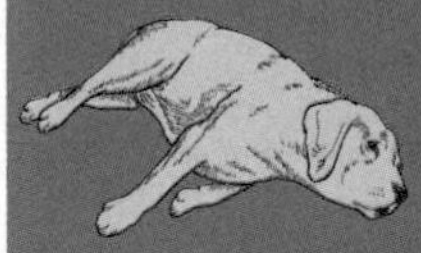	☐ **Constantly groaning or screaming** when unattended ☐ May bite or chew at wound, but unlikely to move ☐ **Potentially unresponsive** to surroundings ☐ **Difficult to distract** from pain	☐ **Cries at non-painful palpation** (may be experiencing allodynia, wind-up, or fearful that pain could be made worse) ☐ May react aggressively to palpation	Moderate to Severe **May be rigid to avoid painful movement** **Reassess analgesic plan**

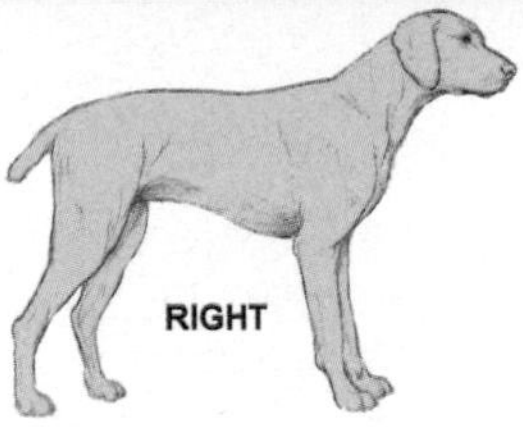

○ Tender to palpation
✕ Warm
■ Tense

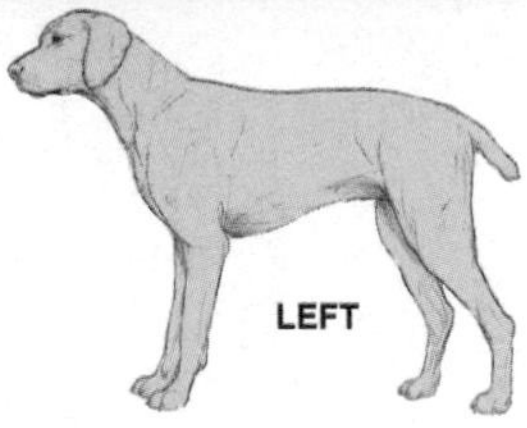

RIGHT   LEFT

Comments _____

© 2006/PW Hellyer, SR Uhrig, NG Robinson   Colorado State University   VETERINARY TEACHING HOSPITAL

FIG. 8.7 Colorado State University Canine Acute Pain Scale. (From https://vetmedbiosci.colostate.edu/vth/wp-content/uploads/sites/7/2020/12/canine-pain-scale.pdf.)

Your Clinic Name Here

Date _____

Time _____

Feline Acute Pain Scale

	Rescore when awake	☐ **Animal is sleeping, but can be aroused - Not evaluated for pain** ☐ **Animal can't be aroused, check vital signs, assess therapy**		
Pain Score	**Example**	**Psychological & Behavioral**	**Response to Palpation**	**Body Tension**
0	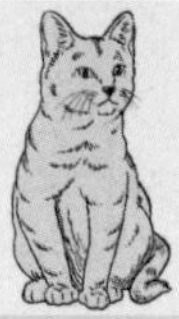	☐ **Content and quiet** when unattended ☐ **Comfortable** when resting ☐ Interested in or **curious** about surroundings	☐ **Not bothered** by palpation of wound or surgery site, or to palpation elsewhere	Minimal
1	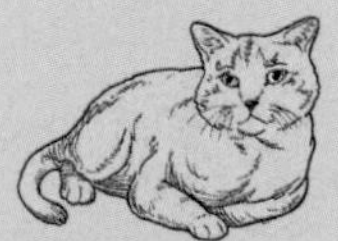	☐ **Signs are often subtle and not easily detected in the hospital setting**; more likely to be detected by the owner(s) at home ☐ Earliest signs at home may be **withdrawal from surroundings or change in normal routine** ☐ In the hospital, may be content or slightly unsettled ☐ **Less interested** in surroundings but will look around to see what is going on	☐ May or may not react to palpation of wound or surgery site	Mild
2	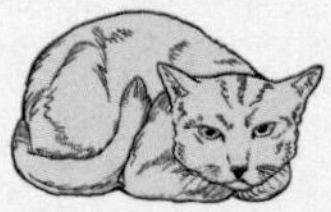	☐ Decreased responsiveness, **seeks solitude** ☐ **Quiet**, loss of brightness in eyes ☐ **Lays curled up or sits tucked up** (all four feet under body, shoulders hunched, head held slightly lower than shoulders, tail curled tightly around body) with eyes partially or mostly closed ☐ **Hair coat appears rough** or fluffed up ☐ May intensively groom an area that is painful or irritating ☐ Decreased appetite, **not interested in food**	☐ **Responds aggressively or tries to escape** if painful area is palpated or approached ☐ Tolerates attention, may even perk up when petted as long as painful area is avoided	Mild to Moderate **Reassess analgesic plan**
3	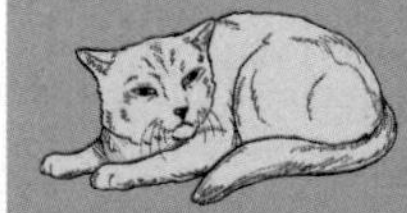	☐ Constantly **yowling, growling, or hissing** when unattended ☐ May bite or chew at wound, but **unlikely to move** if left alone	☐ **Growls or hisses at non-painful palpation** (may be experiencing allodynia, wind-up, or fearful that pain could be made worse) ☐ **Reacts aggressively** to palpation, **adamantly pulls away** to avoid any contact	Moderate **Reassess analgesic plan**
4	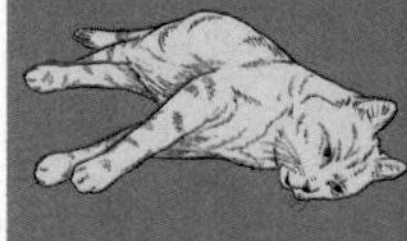	☐ Prostrate ☐ Potentially **unresponsive** to or unaware of surroundings, difficult to distract from pain ☐ Receptive to care (even aggressive or feral cats will be more tolerant of contact)	☐ **May not respond** to palpation ☐ **May be rigid to avoid painful movement**	Moderate to Severe **May be rigid to avoid painful movement** **Reassess analgesic plan**

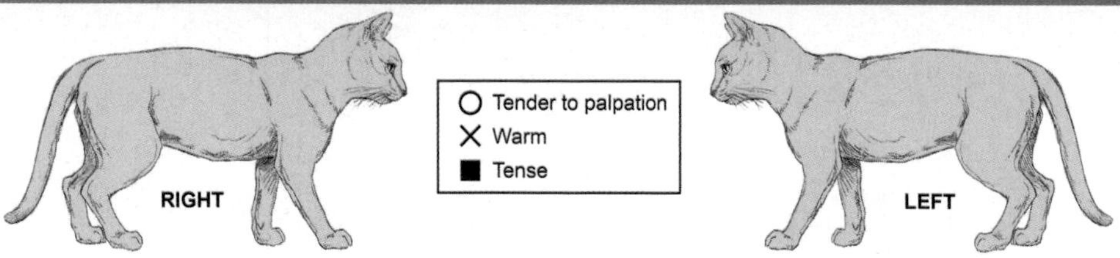

RIGHT   LEFT

○ Tender to palpation
✕ Warm
■ Tense

Comments _____

FIG. 8.8 Colorado State University Feline Acute Pain Scale. (From https://vetmedbiosci.colostate.edu/vth/wp-content/uploads/sites/7/2020/12/feline-pain-scale.pdf.)

Colorado State University

Veterinary Medical Center

Date _____

Time _____

Equine Comfort Assessment Scale

*This scale is designed to be used in the context of the clinical presentation of each animal. If you do not believe the pain scoring criteria to be accurate for this patient, please explain in the comments section below.

Pain Score	Behavior	Clinical Assessment	Postural Features
0	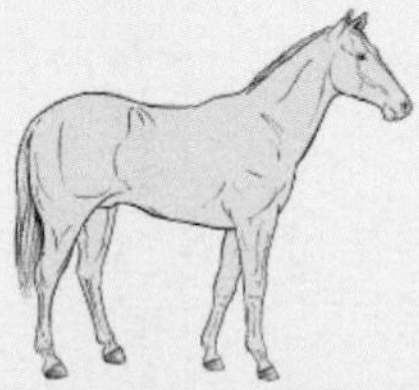 ❑ Responds with interest to gate opening, approach by observer ❑ Takes care in movements around people ❑ Head above withers ❑ Attentive ❑ Moving freely, calmly ❑ Resting comfortably	❑ HR:_____ (usually ≤ 40 bpm) ❑ Eyes: relaxed, normally responsive ❑ Normal muscle tension ❑ No focal areas of heat ❑ Palpation not aversive	❑ No lameness perceptible, bears weight equally ❑ Moves with ease of stride
1	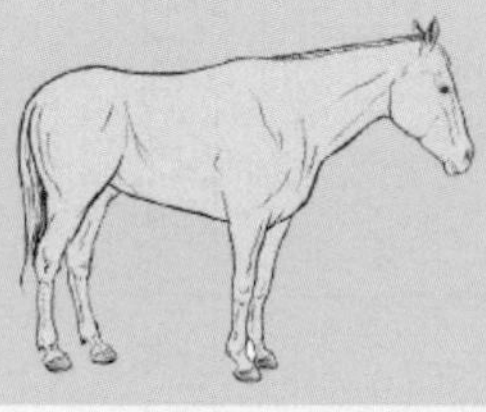 ❑ Head at or above withers ❑ Facing forward and watching ❑ Performs normal behaviors less frequently than expected ❑ Responds with quiet interest to gate opening, approach by observer ❑ Takes care in movements around people	❑ HR:_____ (may be ≤ 40 bpm) ❑ Mild muscle tension ❑ Mild focal areas of heat ❑ Slightly steps, leans or pulls away from palpation, +/- muscle twitching	❑ Lameness difficult to observe, inconsistently apparent ❑ Mild injury or stiffness in movement
2	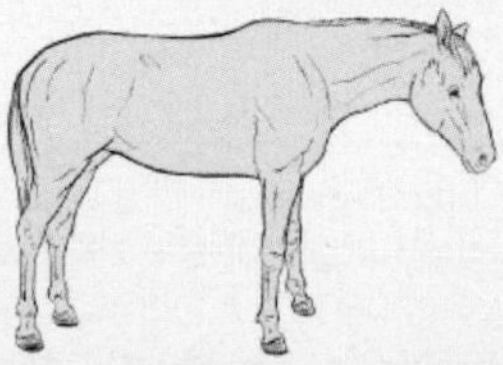 ❑ Head level with withers ❑ Moving slowly about with bedding undisturbed ❑ Mild but more frequent restlessness ❑ Responds to approach ❑ Less enthusiastic, less interested, less interactive ❑ Less careful about movements around people	❑ HR:_____ (may be ≥ 48 bpm) ❑ Tachypnea +/- RR:_____ ❑ Moderate muscle tension ❑ Increasing areas of heat ❑ Palpation more aversive	❑ Lameness apparent only under certain circumstances, favors leg(s) occasionally ❑ Obvious stiffness in movement
3	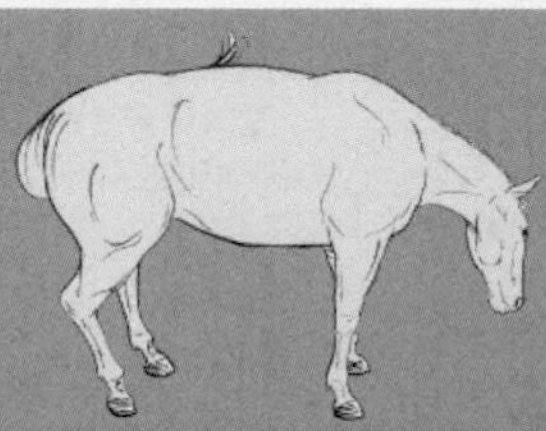 ❑ Head level or below withers ❑ May face back or corner of stall ❑ More vigorous signs of restlessness ❑ Eyes distracted, far away, weary ❑ Minimally reacts to interaction ❑ Stands in one position ❑ Beginning to become internalized ❑ Less careful about movements around people	❑ HR:_____ (may be ≥ 60 bpm) ❑ Tachypnea +/- RR:_____ ❑ Sweating ❑ Severe muscle tension ❑ Widespread areas of heat ❑ Vigorously aversive response to palpation	❑ Moderate lameness, able to bear weight but clearly favors one or more limbs ❑ Obvious discomfort, weight shifting ❑ Arched back ❑ Very stiff movements ❑ Abnormal standing posture
4	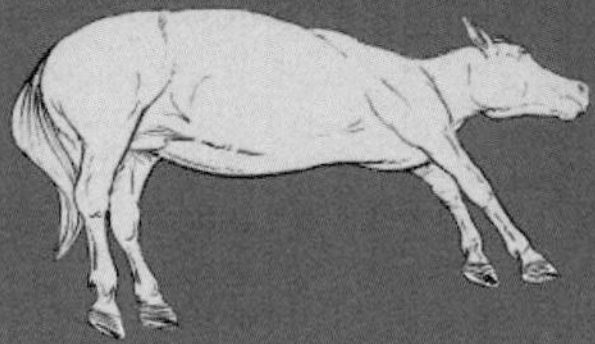 ❑ Head often below withers ❑ Stands in corner or faces wall ❑ Ears back, eyes weary ❑ Frequent signs of severe agitation ❑ Extremely uncomfortable, panicky OR ❑ Extremely internalized/withdrawn ❑ Unwilling to rise ❑ Careless about movements around people	❑ HR:_____ (may be ≥ 70 bpm) ❑ Tachypnea +/- RR:_____ ❑ Profuse sweating ❑ Extreme muscle tension / rigidity +/- fasciculation ❑ Widespread areas of heat ❑ Extremely aversive response to palpation, possibly aggressive	❑ Unable or unwilling to bear weight ❑ May not be able to move ❑ Constant shifting of weight ❑ Very abnormal standing posture OR ❑ In sternal or lateral recumbency

Current Pain Treatment(s):

Comments:_____

_____

_____

FIG. 8.9 Colorado State University Equine Comfort Assessment Scale. (From https://vetmedbiosci.colostate.edu/vth/wp-content/uploads/sites/7/2020/12/equine-pain-scale.pdf.)

Pain score 0-10. Choose one descriptor from each category

Interaction	Awake, willingly interacts, asleep	0	☐
	Awake, responds if encouraged	1	☐
	Awake, reluctant, unwilling	2	☐
Appearance	Asleep, calm	0	☐
	Agitated, vocalizing, looks at injury	1	☐
	Severely agitated, vocalizing, thrashing	2	☐
Posture	Normal, moves easily, asleep	0	☐
	Frequent position changes, guarded gait	1	☐
	Unwilling to lay down, abnormal gait	2	☐
Cardiovascular	HR and/or BP <10% elevated	0	☐
	HR and/or BP 10-20% elevated	1	☐
	HR and/or BP >20% elevated	2	☐
Respiration pattern	Normal	0	☐
	Guarded, mild abdominal	1	☐
	Marked abdominal	2	☐

FIG. 8.10 Categorical numeric rating scale for use in small-animal patients. The observer assigns a score for each category. Observations are performed before the animal is physically touched (e.g., to take a pulse rate). The overall score is used as a guide as to when to treat—for example, the veterinarian in charge may request that analgesics be administered if the pain score is ≥4—or as an assessment of response to treatment (i.e., a score that decreases after therapy).

in posture) or are attributed to aging or other causes (e.g., decreased desire to play in an older animal). Also, subtle signs of pain may be masked when the animal is not in its own environment. Consequently, it is important that owners be taught to recognize signs of pain and be given access to assessment instruments that they can use to help them tell when their pet is in pain. In recent years, several pain scales have been developed to enable both owners and veterinary professionals accurately assess chronic pain, many of which are available online. See Table 8.3 for examples of pain scales designed for assessment of acute and chronic pain in veterinary patients.

Veterinary teaching hospitals and large specialty practices often have their own pain assessment forms that typically combine different types of pain assessment tools in order to assess pain and progression of signs in response to treatment (Fig. 8.11).

Each type of assessment has its limitations. The least complex scales allow quicker assessment but are not as effective at detecting subtle changes. The more complex ones take more time to complete and can seem burdensome, especially if you are not trained to use them. Regardless of the type, the common purpose of these tools is to help determine how much pain the animal is in, to guide selection of appropriate treatments, and to assess patient response. To obtain maximum benefit, a scale should be chosen that is practical and appropriate for the specific circumstances under which it is being used.

Assessing Response to Therapy

After analgesics have been administered, the patient must be periodically checked to determine the response to treatment. The frequency with which pain should be assessed varies widely based on the situation. For instance, animals undergoing major surgery need to be assessed hourly or possibly more frequently during the first few hours of the postoperative period, whereas patients with diseases associated with chronic pain such as arthritis require less frequent evaluation (e.g., monthly or at longer intervals). Effective analgesic treatment causes pain-associated behaviors to gradually recede. Hospitalized patients rest and sleep more easily, and assume normal body positions and postures when asleep and awake. Appetite returns to normal, and appearance will improve as grooming behaviors also return to normal. When awake, animals will be more likely to interact with caregivers rather than ignore them, show aggression, or try to escape. Performance animals will return to form. Fig. 8.12 shows examples of patients that seem comfortable after surgery.

> **TECHNICIAN NOTE** Animals undergoing major surgery need to be assessed hourly or possibly more frequently during the first few hours of the postoperative period, whereas patients with diseases associated with chronic pain such as arthritis require less frequent evaluation.

TABLE 8.3 Pain Scales for Use in Domestic Animals

Name of Scale	Internet Address	Use
Colorado State University Canine Acute Pain Scale	https://vetmedbiosci.colostate.edu/vth/wp-content/uploads/sites/7/2020/12/canine-pain-scale.pdf	Assessment of acute pain in dogs
Colorado State University Feline Acute Pain Scale	https://vetmedbiosci.colostate.edu/vth/wp-content/uploads/sites/7/2020/12/feline-pain-scale.pdf	Assessment of acute pain in cats
Equine Comfort Assessment Scale	https://vetmedbiosci.colostate.edu/vth/wp-content/uploads/sites/7/2020/12/equine-pain-scale.pdf	Assessment of acute pain in horses
Short Form of the Composite Measure Pain Scale (CMPS-SF)	https://www.newmetrica.com/acute-pain-measurement/	Assessment of acute pain in dogs
The Glasgow Composite Measure Pain Scale: CMPS-Feline	https://www.newmetrica.com/acute-pain-measurement/	Assessment of acute pain in cats
The UNESP-Botucatu Multidimensional Composite Pain Scale	http://www.animalpain.com.br/en-us/avaliacao-da-dor-em-gatos.php	Assessment of acute pain in cats
Feline Grimace Scale	https://www.felinegrimacescale.com/	Assessment of acute pain in cats
Canine Brief Pain Inventory	https://www.vet.upenn.edu/research/clinical-trials-vcic/our-services/pennchart/cbpi-tool	Assessment of chronic pain in dogs (by owner)
Feline Musculoskeletal Pain Index	https://cvm.ncsu.edu/research/labs/clinical-sciences/comparative-pain-research/clinical-metrology-instruments/	Assessment of musculoskeletal pain in cats (by owner)

Adapted from Epstein ME, Rodanm I, Griffenhagen G, et al: 2015 AAHA/AAFP pain management guidelines for dogs and cats, *J Feline Med Surg* 17:251–272, 2015.

Pain assessment scores will decrease if analgesic therapy is effective, although it is almost impossible to remove all pain. The goal is to achieve a reduction in the pain score and a more comfortable patient rather than the production of a pain-free patient.

> **TECHNICIAN NOTE** It is often not necessary to spend a lot of time trying to determine if a patient is in pain. Treat for pain and then observe the response to therapy.

PERIOPERATIVE PAIN MANAGEMENT

Preemptive analgesia and multimodal therapy are key to providing successful perioperative analgesia. Multiple receptors and mechanisms have been identified that are responsible for pain and the development of windup. An analgesic plan for moderate to severe pain should make use of several drugs, each having a different mechanism of action. The benefits of multimodal analgesic therapy are that each individual drug dose is reduced, the overall anesthetic drug requirement is reduced, and therefore the risk of toxicity and adverse effects is decreased.

Management of perioperative pain begins in the preoperative period. Premedication (see Chapter 3) offers an opportunity to administer analgesia before surgery (i.e., preemptively). Animals that are in pain before surgery will be in pain after surgery and should be treated for the anticipated severity of postoperative pain. Analgesics can be administered as part of the anesthetic premedication if they also provide or enhance sedation (e.g., opioids, alpha$_2$-adrenoceptor agonists, ketamine). Another modality to provide preemptive analgesia in small animals is the application of a transdermal fentanyl patch (see page 290) at least 6 to 12 hours in advance of anticipated pain. NSAIDs are typically administered preoperatively in large-animal patients and can be administered to small-animal patients preoperatively under certain circumstances when injectable formulations are available and approved for this use.

Intraoperative analgesia may be provided by using local or regional blocks (discussed in Chapter 7), induction and maintenance protocols that include analgesics, by using supplemental analgesic CRIs (see Chapter 9), and by maintaining anesthetic depth at an appropriate level.

Postoperative analgesia is provided by using a variety of agents and techniques that are discussed in more detail later this chapter.

PHARMACOLOGIC ANALGESIC THERAPY

The choice of analgesics is governed by the severity and type of pain and the animal's general condition. The attending veterinarian also selects the route of delivery, which may include injection (subcutaneous [SC], intramuscular [IM], intravenous [IV], intraarticular, epidural, local infiltration), oral administration (per os or PO), or transdermal.

Pharmacologic analgesia can be achieved through a variety of agents. The primary drugs used to treat acute pain are opioids, NSAIDs, and local anesthetics, with use of other analgesics, including alpha$_2$-agonists, ketamine, and gabapentin as needed to achieve adequate pain control. In contrast, treatment of chronic pain usually most often involves use of NSAIDs, gabapentin, amantadine, and anti-Nerve Growth Factor monoclonal antibodies (antiNGF mAb) in combination with a variety of adjunctive treatments, including nutraceuticals, physical therapy, hydrotherapy, and environmental modification. A discussion of commonly used pharmacologic analgesics follows.

Opioids

The pharmacology, mode of action, effects, and use of opioids are discussed in detail in Chapter 3, with an emphasis on their role in premedication. Here, their role as analgesics will be emphasized. Opioids are the oldest analgesics, having been in use for many hundreds of years for this purpose. Despite the development of many other effective analgesic drugs in recent

THE OHIO STATE UNIVERSITY VETERINARY TEACHING HOSPITAL

PAIN MANAGEMENT PLAN

"Pain assessment is considered part of every patient evaluation, regardless of presenting complaint."

PATIENT ID CARD

Date: _____   Department: _____

| Pulse rate: | Temperature: °C / °F | |
| Respiratory rate: | Weight: lbs / kg | Attitude: |

Is pain present upon admission? Y ☐ N ☐   Pain on palpation only? Y ☐ N ☐   Cause of pain:

Signs of pain (describe):   **Descriptors** (Please Circle):

						Restless	Not grooming
Behavior:	Normal ☐	Depressed ☐	Excited ☐	Agitated ☐	Guarding ☐	Aggressive ☐	Agitated	Obtunded
Vocalization:	None ☐	Occasional ☐	Continuous ☐	Other ☐			Trembling	Inappetant
Posture:	Normal ☐	Frozen ☐	Rigid ☐	Hunched ☐	Recumbent ☐	Reluctant to move ☐	Nervous	Biting or Licking area
Gait:	Sound ☐	Lame weight bearing ☐		Lame non-weight bearing ☐	Non-ambulatory ☐			

Other signs of pain: Previous Analgesic History:

Classification of pain: **Anatomical location of pain** (circle):   Comments:

Acute ☐
Acute recurrent ☐
Chronic (>weeks) ☐
Chronic progressive ☐

Superficial ☐
Deep ☐
Visceral ☐

Inflammatory ☐
Neuropathic ☐
Both ☐

Primary hyperalgesia ☐
Secondary hyperalgesia ☐
Central algesia ☐

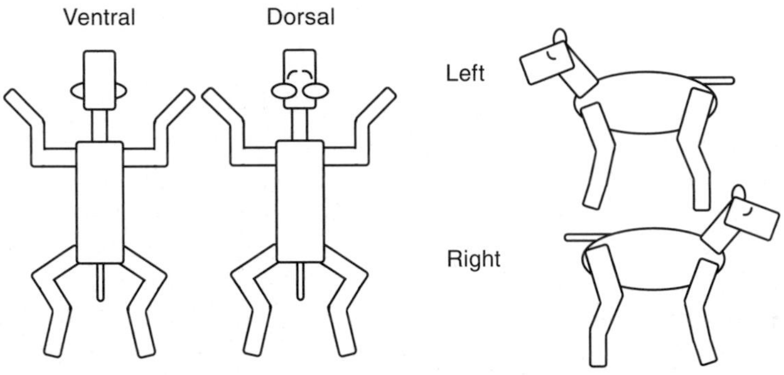

Ventral   Dorsal   Left   Right

VISUAL ANALOGUE SCALE

No Pain   **Worst Possible Pain**

Event	Time(HH:MM):	Date:	Comments:
1			
2			

PAIN THERAPY
(pharmacologic and alternative)

	Date	Dose/Route	Efficacy/Duration	Comments
Current				
Prescribed				

VISUAL ANALOGUE SCALE

No Analgesia   **Complete Analgesia**

Clinician:_____   Release date:_____

FIG. 8.11 The Ohio State pain assessment form. Note that there is a visual analog scale to assess level of pain as well as degree of analgesia after therapy. Complex pain assessment forms or scales are useful for evaluating pain that is subtle, chronic, or difficult to treat. The main drawback of this type of pain assessment tool is that it is time consuming.

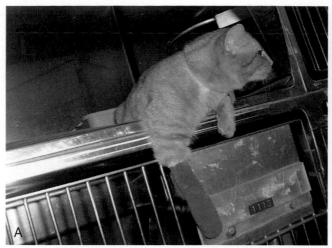
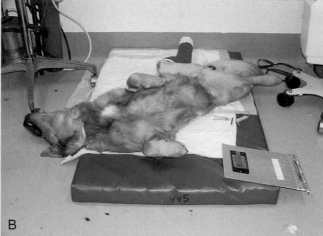

FIG. 8.12 Signs of comfort after surgery. **(A)** One day after surgery for a forelimb wound, this cat was playful and interactive. Analgesia consisted of oral buprenorphine and oral meloxicam. **(B)** One hour after a tibial plateau leveling osteotomy, this Golden Retriever was sleeping on its back and seemed very comfortable. Analgesia consisted of a preoperative morphine epidural and postoperative intravenous carprofen.

years, this important class of drugs still contains many of the first-line agents for the treatment of acute pain.

Opioids provide analgesia through their action on opioid receptors in both the spinal cord and brain as well as in some peripheral tissues such as the synovial membranes of joints. Opioid agonist drugs acting centrally inhibit perception in the brain and central sensitization in the spinal cord.

Doses, routes, and adverse effects of opioids used for postoperative analgesia are given in Table 8.4.

As outlined in Chapter 3, opioids have many specific uses in veterinary anesthesia, including the following:

- Opioids are commonly included in injectable premedications, often in combination with a tranquilizer such as acepromazine or dexmedetomidine. When used preemptively, they diminish windup. The analgesic effect of these preanesthetic mixtures is generally gone by 2 to 4 hours after administration, however, and a single preoperative dose is usually inadequate to prevent or control even moderate pain after surgery.
- At higher doses, opioids can be used in combination with tranquilizers to induce a state of potent sedation (neuroleptanalgesia) that offers considerable analgesia throughout the surgical period and for some time after surgery. (See the discussions of neuroleptanalgesia in Chapter 3 and standing chemical restraint in Chapter 10.)
- Opioids can be used on their own or in combination with other agents (e.g., alpha₂-agonists, NSAIDs, and local anesthetics) to provide postoperative pain control (see later).

Individual opioids vary in their potency, duration, and adverse effects. Mu opioid receptor agonists (e.g., morphine, fentanyl, hydromorphone, and methadone) are generally considered to produce the most potent analgesic effects but are equally likely to induce adverse effects. They are used for moderate to severe pain. Partial mu agonists (e.g., buprenorphine) are less potent analgesics and the degree of sedation is also less pronounced, as are adverse effects on the cardiovascular and respiratory systems. Because of their somewhat weaker analgesic effect compared to full mu agonist drugs, these agents should be reserved for use as preanesthetics and for treatment of mild to moderate pain. Agonist-antagonists (e.g., butorphanol) do not provide adequate analgesia for painful procedures in small animals; however, in large-animal anesthesia they are used for relief of mild to moderate pain.

> **TECHNICIAN NOTE** Mu opioid receptor agonists are generally considered to produce the most potent analgesic effects but are equally likely to induce adverse effects.

In addition to their analgesic properties, many opioids cause some degree of sedation and anxiolysis. If used as sole agents and at high doses, some may induce excitement in patients that are awake, particularly cats and horses.

Common GI effects are characterized by an initial increase in GI activity, including nausea and vomiting (in cats and dogs) and defecation. This is followed by a relative slowdown of the GI tract with the development of ileus, colic in horses, and constipation.

Opioids are metabolized in the liver. Animals with liver disease may have impaired drug metabolism and should receive reduced doses of these agents, with drugs that can be reversed being preferred.

Opioid Agents Used for Moderate to Severe Pain

The potent opioid analgesics most commonly used in veterinary medicine are morphine, hydromorphone, methadone, and fentanyl.

Morphine. Morphine was the first opioid agent used in human and veterinary medicine and is still extensively used in veterinary practice as a preanesthetic and an analgesic. It is a pure agonist with affinity for both mu and kappa opioid receptors (see Chapter 3, page 78). Morphine can be used in cats, dogs, and horses; however, as the likelihood for excitement or dysphoria is higher in cats and horses, it may be prudent to use lower doses

TABLE 8.4 Analgesics

Drug	Species[a]	Route	Dose (mg/kg Unless Otherwise Stated)	Notes
Opioids				
Morphine	Cat	IV (slow), IM, SC	0.2–0.5	Potential for excitement
		CRI	0.1–0.2 mg/kg/h	
		Epidural	0.05–0.1	Use preservative-free drug
	Dog	IV (slow), IM, SC	0.5–1	
		CRI	0.05–0.3 mg/kg/h	Loading dose of 0.05–0.1 mg/kg IV over 5 min; stop if blood pressure drops
		Epidural	0.1	Use preservative-free drug
		PO	2–5	Give bid
	Horse	IV, IM, epidural	0.05–0.1	Potential for excitement, increased locomotor activity (e.g., stall walking), and ileus
	Cattle	IV, IM	0.1–0.5	
		Epidural	0.1	
Hydromorphone	Cat	IV, IM, SC	0.05–0.1	
		CRI	0.01–0.03 mg/kg/h	
	Dog	IV, IM, SC	0.05–0.2	
		CRI	0.01–0.03 mg/kg/h	
Methadone	Dog	IV, IM, SC	1–1.5	
	Horse	IV	0.05–1	Potential for excitement and increased locomotor activity
Fentanyl	Cat	IV	0.001–0.003 (1–3 mcg/kg)	
		CRI	1–4 mcg/kg/h	Higher infusion rate for intraoperative analgesia
		Transdermal patch	2–5 mcg/kg/h	
	Dog	IV	0.002–0.005 (2–5 mcg/kg)	
		CRI	2–10 mcg/kg/h	Higher infusion rate for intraoperative analgesia
		Transdermal patch	2–4 mcg/kg/h	
	Horse	IV	0.001–0.01 (1–10 mcg/kg)	Potential for excitement and increased locomotor activity
		Transdermal patch	0.5–1 mcg/kg/h	
Butorphanol	Cat	IV, IM, SC	0.1–0.4	Can be used to reverse mu agonists
		CRI	0.1–0.2 mg/kg/h	
		PO	0.5–1	
	Dog	IV, IM, SC	0.1–0.4	Can be used to reverse mu agonists
		CRI	0.1–0.5 mg/kg/h	
		PO	0.5–2	
	Horse	IV	0.01–0.04	Potential for ataxia
	Cattle	IV	0.05–0.1	
Buprenorphine	Cat	IV, IM, SC	0.005–0.02	Can be used to antagonize mu agonists
		SC (Simbadol)	0.24 mg/kg once daily (up to 3 days)	Duration of 24 hrs
		Transdermal (Zorbium)	2.7–6.7 mg/kg	Duration of 4 days
		Transmucosal	0.01–0.02	Drip into cheek pouch using 1-mL syringe
	Dog	IV, IM, SC	0.005–0.02	Can be used to antagonize mu agonists
	Horse	IV	0.01–0.04	Potential for ataxia

TABLE 8.4 Analgesics—cont'd

Drug	Species[a]	Route	Dose (mg/kg Unless Otherwise Stated)	Notes
Alpha₂-Adrenoceptor Agonists				
Xylazine	Cat	IV	0.1–0.3	Likely to cause vomiting
		IM, SC	0.2–0.5	
	Dog	IV	0.1–0.2	Likely to cause vomiting
		IM, SC	0.2–0.5	
	Horse	IV	0.5–1	May cause bradycardia, ataxia
		Epidural	0.03–0.05	
	Cattle	Epidural	0.05	
Dexmedetomidine	Cat	IM, SC	10–40 mcg/kg	
	Dog	IM, SC	5–20 mcg/kg	May cause bradycardia
		CRI	0.5–1 mcg/kg/h	
Detomidine	Horse	IV	0.01–0.02	May cause bradycardia, ataxia
		Epidural	0.03–0.06	Sedation, ataxia
	Cattle	Epidural	0.06	
Romifidine	Horse	IV	0.04–0.08	May cause bradycardia
		Epidural	0.08	
Nonsteroidal Antiinflammatory Drugs				All NSAIDs have the ability to cause renal toxicity. COX-2 selective drugs have lower gastrointestinal toxicity than COX-1 selective drugs.
COX-1 Selective NSAIDs				
Aspirin	Cat	PO, every 2–3 days	10 (½ baby aspirin for a 4– 5-kg cat)	Increased bleeding times
	Dog	PO, bid	10–25	Increased bleeding times
Acetaminophen	Dog	PO, tid	5–10	Highly toxic to cats
Flunixin meglumine	Cat	IM once, SC once	0.25	
	Dog	IV sid for three doses IM sid for three doses SC sid for three doses	0.25–1	
	Horse	IV	0.2–1.1	
	Cattle	IV	1	
Ketoprofen	Cat	SC (once)	2	Increased bleeding times
		PO (for 5 days)	0.5–1	Increased bleeding times
	Dog	IV, IM, SC	2	Increased bleeding times
		PO (for 5 days)	0.5–2	Increased bleeding times
	Horse	IV	1.1–2.2	
	Cattle	IV	2	
Ketorolac	Cat	IM, one or two treatments 12 hrs apart	0.25	
	Dog	IV or IM, one to three treatments 12 hrs apart	0.3	
Phenylbutazone	Horse	IV	2–4	Possible GI ulceration
Piroxicam	Dog	PO, sid	0.3	Antineoplastic (bladder tumors)

Continued

TABLE 8.4 Analgesics—cont'd

Drug	Species[a]	Route	Dose (mg/kg Unless Otherwise Stated)	Notes
COX-2 Selective NSAIDs				
Carprofen	Cat	SC	2	GI toxicity possible with chronic use
		PO	1	GI toxicity possible with chronic use
	Dog	IV, IM, SC	2–4	Rarely, liver toxicity
		PO		Rarely, liver toxicity
	Horse	IV	0.5–1.1	
Meloxicam	Cat	SC, sid once, then PO for 4 days[b]	0.1–0.2 (SC), then 0.05 (PO)	For postsurgical pain
		PO, every 3–4 days	0.025	
	Dog	IV, SC, PO, sid	0.1–0.2	
Etodolac	Dog	PO, sid	10–15	Difficult to determine dose accurately in small dogs
Deracoxib	Dog	PO, sid	1–4	
Tepoxalin	Dog	PO, sid	10	Also blocks lipoxygenase
Firocoxib	Dog	PO, sid	5	
Robenacoxib	Cat	PO, sid, ≤3 days	1 (tablet)	Not for use in cats <4 months of age or <5.5 lb in body weight
		SC, sid, ≤3 days	2 (injectable)	
Non-COX, Prostaglandin EP4 Antagonist NSAID				
Grapiprant	Dog	PO, sid	2	
Other Analgesic Drugs				
Ketamine	Dog	CRI	10–20 mcg/kg/h	NMDA antagonist
	Horse	CRI	10–20 mcg/kg/h	NMDA antagonist
Amantadine	Dog	PO, sid	3–5	NMDA antagonist
Dextromethorphan	Dog	PO, sid	0.5–2.0	NMDA antagonist
Amitriptyline	Dog	PO, sid or bid	1–2	Inhibition of neurotransmitter reuptake
Frunevetmab	Cat	SC	1	Monoclonal antibody against nerve growth factor
Gabapentin	Dog	PO, bid	2.5–10	Unknown mechanism; wean off slowly to avoid rebound seizures

[a]Where a species is not listed, no data are available for that specific drug.
[b]Note that treatment with meloxicam for 4 days is off-label. The manufacturer recommends use of a one-time SC dose only.
bid, twice a day; *COX*, Cyclooxygenase; *CRI*, constant rate infusion; *GI*, gastrointestinal; *IM*, intramuscular; *IV*, intravenous; *NSAID*, nonsteroidal antiinflammatory drug; *NMDA*, N-methyl-D-aspartate; *PO*, by mouth; *SC*, subcutaneous; *sid*, once a day; *tid*, three times a day.

initially in these species. Restlessness is seen in some dogs and horses (which manifests as an increase in locomotor activity) shortly after morphine administration, especially in the absence of pain. For this reason, morphine is more commonly administered to horses in combination with sedatives or administered epidurally.

Morphine is an inexpensive and effective option for treatment of moderate to severe pain in most patients. It is effective in treating both visceral and somatic pain and can be given by several routes, including slow IV, IM, SC, intraarticular, and epidural routes, and by spinal injection. Morphine is also available in regular or sustained release tablets for oral use, although efficacy of oral morphine varies considerably among patients.

When morphine is given intravenously, it must not be injected too rapidly, particularly in dogs, as rapid injection may cause release of histamine (characterized by a fall in blood pressure,

flushing, and pruritus). One technique for use in dogs is to draw up a loading dose, which is given slowly intravenously (over 5 minutes) and repeated until the patient appears free of pain or adverse effects occur. Morphine can also be administered intravenously by constant rate infusion (CRI). With this technique, morphine contained in a syringe is slowly administered through an IV catheter by means of a syringe pump.

IM administration of morphine (and other opioids) results in a slightly longer duration of action than IV administration and avoids the risk of hypotension, although IM injection appears to be slightly painful. SC injections cause less patient discomfort (although SC injections have a slightly slower onset of effect). Also, the incidence of excitement, dysphoria, and vomiting in cats is lower when morphine is given by SC injection rather than IM injection.

Although morphine provides potent analgesia and sedation, it is associated with several adverse effects in addition to those mentioned previously. In cats and dogs, there is initial GI stimulation characterized by vomiting, salivation, and defecation. The incidence of vomiting can be reduced by pretreatment with maropitant (see Chapter 3). Morphine also has the potential to cause severe respiratory depression, although this is less common in animals than in human patients. Excitement (particularly in cats given doses >0.1 mg/kg), bradycardia, panting, increased intraocular pressure, increased intracranial pressure, urinary retention, miosis (in dogs), mydriasis (in cats), hypothermia (all species), or hyperthermia (in cats only), are also encountered in some patients after morphine administration. Fortunately, these adverse effects are seldom a significant problem in patients in pain that are treated with analgesic doses.

Morphine has a strong tendency to cause physical dependence (addiction) in humans. It is therefore classified as a Schedule II drug in the United States and is designated as a narcotic in Canada (see Technician Note).

> **TECHNICIAN NOTE: Characteristics and Effects of Morphine**
> - Pure opioid agonist-Schedule II
> - Effective for visceral and somatic pain
> - Duration of action 2–3 hr
> - Given by slow IV, IM, SC, intraarticular, epidural and spinal injection, and CRI
> - Rapid IV injection may cause histamine release with resulting hypotension, pruritus, and flushing
> - Effects include:
>   - Excitement or dysphoria in cats and horses
>   - Restlessness in dogs, especially in the absence of pain
>   - Hypothermia (all species) or hyperthermia (in cats only)
>   - Miosis (dogs) or mydriasis (cats)
>   - Bradycardia
>   - Respiratory depression
>   - Panting in dogs
>   - GI stimulation including vomiting, salivation, and defecation
>   - Colic in horses due to ileus
>   - Urinary retention
>   - Increased intraocular and intracranial pressure

Hydromorphone. Hydromorphone is a pure opioid agonist with a higher potency than morphine and with a similar duration of effect. It can be given via the IV, IM, and SC routes to cats and dogs, and can also be administered as a CRI. Unlike morphine, it does not typically induce histamine release and therefore rarely causes vasodilation. It has less potential to cause excitement in cats compared to morphine. A tranquilizer such as dexmedetomidine, acepromazine, or midazolam may be used concurrently to prevent excitement and supplement the sedative effect of hydromorphone. Otherwise, adverse effects are similar to those seen with morphine: respiratory depression, bradycardia, vomiting, panting in dogs, excessive sedation, and excitement (seen especially at doses >0.2 mg/kg).

Like morphine, hydromorphone can be used as a premedication (IM, alone or in combination with a tranquilizer), as an analgesic (IV, IM, or SC for dogs and cats, repeated every 4 to 6 hours), or as an induction agent for high-risk patients (0.05 to 0.1 mg/kg hydromorphone by slow IV injection followed by 0.05 to 0.2 mg/

kg midazolam drawn into a separate syringe and given intravenously). It is also given by the epidural route and has a similar effect to morphine.

Hydromorphone is classified as a Schedule II drug in the United States and as a narcotic in Canada.

> **TECHNICIAN NOTE: Characteristics and Effects of Hydromorphone**
> - Pure opioid agonist—Schedule II
> - Effective for visceral and somatic pain
> - Given by slow IV, IM, SC, epidural, and CRI
> - Effects are very similar to those of morphine

Methadone. Another synthetic opioid, methadone has similar characteristics to hydromorphone, with the exception that it has the lowest likelihood of causing vomiting in cats and dogs. This drug is also an antagonist at the NMDA receptor (see later), which may make it a favorable choice for treating pain when central nervous system hypersensitivity is present or is likely to develop (e.g., in cases of chronic pain) or in acute pain that has not been treated for several days.

> **TECHNICIAN NOTE: Characteristics and Effects of Methadone**
> - Pure opioid agonist—Schedule II
> - Effective for visceral and somatic pain
> - As compared with morphine: (1) more potent; (2) fewer adverse effects; (3) longer duration of analgesia (4 hr); (4) less vomiting
> - Given by slow IV, IM, SC, and CRI
> - Has NMDA receptor antagonist activity
> - Effects include:
>   - Hyperresponsiveness to sound
>   - Respiratory depression
>   - Panting in dogs
>   - Bradycardia

Fentanyl. Among the most potent analgesics known, fentanyl has a rapid onset and short duration of effect in small animals (onset approximately 2 minutes, duration of effect approximately 20 to 30 minutes after IV injection). It is most commonly administered by CRI or transdermally (see following section). In small-animal patients, fentanyl and midazolam drawn into separate syringes can be used together to induce general anesthesia. When fentanyl is given intravenously, a loading dose is typically administered, followed by a CRI. It can also be given by IM, SC, or epidural injection.

Fentanyl can induce profound sedation, bradycardia, and respiratory depression, and like other mu agonist opioids, it may cause panting (in dogs) or increased sensitivity to sound. Adverse effects of fentanyl are further discussed in the section on transdermal administration later in the chapter.

Fentanyl is sold in combination with the tranquilizer fluanisone under the name Hypnorm (see Chapter 12) in some countries, although it is not available in the United States.

Fentanyl (including transdermal formulations) is a Schedule II drug in the United States and is classified as a narcotic in Canada. The injectable formulation is available in a concentration of 50 mcg/mL.

TECHNICIAN NOTE: Characteristics and Effects of Fentanyl
- Pure opioid agonist—Schedule II
- Effective for visceral and somatic pain
- Duration of action 20–30 min
- Given by IV, IM, SC, epidural and transdermal routes, and CRI
- Effects include:
  - Profound sedation
  - Bradycardia
  - Respiratory depression
  - Panting in dogs
  - Hyperresponsiveness to sound

Buprenorphine. Buprenorphine is a partial mu agonist. It stimulates mu receptors, producing some analgesia, but is less effective than morphine and other pure agonists.

Buprenorphine can be given IV, IM, SC, or by the epidural route. It has a delayed onset of action (15 minutes intravenously and 40 minutes intramuscularly) but provides a longer duration of analgesia than other opioids (6 to 8 hours after IM injection and 18 to 24 hours after epidural injection). The human-label injectable formulation of buprenorphine can also be administered orally to cats and dogs (i.e., buccal or oral transmucosal route); it is important to deliver the drug between the teeth and the cheek so that the drug is not swallowed. Like butorphanol, buprenorphine does not provide adequate analgesia for severe pain (such as orthopedic pain and major soft tissue surgery), but it is useful for mild to moderate pain. It is commonly used to provide analgesia for rodents and other species used in research (see Chapter 12), as well as postoperative analgesia for dogs and cats.

When given at high doses, buprenorphine may induce respiratory depression, which is difficult to reverse with naloxone. Analeptic agents such as doxapram may be somewhat effective in correcting buprenorphine-induced respiratory depression. Intubation and assisted ventilation are necessary in some of these patients because there is a potential for carbon dioxide retention and increased intracranial pressure.

Although buprenorphine has little sedative effect on its own, it can prolong sleep times when given with other agents.

Buprenorphine is a Schedule III drug in the United States. It is relatively expensive and is sometimes provided in ampules that are inconveniently large for small-animal patients. Buprenorphine can, however, be transferred to sterile vials for use on multiple patients.

Most preparations of buprenorphine are not labeled for use in veterinary species. There are two formulations that are labeled for use in cats. Simbadol (Abbott) is approved for subcutaneous injection once daily for up to 3 days for control of postoperative pain in cats. In studies of this preparation, analgesic effects were shown to have a 1-hour onset of action and 24- to 48-hour duration of action. This formulation of buprenorphine is not a sustained release preparation, and the increased duration is due to the high dosage recommended by the manufacturer (0.24 mg/kg). Dysphoria is a possible side effect, and administering a lower dose (e.g., half the recommended dose) may mitigate this. Simbadol has been used off-label in dogs, given IM at 0.005 to 0.02 mg/kg, particularly when standard preparations of buprenorphine have been unavailable. The concentration of buprenorphine in Simbadol (1.8 mg/mL) is high; thus it should not be sent home with owners.

Zorbium (Elanco) is available as a transdermal solution for postoperative pain management in cats. Zorbium is supplied in tubes and is applied between the shoulder blades 1 to 2 hours prior to surgery (similar to topical antiparasitic medications). The drug dries rapidly following application, resulting in absorption by the skin and subsequent slow release into the circulation. A single application provides analgesia lasting 4 days. The concentration of buprenorphine (20 mg/mL) is very high compared to the injectable formulations (usually 0.3 mg/mL or 1.8 mg/mL, depending on the product), so precautions must be taken when administering Zorbium; protective eyewear and impermeable latex or nitrile gloves should be worn, and arms should be covered by wearing a long-sleeved garment, for example, a lab coat. Two different volumes are available: 0.4 mL for cats weighing 1.2 to 3 kg, and 1 mL for cats weighing greater than 3 kg, up to 7 kg. At the time of this writing, Zorbium has not been evaluated in cats weighing less than 1.2 kg; cats that are pregnant, ill, or have chronic diseases; or in cats younger than 4 months.

TECHNICIAN NOTE: Characteristics and Effects of Buprenorphine
- Partial mu agonist—Schedule III
- Effective for mild to moderate visceral and somatic pain
- Duration of action of most preparations is felt to be 6–8 hr after IM injection and 18–24 hr after epidural injection
- The duration of action of the veterinary-label injectable product Simbadol has been shown to be 24–48 hr in cats
- The duration of action of the veterinary-label transdermal product Zorbium has been shown to be 4 days in cats
- Given by IV, IM, SC, transdermal (in the case of Zorbium), and epidural injection
- The human-label injectable formulation may also be given by the oral transmucosal route
- Can be used to reverse sedation and respiratory depression of pure agonists while maintaining some analgesia
- Effects include:
  - Little sedative effect on its own
  - Respiratory depression that is difficult to reverse, especially at high doses

Butorphanol. A synthetic opioid agonist-antagonist, butorphanol was first used in veterinary medicine as a cough suppressant. Butorphanol is widely used as a preanesthetic or sedative (by the SC or IM route alone or in mixtures with dexmedetomidine or acepromazine).

Butorphanol stimulates kappa receptors and antagonizes or blocks mu receptors (see Chapter 3). As such, it is not considered to be effective for treating acute surgical pain in cats and dogs. It is used in horses and ruminants to treat mild to moderate visceral and orthopedic pain.

Butorphanol is available in several concentrations, including 0.5, 2, and 10 mg/mL. Injectable butorphanol may be given via the IV, IM, or SC route. It is potentially toxic to the spinal cord, which limits its use for epidural injection.

The duration of analgesia provided by butorphanol may be short (as little as 1 hour in dogs after IM or SC injection, which limits its usefulness for the treatment of pain). To avoid frequent readministration, butorphanol can be given as a CRI (in IV fluids or by syringe pump) after a loading dose.

Butorphanol produces less sedation, dysphoria, and respiratory depression than most opioids. Although moderate doses of butorphanol may cause some respiratory depression, higher doses do not depress respiration further (a phenomenon known as the *ceiling effect*). Heart rate, blood pressure, and cardiac output may be decreased after the administration of butorphanol; however, the effect is less than that of morphine, and pretreatment with atropine is not usually required. Panting, vomiting, and histamine release, effects associated with some opioid agonists, are seldom seen with this drug.

Butorphanol can be used as an antagonist to partially reverse respiratory depression and sedation induced by mu agonist opioids such as morphine or fentanyl, although the anesthetist must be aware that it will also partially reverse the analgesic effect of these drugs. The dose used for reversal is up to 0.4 mg/kg, administered intravenously to effect in increments of 0.01 to 0.05 mg/kg every 3 to 5 minutes. The antagonistic effect of butorphanol is less predictable and less potent than that of naloxone and can be overridden by subsequent administration of high doses (two to three times the normal dose) of morphine.

Butorphanol is classified as a Schedule IV drug in the United States. In Canada, it is classified as a controlled drug.

TECHNICIAN NOTE: Characteristics and Effects of Butorphanol
- Opioid agonist antagonist—Schedule IV
- Not effective for acute pain in small animals
- Effective for mild to moderate visceral and somatic pain in large animals
- Duration of action short (as little as 1 hr after IM or SC injection in dogs)
- Given by IV, IM, SC injection, and by CRI
- Injectable formulation is available in multiple concentrations
- Can be used to reverse sedation and respiratory depression of pure agonists while maintaining some analgesia
- Effects include:
  - Less sedation, dysphoria, cardiac depression, and respiratory depression than opioid agonists

---

Nalbuphine. Nalbuphine is a kappa agonist and mu antagonist like butorphanol, but its antagonist properties are greater. It is currently the only injectable opioid agent for veterinary use that is not classified as a controlled drug in the United States. It is a weak analgesic and sedative and can be used as a reversal agent for opioid agonists. Bradycardia, respiratory depression, and sedation are uncommon with this agent.

Use of Opioid Injections to Treat Postoperative Pain

Opioids can be administered by a variety of routes for prevention or treatment of postoperative pain. In many practices, opioids are given by IM or SC injection, preferably before the animal regains consciousness from anesthesia. Injections may be repeated as necessary to prolong the analgesic effect (see Table 8.4 for information on dose and duration).

From the standpoint of analgesia, one major disadvantage of opioid agents is their relatively short duration of effect when given via the SC or IM route. Morphine offers 2 to 3 hours of analgesia for severe pain and 4 to 6 hours for moderate or mild pain; hydromorphone, 2 to 4 hours; fentanyl, approximately 20 minutes; and butorphanol, 1 to 2 hours in dogs and up to 4 hours in cats. Repeat injections can be given but are expensive, require hospitalization, are uncomfortable for the patient, and create peak-and-trough blood levels instead of a constant, effective blood concentration.

A second disadvantage of opioid use is the potential for adverse effects such as respiratory depression, bradycardia, excitement (usually exhibited as apprehension, hypersalivation, and mydriasis), excessive sedation, panting, increased sensitivity to sound, urinary retention, and GI effects. These adverse effects are seldom severe when analgesic dosages are used. However, it is advisable to avoid opioid use or to use them with caution in high-risk patients, such as those with hypotension, hepatic disease, preexisting respiratory difficulties, CNS disorders such as head injuries or increased intracranial pressure, or altered bowel motility.

Both disadvantages of opioids—their short duration and potential for adverse effects—may be partially overcome by giving these drugs by routes other than IM or SC injection. Alternative routes for opioid administration include constant rate infusion, epidural injection, transdermal application, and intraarticular administration. When used by these alternative routes, opioids may produce effective, economical, and long-acting analgesia, with minimal adverse effects. However, use of opioids by these routes constitutes off-label use in many animal species, and informed consent should be obtained from the animal's owner.

Intravenous Infusion of Opioids

Morphine, fentanyl, hydromorphone, methadone, and butorphanol can be given intravenously by CRI. This is sometimes the only method of analgesic delivery that is effective in constant, unremitting pain. Animals are given an initial loading dose (e.g., 0.1 mg of morphine per kilogram intravenously every 3 to 5 minutes) until the desired effect is achieved. The same dose is then given over 4 hours through a constant flow of IV fluids.

Ideally, a CRI should be administered using an automated infusion pump or syringe pump. Practices that lack this type of specialized equipment can deliver opioid analgesics continuously in IV fluids by adding an opioid directly to a bag of fluids and using a burette to carefully control the infusion rate. When preparing a CRI, it is important to gently rotate the bag or syringe containing the drug/diluent mixture several times to ensure it is adequately mixed (see Table 8.4 for doses and Chapter 9, Boxes 9.7, 9.8, and 9.9, for instructions on preparing CRIs).

Patients must be frequently monitored for signs of inadequate pain control (in which case the rate of administration should be increased) or excessive sedation, dysphoria, respiratory depression, bradycardia, panting, and other signs that indicate an excessive dose. If these signs are present, the rate of administration should be decreased. The duration of pain control (for morphine) is 30 minutes past the discontinuation of the IV fluids. If morphine is inadequate to control pain, lidocaine also can be added to the fluids and infused at 2–3 mg/kg/h (dogs only). For severe pain, morphine, lidocaine, and ketamine can be coinfused as a combination referred to as "MLK" (Procedure 8.1).

PROCEDURE 8.1 **Procedure for Adding Morphine, Lidocaine, Ketamine to Intravenous Fluids to Provide Analgesia for Dogs During Surgery**

1. Add the following amounts of drugs to a 500-mL bag of crystalloid fluids:
   - 1.6 mL of morphine 15 mg/mL (24 mg morphine)
   - 15 mL of lidocaine 20 mg/mL (300 mg lidocaine)
   - 0.6 mL of ketamine 100 mg/mL (60 mg ketamine)
2. Remember to mark the bag of fluids using an appropriate additive label.
3. Administer the fluids at 5 mL/kg/h during surgery.[a] The infusion rates will be:
   - Morphine 0.24 mg/kg/h
   - Lidocaine 3 mg/kg/h
   - Ketamine 0.6 mg/kg/h
4. Important points to remember when administering the combination:
   - A fluid bag containing this combination should not be used to administer fluid boluses

- Lidocaine takes several hours to reach an effective concentration; therefore 2 mg/kg IV should be administered at the start of the anesthetic period or given before IV induction
- The effects of the combination will usually last for 1 hr after termination of the infusion, sometimes delaying recovery. Turning the infusion off before postoperative radiographs or bandage application will decrease time spent in recovery.
- Particular care should be taken when administering this combination to small dogs to prevent overdose. Use of a smaller bag of fluids, a Buretrol, or an infusion pump is recommended.

[a]If fluids are being delivered at lower rates, then the amount of drugs added will have to be adjusted (e.g., if fluids are given at a rate of 2.5 mL/kg/h), the amount of each drug to be added would be doubled.

Intraarticular Use of Opioids

Opioids may be given by the intraarticular route, particularly after elbow or stifle surgery. In this technique, 0.1 to 0.3 mg/kg of morphine is diluted in a volume of saline equivalent to 1 mL/10 kg body weight and instilled into the joint with a sterile catheter immediately after closure of the joint capsule. This technique provides 8 to 12 hours of postoperative analgesia.

Epidural Use of Opioids

With the instillation of a small dose of an opioid or other analgesic into the epidural space at the lumbosacral junction, it is possible to achieve excellent and long-lasting analgesia of the hindlimbs, abdomen, caudal thorax, pelvis, and tail. Currently, preservative-free morphine is the opioid most commonly used for epidural analgesia. Local anesthetics such as lidocaine may impair movement, urination, and defecation, and may cause a sympathetic blockade if the drug diffuses too far cranially, which may result in severe hypotension. Occasionally, morphine and local anesthetics are used epidurally in combination. Morphine is also sometimes combined with an alpha2-agonist for epidurals in large-animal patients.

Morphine given by the epidural route offers more profound analgesia for a longer time than when given by other routes, and pain relief will last beyond the surgical procedure. Epidural morphine has a direct, long-lasting effect on the pain receptors in the spinal cord, but it does not reach high concentrations in the bloodstream because of low fat solubility. Adverse effects such as sedation (dogs), excitement (cats), respiratory depression, and nausea are therefore rare, although urinary retention and pruritus may be seen.

To achieve preemptive analgesia for postoperative pain, epidural morphine should be given after induction but before the surgical procedure. Epidural morphine is significantly less effective when administered in the postoperative period. Preservative-free morphine is preferred because the preservatives typically found in morphine preparations (formaldehyde and phenol) are potentially neurotoxic.

The technique for epidural morphine administration is similar to epidural administration of lidocaine (see Procedure 7.3). Normally, the animal is anesthetized or deeply sedated and is positioned in sternal recumbency with the head slightly elevated and the hindlimbs pulled forward to open the lumbosacral space. An epidural puncture is performed. Once it has been determined that the needle is in the epidural space, morphine is injected over 30 to 60 seconds. Ideally, a single-dose vial of preservative-free morphine should be used, diluted with sterile saline to a volume of 0.3 mL/kg. The recommended maximum volume that should be injected is 0.45 mL/kg. Onset of analgesia is approximately 20 to 60 minutes after injection, and analgesia lasts 6 to 24 hours. If more prolonged analgesia is required, an epidural catheter can be used to instill morphine into the epidural space over a longer period (hours to days).

Although epidural analgesia is regarded as a safe procedure, it should not be undertaken in animals with septicemia, local infections in the lumbosacral space, bleeding disorders, spinal trauma, or neurologic disease of the spinal cord. Local anesthetics should not be administered by the epidural route to hypotensive patients. It is relatively difficult to administer epidural anesthetics to obese animals. Epidural hematomas and abscesses may result from improper needle placement or unsterile technique. Urinary retention may occur in the first 24 hours after surgery, and the bladder should be monitored closely in all patients that have received epidural analgesics. Urinary catheterization may be necessary in some patients. Pruritus, delayed respiratory depression, sedation, vomiting, and nausea have been reported in human patients but are uncommon in dogs. These symptoms, if they occur, can be treated with naloxone hydrochloride (0.01 mg/kg IV). Animals that have received epidural morphine and are recumbent should be repositioned every 2 to 4 hours because normal sensation may be absent. Failure to reposition animals may result in pulmonary atelectasis or prolonged pressure on superficial nerves, leading to temporary or permanent loss of function.

Transdermal Use of Opioids

Transdermal patches containing fentanyl are another convenient option for long-term opioid administration. Fentanyl patches have been used for many years in the treatment of severe pain in human patients. The analgesic effect of a fentanyl patch is thought to be comparable to that of IM hydromorphone, but the duration of analgesia is considerably longer.

A patch consists of a reservoir of fentanyl enclosed in plastic. The patch is applied to the clipped skin of the animal and is left in place for several days (Procedure 8.2). Patches come in different

PROCEDURE 8.2 Applying a Fentanyl Patch

1. Various locations can be used for patch application, including the lateral thorax, dorsal neck (commonly used in small animals), or upper part of the limb (commonly used in horses). Any location that is hard for the animal to reach with its mouth or limb will work. Once applied, the patch should not contact sources of external heat.
2. The skin is clipped, taking care not to nick the skin (which may result in the fentanyl being absorbed too rapidly). If soiled, the skin can be cleansed with water (only) and dried thoroughly.
3. The patch is removed from its protective backing and should be handled by its edges only, or gloves should be worn to avoid contact with the patch membrane.
4. The adhesive side of the patch is applied to the shaved skin and held in place for 1–2 min. If the patch does not adhere to the skin, a Tegaderm (3M) transparent dressing or other light dressing can be placed over the fentanyl patch. Skin staples can also be used to secure the patch if it is placed while the animal is anesthetized, taking care not to puncture the drug chamber (Fig. 1). Tissue adhesive should not be used to attach the patch to the patient because it alters the absorption of the fentanyl. If necessary, the patch may be covered with bandage material to prevent removal by the patient (particularly dogs[a]).
5. The patch remains in place for several days, during which time the fentanyl is gradually absorbed. Blood levels remain at therapeutic levels for approximately 5 days in cats and 3 days in dogs, although there is considerable variation in duration and effectiveness among patients.
6. At the end of this time, the patch should be peeled off and disposed as medical waste. If the patient has been discharged in the interim, it is advisable that the patient return to the clinic for patch removal and assessment.
7. If a longer duration of analgesia is required, a new patch can be applied at a separate clipped site.
8. Fentanyl patches can be used in other species, following similar directions as for dogs. Fig. 2 shows a fentanyl patch applied to a horse's forelimb.

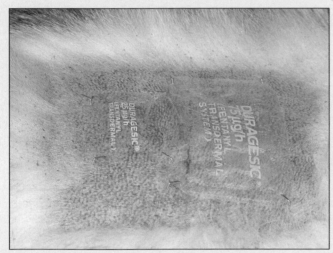

FIG. 1 Fentanyl patch applied to the skin of a dog and secured using skin staples. Care should be taken not to place the staples through the drug reservoir chamber.

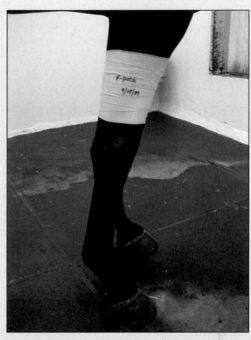

FIG. 2 Fentanyl patch secured to the forelimb of a horse with Elastikon bandage. Note the writing on the bandage, which communicates to the caregivers that a patch is underneath and when it was applied.

[a]Accidental ingestion of the patch produces no signs in dogs or cats if the patch reaches the stomach or intestines intact because any fentanyl absorbed is metabolized rapidly by the liver. However, overdose may occur after oral absorption (e.g., if a patch is chewed and punctured).

sizes that deliver different amounts of fentanyl each hour. A 12.5-mcg/h patch is useful in animals weighing less than 4 kg. The 25-mcg/h patch is used in cats and in dogs weighing 4 to 6 kg. A 50-mcg/h patch is used in dogs weighing 7 to 20 kg; a 75-mcg/h patch is used in dogs weighing 21 to 30 kg; and dogs that weigh more than 30 kg receive a 100-mcg/h patch (Table 8.5). Large-animal patients may require several patches for effective plasma levels of fentanyl to be reached. Patches should not be cut or trimmed because this will cause erratic drug release and possible human exposure. In patients showing signs of inadequate pain control 24 hours after patch application, a second patch or another analgesic agent can be added.

Because fentanyl is absorbed through the skin relatively slowly, there is a delay of 4 to 12 hours in cats and 12 to 24 hours in dogs before therapeutic blood levels are achieved. To achieve preemptive analgesia, apply the patch at least 6 hours before the start of surgery in cats and at least 12 hours before the start of

TABLE 8.5 Choosing an Appropriate Fentanyl Transdermal Patch

Body Weight (kg)	Fentanyl Transdermal Patch Delivery Rate
<4 kg	12.5-mcg/h
4–6 kg	25-mcg/h
7–20 kg	50-mcg/h
21–30 kg	75-mcg/h
>30 kg	100-mcg/h
Large animals	May need multiple patches depending on the patient size

surgery in dogs. If application of the patch is delayed until after surgery, it is necessary to provide the patient with another opioid (e.g., morphine, hydromorphone, or methadone) or an NSAID such as meloxicam, ketoprofen, or carprofen until the patch takes effect. Butorphanol or buprenorphine should not be used concurrently with a fentanyl patch because either may partially block the opioid receptors, reducing the analgesic effect.

Many types of patients benefit from a fentanyl patch, including postoperative patients (e.g., after onychectomy, orthopedic procedures, or abdominal surgery) and those that have trauma, burns, cancer, or painful abdominal conditions such as pancreatitis.

Recent studies have shown considerable variation among animals in the concentration of fentanyl absorbed from a transdermal patch. One study showed that a 50-mcg/h patch in dogs delivered as little as 13.7 and as much as 49.8 mcg/h. Patients should be observed for signs of breakthrough pain (which may indicate a low plasma fentanyl concentration) and supplemented with morphine, methadone, hydromorphone, or an NSAID as required.

Excessively high plasma fentanyl concentrations may develop in some patients. If this occurs, the most common signs are ataxia and sedation in dogs and dysphoria and disorientation in cats. Affected cats appear fearful or excited, are hypersensitive to sound, and may have widely dilated pupils. Panting is also a problem in some animals. Treatment, if necessary, consists of removing the patch and/or giving a narcotic antagonist (e.g., naloxone or butorphanol).

There have been some reports of death caused by respiratory failure when human patients self-administered more than one patch at a time, but respiratory depression is uncommon in veterinary patients with fentanyl patches. Respiratory depression may be seen in trauma patients, particularly in animals with CNS signs. Other adverse effects reported in human patients include constipation, physical dependence, muscle rigidity, miosis, mood changes, bradycardia, and bronchoconstriction. Use of fentanyl patches is not recommended in human patients with respiratory disease, increased intracranial pressure, impaired consciousness, or bradycardia, hepatic or renal dysfunction, or brain tumors; these recommendations may also hold true for animals. Some patients may exhibit a mild transient dermatitis at the patch site after removal, and delayed hair regrowth at the patch site is common.

Transdermal patches may release excessive amounts of fentanyl if they are heated, and fentanyl overdoses have been reported in human beings who lie under electric blankets while wearing a patch. It is therefore suggested that fentanyl patches be avoided in animals with fevers and that patch contact with hot water bottles and other external sources of heat be avoided.

There is some concern regarding the potential for abuse by adult people or ingestion of a patch by a child or pet. For this reason, the manufacturer does not support the use of fentanyl patches in animals. Some veterinarians address this concern by using the patch only on hospitalized animals or by carefully selecting and educating owners before discharging an animal that is wearing a patch.

Nonsteroidal Antiinflammatory Drugs

NSAIDs, also called *nonsteroidal antiinflammatory analgesics* or NSAAs, are a large group of agents that have been used for many years to control minor pain in human beings and animals. The NSAID group includes such common drugs as acetylsalicylic acid (aspirin) and acetaminophen, and newer agents such as robenacoxib, carprofen, meloxicam, ketoprofen, tolfenamic acid, firocoxib, and grapiprant. Dose and toxicity information for individual NSAID agents are summarized in Table 8.4.

Newer and more powerful NSAIDs such as ketoprofen, meloxicam, robenacoxib, and carprofen are commonly used for postoperative analgesia after procedures as diverse as ovariohysterectomy and fracture repair. NSAIDs are also useful for treatment of dental pain, panosteitis, osteoarthritis, meningitis, mastitis, and other painful medical conditions because of their strong antiinflammatory action.

NSAIDs have several beneficial effects on animal patients, including the following:

- All NSAIDs appear to be effective analgesics for somatic (musculoskeletal) pain and require approximately 30 to 60 minutes to achieve full analgesic effect, regardless of the route of administration.
- NSAIDs have potent antiinflammatory properties. This, combined with their analgesic effect, is the basis for the widespread use of drugs such as carprofen and robenacoxib in the treatment of osteoarthritis, panosteitis, hypertrophic osteodystrophy, and muscular pain.
- Some NSAIDs are antipyretic (reduce fevers).

Mechanism of Action

The clinical effects of NSAIDs (with the exception of grapiprant—see below) stem chiefly from their inhibition of prostaglandin synthesis. Prostaglandins (often abbreviated PGs) are a group of extremely potent chemicals that are normally present in all body tissues and are involved in the mediation of pain and inflammation following tissue injury. Prostaglandins are also responsible for a variety of homeostatic ("housekeeping") processes, including maintenance of normal GI, reproductive, renal, and ophthalmic function. Most NSAIDs prevent pain and inflammation by inactivating the enzyme cyclooxygenase (COX), which catalyzes one of the steps in the production of prostaglandins. There are two important COX isoenzymes that vary in importance from tissue to tissue. COX-1 is normally present in most tissues, whereas COX-2 is present in some, such as the central nervous system, kidney, reproductive organs, and eyes. COX-2 is inducible (i.e., not normally present, but is produced under certain circumstances), particularly during tissue damage and inflammation. Inhibition of both COX isoenzymes but particularly COX-2 has been linked to analgesic effects. Most NSAIDs inhibit both COX-1 and COX-2, although the ratio of COX-1 to COX-2 inhibitory effects of individual NSAIDs varies considerably. Drugs that are COX-2 selective (carprofen, meloxicam, deracoxib, rebenacoxib) or specific (firocoxib) are less likely to interfere with intestinal barrier function and produce GI ulceration; however, all NSAIDs have the potential to be nephrotoxic.

The relative effect of an NSAID on these enzymes will determine both the analgesic potency and the severity and type of adverse effects after the administration of that particular drug (see the separate section on adverse effects).

Although most NSAIDs are active against prostaglandins in peripheral tissues only, others also have effects on prostaglandin synthesis in the brain and spinal cord and are therefore said to act both centrally and in the peripheral tissues.

As a group, NSAIDs are well absorbed orally, and many are available in tablet or liquid form. Injectable NSAIDs are also available and can be given at the end of surgery to provide 24 hours of pain relief. Some NSAIDs, for example, carprofen and robenacoxib, can also be used before surgery in selected patients to achieve preemptive analgesia. If long-term analgesia is required, injections can be repeated in some cases, or tablets can be dispensed.

All NSAIDs are eliminated by metabolism and conjugation within the liver, followed by renal or biliary elimination. The NSAID group of drugs is unusual in that there is significant variation in duration of effect between species. For example, the plasma half-life of aspirin is 1 hour in the horse, 8 hours in the dog, and 38 hours in the cat. The prolonged half-life of aspirin in the cat is a result of the low levels of the enzyme glucuronyl transferase (one of the enzymes that metabolizes salicylate NSAIDs, such as aspirin) in that species. There is also significant variation among species in the toxicity of particular NSAIDs. For example, acetaminophen is extremely toxic in cats but can be a useful agent in dogs. Similarly, ibuprofen is considered safe for use in humans but has significant toxicity in dogs and cats. Because of this variation, the safety of any NSAID in one species does not imply that it can be used with impunity in all species (see Table 8.4 for dosages and cautions for specific agents). In particular, it cannot be assumed that dosages and administration schedules that are appropriate for dogs can be safely used in cats.

NSAIDs have some advantages over opioids: they are not subject to the storage, handling, and record-keeping regulations that govern narcotics; they have little abuse potential; and they are effective when given orally. Unlike opioids, NSAIDs have a negligible effect on the cardiovascular and respiratory systems. NSAIDs also do not depress the CNS and therefore lack the sedative effect of opioids. When used in healthy patients according to label directions, they provide effective and safe relief for mild to moderate pain. They frequently provide adequate analgesia in large animal species for severe pain and are generally well tolerated in adult animals.

Adverse Effects

Unfortunately, NSAIDs as a group have a significant potential for toxicity in small animal patients. Most people who work in veterinary hospitals are aware of the toxicity of acetaminophen in cats. A single 325-mg capsule may cause acute liver damage within 4 hours of ingestion because of the formation of toxic metabolites within the liver. Many NSAIDs are safe for use in healthy animals but can have serious toxic effects in animals that are dehydrated or hypotensive.

Many of the adverse effects of NSAIDs are attributable to the fact that they reduce not only the production of the prostaglandins that mediate pain, inflammation, and fever but also those that are beneficial. Pharmaceutical companies have attempted to formulate NSAIDs that will prevent the production of harmful prostaglandins while preserving the production of beneficial prostaglandins. Theoretically, this can be achieved if the NSAID inhibits the enzyme COX-2 (which is active in damaged or inflamed tissues and synthesizes the prostaglandins that cause pain) but does not affect COX-1 (which synthesizes the prostaglandins that help maintain normal physiologic functions such as protection of the gastric mucosa and modulation of blood flow to the kidney). In theory, it is also possible to produce NSAIDs that have more than 1000-fold specificity for COX-2 over COX-1 and are therefore extremely safe for use in terms of their GI adverse effects. However, the drugs currently available do not have this degree of specificity, and the COX-2 isoenzyme is important for normal function in some organs, such as the kidney, eye, reproductive tract, and the GI tract. Further confusing the picture, an agent that has pronounced specificity for COX-2 in one species does not necessarily show the same specificity in another species.

One example of a beneficial prostaglandin that is adversely affected by many NSAIDs is prostaglandin E_2 (PGE_2), which is normally present within the stomach mucosa and helps reduce gastric acid secretion and promotes mucus production. When PGE_2 levels are reduced by the administration of an NSAID, gastric acid secretion increases and mucus production decreases, which sometimes leads to the production of stomach ulcers. Up to 50% of dogs treated with aspirin have mild stomach ulceration within a few days of treatment, which may result in vomiting, GI bleeding, and inappetence, but more often is not clinically apparent. Occasionally, animals with GI ulceration resulting from NSAID use may undergo a sudden episode of life-threatening hemorrhage. In dogs, ulcerogenic potential appears to be high for ketoprofen, naproxen, ibuprofen, flunixin, and piroxicam, and use of these agents for prolonged periods (over 5 days) is associated with a high incidence of adverse effects. Meloxicam and carprofen have less ulcerogenic activity in dogs and are preferred for long-term use, as in dogs with osteoarthritis.

It is helpful to administer oral NSAIDs with a meal to dilute the drug that is present in the stomach. The synthetic prostaglandin misoprostol, which is given orally at a dose of 2 to 4 mg/kg tid, is a GI protectant, which can be prescribed. Histamine-2 (H_2)–receptor antagonists such as famotidine or ranitidine are also helpful in treatment of stomach ulcers.

Another potential adverse effect of NSAIDs is renal toxicity. The prostaglandins PGE_2 and prostacyclin normally maintain adequate blood flow within the kidney. In anesthetized animals and other animals that are prone to hypotension (such as trauma patients), these prostaglandins play a vital role in maintaining renal blood flow. By blocking prostaglandin synthesis, NSAIDs have the potential to decrease renal blood flow in these patients, leading to renal hypoxia. Dogs are apparently very susceptible to development of renal failure when blood pressure decreases, and there are several reports of acute renal failure after the administration of NSAIDs during anesthesia. To avoid the risk of renal damage in anesthetized patients, the use of NSAIDs should be postponed until after anesthesia, and preemptive or intraoperative use is not advised unless the patient is receiving intraoperative IV fluids and arterial blood pressure monitoring is available. Some NSAIDs are approved for preoperative use (e.g., carprofen and robenacoxib); however they should be used cautiously or avoided in patients that are hypotensive or have preexisting renal disease. Fortunately,

NSAID-induced renal insufficiency is usually reversible (particularly in young, healthy patients) with the administration of IV fluids. It is much more difficult to reverse in geriatric patients or in patients with preexisting renal failure. It is a prudent practice to screen geriatric patients for renal disease before anesthesia (by determining values for blood urea nitrogen, creatinine, and/or urine specific gravity) and to avoid NSAIDs in patients with decreased renal function.

Another potential adverse effect of NSAIDs is impaired platelet aggregation, which can lead to prolonged bleeding times. This effect may be beneficial in some circumstances (e.g., by lowering the risk of stroke in human patients who regularly take aspirin). However, there is a potential for increased bleeding in patients that are given NSAIDs before or during surgery. As with the potential for renal toxicity, this concern can be minimized by postponing the use of NSAID agents until after surgery has been completed. If preemptive use of an NSAID is indicated, carprofen can be used (in the dog) because it has been shown to have less renal toxicity and platelet-inhibiting effect than some other NSAID agents.

Liver damage appears to be associated with the use of NSAID agents in some patients. Carprofen has been extensively studied in this regard and, although the incidence of liver disease is low, this is a recognized adverse effect of this drug. Hepatocellular toxicosis appears to be most common in Labrador Retrievers and may be evident as soon as 2 weeks after initiation of treatment. Monitoring bile acid levels appears to be a sensitive method of detecting early signs of toxicity.

NSAIDs may antagonize the action of several drugs commonly prescribed for cardiac disease and hypertension, including angiotensin-converting enzyme (ACE) inhibitors and some diuretics.

As with most drugs, there is great variation among individual patients in the potency, duration, and adverse effects produced by NSAIDs. When used for postoperative pain control, NSAIDs are safe to use in well-hydrated young to middle-aged animals with normal renal and hemostatic function. NSAIDs should be used with care or avoided entirely in dehydrated patients and in animals with coagulopathies or liver or kidney dysfunction. Because of the potential for GI ulceration, these agents should be avoided in patients with GI disorders and in patients that are receiving corticosteroids (which also contribute to ulcer formation). Animals that have low blood pressure, congestive heart failure, or hemostatic disorders such as thrombocytopenia are generally high-risk candidates for NSAID therapy. Patients with trauma should not receive NSAIDs unless they are in stable condition with no indication of hemorrhage, they are receiving IV fluids, and general anesthesia is not anticipated within the next 48 hours. For some patients (e.g., geriatric patients and patients with renal disease), NSAIDs should be used only in conjunction with IV fluids and blood pressure monitoring. Opioids appear to be a safer therapeutic option in these patients.

Grapiprant (Galliprant [Elanco]) is classified as an NSAID that does not inhibit COX. This non-COX NSAID works by antagonizing the EP4 prostaglandin receptor and is licensed for treating osteoarthritis in dogs. Possible side effects of grapiprant include vomiting, soft stool, lethargy, and hypoproteinemia. It is not possible to accurately dose dogs weighing less than 3.6 kg due to the tablet formulations available.

TECHNICIAN NOTE: Characteristics and Effects of NSAIDs

- These agents vary widely in terms of indications, adverse effects, and use
- All NSAIDs are effective for somatic pain. Newer NSAIDs are effective for both visceral and somatic pain
- May be given by oral and/or parenteral routes (IV, IM, SC) depending on the specific agent
- Most NSAIDs have antiinflammatory and analgesic effects
- Generally safe to use in well-hydrated young to middle-aged animals with normal renal and hemostatic function
- Use with care or avoid entirely in dehydrated patients and in animals with coagulopathies or liver or kidney dysfunction
- Avoid in patients with GI disorders and in patients that are receiving corticosteroids
- Animals with low blood pressure, congestive heart failure, or hemostatic disorders such as thrombocytopenia are generally at high risk for NSAID therapy
- Effects include:
  - GI toxicity due to increased gastric acid production and decreased mucus production. Signs may include vomiting, bleeding, inappetence, and melena, or may be absent.
  - Decreased platelet aggregation with prolonged bleeding time
  - Renal toxicity due to decrease in blood flow
  - The risk of adverse effects is increased if the patient is dehydrated or hypotensive
- For some patients (e.g., geriatric patients and patients with renal disease), NSAIDs should be used only in conjunction with IV fluids and blood pressure monitoring
- Do not use these agents intraoperatively unless the patient is hydrated, is receiving intravenous fluids, and arterial blood pressure is monitored
- Patients with trauma should not receive NSAIDs unless they are in stable condition with no indication of hemorrhage, they are receiving IV fluids, and general anesthesia is not anticipated within the next 48 hr
- Most NSAIDs work by inhibiting cyclooxygenase (COX), an enzyme involved in the production of prostaglandins
- Grapiprant is a non-COX prostaglandin E_2 EP4 receptor antagonist NSAID used to treat osteoarthritis in dogs

---

Local Anesthetics

Local anesthetic agents have long been used to allow surgical procedures to be performed in conscious animals, but their use in preventing or treating postoperative pain is more recent. The presence of local anesthetic blocks sodium channels, which prevents transduction and transmission of noxious stimuli into nerve impulses peripherally (local blocks) as well as centrally (if administered by epidural). Local anesthetic can be sprayed or injected at the site of an injury or a surgical site or infiltrated around nerves supplying the affected area. They can also be used to desensitize an entire region, as with epidural administration or IV infusion. Local anesthetics have many advantages, including complete anesthesia of the affected area, low toxicity (when given at the appropriate dose), and rapid onset of action. Unfortunately, the duration of action is relatively short, and the danger of CNS and cardiac toxicity limits repeated use. The use of local anesthetics for pain control is discussed in detail in Chapter 7.

Other Analgesic Agents

Opioids, NSAIDs and local anesthetics are the mainstays of postoperative pain control; however, other agents may be useful in some circumstances. These include alpha$_2$-adrenoceptor agonists, ketamine, gabapentin, amantadine, and frunevetmab.

Alpha$_2$-Adrenoceptor Agonists

The pharmacology, mode of action, effects, and use of alpha$_2$-adrenoceptor agonists (also referred to as alpha$_2$-agonists) are discussed in detail in Chapter 3, page 74 with emphasis on their role as sedatives. Here, the analgesic properties of these agents will be emphasized. Although alpha$_2$-adrenoceptor agonists such as xylazine and dexmedetomidine provide good analgesia by activating alpha$_2$-adrenergic receptors both centrally and in the periphery, their use for pain control in small animals is limited by three factors: (1) the short duration of their analgesic effect (in the case of xylazine, 30 to 60 minutes and for dexmedetomidine, 30 to 90 minutes); (2) the profound sedative effect of these agents; and (3) the potential for serious adverse effects (respiratory depression, vomiting, bradycardia, atrioventricular block, and hypotension, which may be exacerbated by opioids). It is difficult to determine the quality or duration of analgesia in some patients because the sedative effect of these drugs remains even after the analgesic effect has worn off and may mask signs of persistent pain. In dogs and cats, these agents should be used only for young to middle-aged, healthy patients. However, when used in low doses (e.g., xylazine at 0.1 mg/kg IV, IM, SC; and dexmedetomidine at 0.001 to 0.005 mg/kg IV, IM, SC), these agents appear to potentiate the effect of opioids and may contribute to the quality of analgesia in the postoperative period. Butorphanol and dexmedetomidine in combination appear to provide effective analgesia and sedation for minor clinical procedures.

Recently, alpha$_2$-adrenoceptor agonists have been shown to produce significant analgesia when administered by the epidural route (alone or in combination with opioids and other agents). Dexmedetomidine (0.005 mg/kg) can be added to morphine to prolong the duration of epidural analgesia.

The analgesic effect of xylazine is antagonized by yohimbine, and the analgesic effect of dexmedetomidine is antagonized by atipamezole.

Alpha$_2$-adrenoceptor agonists (xylazine, detomidine, romifidine) are commonly administered to horses to provide sedation, muscle relaxation, and analgesia. The degree of sedation provided is typically less than seen in small animals and horses typically remain standing, although they may become ataxic. Analgesia provided by these agents is adequate for moderately to severely painful diseases or procedures. Cardiovascular adverse effects such as bradyarrhythmias (including second-degree atrioventricular block), initial hypertension, and ultimately hypotension, are commonly seen. Heavy sedation should be induced cautiously in horses with preexisting upper airway stridor, as lowering of the head, which results in congestion of the nares and nasal passages, combined with relaxation of the upper airway and pharyngeal muscles, may lead to respiratory obstruction in these patients.

Alpha$_2$-adrenoceptor agonists cause decreased gut motility, which may lead to gas distension and colic postoperatively. Alpha$_2$-adrenoceptor antagonists (yohimbine, atipamezole) can be used to reverse these unwanted effects; however, analgesia and sedation will also be reversed. Use of these agents may even result in excitement.

Ketamine

Ketamine is a dissociative injectable anesthetic (see Chapter 3) that has become popular as an adjunct to more potent analgesics (opioids, local anesthetics, alpha$_2$-agonists) because it blocks the NMDA receptors in the CNS at the level of the spinal cord. Antagonism of the NMDA receptors is important in preventing central sensitization or windup. The dose of ketamine needed to antagonize these receptors is much lower than that required to induce anesthesia. Ketamine can be administered as IV boluses or as a CRI. Ketamine alone does not typically provide sufficient analgesia; therefore it is most commonly administered in conjunction with other drugs. A commonly used approach to provide intraoperative analgesia for painful orthopedic surgery in healthy dogs is to coinfuse MLK. (See Table 8.4 and Procedure 8.1.)

Ketamine should be avoided or used with extreme caution in patients with hypertrophic cardiomyopathy or in cats with compromised renal function. Adverse effects of ketamine are dose related and rarely seen at analgesic dosages but may include tachycardia, increased blood pressure, increased intraocular and intracranial pressure, seizures and postoperative delirium, and salivation.

Orally administered NMDA antagonists include amantadine and dextromethorphan.

Gabapentin

Gabapentin is an anticonvulsant that is also used as an analgesic adjunct for neuropathic pain and hypersensitivity, including allodynia. It is similar structurally to GABA (gamma-aminobutyric acid) and appears to work by preventing influx of calcium into the cells. It may be useful in dogs and cats for chronic musculoskeletal pain that is unresponsive to NSAIDs and for postsurgical pain, although there are currently few studies supporting this assertion.

Gabapentin has few adverse effects other than drowsiness. The liquid form of this drug should not be used because it contains xylitol, which is potentially toxic to dogs and cats.

Amantadine

Amantadine is a NMDA receptor antagonist that was originally used as an antiviral agent in human patients. It may be useful as an analgesic adjunct for neuropathic pain and central hypersensitivity as well as chronic pain associated with musculoskeletal disease. It has a narrow therapeutic index. Side effects include agitation and GI upset.

Frunevetmab

Frunevetmab (Solensia) has recently become available for clinical use in cats with chronic osteoarthritis as a monthly injection. Frunevetmab has a unique mechanism of action in that it is a monoclonal antibody that binds to nerve growth factor (NGF), a mediator that enhances pain signaling within the nociceptive pathway. This neutralizes the activity of NGF, providing relief from the chronic pain of osteoarthritis. At the time of this writing, this drug has only been available for a few months and is only licensed for use in cats. As such, we consider it prudent to review the relevant literature on a regular basis for to remain current regarding this drug.

Corticosteroids

These drugs (e.g., prednisone, dexamethasone) have strong antiinflammatory properties which, as with the NSAIDs, act by decreasing prostaglandin activity. Corticosteroids should not be used concurrently with NSAIDs, as both drug classes are ulcerogenic. Other long-term adverse effects include immunosuppression and development of hyperadrenocorticism.

Tramadol

Tramadol is a nonopiate drug that is given orally and has weak agonist activity at the mu receptor. One of its metabolites, O-desmethyltramadol, has six times the activity of the parent compound at the mu receptor. Unfortunately, metabolism of tramadol in dogs does not produce O-desmethyltramadol and it is no longer considered a useful mu opioid agonist in this species. There may be analgesic benefit in cats since metabolism in this species does produce O-desmethyltramadol. Tramadol may be useful as an analgesic adjunct in chronic pain where NSAIDs are not effective enough on their own, since an additional mechanism of tramadol is inhibition of norepinephrine and serotonin reuptake, which also promotes analgesia. Consequently, tramadol should not be administered with other norepinephrine and serotonin reuptake inhibitors (e.g., amitriptyline).

Tranquilizers

Although acepromazine, diazepam, and other tranquilizers are not considered to be analgesics, they may potentiate the effect of opioids in some patients. Possible explanations for this include the fact that pain appears to be intensified in anxious patients, and drugs that cause CNS depression also alter pain perception by the brain. Most animals that have received adequate analgesia but seem restless may become calmer after administration of acepromazine (0.01 to 0.05 mg/kg SC, IM, or IV) or diazepam (0.2 mg/kg IV). Tranquilizers are also useful in cats that develop excitement/mania and in horses that show excitement/excessive stall pacing after opioid administration. Because tranquilizers have no analgesic effect, they should never be used as a substitute for opioids or other analgesic agents. Acepromazine should be used with caution in patients with blood loss, dehydration, or low blood pressure. Note that use of an alpha$_2$-agonist to counter restlessness or excitement in the postoperative period is common and will contribute to analgesia.

Other Analgesic Adjuncts

There are a number of other drug classes including antidepressants, antianxiety drugs, and biphosphonates that have a role in pain management. Many of these agents are used with first-line analgesics for specific types of pain, such as neurogenic pain or cancer pain that is difficult to control. The reader is directed to an analgesia textbook for more information about these drugs.

Multimodal Therapy

Because there are several mechanisms by which pain is produced, it is often helpful to use more than one type of analgesic to relieve pain, whether acute or chronic. Multimodal therapy (also known as *combination* or *balanced analgesia*) may be more successful than treatment with any single agent because pain perception is affected at several points along the pain pathway and different mechanisms are targeted. For example, it has been shown in human patients that the use of piroxicam (an NSAID) and buprenorphine (an opioid) together provides analgesia that is superior to that with use of either agent alone. The concurrent use of NSAIDs with opioids may allow a 20% to 50% reduction in the opioid dose.

One familiar example of combination therapy is a mixture of acetaminophen and codeine, which is an effective oral treatment for moderate to severe pain in the dog. When given orally at a dose rate of 10 mg of acetaminophen per kilogram and 0.5 to 1 mg of codeine per kilogram every 6 to 12 hours, the combination is safe in healthy dogs for up to 5 days. If necessary, the codeine can be supplemented up to 4 mg/kg. Constipation and sedation are common adverse effects of this drug combination, and the diet should be supplemented with a fiber source such as bran or psyllium. Acetaminophen-codeine should never be given to cats and should also be avoided in dogs with hepatic disease.

When treating acute pain, opioids and NSAIDs may be given to a patient simultaneously or at different times. For example, a fentanyl patch may be applied to a cat and a dose of meloxicam given at the same time to provide analgesia during the lag time when the patch has not yet taken effect. Alternatively, a dog undergoing an orthopedic operation can be premedicated with morphine (0.2 to 0.3 mg/kg IM) followed by administration of an injectable NSAID (such as meloxicam or carprofen) at the end of the operation and followed up with an NSAID given orally for 3 days. This type of "balanced analgesia" allows the use of relatively modest doses of analgesics with a low risk of adverse effects, yet achieves effective pain relief in many patients.

Coinfusion of MLK is another type of combination therapy that is easily administered in IV fluids during surgery. Benefits include multimodal analgesia provided by three different mechanisms of action and decreased inhalant anesthetic requirement. Problems encountered with MLK include delayed recovery from anesthesia and decreased accuracy of administration, especially with smaller patients. Delayed recovery can be avoided by decreasing the infusion rate until the patient is awake. Use of infusion pumps or burettes increases accuracy of delivery to smaller patients.

See Protocols 8.1–8.7 for examples of multimodal perioperative analgesia therapies for commonly performed surgeries.

PROTOCOL 8.1 Example of a Multimodal Pain Management Protocol for a Cat Undergoing Ovariohysterectomy (Spay) or Castration

Preemptive Analgesia
- IM buprenorphine and a tranquilizer (premedication)
- ªIntraperitoneal lavage (spay) or testicular block (castration)

Postoperative Analgesia
- Transdermal buprenorphine (Zorbium) once prior to discharge
- Send home with NSAIDs for 2–3 days (only those approved for this duration); reassess if the cat seems to be in pain

ª2020 AAHA Anesthesia and Monitoring Guidelines for Dogs and Cats (https://aaha.org/anesthesia). Testicular block—figure 3, page 10; Intraperitoneal lavage—figure 4, page 11.
IM, Intramuscular; *NSAID,* nonsteroidal antiinflammatory drug.

PROTOCOL 8.2 Example of a Multimodal Pain Management Protocol for a Cat Undergoing Onychectomy (Declaw)

Preemptive Analgesia
- IM buprenorphine and a tranquilizer (premedication), with or without ketamine (premedication or total injectable anesthesia)
- Three-point block with local anesthetic (see Chapter 7, page 248)

Postoperative Analgesia
- Transdermal buprenorphine (Zorbium) once prior to discharge
- Send home with NSAIDs for 2–3 days (only those approved for this duration); reassess if the cat seems to be in pain

IM, Intramuscular; *NSAID,* nonsteroidal antiinflammatory drug.

PROTOCOL 8.3 Example of a Multimodal Pain Management Protocol for a Dog Undergoing Ovariohysterectomy (Spay) or Castration

Preemptive Analgesia
- IM morphine or hydromorphone and a tranquilizer (premedication)
- ªIntraperitoneal lavage (spay) or testicular block (castration)

Postoperative Analgesia
- Injectable NSAID after anesthesia
- Buprenoprhine IM after anesthesia
- Send home with NSAIDs for 2–3 days; reassess if the dog seems to be in pain

ª2020 AAHA Anesthesia and Monitoring Guidelines for Dogs and Cats (https://aaha.org/anesthesia). Testicular block—figure 3, page 10; Intraperitoneal lavage—figure 4, page 11.
IM, Intramuscular; *NSAID,* nonsteroidal antiinflammatory drug.

PROTOCOL 8.4 Example of a Multimodal Pain Management Protocol for a Dog Undergoing Surgery to Repair a Fractured Bone

Preemptive Analgesia
- NSAID SC before surgery unless contraindicated
- IM morphine and a tranquilizer (premedication)

Intraoperative Analgesia
- Morphine, lidocaine, ketamine constant rate infusion (CRI)

Postoperative Analgesia
- IM morphine every 4–6 hr for the first 12–24 hr
- Start oral NSAID therapy once the patient is alert enough to eat
- Send the dog home with NSAIDs for 3–5 days; reassess earlier if the dog seems to be in pain

IM, Intramuscular; *NSAID,* nonsteroidal antiinflammatory drug; *SC,* subcutaneously.

PROTOCOL 8.5 Example of a Multimodal Pain Management Protocol for a Cat Undergoing Multiple Dental Extractions

Preemptive Analgesia
- IM hydromorphone and a tranquilizer (premedication)

Intraoperative Analgesia
- Dental nerve blocks with bupivacaine (see Chapter 7)

Postoperative Analgesia
- Administer transdermal buprenorphine (Zorbium), then send the cat home with NSAIDs; reassess if the cat seems to be in pain

IM, Intramuscular; *NSAID,* nonsteroidal antiinflammatory drug; *OTM,* oral transmucosal.

PROTOCOL 8.6 Example of a Multimodal Pain Management Protocol for a Dog Undergoing Chain Mastectomy

Preemptive Analgesia
- IM methadone and a tranquilizer (premedication)

Intraoperative Analgesia
- Fentanyl CRI 5–10 mcg/kg/h

Postoperative Analgesia
- IV methadone every 3–4 hr for 12–24 hr or CRI fentanyl 1–5 mcg/kg/h
- Send the dog home with NSAIDs for 3 days; reassess earlier if the dog seems to be in pain

CRI, Constant rate infusion; *IM,* intramuscular.

PROTOCOL 8.7   Example of a Multimodal Pain Management Protocol for a Horse Undergoing Bilateral Stifle Arthroscopy

Preemptive Analgesia
- NSAID IV before surgery unless contraindicated
- Alpha$_2$-agonist and butorphanol as premedication

Intraoperative Analgesia
- Lidocaine infusion

Postoperative Analgesia
- Butorphanol as needed
- Oral NSAID therapy, which can be continued at home; reassess if the horse seems to be in pain

---

IV, Intravenously; *NSAID,* nonsteroidal antiinflammatory drug.

HOME ANALGESIA

There are several options for pain relief in dogs and cats discharged from the hospital. Meloxicam, carprofen, other NSAIDs, and now frunevetmab in cats, are commonly prescribed for long-term therapy of osteoarthritis and other chronic painful conditions. Tylenol with codeine (dogs only) is also available in tablet form and is suitable for treatment of mild to moderate chronic pain.

Transdermal buprenorphine (Zorbium) administered to cats prior to discharge from the clinic, is effective for 4 days following a single dose, and so is a good option to control postoperative pain.

NURSING CARE

Visits to the clinic for outpatient care or hospitalization can be extremely stressful for veterinary patients. Patients that are anxious, stressed, or fearful often will not eat, sleep, or eliminate normally. These alterations in normal behavior in turn impair healing and can lead to hyperalgesia and other negative consequences.

Patient stress, discomfort, and pain can be reduced through interventions such as optimization of the patient's environment, use of gentle handling techniques, and nutritional interventions that can be performed or coordinated by the veterinary technician. Although interventions of this type are all too often not addressed, in some cases, they can be a significant factor influencing patient outcomes.

Optimization of the patient's environment when hospitalized is a simple but important component of reducing patient stress. This refers to taking steps to ensure that the patient feels as comfortable and unafraid as possible. Providing conscientious nursing care, including keeping the animal and its cage or stall clean and dry, affording ample opportunity for defecation and urination (including bladder expression or catheterization if necessary), providing comfortable bedding and quiet surroundings, and gently reassuring the patient can all significantly affect the way the patient responds. Also, treatments and monitoring should be scheduled so that the patient is not disturbed unnecessarily.

Other interventions that optimize the environment include positioning the patient so that it does not lie on a surgery site or traumatized area. Some patients benefit from being turned every 2 to 3 hours. Unconscious animals may require the application of ophthalmic ointment to prevent corneal drying.

Anxious patients may benefit from having a blanket, towel, an article of the owner's clothing, or toy from home with them. When appropriate, allowing the owner to visit can increase the patient's sense of security, and owners are often much more successful in coaxing a patient to eat that otherwise would not.

Cats and dogs should be separated, noise should be minimized, and ideally, patient cages should be positioned so that animals are not able to see one another. Cats should not be housed in bottom row cages because many cats feel more vulnerable when they are near the floor. Attention to these and other similar interventions can significantly decrease the amount of stress the patient feels.

Use of gentle handling techniques is another intervention that is very beneficial when working with patients that are in pain. In busy clinics, when employees feel overwhelmed and overburdened with patient care duties, the likelihood that patients are handled with unnecessary roughness or excessive restraint increases. Attention to and awareness of how one approaches these patients and handles them is therefore helpful to avoid placing more stress on patients that are experiencing the baseline stress inherent in being hospitalized. The AAFP and ISFM Feline-Friendly Handling Guidelines, published in the Journal of Feline Medicine and Surgery in 2011, addresses these and other issues related to handling cats that reduce pain and fear in hospitalized feline patients.

NONPHARMACOLOGIC THERAPIES

There are many nonpharmacologic analgesic therapies that may be used along with drugs to help manage both acute and chronic pain. These therapies vary widely in terms of the amount of evidence that exists supporting their effectiveness.

For instance, many experts recognize acupuncture as a safe and effective method of pain control, and there are evidence-based studies that strongly support its value in treating both acute and chronic pain. Physical rehabilitation is commonly used postoperatively for patients undergoing orthopedic surgery to enhance recovery, restore function, and reduce pain, and is considered by some surgeons as essential to achieving good results. It is also used to manage pain associated with chronic orthopedic disorders.

Other nonpharmacologic methods of pain control that may be effective in some situations include massage therapy, application of cold (for acute injuries) or heat (for chronic injuries), physiotherapy, laser therapy, magnetic therapy, and homeopathic or herbal remedies such as Bach flower remedies.

TABLE 8.6 Nonpharmacologic Modalities

Nonpharmacologic Modality	Common Indications	Proposed Mechanism of Pain Relief
Acupuncture (insertion of needles through the skin at specific acupuncture points)	• Treatment of acute and chronic pain • Treatment of a wide variety of medical conditions	• In Traditional Chinese Veterinary Medicine, acupuncture is felt to restore the balance of body energy or "qi" (pronounced "chi") through stimulation of specific points along pathways called "meridians" • Causes a complex set of effects on a variety of body systems including the nervous, endocrine, and immune systems, including release of natural internal opioids and blockage of pain transmission
Physical therapy and rehabilitation (use of a variety of techniques including therapeutic exercises, underwater treadmill, and message)	• Reduction of pain and disability following orthopedic surgery • Treatment of chronic pain from osteoarthritis	• Effects result from reduction of disability and restoration of normal function as well as other benefits such as release of natural internal opioids
Therapeutic laser therapy (low-level laser therapy or "cold laser") (application of laser light by contact or noncontact in a perpendicular orientation to the skin)	• Treatment of chronic pain from osteoarthritis • Relief of pain from surgical or traumatic wounds • Promotion of healing and reduction of inflammation	• Proposed mechanisms include absorption of light by mitochondria and increased production of adenosine triphosphate (ATP) • Other proposed mechanisms include blockage of pain transmission, release of natural internal opioids, and stimulation of acupuncture points
Pulsed magnetic field therapy (PMFT)	• Relief of musculoskeletal pain	• Analgesic effects felt to be due to normalization of disturbed electrical fields
Cryotherapy (application of cold)	• Relief of pain in the immediate period following injury	• Numerous mechanisms, including reduction of inflammation, raising the pain threshold, and decreasing muscle spasm
Thermotherapy (application of heat)	• Relief of chronic pain, especially pain resulting from muscle spasm	• Numerous mechanisms, including increase in blood flow and reduction of muscle tone
Transcutaneous Electrical Nerve Stimulation (TENS) (application of low-level electrical current via surface electrodes)	• Primarily, relief of pain arising from chronic conditions	• Mechanism of action unknown; may involve release of natural internal opioids and blockage of pain transmission
Extracorporeal Shock Wave Treatment (ESWT) (application of high-energy, high-amplitude acoustic pressure waves)	• Relief of pain from chronic osteoarthritis.	• Mechanism of action unknown; may involve reduction of inflammation, and inhibitory effect on pain signals
Therapeutic ultrasound (application of penetrating ultrasound waves to the skin)	• Relief of pain from osteoarthritis, muscle spasm, tendonitis, and scar tissue • Stimulation of wound healing	• Mechanisms of action may include increased blood flow, muscle relaxation, reduction of inflammation, and increased pain threshold

Generally, these methodologies are used in conjunction with and as an adjunct to pharmacologic therapy. The effectiveness of some of these therapies has not been demonstrated in controlled studies. (See Table 8.6 for a summary of the common indications and proposed mechanisms of action for each of these modalities.)

Practitioners who have an interest in using one of these nonpharmacologic methods should receive training that includes information about indications, precautions, and limitations, and should have knowledge regarding how strong the evidence is that the modality is effective. There are many opportunities to attend professional training and continuing education for acupuncture, physical therapy, and a variety of other nonpharmacologic therapies. If the practitioner is not trained, patients that may benefit from one of these modalities should be referred to another practitioner experienced in its use.

KEY POINTS

1. The veterinary technician or nurse forms a vital part of the veterinary caregiving team. Through an understanding of pain physiology, pain-associated behaviors, pain assessment tools, analgesic drug pharmacology, and communication skills, the technician contributes significantly to the comfort and welfare of patients.

2. Pain assessment is an essential part of every patient evaluation, regardless of presenting complaint.

3. Pain is a complex, individual experience that has been defined as an aversive sensory and emotional experience that elicits protective motor actions, results in learned avoidance, and may modify species-specific behavior traits, including social behavior.

4. Untreated pain can negatively affect a patient's behavior, physiology, metabolism, and immune system, causing poor performance, weight loss, delayed wound healing, increased susceptibility to infection, and patient suffering.

5. Physiologic pain normally occurs in response to a noxious stimulus where there is a possibility of or actual tissue injury and is a protective mechanism.

6. Pathologic pain is due to malfunction of or damage to the nervous system and is a type of pain that is amplified and persistent. It serves no useful function but causes suffering.

7. The pain pathway consists of the following four components: transduction, transmission, modulation, and perception.

8. Peripheral hypersensitivity or primary hyperalgesia is caused by the presence of inflammation.

9. Central hypersensitivity or secondary hyperalgesia ("windup") is caused by changes to neurons in the spinal cord.

10. The practice of administering analgesics before surgery to decrease analgesic requirements and minimize central nervous system sensitization is called preemptive analgesia.

11. The practice of administering several analgesic drugs that work via different receptor mechanisms is called multimodal analgesia.

12. Pain assessment tools can be used to assess pain and response to analgesic therapy.

13. Several validated species-specific pain assessment tools are available for assessment of both acute and chronic pain.

14. Opioid receptor agonists such as morphine, hydromorphone, methadone, and fentanyl are currently among the most effective drugs for treating acute pain.

15. Potential side effects of the mu-agonist opioids include sedation, respiratory depression, vomiting, defecation, gastrointestinal (GI) ileus, pruritus, excitement, hyperthermia, and dysphoria.

16. The partial agonist opioid buprenorphine has a long duration of action but may not provide sufficient analgesia for severe acute pain. It has been shown to provide good analgesia in rodents.

17. Agonist-antagonist opioid drugs such as butorphanol have a short duration of action and are not as effective at treating severe pain but have fewer side effects and are used extensively in large animals.

18. Nonsteroidal antiinflammatory drugs decrease inflammation by inhibiting prostaglandin synthesis or by blocking its effects and are commonly used to provide analgesia postoperatively.

19. The side effects of NSAIDs include liver and renal toxicity, increased bleeding times, and GI ulceration.

20. Local anesthetics provide analgesia via their sodium channel blocking activity and can be administered locally, epidurally, or, in the case of lidocaine, as a constant rate infusion.

21. Alpha$_2$-adrenoceptor agonists are effective analgesics; however, because of their side effects in small animals and ruminants, they are more commonly used for this purpose in horses.

22. Ketamine antagonizes NMDA receptors in the spinal cord, preventing central sensitization.

23. Corticosteroids have potent antiinflammatory activity and because they act by the same mechanism as NSAIDs, should not be used concurrently with drugs of that class.

24. Frunevetmab is a monoclonal antibody against nerve growth factor and is licensed for monthly injection to treat osteoarthritic pain in cats.

25. Gabapentin and amantidine are adjunctive agents that are used with other analgesics for specific purposes such as treatment of neuropathic pain and hypersensitivity.

26. Providing appropriate nursing care to the hospitalized animal is an important part of ensuring that a patient is comfortable when its pain is being treated.

27. Nonpharmacologic therapies, such as acupuncture, physical therapy, and therapeutic laser, may effectively treat pain by a variety of mechanisms such as stimulating the release of endorphins.

REVIEW QUESTIONS

1. *Idiopathic pain* is defined as:
   a. Pain that is caused by cancer
   b. Pain that is of unknown cause
   c. Pain that is caused by inflammation
   d. Pain that is caused by injury to nerves

2. *Pathologic pain* is defined as:
   a. Pain that is caused by cancer
   b. Pain that is of unknown cause
   c. Pain that is prolonged and exaggerated
   d. Pain that is not associated with tissue injury

3. An ovariohysterectomy, which involves surgically incising the skin and abdominal wall and excising the uterus and ovaries, has the following components of pain:
   a. Somatic pain only
   b. Visceral pain only
   c. Both somatic and visceral pain
   d. Neither somatic nor visceral pain

4. The process by which thermal, mechanical, or chemical noxious stimuli are converted into electrical signals called *action potentials* is:
   a. Perception
   b. Modulation
   c. Transduction
   d. Transmission

5. In the spinal cord, pain impulses can be altered by neurons that either suppress or amplify nerve impulses. This process is known as:
   a. Perception
   b. Modulation
   c. Transduction
   d. Transmission

6. Where in the pain pathway does secondary sensitization or "windup" occur?
   a. Brain
   b. Spinal cord
   c. Visceral pain receptors
   d. Peripheral pain receptors
7. Which of the following statements regarding multimodal analgesic therapy is NOT true?
   a. The dose of each drug is decreased when several drugs are used
   b. Each drug used may target one or more steps in the nociceptive pathway
   c. Drugs should be chosen that have different mechanisms of action
   d. Side effects are generally increased when using several analgesics concurrently
8. Which of the following drug combinations is an example of multimodal analgesic therapy?
   a. Dexmedetomidine, sevoflurane
   b. Acepromazine, ketamine, isoflurane
   c. Acepromazine, morphine, isoflurane
   d. Dexmedetomidine, morphine, ketamine
9. Which one of the following analgesic plans targets all four steps of nociception by using three different classes of analgesic agents?
   a. Morphine IM, fentanyl CRI, lidocaine nerve block
   b. Methadone CRI, morphine IM, bupivacaine nerve block
   c. Morphine IM, ketamine CRI, lidocaine nerve block
   d. Ketamine CRI, lidocaine CRI, and bupivacaine nerve block
10. Treating pain does not improve wound healing.
    True
    False
11. Administering analgesics before tissue injury is known as:
    a. Premedication
    b. Local analgesia
    c. Multimodal analgesia
    d. Preemptive analgesia
12. Which of the following is *not* a potential side effect of opioid administration in cats and dogs?
    a. Vomiting
    b. Dysphoria
    c. Renal failure
    d. Respiratory depression
13. Which of the following is the mechanism of action of nonsteroidal antiinflammatory drugs?
    a. They block sodium channels
    b. They are alpha$_2$-receptor agonists
    c. They inhibit prostaglandin synthesis or action
    d. They are mu-opioid receptor agonists
14. Which of the following is *not* a potential side effect of NSAID administration?
    a. Liver damage
    b. Kidney damage
    c. Gastrointestinal ulcers
    d. Respiratory depression
15. A pain scale can be used to assess pain as well as response to analgesic therapy.
    True
    False

SELECTED READINGS

Gaynor JS, Muir WW III: *Handbook of veterinary pain management*, ed 3, St. Louis, 2015, Elsevier.

Goldberg ME, Shaffran N: *Pain management for veterinary technicians and nurses*, ed 1, Ames, IA, 2015, John Wiley & Sons, Inc.

Gruen ME, Lascelles BDX, Colleran E, et al: 2022 AAHA pain management guidelines for dogs and cats, *J Am Anim Hosp Assoc* 58:55–76, 2022.

Lerche P, Muir WW III: Peri-operative pain management in horses. In Muir WW III, Hubbell JAE, editors: *Equine anesthesia*, ed 2, St. Louis, MO, 2008, Mosby.

Rodan I, Sundahl E, (co-chairs), et al: AAFP and ISFM feline-friendly handling guidelines, *J Feline Med Surg* 13:364–375, 2011.

Shaffran N, Grubb T: Pain management. In Beal AD, Samples OM, editors: *Clinical textbook for veterinary technicians and nurses*, ed 10, St. Louis, MO, 2022, Elsevier.

Sparkes A (Panel Chair), Heiene R, Lascelles B, et al: ISFM and AAFP consensus guidelines long-term use of NSAIDs in cats, *J Feline Med Surg* 12:521–538, 2010.

Steagal PV, Monteiro BP: Acute pain in cats: recent advances in clinical assessment, *J Feline Med Surg* 21:25–34, 2019.

Canine and Feline Anesthesia

LEARNING OBJECTIVES

When you have completed this chapter, you will be able to:

- Describe anesthetic techniques commonly used in small-animal practices.
- List strategies used to minimize adverse effects when selecting an anesthetic protocol.
- Describe how different methods of anesthetic induction and maintenance influence the dynamics of an anesthetic event.
- Prepare a small-animal patient, anesthetic equipment, and anesthetic agents and adjuncts for general anesthesia.
- Describe induction of general anesthesia by intravenous (IV) injection of a short-acting agent by mask or chamber induction or by intramuscular (IM) injection.
- Explain cautions and risks associated with each method of anesthetic induction and strategies to maximize patient safety.
- List reasons for, advantages of, and potential complications of endotracheal intubation.

- Explain how to do each of the following: (1) select and prepare an endotracheal tube (ETT) for placement, (2) place an ETT in a dog or cat, (3) check for proper placement, (4) inflate the cuff, (5) minimize laryngospasm, and (6) extubate a patient during anesthetic recovery.
- Describe maintenance of general anesthesia by administration of an inhalant agent, repeat IV boluses of a short-acting anesthetic, constant rate infusion (CRI), or concurrent use of an inhalant and supplemental injectable agent.
- List principles of providing for patient positioning, comfort, and safety during anesthetic maintenance.
- List factors that affect patient recovery from anesthesia, the signs of recovery, appropriate monitoring during recovery, and oxygen therapy during recovery.
- Describe general nursing care during the postanesthetic period.

KEY TERMS

Anatomic dead space
Anesthetic induction
Anesthetic maintenance
Anesthetic protocol
Anesthetic recovery

Central nervous system (CNS)
    vital centers
Hypostatic congestion
Laryngospasm
Mechanical dead space

Pneumomediastinum
Pneumothorax
Stridor
Titration
Total intravenous anesthesia

INTRODUCTION TO CANINE AND FELINE ANESTHESIA

Small-animal[a] patients are restrained and anesthetized by means of a variety of techniques including general anesthesia, sedation, neuroleptanalgesia, and local and regional anesthesia. Of these options, general anesthesia is most commonly used for several reasons. The immobilization and unconsciousness associated with general anesthesia enable most procedures to be performed more quickly and safely than is possible with alternative techniques. General anesthetics also produce analgesia during the period of unconsciousness and, if used along with analgesics as a part of a balanced protocol, during the preoperative and postoperative periods as well. In addition, general anesthetic procedures can be performed with readily available resources and at a reasonable cost. In dogs and cats, general anesthesia is induced and maintained using balanced protocols, inhalants, intramuscular (IM) protocols, and total intravenous (IV) techniques.

Mild to heavy sedation and neuroleptanalgesia are also frequently used to facilitate diagnostic and therapeutic procedures in small animals that are frightened, aggressive, or in pain. Box 9.1 lists some of the procedures commonly performed with patients under sedation or neuroleptanalgesia. Box 9.2 shows American College of Veterinary Anesthesia and Analgesia (ACVAA) monitoring guidelines for sedated patients.

Although less frequently employed than general anesthesia, sedation, or neuroleptanalgesia, local and regional techniques are used along with general anesthesia in small animals to provide additional analgesia for many procedures including dental, elective, abdominal, and orthopedic. Neuromuscular blocking agents are rarely used in general practice but are sometimes used to provide muscle relaxation for ocular and orthopedic procedures in veterinary schools and referral practices.

---

[a]Veterinary practices that provide health care services for dogs and cats are traditionally referred to as *small animal* or *companion animal practices,* although many other species, traditionally referred to as *exotic animals,* may also be served by these clinics. The term *exotic animals* includes mammals referred to as *pocket pets* or *small exotic mammals* (rabbits, ferrets, guinea pigs, hamsters, gerbils, rats, and mice), birds, reptiles, amphibians, and fish. Although any of these species rightfully can be classified as small animals, in this chapter the term *small animal* will be used specifically in reference to dogs and cats.

BOX 9.1 Examples of Procedures Commonly Performed Under Sedation or Neuroleptanalgesia

- Radiographic studies
- Ultrasonographic studies
- Transtracheal washes
- Otic examination, flushing, and treatment
- Blood draws
- Wound treatment
- Bandage and splint application
- Toenail trimming
- Grooming
- Orogastric intubation
- Urinary catheterization

BOX 9.2 American College of Veterinary Anesthesia and Analgesia Monitoring Guidelines for Sedation Without General Anesthesia

The objective of the American College of Veterinary Anesthesia and Analgesia (ACVAA) monitoring guidelines for sedated patients is "to ensure adequate oxygenation and hemodynamic stability in the obtunded patient." To accomplish this, the ACVAA makes the following recommendations:

Intermittent monitoring of basic respiratory and cardiovascular parameters in the heavily sedated animal should be routine. Supplemental oxygen, an endotracheal tube, and materials for IV catheterization should always be readily available. Particular attention should be paid to brachycephalic breeds that are particularly at risk for airway obstruction under heavy sedation.

PREPARATION FOR AN ANESTHETIC PROCEDURE

The veterinary technician or nurse in any busy small-animal practice routinely has a constant stream of demands from the time of arrival to the end of the day. In order to function effectively in this environment, they must manage time efficiently so that the most pressing patient needs are met first. After essential tasks have been managed, often, little time is left for less critical needs such as preparation. The technician or nurse must resist the temptation to limit or eliminate this important step, however, because incomplete preparation often results in complications ranging from mild to life-threatening, especially in anesthetized animals that are not young and healthy. Any time saved by abbreviating preparation is often offset managing

---

PROCEDURE 9.1   Preparation for General Anesthesia in a Dog or Cat

One to Several Days Prior to the Procedure

1. Assist the attending veterinarian in acquisition of a minimum patient database (MPD). (See Chapter 2 for a discussion of acquisition of the MPD.)
2. Prepare prescribed anxiolytic drugs (such as gabapentin for cats and gabapentin or trazodone for dogs) for administration at home during the hours before leaving for the hospital.
3. Educate the client regarding fasting instructions, administration of anxiolytics, and administration of ongoing medications.

Upon Arrival at the Hospital on the Day of the Procedure

1. Use low-stress handling techniques to minimize fear, anxiety, and stress. This is especially important for cats (see AAFP and ISFM Feline-Friendly Nursing Care Guidelines[a] and Feline-Friendly Handling Guidelines[b] for more information about these techniques as they apply to cats).
2. Assess, prepare, and weigh the patient. (See Chapter 2 for a discussion of patient assessment, preparation, and stabilization.)
3. Determine the protocol (anesthetic agents, doses, and routes and sequence of administration).
4. Calculate the volume of each agent to give (preanesthetic, induction, maintenance, and analgesic agents) and fluid administration rates.
5. Calculate the oxygen flow rates (see Chapter 4, page 150). (See Table 9.2 for a quick reference oxygen flow rate chart for partial rebreathing systems and Table 9.3 for a quick reference oxygen flow rate chart for nonrebreathing systems.)
6. Prepare equipment required to administer drugs (scales, syringes, needles, anesthetic agents and adjuncts, reversal agents, emergency cart, controlled substance log, and tape and permanent marker to label syringes).
7. Prepare fluid administration equipment (clippers, antiseptic scrub and rinsing agent, catheters, tape, normal saline, catheter cap, administration and extension set, fluids).
8. Prepare equipment for endotracheal intubation (see Fig. 9.11).
9. Prepare monitoring equipment, including anesthesia record, stethoscope, monitors, and probes (see Chapter 6).
10. Choose an appropriate breathing circuit for the patient that minimizes dead space to no more than 2–3 mL/kg body weight (see Chapter 4, page 108 for a discussion of dead space).
11. Both rebreathing and nonrebreathing circuits should ideally be outfitted with a pressure manometer and a safety pressure relief valve either separate from or built into the adjustable pressure limiting (APL) valve. A high-pressure alarm may also be used to warn of excess pressure in the breathing circuit (see Chapter 4, page 137).
12. Assemble and test the anesthetic machine. This should include a low-pressure leak test and a test of the integrity of the inner tube of a Bain coaxial circuit (if used) (see Chapter 4, Procedures 4.1 and 4.2).

[a]Carney HC, Little S, Brownlee-Tomasso D, et al: AAFP and ISFM feline-friendly nursing care guidelines, *J Feline Med Surg* 14:337–349, 2012.
[b]Rodan I, Sundahl E, Carney H, et al: AAFP and ISFM feline-friendly handling guidelines, *J Feline Med Surg* 13:364–375, 2011.

---

problems that could have been prevented had it been given due attention. The reader is referred to Chapter 2 for a detailed discussion of the essentials of preparation. Procedure 9.1, shows a summary of the steps required to prepare for general anesthesia in a small animal patient.

> **TECHNICIAN NOTE** Incomplete preparation for an anesthetic procedure often results in complications ranging from mild to life-threatening, especially when anesthetic procedures are performed in animals that are not young and healthy. Any time saved by abbreviating preparation is often offset managing problems that could have been prevented.

SELECTING A PROTOCOL

An **anesthetic protocol** is a list of the anesthetics and adjuncts prescribed for a particular patient, including dosages, routes, and order of administration. The attending veterinarian commonly selects anesthetic protocols, although they may authorize an experienced technician or nurse to suggest a protocol, which then must be approved before administration. A suitable protocol takes into account the minimum patient database, the patient's physical status class, and the procedure to be performed. Specific drug choices are also influenced by training, clinical experience, and personal preference, and therefore vary widely among attending veterinarians.

> **TECHNICIAN NOTE** Double-check all injectable drug doses before administration and ensure that the concentration of an agent drawn into a syringe is the same as that used for drug calculations.

When the protocol is known, drug doses, oxygen flow rates, and fluid administration rates must be calculated and checked *carefully* by the veterinary technician or nurse to ensure that the correct drugs and amounts are prepared. Box 9.3 shows the steps required to calculate the doses of most injectable drugs. Ill, geriatric, pediatric, or otherwise compromised patients (physical status class PS3 to PS5) require use of modified protocols based on the patient's primary condition. (See Chapter 13 for recommendations regarding class PS3 to PS5 small-animal patients.) Management of these cases can be quite challenging and requires customization of the anesthetic protocol by the attending veterinarian.

> **TECHNICIAN NOTE** Always label all syringes containing injectable agents with patient identification, the name of the drug, and the drug concentration if more than one concentration is available.

As discussed in the chapter on monitoring, anesthesia affects **central nervous system (CNS) vital centers**. Every anesthetized patient is at risk for potentially serious adverse effects such as hypotension, hypoventilation, hypoxemia, and hypothermia because of the actions of anesthetics and adjuncts on these centers. When choosing the protocol and preparing the agents, the anesthetist can use a number of strategies to minimize these adverse effects as follows:

- Unless the procedure must be performed immediately for the patient's well-being, correct significant physiologic abnormalities such as dehydration, hypotension, and anemia before anesthesia.

BOX 9.3 Dosage Calculations for Injectable Drugs

With the exception of a constant rate infusion (CRI), the volume of most injectable agents to be administered is calculated using the following standard formula:

$$\text{Volume (mL)} = \frac{\text{Patient body weight (kg or lb)} \times \text{Prescribed dose (mg or mcg/kg or lb body wt)}}{\text{Drug concentration (mg or mcg/mL)}}$$

The prescribed dose is the amount of the agent prescribed by the veterinarian in milligrams or micrograms per unit of body weight. The drug concentration is found on the drug vial label and is most often expressed in milligrams or micrograms per milliliter. For prevention of errors when this calculation is performed, all units of measure must match. (All patient body weight units must be converted to either kilograms or pounds, and the prescribed dose and drug concentration units must be converted to either milligrams or micrograms.)

Example

How much propofol should you draw up to induce a 20-lb mixed-breed dog for a COHAT? The prescribed dose is 5 mg/kg body weight and the drug concentration is 10 mg/mL.

$$\text{Patient body weight (kg)} = 20\,\text{lb} \times \frac{1\,\text{kg}}{2.2\,\text{lb}} = 9.1\,\text{kg}$$

$$\text{Volume (mL)} = \frac{9.1\,\text{kg} \times 5\,\text{mg/kg}}{10\,\text{mg/mL}} = 4.55\,\text{mL}$$

- Base the anesthetic protocol on results of the minimum patient database. Do not use a single standard protocol for all patients.
- Use a balanced protocol consisting of multiple agents. This approach reduces the required dose of any one agent, thus minimizing the adverse effects of all agents.
- Double-check all injectable drug doses before administration and ensure that the concentration of an agent drawn into a syringe is the same as that used for the drug calculations.
- Label all syringes containing injectable anesthetic agents with the patient identification, the name of the drug, and the drug concentration if more than one concentration is available.
- Administer no more than the minimum dose of drug needed to achieve the desired level of anesthesia.
- Unless told otherwise, administer all IV agents to effect (see page 313).

SUMMARY OF A GENERAL ANESTHETIC PROCEDURE

In order to give anesthetic agents safely, it is important to have a clear understanding of the dynamics of an anesthetic procedure. The word *dynamics* refers to the changes in the patient's level of consciousness over time, including when, how extensively, and how quickly these changes occur. Armed with this understanding, the anesthetist is able to administer agents effectively, detect adverse reactions rapidly, and recognize and respond to patient needs quickly. An anesthetist without this knowledge is unable to make sound decisions, differentiate normal from abnormal responses, or react rapidly enough to protect the patient.

The protocol is the primary determinant of these dynamics. The agent used and the route of administration affect how quickly the patient becomes unconscious and awakens and the amount of control the anesthetist has over anesthetic depth. For instance, when given intramuscularly, most drugs begin to act, reach peak effect, and wear off relatively slowly, and they afford the anesthetist very little control over anesthetic depth. In contrast, the commonly used inhalant agents act, reach peak effect, and are eliminated relatively quickly, and they give the anesthetist excellent control. The dynamics for each of the commonly used protocols are summarized in the following sections.

> **TECHNICIAN NOTE** Once an IM injection has been given for anesthetic induction, the anesthetist has little control over changes in depth or the peak effect. If the depth is inadequate, the anesthetist can give additional drug, but if the depth is excessive, the anesthetist can only monitor and support the patient until the agent is metabolized and the patient recovers naturally unless reversal agents are available for one or more of the drugs used.

Anesthetic Induction With an Intramuscular Agent or Combination

When anesthetics or adjuncts are administered by IM injection, anesthetic depth gradually increases after injection (typically over 5 to 20 minutes) and after peak effect, gradually decreases as the agent is metabolized (typically over 30 to 60 minutes or longer). Once the injection has been given, the anesthetist has little control over changes in depth or the peak effect. If the depth is inadequate, the anesthetist can give additional drug, but if depth is excessive, the anesthetist can only monitor and support the patient until the agent is metabolized and the patient recovers naturally. The only exception to this is when using opioids, benzodiazepines, and alpha$_2$-agonists. In these cases, the anesthetist can decrease anesthetic depth rapidly by administering the corresponding antagonist (reversal agent) (Fig. 9.1).

Anesthetic Induction With an Intravenous Injection of a Short-Acting Agent to Effect

Anesthetic induction with an IV injection of a short-acting agent to effect is a technique used for short procedures that require less than 10 minutes of anesthesia, such as removal of a Steinman bone pin, examination of the pharynx and larynx, or changing of a bandage. Propofol, alfaxalone, or etomidate may be used this way. When anesthesia is induced by IV injection, anesthetic depth typically increases rapidly over 15 seconds to a few minutes after the initial injection, then decreases gradually over 10 to 20 minutes. When using this technique, the anesthetist controls the peak effect and can increase anesthetic depth rapidly by giving additional boluses of the drug. However, as with IM anesthesia, there is little control over duration because anesthetic depth only decreases as the drug is naturally metabolized or redistributed (Fig. 9.2).

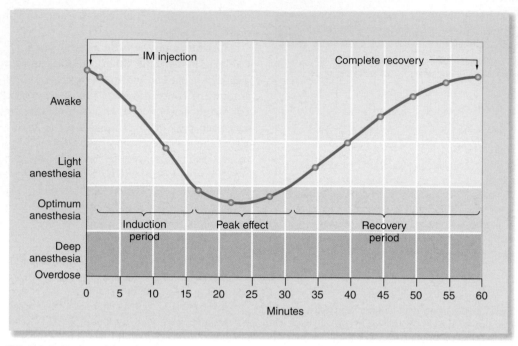

FIG. 9.1 Induction with an intramuscular *(IM)* agent or combination. When this route is used, anesthetic induction is gradual, with peak effect about 15 to 20 minutes after a single IM injection. Recovery is even more gradual as the agent is metabolized or redistributed.

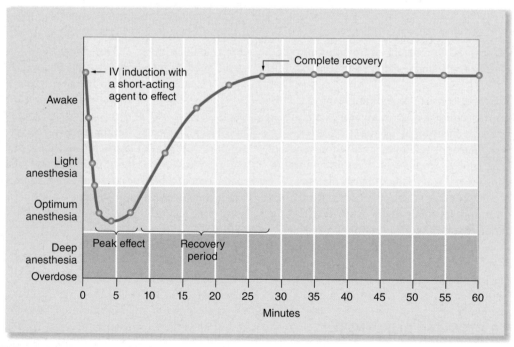

FIG. 9.2 Induction with an intravenous *(IV)* injection of a short-acting agent to effect. Anesthetic induction is very rapid, peak effect is short, and recovery is gradual but relatively rapid as the agent is metabolized or redistributed.

TECHNICIAN NOTE When inducing anesthesia with IV injection of a short-acting agent, the anesthetist can increase the depth rapidly by giving incremental boluses but—as with IM administration—if the patient is deeply anesthetized, the anesthetist can only support the patient and wait until the agent is metabolized or redistributed and the anesthetic depth naturally decreases.

Total Intravenous Anesthesia by Intravenous Boluses of a Short-Acting Agent

With **total intravenous anesthesia** (TIVA) using IV boluses of a short-acting agent, anesthesia is induced as previously described and then is maintained by giving additional boluses approximately every 3 to 8 minutes as needed to maintain surgical anesthesia. This technique is acceptable for noninvasive procedures of short to moderate length but is somewhat cumbersome for major surgeries because it is challenging to keep the patient at an optimum anesthetic depth even with constant monitoring. Propofol is the agent most commonly used to provide TIVA, although alfaxalone and etomidate are alternatives. With this technique, the anesthetist can increase the depth rapidly by giving incremental boluses but, as with IM administration, if the patient is deeply anesthetized, the anesthetist can only support the patient and wait until the agent is metabolized and the anesthetic depth naturally decreases (Fig. 9.3).

Total Intravenous Anesthesia by Constant Rate Infusion

TIVA by constant rate infusion (CRI) is similar to TIVA by bolus injections, except that anesthesia is maintained by infusing small amounts of anesthetic constantly with a syringe pump. Although similar in effect to maintenance with bolus injections, this technique moderates and slows down changes in depth by avoiding sudden infusion of a large amount of drug. Instead, only the amount needed to maintain anesthesia is infused on a continuous basis for the duration of the procedure (Fig. 9.4).

Induction and Maintenance With an Inhalant Agent

The use of an inhalation agent for induction and maintenance differs from injection techniques in several respects. Anesthetic induction with the commonly used inhalant agents is usually faster than IM induction but slower than IV induction (between approximately 3 and 8 minutes with isoflurane or sevoflurane). Also, the anesthetist has excellent control over depth

and can either increase or decrease depth relatively rapidly by changing the vaporizer dial setting. With inhalant agents, however, there is a delay between the time the dial setting is changed and the time it takes for the patient's anesthetic depth to change because it takes at least several minutes for the new concentration to fill the breathing circuit, reach the patient's lungs, and equilibrate with the blood and CNS.

> **TECHNICIAN NOTE** With inhalant agents, there is a delay between when the dial setting is changed and when the anesthetic depth changes. For this reason, vaporizer setting adjustments must be anticipated as much as possible through close monitoring.

The time required for anesthetic depth to change is influenced by a number of factors including the patient's respiratory drive, the agent used, the carrier gas flow rate, the type of breathing circuit, and the volume of the breathing circuit. For this reason, vaporizer setting adjustments must be anticipated as much as possible through close monitoring. In general, if a patient's anesthetic depth is significantly light or deep, larger dial changes are warranted; whereas if the patient's anesthetic depth is slightly light or deep, more subtle changes are needed. The anesthetist will develop a feel for the exact amount to change the dial setting in any given circumstance through experience (Fig. 9.5).

Intravenous Induction and Maintenance With an Inhalant Agent

IV induction and maintenance with an inhalant agent is the most commonly used method of inducing and maintaining general

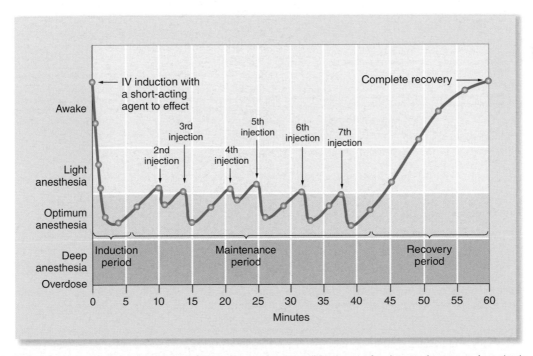

FIG. 9.3 Total intravenous anesthesia (TIVA) using intravenous *(IV)* boluses of a short-acting agent. Anesthetic induction is very rapid, peak effect is short, and surgical anesthesia is maintained with administration of repeat boluses every 3 to 8 minutes to effect. As with a single injection, recovery is gradual after the final bolus but relatively rapid as the agent is metabolized or redistributed.

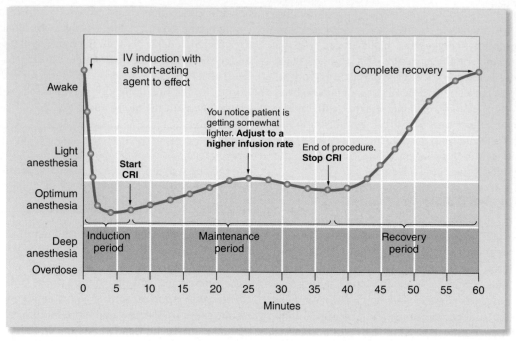

FIG. 9.4 Total intravenous anesthesia (TIVA) by constant rate infusion *(CRI)*. Anesthetic induction is very rapid, peak effect is short, and surgical anesthesia is maintained with a CRI. The rate of infusion is adjusted based on assessment of the anesthetic depth. After discontinuation of the CRI, recovery is gradual but relatively rapid as the agent is metabolized or redistributed.

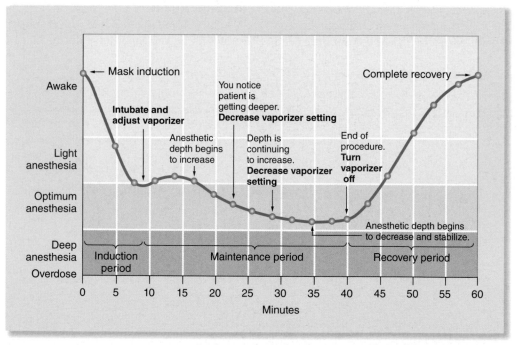

FIG. 9.5 Induction and maintenance with an inhalant agent. Induction is relatively rapid but gradual. Anesthesia is maintained by continued administration of the inhalant agent. The percentage administered is adjusted on the basis of assessment of the anesthetic depth. After discontinuation of the agent, recovery is gradual but relatively rapid as the agent is exhaled. Note that there is a delay after any change in the vaporizer setting. This is typical of inhalant anesthesia because of the time required for the concentration of the agent in the breathing circuit to reach the dialed concentration.

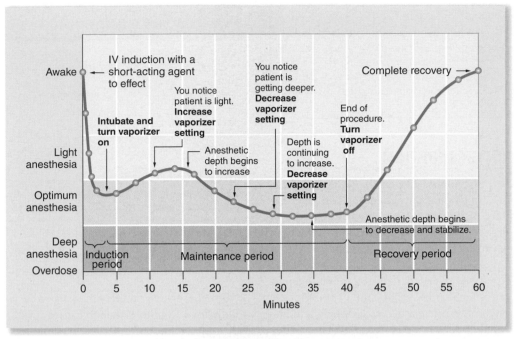

FIG. 9.6 Intravenous *(IV)* induction and maintenance with an inhalant agent. This method has features of induction with an IV injection of a short-acting agent to effect and induction and maintenance with an inhalant agent. Anesthetic induction is very rapid, and the dynamics of maintenance are identical to those shown in Fig. 9.5.

PROCEDURE 9.2 Sequence of Events for Induction of General Anesthesia With an Intravenous Agent and Maintenance With an Inhalant Agent in a Small Animal Patient

1. Administer premedications IM approximately 15–20 min or IV approximately 5–10 min before anesthetic induction.
2. Place an intravenous catheter, attach a fluid administration set, and begin fluid administration.
3. Administer the induction agent.
4. Check the patient's readiness for intubation.
5. Place and secure the endotracheal tube.
6. Check the patient's vital signs.
7. Turn on the oxygen and connect the endotracheal tube to the breathing circuit.
8. Inflate the endotracheal tube cuff.
9. Turn the vaporizer on to the appropriate setting.
10. Determine the patient's anesthetic depth and commence regular monitoring.
11. Position and secure the patient for the procedure, giving attention to padding, maintenance of an open airway, unrestricted blood flow, and unrestricted chest excursions.
12. Attach monitoring devices.
13. Continue to monitor and adjust the anesthetic and oxygen levels as needed until completion of the procedure.

---

anesthesia in small animal patients. It has dynamic elements of both IV and inhalant administration, as illustrated in Fig. 9.6, including rapid induction, good control over both increases and decreases in anesthetic depth, and a relatively rapid recovery. The sequence of events associated with this technique is summarized in Procedure 9.2.

> **TECHNICIAN NOTE** With inhalant agents, if a patient's anesthetic depth is significantly light or deep, larger dial changes are warranted, whereas if the patient's anesthetic depth is slightly light or deep, more subtle changes are needed.

EQUIPMENT PREPARATION

During a typical anesthetic induction, many events occur in rapid succession. Anesthetic agents are administered; the patient becomes unconscious and recumbent; the endotracheal tube is placed, secured, cuffed, and attached to the machine; the anesthetic vaporizer is turned on; the patient is positioned and monitored; and adjustments are made as needed, all within the first few minutes. Because these events follow one another so rapidly, the technician or nurse does not have the luxury of leaving the patient to locate equipment. For this reason, all equipment must be carefully gathered, checked, and organized before commencement of the procedure.

Unless IM or total IV techniques are used, most small animal patients are anesthetized with inhalant anesthetics delivered by means of a small animal anesthesia machine outfitted with a rebreathing circuit. Patients weighing less than 3 kg require a nonrebreathing circuit, and patients between 3 and 7 kg can be anesthetized with either a rebreathing circuit with pediatric breathing tubes or with a nonrebreathing circuit. Equipment required to intubate the patient, give injections, and administer fluids is also required—as is, especially if surgery will be performed, equipment designed to prevent hypothermia. A crash cart containing emergency equipment and drugs should also always be available.

TECHNICIAN NOTE Most small-animal patients weighing 3 kg or more are anesthetized by means of a small-animal anesthesia machine outfitted with a rebreathing circuit. Patients weighing less than 3 kg require a nonrebreathing circuit, and patients between 3 and 7 kg can be anesthetized with either a rebreathing circuit with pediatric breathing tubes or with a nonrebreathing circuit.

PREMEDICATION OR SEDATION

Premedication refers to the administration of anesthetic agents and adjuncts to calm and prepare the patient for anesthetic induction. Preanesthetic medications are chosen specifically to produce a set of desired effects such as anxiolysis, sedation, cholinergic blockade, analgesia, and muscle relaxation.

Anxiolytics are typically prescribed to be given orally at home before the owner transports the patient to the clinic. Gabapentin is commonly used for cats and either gabapentin or trazodone is used for dogs, although other agents such as dexmedetomidine oromucosal gel (labeled for use in dogs) may also be used for some patients. Gabapentin and trazodone are typically given between 1 and 3 hours before leaving for the hospital. See Protocol 9.1 for example anxiolytic protocols commonly used in physical status class (PSC) P1 and P2 dogs and cats.

Tranquilizers, alpha$_2$-agonists, opioids, dissociatives, and anticholinergics are often given intramuscularly after arrival at the hospital to further premedicate patients prior to anesthetic induction. These agents may be used alone or in combination to produce the desired degree of sedation ranging from light to deep. The level of sedation may be changed by doing one or more of the following:

1. Increasing or decreasing the dose of the drug or drugs in a combination
2. Choosing drugs with more or less profound effects (e.g., for increased sedation, choose an alpha$_2$-agonist instead of a benzodiazepine tranquilizer, or choose an opioid agonist as opposed to an opioid agonist-antagonist)
3. By adding or subtracting an additional anesthetic drug such as a dissociative or alfaxalone.

PROTOCOL 9.1 Anxiolytic Protocols for Physical Status Class P1 and P2 Dogs and Cats

Dogs
1. **Gabapentin[a] (PO):** Gabapentin 20–40 mg/kg 2–3 hrs before leaving for the hospital
2. **Trazodone[a] (PO):** Trazodone 3–7.5 mg/kg 1–2 hrs before leaving for the clinic

Cats
1. **Gabapentin (PO):** Gabapentin 50–100 mg/cat (up to 150 mg in large cats) 2–3 hrs before leaving for the hospital

Note that the same drugs may be used for patients with physical status class (PSC) P2, but doses may need to be lower.
[a]Dosages from Grubb T, Sager J, et al: 2020 AAHA anesthesia and monitoring guidelines for dogs and cats, *J Am Animal Hospital Assoc* 56(2):1–24, 2020.

BOX 9.4 Drug Choices Commonly Used to Produce Various Levels of Sedation

Light Sedation
- Opioid agonist-antagonist (A/A) given alone
- Tranquilizer given alone
- Combination of opioid A/A and benzodiazepine tranquilizer

Moderate Sedation
- Combination of opioid partial agonist (PA) or A/A and acepromazine
- Combination of opioid PA or A/A and dexmedetomidine

Deep sedation
- Combination of the following: (1) alfaxalone or ketamine; (2) opioid A, PA, or A/A; and (3) benzodiazepine or dexmedetomidine

Note that many combinations in addition to the ones shown here are used depending on the attending veterinarian's preference.
A, Agonist; *A/A,* agonist/antagonist; *PA,* partial agonist.

Box 9.4 gives examples of drugs and combinations commonly used in both dogs and cats to produce light, moderate, and deep sedation.

Realize that many factors including patient signalment, physical status class, and concurrent drug use will influence the effect any given drug or combination will have. Clinical judgment must therefore be used to determine the most appropriate protocol and dose to use for any given patient, and great care should be used when administering these agents to patients with preexisting disease, neonatal patients, and geriatric patients. No matter what protocol or dose is used, the patient must be watched closely for untoward effects that may require intervention (e.g., administration of reversal agents for excessive cardiovascular depression, oxygen therapy if SpO$_2$ is low, or endotracheal intubation and ventilation if respiratory depression is severe).

See Protocols 9.2 and 9.3 for example preanesthetic and sedative protocols in PSC P1 and P2 dogs and cats respectively.

TECHNICIAN NOTE When administering preanesthetic medications, clinical judgment must be used to determine the most appropriate protocol and dose to use for any given patient. Great care should be used when administering these agents to patients with preexisting disease, neonatal patients, and geriatric patients. No matter what protocol or dose is used, the patient must be watched closely for untoward effects that may require intervention.

After IM injection of preanesthetic medications, the patient should be placed in a location that is quiet but permits close observation until the agent takes effect (for many drugs given intramuscularly, about 15 to 20 minutes). If the patient is excited or stimulated during this time, the beneficial effects of the drugs may be diminished. Especially if the patient is heavily sedated, observation every few minutes is paramount to permit prompt intervention in the event that the patient experiences complications. Once the patient is adequately sedated, anesthetic induction should immediately follow or, as an alternative, these protocols can be used alone to provide sedation for diagnostic and therapeutic procedures or induction of general anesthesia.

PROTOCOL 9.2 Premedication and Sedative Protocols for Physical Status Class P1 And P2 Dogs

Protocols for Premedication or Light–Moderate Sedation

1. **Acepromazine (IM):** Acepromazine 0.01–0.05 mg/kg IM with a maximum dose of 3 mg *(not for use in old or debilitated patients, or in sensitive breeds).*
2. **Dexmedetomidine (microdose) (IM):** Dexmedetomidine 0.0015–0.003 mg/kg IM *(equivalent to 1.5–3 mcg/kg).*
3. **Butorphanol and midazolam (IM/IV):** Butorphanol 0.2–0.4 mg/kg and midazolam 0.2 mg/kg and IM/IV *(halve the doses for IV administration; can use hydromorphone 0.1 mg/kg in place of butorphanol).*
4. **Hydromorphone (IM/IV):** Hydromorphone 0.05–0.1 mg/kg IM or IV.
5. **"TTDex"[a] (Telazol–butorphanol [Torbugesic]–dexmedetomidine) (IM):** Add 2.5 mL butorphanol (10 mg/mL) and 2.5 mL dexmedetomidine (0.5 mg/mL) to 1 vial of Telazol powder. The final mixture contains 50 mg tiletamine, 50 mg zolazepam, 0.25 mg dexmedetomidine, and 5 mg butorphanol per mL of the mixture. Give at a rate of 0.005 mL/kg for light sedation; up to 0.04 mL/kg IM for moderate anesthesia. *Note that it is important to measure the doses in this combination very carefully.*

Protocols for Premedication or Moderate–Deep Sedation (for Minor Procedures Such as Radiography or Grooming)

1. **"BAG" (IM/IV):** Butorphanol 0.2 mg/kg, acepromazine 0.05 mg/kg, and glycopyrrolate 0.005 mg/kg mixed in one syringe and given IM or IV (as an alternative, mix 1 mL acepromazine [10 mg/mL], 4 mL butorphanol [10 mg/mL], and 5 mL glycopyrrolate [0.2 mg/mL], and give this mixture at a volume of 0.5 mL per 10 to 20 lb of body weight [4.5 to 9 kg]).
   (Can use buprenorphine 0.01 mg/kg in place of butorphanol to make a combination referred to as **"Super BAG."**)
2. **Butorphanol and dexmedetomidine (IM):** Butorphanol 0.2–0.4 mg/kg and dexmedetomidine 0.005–0.01 mg/kg IM *(can use hydromorphone 0.1 mg/kg in place of butorphanol).*
3. **Dexmedetomidine–ketamine (IM/IV):** Dexmedetomidine 0.015 mg/kg and ketamine 3 mg/kg IM *(halve the doses for IV administration; do not reverse the dexmedetomidine until at least 40 min later).*
4. **"Doggie Magic" (ketamine–butorphanol–dexmedetomidine) (IM):** Use the chart provided on the package insert to dose dexmedetomidine at 125–375 mcg/m². Mix an equal volume of butorphanol (10 mg/mL) and an equal volume of ketamine (100 mg/mL) in the same syringe. This equates to approximately 0.1–0.3 mL of each drug (when using Dexdomitor [0.5 mg/mL]) for a dog weighing 5.1–10 kg. Administer IM. *(Note that using doses based on a dexmedetomidine dose of 125 mcg/m² will produce light to moderate sedation. Higher doses will produce increasingly profound sedation or even general anesthesia.)*
5. **Telazol[a] (IM/IV):** Telazol 3 to 10 mg/kg IM (for aggressive patients); or 1 to 4 mg/kg **IV to effect** (higher doses may be needed for unsedated patients). *(Note that this drug may result in light general anesthesia and may result in rough recovery in unsedated patients.)*

[a]Dosages from Grubb T, Sager J, et al: 2020 AAHA anesthesia and monitoring guidelines for dogs and cats, *J Am Animal Hospital Assoc* 56(2):1–24, 2020.

PROTOCOL 9.3 Premedication and Sedative Protocols for Physical Status Class P1 and P2 Cats

Protocols for Premedication or Light–Moderate Sedation

1. **Butorphanol[a] (IM/IV):** Butorphanol 0.2–0.4 mg/kg IM/IV.
2. **Dexmedetomidine (IM):** Dexmedetomidine 0.003–0.01 mg/kg IM.
3. **Butorphanol and acepromazine[a] (IM):** Butorphanol 0.4 mg/kg and acepromazine 0.025–0.1 mg/kg (up to a maximum dose of 1 mg) IM.
4. **Butorphanol and midazolam[a] (IM/IV):** Butorphanol 0.2–0.4 mg/kg and midazolam 0.2 mg/kg IM/IV.

Protocols for Premedication or Moderate–Deep Sedation (for Minor Procedures Such as Radiography or Grooming)

1. **Hydromorphone and acepromazine (IM):** Hydromorphone 0.05–0.1 mg/kg and acepromazine 0.025–0.1 mg/kg (up to a maximum dose of 1 mg) IM.
2. **Butorphanol and dexmedetomidine (IM):** Butorphanol 0.4 mg/kg and dexmedetomidine 0.003–0.01 mg/kg *(can use buprenorphine 0.01 mg/kg in place of butorphanol).*

3. **Dexmedetomidine and ketamine[a] (IM):** Dexmedetomidine 0.01–0.02 mg/kg and ketamine 1–2 mg/kg IM.
4. **"Kitty Magic" (ketamine–butorphanol–dexmedetomidine) (IM):** Ketamine 2.2–4.4 mg/kg, butorphanol 0.22–0.44 mg/kg, and dexmedetomidine 0.011–0.022 mg/kg mixed in the same syringe. This equates to 0.1–0.2 mL of each drug (when using Dexdomitor [0.5 mg/mL]) for an average-sized (4.5-kg) cat. Administer IM. *(Note that the higher end of the dose may result in light general anesthesia.)*
5. **Butorphanol, midazolam, and alfaxalone[a] (IM):** Butorphanol 0.2–0.4 mg/kg, midazolam 0.2 mg/kg, and alfaxalone 1 to 2 mg/kg IM.
6. **Telazol[a] (IM/IV):** Telazol 3 to 10 mg/kg IM *(for aggressive patients)*; or 1 to 4 mg/kg **IV to effect** (higher doses may be needed for unsedated patients). *(Note that this drug may result in light general anesthesia and may result in rough recovery in unsedated patients.)*

[a]Dosages from Grubb T, Sager J, et al: 2020 AAHA anesthesia and monitoring guidelines for dogs and cats, *J Am Animal Hospital Assoc* 56(2):1–24, 2020.
IM, Intramuscular; *IV,* intravenous.

TECHNICIAN NOTE After IM injection of preanesthetic medications, the patient should be placed in a location that is quiet but that permits close observation until the agent takes effect (for many drugs given intramuscularly, about 15–20 min). If the patient is excited or stimulated during this time, the beneficial effects of the drugs may be diminished.

ANESTHETIC INDUCTION

Anesthetic induction is the process by which an animal loses consciousness and enters surgical anesthesia. The goal of anesthetic induction is to take the patient from consciousness to stage III anesthesia smoothly and rapidly so that an endotracheal tube or supraglottic airway device (SGAD) can be placed. During any induction, the patient passes through the excitement stage and therefore may show signs of incoordination or struggling, followed by progressive relaxation and unconsciousness. Excitement and struggling during induction hamper restraint, increase the risk of inadvertent perivascular drug injection, and predispose the patient to traumatic injury, vomiting, cardiac arrhythmias, and other adverse effects, and so should be minimized through administration of preanesthetic medications.

> **TECHNICIAN NOTE** During anesthetic induction, the patient should be sufficiently anesthetized to permit intubation but should generally be kept in a light plane of anesthesia until the tube or SGAD is placed.

During induction, the patient should be sufficiently anesthetized to permit intubation, but should generally be kept in a light plane of anesthesia until the tube or SGAD is placed. At this point, anesthetic depth can be adjusted as needed. Induction is most commonly accomplished by IV or IM administration of injectable agents, or less commonly, by administration of inhalant agents via a mask or chamber. IM administration of injectable agents in combination is frequently used in animal shelters to induce and maintain anesthesia in patients undergoing routine procedures such as spays and castrations. Of these techniques, IV induction has the advantage of producing unconsciousness within seconds to a few minutes at most. Therefore most animals that undergo induction by this method pass through the excitement stage quickly, allowing rapid control of the airway. In contrast, mask or chamber induction typically takes at least 5 to 10 minutes, increasing the likelihood of undesirable effects. Induction after IM injection typically takes about 10 to 20 minutes but results in smooth, gradual CNS depression with little apparent excitement. What follows is a description of specific techniques used to induce anesthesia.

Intravenous Induction

Agents commonly used to induce general anesthesia in dogs and cats by IV injection include: (1) propofol, (2) alfaxalone, (3) etomidate, (4) a mixture of ketamine and either midazolam or diazepam (usually a 1:1 ratio by volume), and (5) neuroleptanalgesics (combination of an opioid and tranquilizer), as well as various other combinations containing dissociatives, tranquilizers, and opioids. Protocol 9.4 lists common IV induction protocols in PSC P1 and P2 dogs and cats.

To induce general anesthesia by the IV route, a volume of the agent to be administered is calculated, based on a prescribed dose, and drawn into a syringe. The agent is then injected directly into the vein or into a winged-infusion set or indwelling catheter *to effect* until the patient can be intubated or until the patient is at an adequate plane of anesthesia for completion of the planned procedure.

> **TECHNICIAN NOTE** The term "to effect" means that only the amount of injectable anesthetic necessary to produce unconsciousness is given, rather than administering the entire dose calculated on a milligram per kilogram basis.

The term "to effect" means that only the amount of injectable anesthetic necessary to produce unconsciousness is given, rather than administering the entire dose calculated on a milligram per kilogram basis. This technique is necessary because the amount of drug needed to induce or maintain anesthesia cannot be precisely predicted for a given patient and most anesthetic agents have narrow therapeutic indices.

PROTOCOL 9.4 Intravenous Induction Protocols for Physical Status Class P1 and P2 Dogs and Cats

1. **Propofol (IV to effect):** Propofol 6–8 mg/kg IV to effect if not premedicated or 2–4 mg/kg IV after premedication. *(Note: adding 0.2–0.4 mg/kg midazolam or diazepam will reduce the dose required.)*
2. **Alfaxalone[a] (IV to effect):** Alfaxalone 1–3 mg/kg IV to effect (dogs); 2–5 mg/kg IV to effect (cats): As with any IV anesthetic, the total amount needed is significantly influenced by the use of premedication and therefore may be more or less than the listed doses.
3. **Etomidate[a] (IV to effect):** Etomidate 1–3 mg/kg IV to effect. *(Note: 0.2–0.4 mg/kg midazolam or diazepam may be given IV 30 sec before etomidate to reduce adverse effects as well as the dose required.)*
4. **Ketamine and midazolam (IV to effect):** Ketamine 5.5 mg/kg IV and midazolam 0.28 mg/kg IV mixed in the same syringe. *(Equivalent to 1 mL of the mixture per 20 lb of body weight.)* An equivalent volume of diazepam can be substituted for midazolam. Butorphanol 0.1–0.2 mg/kg or hydromorphone 0.1 mg/kg can be given IV before induction in a separate syringe for additional analgesia.
5. **Midazolam and hydromorphone (IV to effect) (this protocol is intended for older or compromised patients):** Midazolam 0.2 mg/kg (maximum dose of 5 mg) IV alternating with hydromorphone 0.1 mg/kg IV. Use separate syringes. Administer boluses of each agent alternately until the patient can be intubated. May need more to allow intubation. *(Diazepam may be substituted for midazolam at the same dose; fentanyl at a dose of 2 mcg/kg may be substituted for hydromorphone.)*
6. **Ketamine and propofol ("Ketofol") (IV to effect):** Ketamine 2 mg/kg and propofol 2 mg/kg. Give the mixture IV to effect.

[a]Dosages from Grubb T, Sager J, et al: 2020 AAHA anesthesia and monitoring guidelines for dogs and cats, *Journal of the American Animal Hospital Association* 56(2):1–24, 2020.
IM, Intramuscular; *IV,* intravenous.

For example, the amount of propofol required to induce anesthesia in a quiet, older dog may be one-quarter to one-half of the dose required for an active, young dog of equivalent body weight. Similarly, a cat with a urinary obstruction may be deeply anesthetized after receiving a very small dose of ketamine, whereas a healthy cat may require several times more to reach an equivalent depth. The drugs used for premedication also affect the dose of general anesthetic required. For example, a patient that has not received any premedication may require two or three times as much as a patient that has been premedicated with a neuroleptanalgesic combination to reach a comparable plane of anesthesia.

For these reasons, IV drugs are given as a series of bolus injections and discontinued when the desired depth is reached—a process known as titration. A competent anesthetist monitors the patient closely and alters the amount of anesthetic given to suit the patient's requirements rather than relying solely on a calculated dose. (See Procedure 9.3 for IV induction techniques in dogs and cats.)

After induction with the commonly used IV injectable agents, the duration of anesthesia varies but is usually no more than 10 to 20 minutes. If more than 20 minutes is required, anesthesia is maintained with inhalation anesthetics or administration of propofol, alfaxalone, or etomidate by repeat boluses or CRI. This is not recommended with other injectable agents such as

PROCEDURE 9.3 Intravenous Induction for a Dog or Cat

Although each intravenous (IV) agent or combination is given somewhat differently, all intravenously administered general anesthetics should be given to effect so that the patient receives only the minimum amount necessary to induce anesthesia.

Giving an IV Anesthetic to Effect

Give an initial bolus of one-quarter to one-half the calculated dose. Immediately after giving the initial bolus, check the heart rate and respiratory rate to be sure the patient is stable and is breathing (while keeping in mind that a brief period of apnea is a common adverse effect of some intravenous anesthetics). As soon as the patient relaxes, remove the muzzle and any other restraint devices. Continue monitoring and give additional boluses as necessary until the patient has passed through stage II. When signs of readiness for intubation are present, intubate the patient and take the steps necessary to bring the patient to surgical anesthesia.

During this process, there must be interplay between administration of the drug and patient monitoring. Give the initial dose; then rapidly check the vital signs, pedal reflex, palpebral reflex, and jaw tone; give more if needed; check again; and so on, until the patient is in a plane of anesthesia sufficient to permit intubation. After the initial dose, subsequent doses should generally be about one-fifth to one-tenth the calculated dose.

- **Propofol:** Give propofol slowly at a rate of one-quarter to one-half the calculated dose every 30 sec to effect. A more rapid injection rate may be helpful for uncooperative patients but is more likely to induce apnea. If the injection is too slow, excitement may be seen.
- **Alfaxalone:** Give alfaxalone slowly at a rate of one-quarter the calculated dose every 15 sec to effect.
- **Etomidate:** Give rapidly to effect after premedication with a tranquilizer or concurrently with IV midazolam or diazepam (use a separate syringe if diazepam is chosen). Some anesthetists recommend administering it via the port of a fluid administration set with the fluids running to reduce adverse effects.
- **Ketamine–midazolam** and other **ketamine–tranquilizer mixtures:** Give slowly to effect over 60–120 sec. Slow injection minimizes the adverse effects of these combinations, which may take as long as 2 min to reach peak effect. Therefore an overly rapid injection rate may result in overdose. If a bolus injection technique is preferred, one-third to one-half the calculated dose can be given over 15–30 sec, with further increments every 30–60 sec until the desired depth is reached.
- **Neuroleptanalgesic combinations** (e.g., hydromorphone and midazolam): Give an IV bolus of midazolam followed by a bolus of hydromorphone. Some patients may require an additional bolus of each drug to allow intubation and occasionally, may require a third bolus.

---

ketamine and midazolam because if such drugs are given in this way, large amounts of anesthetic may accumulate in the body and prolong recovery.

Induction With Inhalation Agents

Inhalation agents commonly used to induce general anesthesia in dogs and cats include isoflurane and sevoflurane. These agents are administered by means of a face mask or anesthetic chamber. Protocol 9.5 shows inhalant induction protocols in PSC P1 and P2 dogs and cats.

Mask Induction

Mask induction involves administration of an inhalant anesthetic such as isoflurane or sevoflurane via a face mask. This method of induction is feasible only with the use of inhalation anesthetics with a low blood–gas solubility coefficient such as isoflurane or sevoflurane because the rapid induction time associated with these agents results in passage through stage II anesthesia quickly enough to minimize excitement. For some patients in critical condition, induction by mask may be safer than induction with injectable agents because the anesthetist can decrease anesthetic depth or discontinue the agent by adjusting the vaporizer setting if problems arise.

PROTOCOL 9.5 Inhalant Induction Protocols for Physical Status Class P1 and P2 Dogs and Cats

1. **Isoflurane:** Administer isoflurane at 3%–5% by mask or chamber.
2. **Sevoflurane:** Administer sevoflurane at 4%–5% by mask or chamber.

Patients should receive rates at the lower end of these ranges if preanesthetic medications have been administered.

TECHNICIAN NOTE Successful mask induction requires skillful restraint (enough to prevent operator and patient injury but not so much as to restrict chest excursions or the airway). Mucous membrane color and refill time as well as ocular indicators of anesthetic depth are not easily observed, although monitoring requirements are no different with this method of induction.

Mask induction is challenging for several reasons and is associated with higher risk than most other induction techniques. Many patients struggle, necessitating skillful restraint (enough to prevent operator and patient injury but not so much as to restrict chest excursions or the airway). The fear associated with passage through stage I and the excitement associated with passage through stage II cause release of epinephrine and other catecholamines, which can predispose the patient to cardiac arrhythmias, hypotension, and other adverse effects. Also, mucous membrane color and refill time as well as ocular indicators of anesthetic depth are not as easily observed because the mask partially obscures the eyes and muzzle, although monitoring requirements are no different with this method of induction.

The mask should be carefully fitted before commencement of mask induction. There should be a reasonably tight seal between the muzzle and the rubber gasket without constriction of the tissues or discomfort. The mask should be long enough to accommodate the full length of the patient's muzzle (so that the nares do not press against the end of the mask when the muzzle is fully inserted) but not too long. Be aware that higher oxygen flow rates are required than when an endotracheal tube is used. The technique for mask induction is described and illustrated in Procedure 9.4.

PROCEDURE 9.4 Mask Induction for a Dog or Cat

1. Use either a malleable black rubber mask or a clear plastic mask with a rubber diaphragm for mask induction. The mask should fit tightly on the animal's face to minimize leakage of gas and should not be any larger than necessary in order to minimize dead space.

2. Connect the mask to the Y-piece of a rebreathing circuit or the patient connector of a nonrebreathing circuit and hold it in place over the animal's muzzle (Fig. 1).

3. Give 100% oxygen for 2–3 min to allow the patient to adjust to the mask and to increase the amount of oxygen in the blood. The oxygen flow rate should

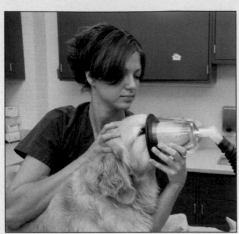

FIG. 1 Mask induction. Note the good fit of the mask around the muzzle to minimize leakage.

ideally be set at 30 times the patient's tidal volume (1–3 L/min for patients weighing ≤ 10 kg and 3–5 L/min for patients weighing > 10 kg) because higher flow rates help speed induction.

4. Set the anesthetic vaporizer to deliver 0.5% isoflurane or 1% sevoflurane. Sevoflurane is less pungent than isoflurane and better accepted.

5a. Gradually increase the concentration of anesthetic by small increments (0.5% every 30 sec for isoflurane and 1% every 30 sec for sevoflurane) until an anesthetic concentration of 3%–5% for isoflurane or 4%–5% for sevoflurane is reached. This is higher than the maintenance level but allows a rapid uptake of the anesthetic and faster induction. The slow increase helps reduce struggling, prevents cardiac arrhythmias, and allows the animal to become accustomed to the smell of the anesthetic. This method is often well accepted by premedicated cats and dogs, although some struggling may be seen after 2–3 min when isoflurane is given, corresponding to stage II excitement. Most patients reach stage III, plane 1, in about 5–10 min, depending on the agent used.

5b. Other anesthetists suggest increasing the vaporizer setting to the induction level immediately, especially if the patient is difficult to handle, to minimize the time spent in stage II. If the patient struggles, the anesthetist must observe the patient closely for cyanosis, hypotension, or other problems, and must be ready to act quickly if the patient becomes compromised.

6. As soon as the patient is in lateral recumbency, assess readiness for intubation and adjust the anesthetic level as appropriate, then place an endotracheal tube. From this point on, the patient is managed much the same as for intravenous induction.

There are several cautions associated with mask induction of which the anesthetist must be aware:

- Mask induction may result in significant exposure of personnel to waste anesthetic gas, because no matter how well the mask is fitted, some leakage is inevitable. Therefore adequate room ventilation is necessary to prevent excess inhalation of waste gas (see Chapter 5).

- If the animal resists mask induction, struggling may cause the release of epinephrine, which predisposes the patient to potentially fatal cardiac arrhythmias and hypotension. To avoid this, induce anesthesia by mask only in calm or sedated patients.

- Because of the longer induction time compared with IV administration, mask induction is not appropriate for patients with poor respiratory function (e.g., upper airway disease or obstruction, difficult breathing because of brachycephalic conformation, diaphragmatic hernia, pleural effusion, or pulmonary edema), unfasted patients, or patients at risk for vomiting or regurgitation during induction. These patients must be intubated immediately to prevent serious adverse effects and permit rapid control of the airway and ventilatory support.

- The anesthetist must ensure that the airway is kept open at all times during mask induction. The mask must not occlude the patient's nostrils, as might happen with a cat or brachycephalic patient if the mask is too small or tight. The anesthetist must not compress the airway or chest during restraint.

- Masks are a significant source of dead space, especially if not well fitted to the patient's muzzle, and so can result in rebreathing of carbon dioxide.

Although a mask can be used to maintain anesthesia, the anesthetist is not able to protect the airway, prevent aspiration, provide ventilatory support, or observe respirations as readily as when a tube is present. For these reasons, most anesthetists intubate the patient immediately after induction.

Chamber Induction

Chamber induction involves placing the patient in a closed chamber infused with anesthetic gas. This technique is feasible only for patients small enough to fit comfortably into a chamber (typically those weighing less than 5 to 7 kg) and is therefore primarily used for small patients that are aggressive or difficult to handle.

> **TECHNICIAN NOTE** During chamber induction, it is impossible to assess most monitoring parameters accurately. Thus, the anesthetist must be vigilant and prepared to act quickly if the patient shows signs of compromise.

Most chambers are small, clear boxes that resemble a 5-gallon aquarium (Fig. 9.7). The chamber should be examined before induction. A tight-fitting lid and two ports (one for entry of fresh gas and another for exit of excess gas) are required. Although there is more than one way to supply oxygen and anesthetic gases to a chamber, a common way is to remove the Y-piece from the corrugated breathing tubes of a rebreathing circuit and attach the inspiratory tube to one chamber port and

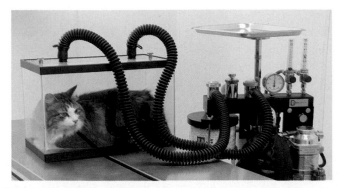

FIG. 9.7 Anesthetic chamber attached to the corrugated breathing tubes of a rebreathing circuit in place of the Y-piece.

PROCEDURE 9.5 Chamber Induction for a Dog or Cat

1. Place the conscious animal inside an anesthetic chamber. The chamber should be large enough for the patient to lie down with its neck extended. If the patient can be handled, an ophthalmic lubricant should be applied before the patient is placed in the induction chamber.

2. Remove the Y-piece of a rebreathing circuit and attach one corrugated hose to each port of the chamber.

3. Deliver a mixture of oxygen at 5 L/min and isoflurane at 3%–5% or sevoflurane at 4%–5%.

4. During passage through stages I and II, patients typically exhibit fear and agitation. The patient may attempt to escape or vocalize. Gradually, with the onset of anesthesia, the patient will become increasingly depressed and immobile.

5. As soon as the patient can no longer stand, rock the chamber gently to assess the patient's status. Initially, the patient will respond by righting itself until anesthesia is of sufficient depth to prevent purposeful movement. When the patient is immobile enough to allow it to be safely handled, remove it from the chamber, place a mask, and proceed as with mask induction.

6. To minimize exposure to waste anesthetic gas:
   - Ideally, enlist the help of two people (one to open, close, and manage the chamber and one to hold the patient) so that the waste gas can be managed without compromising patient safety.
   - Check that the lid is properly sealed before commencing chamber induction.
   - Perform chamber induction in an area that is well ventilated (with at least 15 air changes per hour).
   - Avoid opening the chamber any more often than necessary.
   - Turn the vaporizer off before removing the lid.
   - Ideally, before removing the lid, run pure oxygen to scavenge as much waste gas as possible. This is often not possible, however, because of the need to check vital signs rapidly, ensure a patent airway, and perform endotracheal intubation.
   - Remove the patient quickly, immediately replace the lid, and continue to run pure oxygen at a rate of 5 L/min for at least 2–3 min to purge waste gas from the system.

the expiratory tube to the other port. Place the patient in the chamber, close the lid, and proceed, following the instructions summarized in Procedure 9.5 and illustrated in Fig. 9.7.

TECHNICIAN NOTE Anesthetic chambers allow the induction of anesthesia in even the most uncooperative animal but are associated with complications from stress, trauma, vomiting, airway blockage, and other issues.

Anesthetic chambers allow the induction of anesthesia in even the most uncooperative animal but are associated with complications from stress, trauma, vomiting, airway blockage, and other issues including the following:

- Given that it is impossible to assess most monitoring parameters accurately while the patient is inside a chamber, the anesthetist must be vigilant and prepared to act quickly if the patient shows signs of compromise.
- As with mask induction, there is some risk of regurgitation or vomiting, especially with a nonfasted patient. Because the airway is unprotected, aspiration of stomach contents may occur.
- There is considerable risk of exposure of hospital personnel to waste anesthetic gas, particularly when removing the patient from the chamber. The chamber must be equipped with a scavenger and ideally, the anesthetic gas should be evacuated before the chamber is opened so that waste gas exposure can be avoided. This is often not possible in a clinical setting, however, because of the need to remove the patient quickly.
- As with induction by mask, epinephrine release will predispose the patient to cardiac arrhythmias and hypotension.
- As with mask induction, chamber induction is not appropriate for patients in which rapid control of the airway is required.

For these reasons, chamber induction should be only used as a last resort in situations where other induction techniques are not feasible.

Intramuscular Induction

Agents commonly used to induce general anesthesia in dogs and cats by IM injection include neuroleptanalgesic combinations and various combinations of tranquilizers, dissociatives, and opioids when given at doses higher than that used for sedation.

The following protocols are examples of IM combinations from Protocols 9.2 and 9.3 that can be used to induce general anesthesia in PSC P1 and P2 dogs and cats when the higher doses within the indicated range are used:

- Telazol (IM)
- "TTDex" (Telazol–butorphanol–dexmedetomidine) (IM) (dogs only)
- "Doggie Magic" or "Kitty Magic" (ketamine–butorphanol–dexmedetomidine) (IM)

IM induction is useful for animals in which IV injections are difficult, such as ferrets and very young puppies and kittens. IM induction using restraint equipment such as the EZ Nabber (Campbell Pet Company) (Fig. 9.8) or the Wild Child Chamber (MAI Animal Health) (Fig. 9.9), is necessary to induce anesthesia in extremely aggressive domestic animals. IM induction is also standard in animals that are difficult to approach or impossible to handle or for which IV or mask induction is not feasible, such as wild animals and captive animals in zoos. In these animals, dissociative-tranquilizer mixtures, neuroleptanalgesics, or ultrapotent opioids (particularly etorphine and thiafentanil) are usually administered by means of a blowpipe or tranquilizing gun.

Induction by IM injection differs from IV induction in several important respects.

- IM injections cannot be titrated or given to effect. Usually, the entire calculated dose is given at once.

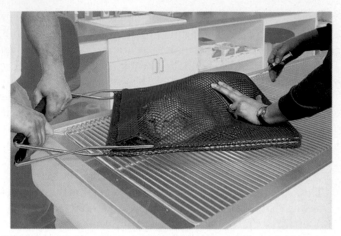

FIG. 9.8 EZ Nabber (Campbell Pet Company). As shown in this photo, the patient is restrained in sternal recumbency between the two mesh jaws of the EZ Nabber by squeezing the two handles together, and an IM injection is given by passing the needle through the mesh. (From EZ Nabber, Campbell Pet Company: https://www.campbellpet.com/products/ez-nabber?variant=42686437331.)

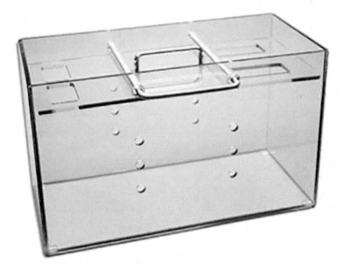

FIG. 9.9 Wild Child Chamber (MAI Animal Health). Note that this restraint chamber is constructed such that the patient can be restrained in sternal recumbency by gently lowering the top and locking it into position over the patient's back with the horizontal U-shaped steel bar. An IM injection can then be safely given through one of the rectangular holes in the top. (From Wild Child Chamber (MAI Animal Health): https://www.maianimalhealth.com/en/product/products-by-brand-mcculloch-medical/wild-child-chamber-17-x-10-12-x-8–55220.)

- In general, the dose for IM injection is about twice the corresponding IV dose.
- Drugs administered by the IM route require more time to reach a high enough concentration in the brain to induce anesthesia. IM induction is therefore characterized by a relatively slow onset of anesthesia (typically 10 to 20 minutes) compared with IV induction. Occasionally, if drugs are deposited in a fascial plane between muscles or in subcutaneous (SC) tissue, slow or incomplete absorption may result in an even longer induction or a blunted effect.

- After peak effect, if the patient's depth of anesthesia is still inadequate, additional drug must be given or an inhalant agent must be administered with a mask until the patient can be intubated. (Remember that some drugs such as propofol and etomidate *must not* be given intramuscularly.)
- IM induction is characterized by a lengthy recovery period because the animal requires considerable time to metabolize the relatively large dose of drug given by this route.

The differences between IM and IV administration are illustrated by the use of ketamine in cats. When ketamine is given IV at a dose of 5 mg/kg, induction of anesthesia occurs in less than 1 to 2 minutes. Alternatively, the drug can be given IM at a dose of 15 mg/kg, inducing anesthesia in 5 to 10 minutes. Recovery from IV ketamine administration usually begins in 10 to 15 minutes, and healthy animals often appear fully recovered within 1 to 2 hours. In contrast, complete recovery from IM ketamine administration may require several hours or more.

Other Induction Techniques

Oral administration of certain anesthetics (most notably ketamine) has occasionally been used in circumstances in which injection is dangerous or difficult, such as induction of anesthesia in feral cats. However, in recent years, alternative techniques have made this practice unnecessary in most cases.

Other routes of administration for injectable agents include the SC, rectal, and intraperitoneal routes. For dogs and cats, these routes are too slow or impractical for routine use.

ENDOTRACHEAL INTUBATION

After induction of general anesthesia, an ETT is usually placed in the patient's airway, although placement of an SGAD is an alternative method of securing the airway (*see* page 325 *for a description of this technique*). An endotracheal tube conducts air or anesthetic gases directly from the breathing circuit to the trachea, bypassing the nasal passages and pharynx (Fig. 9.10). Placement of an endotracheal tube is especially beneficial for maintaining anesthesia with inhalant anesthetics but also offers several key advantages, even when anesthesia is maintained with injectable protocols.

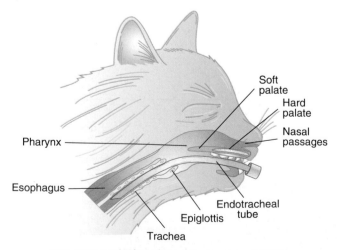

FIG. 9.10 Intubation of the cat, showing anatomy.

- When properly maintained, an endotracheal tube helps to maintain an open airway, decreasing the likelihood of airway obstruction caused by patient position, collapse of pharyngeal tissues, foreign material, or any other cause. Because of the importance of maintaining a patent airway, it is customary to leave the tube in place throughout anesthesia and into the recovery period until the animal regains the swallowing reflex.
- Intubation allows more efficient delivery of anesthetic gas to the animal than does a mask. Because gas flow rates can be lowered, intubation results in reduced exposure of hospital personnel to waste anesthetic gas and is more economical.
- Use of an endotracheal tube with an inflated cuff reduces the risk of aspiration of vomitus, blood, saliva, or other material that may be present in the oral cavity or breathing passages. This material may accumulate during any procedure; however, the risk of aspiration is particularly high during oral surgery or dentistry and in patients that have not been fasted.
- An endotracheal tube of the correct diameter and length will improve efficiency of gas exchange by reducing the amount of anatomic dead space. Anatomic dead space is composed of the portions of the breathing passages that contain air but in which no gas exchange can occur (i.e., the mouth, nasal passages, pharynx, trachea, and bronchi). With the anatomic dead space minimized (due to the fact that the inner diameter of the ETT is less than the inner diameter of the mouth, pharynx, and trachea), the endotracheal tube ensures that a larger proportion of the gas delivered to the patient reaches the exchange surface in the alveoli.
- The anesthetist can support ventilation in intubated patients by manual or mechanical means. *Manual ventilation* refers to forced delivery of oxygen and anesthetic gases by squeezing the reservoir bag of the anesthetic machine. *Mechanical ventilation* refers to use of a mechanical ventilator to achieve the same result. Manual and mechanical ventilation are discussed in detail in Chapter 7. Because of the respiratory depression associated with anesthesia, periodic manual or mechanical ventilation is necessary for most anesthetized patients to ensure adequate gas exchange. Intermittent mandatory manual or mechanical ventilation is required for patients that have been given neuromuscular blocking agents or when the thoracic cavity is open.
- Endotracheal intubation followed by manual or mechanical ventilation is also essential for patients in respiratory or cardiac arrest. For this reason, it is advisable to have a laryngoscope and an endotracheal tube of the correct size readily available for all anesthetized patients, even if endotracheal intubation is not planned.

Equipment for Endotracheal Intubation

The following equipment is required to perform endotracheal intubation (Fig. 9.11):
- Appropriately sized endotracheal tubes (at least three of slightly different diameters)
- Small amount of sterile, water-soluble lubricant
- 2-foot length of IV tubing, rolled gauze, or other tie to secure the tube

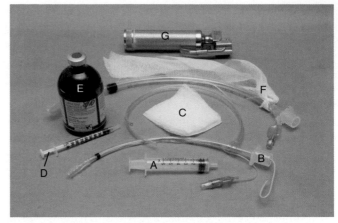

FIG. 9.11 Intubation equipment. *A,* Cuffing syringe; *B,* 4-mm internal diameter (ID), polyvinyl chloride (PVC) endotracheal tube (ETT) with stylette and intravenous (IV) tubing tie; *C,* 3 × 3 gauze sponge; *D,* 1-mL syringe containing 0.1 mL of injectable lidocaine; *E,* 2% lidocaine injectable solution; *F,* 8-mm ID PVC ETT with gauze tie; *G,* laryngoscope (optional). A small amount of sterile, water-soluble lubricant should also be available.

- Gauze sponge to grasp the tongue
- 6- or 12-mL syringe for dogs or a 3-mL syringe for cats to inflate the cuff
- Good examination light
- Stylette (a blunt, bendable rod, often made of metal, which is placed inside the tube to stiffen it); used for narrow-diameter tubes (most commonly when intubating cats) or for any other tube that requires additional support
- Lidocaine injectable solution to control **laryngospasm** (in cats only)
- Laryngoscope with an appropriately sized blade if desired

> **TECHNICIAN NOTE** When preparing for endotracheal intubation, select at least three tubes of slightly different diameters so that you are prepared if your first choice does not fit. Ideally the endotracheal tube should extend from the tip of the nose to the thoracic inlet.

Selecting an Endotracheal Tube

Endotracheal tubes are available in a wide variety of diameters and lengths. The tube must be of a diameter that is small enough to allow placement without causing trauma to the trachea but large enough to produce a seal when the cuff is inflated. Using the largest diameter that will safely fit affords the advantage of maximizing the size of the airway, which is especially important in cats to minimize the risk of complications such as resistance to movement of gases and obstruction of the tube. It must be of sufficient length to reach the thoracic inlet when fully inserted but must not be so long as to reach the mainstem bronchi or to extend beyond the end of the muzzle when inserted the correct distance.

At least three tubes of slightly different diameters should be selected so that you are prepared if your first choice does not fit. The size required by any given patient is influenced by species, conformation, and breed. For instance, cats require tubes of smaller diameter than dogs of comparable body weight. Most brachycephalic breeds require a tube several sizes smaller than mesocephalic or dolichocephalic breeds. An obese patient will require a smaller tube, and an emaciated patient will require a larger tube than a patient of normal conformation that weighs the same.

In view of these variations, the following guidelines can be used to estimate the proper size based on patient body weight. Most adult cats require a 3.5- to 4.5-mm tube, although kittens may require a 2.5- to 3.0-mm tube and very large domestic cats may need up to a 5.0-mm tube. A dog weighing 20 kg will generally require a 9.5- to 10-mm tube. The size should be increased or decreased by approximately 1 mm for each 5 kg of body weight over or under 20 kg. For example, a 7.5- to 8-mm tube should be prepared for a 10-kg patient and a 10.5- to 11-mm tube should be prepared for a 25-kg patient. This guideline applies to canine patients weighing about 10 to 40 kg. (See Table 9.1 for size recommendations.)

Next, determine if the tube is the appropriate length. The endotracheal tube should ideally extend from the tip of the nose to the thoracic inlet. If it is too short, it may not be long enough to reach the trachea at all. If the tube is too long, one of two problems may occur. If inserted too far, the beveled end may advance into only one mainstem bronchus, thus supplying only one lung with oxygen and anesthetic. If inserted only to the thoracic inlet, the portion of the tube extending from the mouth will increase mechanical dead space (Fig. 9.12). Either situation predisposes the patient to hypoventilation and hypoxemia. If a tube of the appropriate length is unavailable, the machine end of the tube can be trimmed, with care being taken to avoid cutting into the cuff inflation apparatus. Endotracheal tubes are further discussed in Chapter 4.

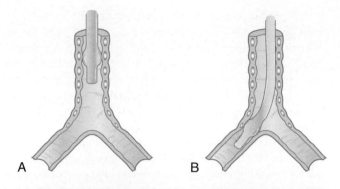
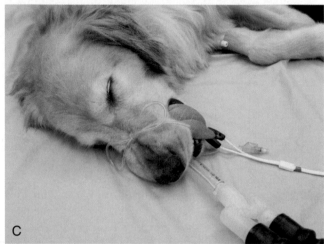

FIG. 9.12 (A) Endotracheal tube placed at the correct distance in the trachea. **(B)** Endotracheal tube advanced too far into the trachea and into the mainstem bronchus. **(C)** Endotracheal tube extending beyond the nasal planum, which increases mechanical dead space.

TABLE 9.1 Recommended Endotracheal Tube Sizes	
Species and Body Weight (kg)	**Tube Size (Internal Diameter [mm])**
Cat	
1	2.5–3
2–4	3.5–4
5 or greater	4–5
Dog	
2	5
4	5.5–6
7	6.5–7
10	7.5–8
15	8.5–9
20	9.5–10
25	10.5–11
30	11.5–12
40	13–14

Preparing the Tube

Before an endotracheal tube is used, it must be checked for integrity. It should be clean, sanitized, and free of blockages, holes, deterioration, or other damage. The connector must be securely attached and the cuff must inflate and hold pressure after the syringe has been detached from the valve. A soft or narrow tube may require use of a stylette that does *not* extend beyond the patient end of the tube to stiffen it during placement. The tube should be lubricated with a small amount of sterile water-soluble lubricant or with the patient's saliva immediately before placement. The use of water-soluble lubricant acts to improve the seal provided by the cuff and so provides increased protection of the airway.

Intubation Procedure

Successful endotracheal tube placement requires knowledge of the anatomy of the pharynx and larynx, including the glottis, epiglottis, vocal folds, and soft palate. (See Fig. 9.13 for a review of the anatomy.) Careful restraint, positioning, and lighting are necessary to maximize visibility of the larynx. Very subtle differences in these factors can make the difference between success and failure. This is especially true in cats. If you cannot easily see the larynx, insist that your assistant alter the position of the patient, the way the head is held, or the lighting until you

TABLE 9.2 Small Animal Oxygen Flow Rate Quick Reference Chart (When Using a Rebreathing System)

Weight (kg)	Maintenance (L/min)[a] (based on 20–40 mL/kg/min; minimum of 0.5 L/min)[b]	Induction, Recovery, and Changes in Anesthetic Depth (L/min) (based on 50–100 mL/kg/min; minimum of 0.5 L/min and maximum of 5 L/min)[b]	Emergency (L/min) (based on 200–300 mL/kg/min; maximum 5 L/min)[b]
3–4	0.5	0.5	0.8
5–6	0.5	0.5	1.5
7–10	0.5	0.7	2
11–15	0.5	1	3
16–20	0.5	1.5	4
21–25	0.8	2	5
26–40	1	2.5	5
41–60	1.5	4	5
61–80	2	5	5
81–100	3	5	5
101–150	4	5	5

[a]Partial rebreathing maintenance flow rates.
[b]Note that suggested flow rates in this table are within the listed range; however, the optimum oxygen flow rate for each patient must be tailored to its unique needs.

TABLE 9.3 Small Animal Oxygen Flow Rate Quick Reference Chart (When Using a Nonrebreathing System)

Weight (kg)	OXYGEN FLOW RATES (L/min)[a]	
	Mapleson A (Magill)[b] Modified Mapleson A (Lack)[b] (based on 100–200 mL/kg/min; minimum of 0.5 L/min)[a]	Modified Mapleson D (Bain Coaxial With no Rebreathing) Mapleson E (Ayre's T-piece) Mapleson F (Norman Mask and Jackson–Rees) (based on 200–400 mL/kg/min; minimum of 0.5 L/min)[a]
1	0.5	0.5
2	0.5	0.8
3	0.5	1
4	0.8	1.5
5–6	1	2
7	1.3	2.5

[a]Note that suggested flow rates in this table are within the listed range; however, the optimum oxygen flow rate for each patient must be tailored to its unique needs. When using a nonrebreathing system, a capnograph should be used on all patients to confirm that inspired CO_2 is less than 5 mmHg. Values exceeding this amount indicate inadequate oxygen flow. If capnometry is not available, the anesthetist should err on the side of the higher end of the range for oxygen flow rates when using a nonrebreathing system.
[b]Controlled ventilation is not recommended with these systems.

can. A failure to do this frequently results in delay, frustration, and inability to intubate the patient successfully. A little time spent optimizing these factors is well worth the effort.

Endotracheal intubation is performed in essentially the same way in both dogs and cats, although it is typically more challenging in cats because of the smaller size of the larynx, decreased visibility, and the predisposition to laryngospasm typical of feline patients.

TECHNICIAN NOTE Readiness of the patient for endotracheal intubation is characterized by:
- Unconsciousness
- Lack of voluntary movement
- Absent pedal reflex
- Sufficient muscle relaxation to allow the mouth to be held open
- No swallowing when the tongue is grasped.

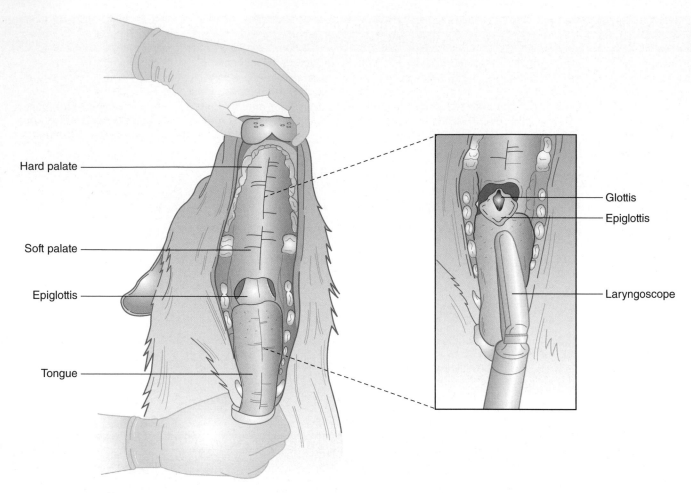

FIG. 9.13 Anatomy of the pharynx. When the epiglottis is depressed, the glottis is exposed *(see inset)*. The endotracheal tube is then advanced through the glottis.

First, prepare the necessary equipment, and prepare the patient for anesthetic induction. Induce anesthesia by IV or IM injection, mask, or chamber until the patient is in a state of readiness for intubation. This requires administration of anesthetic, combined with careful monitoring, until the patient passes through stage II. Readiness for intubation is characterized by unconsciousness, a lack of voluntary movement, an absent pedal reflex, sufficient muscle relaxation to allow the mouth to be held open, and no swallowing when the tongue is grasped. As soon as the patient reaches this point, proceed with intubation.

In most cases, intubation must be performed rapidly and efficiently because the window for successful intubation is short (typically 1 to 2 minutes with injectable protocols and often less than a minute with inhalation protocols). Immediately after intubation, place the patient in lateral recumbency, secure the tube, turn on the oxygen, attach the breathing circuit, cuff the tube, turn on the anesthetic vaporizer, and immediately start monitoring.

With typical protocols (assuming the patient has not been overdosed), many patients are in light stage III anesthesia after intubation, although the stage and plane vary between cases. If the patient is in light stage III anesthesia (as characterized by one or two forceful exhalations immediately after tube placement, strong jaw tone, present palpebral reflex, and in some cases spontaneous movement, swallowing, or chewing), use high oxygen flow and keep the inhalant anesthetic agent on induction level (3% to 5% isoflurane or 4% to 5% sevoflurane) until the patient begins to enter a deeper plane, then immediately decrease the vaporizer setting to a safe level while continuing to monitor. Adjustments are then made in response to monitoring parameters. As soon as the patient's condition is stable, attach any mechanical monitoring devices and prepare the patient for the procedure. Details of the intubation procedure are given and illustrated in Procedure 9.6.

TECHNICIAN NOTE Inadvertent misplacement of the endotracheal tube in the esophagus is common and sometimes not detected because air may appear to move in and out of the tube and reservoir bag, even if the tube is not in the trachea. This will result in an inability to keep the patient anesthetized and possible airway blockage and hypoxemia.

PROCEDURE 9.6 Intubation Procedure for a Dog or Cat

1. Place the patient in sternal recumbency.[a]
2. Have an assistant grasp the patient's maxilla behind the canine teeth, extend the neck, and raise the head so that the head and neck are in a straight line. Be sure the lips and whiskers are pulled dorsally and out of the line of sight. The neck should be propped upright and not allowed to sag. The assistant should not push on the ventral aspect of the neck, head, or throat because this may obscure the view, making intubation difficult.
3. Grasp the tongue with a gauze sponge and open the mouth fully by firmly pulling the tongue out and down (Fig. 1A [dog]; and Fig. 2A [cat]). A mouth gag can be used to hold the mouth open.
4. Adjust the light so that the larynx is well illuminated (Fig. 1B [dog]).
5. If necessary, use the tube or laryngoscope gently to displace the epiglottis ventrally or the soft palate dorsally until the glottis can be visualized[b] (Fig. 1C [dog]; and Fig. 2B [cat]). When using a laryngoscope, press down on the base of the tongue below the epiglottis to aid in visualizing the glottis.
6. Gently insert the tube past the vocal folds using a rotating motion, but *never force the tube!* (Fig. 2C [cat]) If the tube is too large to pass easily, exchange the tube for one of smaller diameter.

7. After the tube has been placed, gently transfer the patient into lateral recumbency.
8. Check the tube to ensure that it is in the trachea. Then check that it is inserted to an appropriate distance and is oriented to match the natural curve of the trachea.
9. Secure the tube in place with a tie (e.g., length of used IV administration set tubing, hard roll gauze, shoelace, or commercial tie designed for this purpose).
10. Position the tongue so that it hangs loosely from the mouth and is not compressed by the tie.
11. Turn on the oxygen flowmeter(s).
12. Connect the endotracheal (ET) tube connector to the breathing circuit.
13. Inflate the cuff and check for leaks.
14. Turn on the anesthetic vaporizer and select the appropriate setting (if maintaining with an inhalant agent).
15. Commence regular monitoring.
16. Ensure a patent airway by checking the position of the patient and tube. The neck and tube should assume a gentle natural curve.

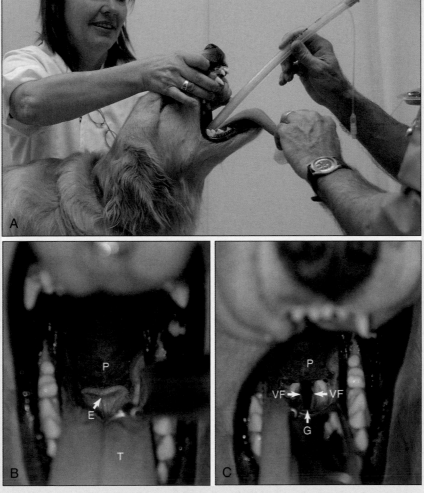

FIG. 1 (A) Proper position for endotracheal intubation in a dog. **(B)** The anatomy of the pharynx and larynx: *E*, epiglottis, which in this view is covering the glottis; *P*, palate; *T*, tongue. **(C)** In this view, the epiglottis has been displaced ventrally with a laryngoscope blade. The glottis *(G)* is visible as the dark, oval opening between the vocal folds *(VF)*, which move apart when the patient inhales and relax as the patient exhales.

Continued

PROCEDURE 9.6   Intubation Procedure for a Dog or Cat—cont'd

FIG. 2 **(A)** Proper positioning for endotracheal intubation in a cat. Note that the assistant uses the fourth and fifth fingers of the hand to grasp the back of the head so that it can be extended upward and toward the anesthetist. This position ensures an optimal view of the larynx. **(B)** The anatomy of the pharynx and larynx: *E,* epiglottis; *G,* glottis; *VF,* vocal folds. **(C)** The endotracheal tube is advanced into the glottis.

ᵃSome anesthetists prefer to position the patient in dorsal recumbency. If this position is used, a laryngoscope held with the handle up is used to displace the epiglottis against the base of the tongue.

ᵇSome anesthetists prefer to intubate dogs blindly (by feel). The patient is placed in lateral recumbency and the tube is passed along the roof of the mouth, over the epiglottis, and into the trachea. If this technique is used, care must be taken to prevent trauma to the delicate tissues of the pharynx and larynx.

Checking for Proper Placement

The entrance to the esophagus lies just dorsal to the entrance to the trachea and although difficult to see, easily accommodates the endotracheal tube. Inadvertent misplacement in the esophagus is common and sometimes not detected because air may appear to move in and out of the tube and reservoir bag even if the tube is not in the trachea. This will result in an inability to keep the patient anesthetized and possible airway blockage and hypoxemia. The following techniques may be used to confirm proper placement in the trachea.

- Revisualize the larynx and confirm that the tube is in the correct location
- Watch for expansion and contraction of the reservoir bag as the animal breathes
- Feel for air movement from the tube connector as the patient exhales or when light, quick pressure is applied to the chest wall
- Watch for fogging of the tube with condensation during exhalation
- Check that the motion of the unidirectional valves coincides with breathing. The inhalation valve should open as the patient inhales and the exhalation valve should open when the patient exhales.
- Connecting a capnograph to the endotracheal tube will reveal an appropriate waveform and end-tidal CO_2 level if the animal is correctly intubated
- Palpate the neck. The trachea is the only naturally firm structure in the neck. If the tube is inside the trachea, only the trachea will be palpable. If the tube is in the esophagus, both the tube and trachea may be palpable. It is not always easy to feel the tube, however, so mastery of this technique requires practice.
- The ability of the patient to vocalize (growl, whine, or cry) indicates a misplaced tube. This is because vocalization requires the vocal cords to vibrate together, which is impossible if the tube is properly placed.
- Many patients, especially if in a light plane of anesthesia, will cough or exhale forcefully during intubation. This is indicative of proper placement, although not all patients exhibit this sign, especially if the anesthetic plane is moderate to deep.

(See Case Presentation 9.1 for an example of the importance of checking the tube for proper placement.)

CASE PRESENTATION 9.1

Julia, a registered veterinary technician, was assigned to prepare for surgery the left rear limb of Caesar, a 42-kg, 6-year-old, male German Shepherd that was undergoing repair of his left cranial cruciate ligament. The patient had been premedicated with 4.0 mg hydromorphone and 0.3 mg dexmedetomidine administered by intramuscular (IM) injection, and anesthesia was induced 15 min later with 180 mg ketamine and 9 mg diazepam by intravenous (IV) injection. A 12-mm internal diameter (ID) endotracheal tube (ETT) was placed and cuffed, and Caesar was placed on 2.5% isoflurane and an oxygen flow rate of 2.5 L/min. At that time, he was assessed to be in stage III surgical anesthesia.

Twenty minutes into the surgical preparation, Julia noticed subtle voluntary movement of Caesar's limbs and shivering, and immediately became concerned that Caesar's anesthetic depth was no longer adequate. A rapid assessment revealed a brisk pedal reflex, swallowing movements, an HR of 170 bpm and an RR of 40 breaths/min.

1. ***What are some possible causes of this sudden change in anesthetic depth?***
2. ***What should Julia do first?***

TECHNICIAN NOTE A capnograph can be used to confirm proper endotracheal tube placement. An appropriate waveform and end-tidal CO_2 level indicate that the tube is properly placed, whereas a "flat line" indicates incorrect placement.

Securing the Tube

The tube is secured in place with a 2-foot-long (60 cm) piece of IV administration set tubing, hard roll gauze, shoelace, or commercial tie designed for this purpose. Tie gauze or a shoelace around the tube near the connector using a surgeon's throw, or IV tubing around the tube using a half-hitch or lark's head knot (Fig. 9.14). Do not place the tie around pilot line (the small tube supplying the pilot balloon). Be sure that the tie is secure enough that it does not slide up or down the tube but not so tight that it compresses the tube, then tie the loose ends over the nose for dolichocephalic dogs or behind the head for cats and brachycephalic dogs with a bow or quick release knot. When properly secured, the tube should not move in or out when manipulated.

Cuff Inflation

Immediately after successful intubation, the cuff of the endotracheal tube must be gently inflated until a seal is formed between the trachea and the cuff. Cuff inflation prevents leakage of anesthetic gases and inhalation of room air, which will result in a variety of complications including contamination of the surgery suite with waste gases and difficulty keeping the patient anesthetized. To inflate the cuff, first extend the patient's head to straighten the airway. Attach an air-filled 6- or 12-mL syringe (dogs) or 3-mL syringe (cats) to the valve port. Have an assistant close the popoff valve and gently compress the reservoir bag, watching the pressure manometer. Listen for gas leakage around the tube, which may sound like a soft hiss or gurgling. For dogs, slowly inflate the cuff until the leaking just ceases at a pressure of 18 to 20 cm H_2O but resumes at higher pressures. In cats, the current standard is to use a 3-mL syringe to sequentially add air in 0.5-mL increments until no leak is heard up to 16 to 18 cm

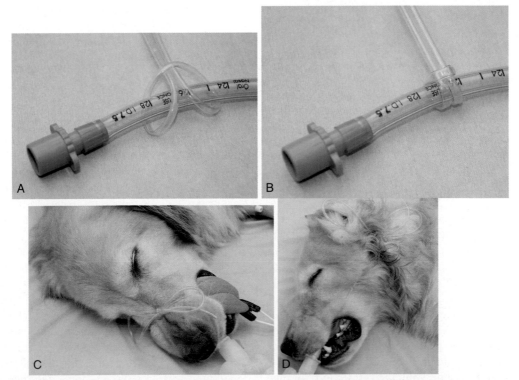

FIG. 9.14 (A) Endotracheal tube (ETT) with intravenous (IV) tubing tie showing the lark's head knot. **(B)** ETT with the lark's head knot pulled tight to prevent the tube from slipping. **(C)** ETT IV tubing tie firmly secured around the nose of a dolichocephalic animal to prevent movement. **(D)** ETT IV tubing tie secured around the back of the head. Used for cats, brachycephalic dogs, and possibly for patients undergoing a COHAT.

H_2O.[b] Avoid overinflation of the cuff, which can result in a variety of mild to serious complications. Inflation should be checked again after 15 or 30 minutes of anesthesia because tracheal diameter may increase as a result of muscle relaxation, or a slow, undetected leak in the cuff or pilot line may cause the cuff to deflate. Even when using care, it can be challenging to achieve the level of cuff inflation required to produce a safe but reliable seal. An ETT cuff pressure manometer such as the Anapnoguard (AG) Cuffill Device (Hospitech Respiration Ltd.) (see Chapter 4, Fig. 4.8), can be used to check that inflation is at the desired level.

Some anesthetists suggest use of a specific volume of air to inflate the cuff or to estimate the inflation by palpating the pilot balloon. These recommendations are very inaccurate indicators of appropriate cuff inflation and in fact, are potentially dangerous because the volume necessary to seal the cuff depends on the relationships among the external diameter of the tube, the internal diameter of the trachea, and the size and type of the cuff, and is thus somewhat different for every patient and anesthetic procedure.

> **TECHNICIAN NOTE** For dogs, slowly inflate the cuff until the leaking just ceases at a pressure of 18–20 cm H_2O but resumes at higher pressures. In cats, use a 3-mL syringe to sequentially add air in 0.5 mL increments until no leak is heard, up to 16–18 cm H_2O. Inflation should be checked again after 15 or 30 min of anesthesia because tracheal diameter may increase as a result of muscle relaxation, or a slow, undetected leak in the cuff or pilot line may cause the cuff to deflate.

Laryngospasm

Laryngospasm is a reflex closure of the glottis in response to contact with any object or substance. This reflex will cause the glottis to close forcibly during intubation. This complication is most commonly encountered in cats (also in swine and small ruminants), especially when under a light plane of anesthesia. It is extremely difficult to place a tube in a patient experiencing laryngospasm because the glottis closes as soon as it is touched with the tube and cannot be forced open without damaging the larynx.

> **TECHNICIAN NOTE** Particular care should be used when intubating cats, which have a narrow glottis that is easily traumatized. Irritation of the larynx during intubation causes laryngospasm, which can occlude the airway if severe.

Laryngospasm is frustrating, makes successful intubation difficult, and in extreme cases, causes hypoxemia and cyanosis. If the patient becomes cyanotic, immediately release the tongue and administer oxygen by mask. In most cases, the cyanosis will quickly resolve. Laryngospasm can be prevented by using one or more of the following strategies.

- Apply no more than 0.1 to 0.2 mL of 2% injectable lidocaine directly to the glottis before placement. Do this by dripping 2 to 4 drops on the arytenoid cartilages with a tomcat catheter attached to a 1-mL syringe. Wait 30 to 60 seconds for the lidocaine to take effect before attempting intubation.

[b]Robertson SA, Gogolski SM, Pascoe P, et al: AAFP feline anesthesia guidelines, *J Feline Med Surg* 20:602–634, 2018.

- Be sure the patient is adequately anesthetized before attempting to intubate the patient because increased anesthetic depth decreases the incidence and severity of laryngospasm.
- Prepare carefully, wait for the glottis to open before attempting placement, and try to get the tube in the first time. Repeat attempts worsen laryngospasm.
- *Never force the tube!* This can lead to severe and potentially life-threatening complications, including tracheal rupture, **pneumothorax**, and **pneumomediastinum**.

> **TECHNICIAN NOTE** When intubating a cat, prepare carefully, ensure that the patient is adequately anesthetized, wait for the glottis to open before attempting placement, and try to get the tube in the first time. *Never force the tube!* This can lead to severe and potentially life-threatening complications including tracheal rupture, pneumothorax, and pneumomediastinum.

Complications of Intubation

A number of hazards are associated with endotracheal intubation (Box 9.5). Most are associated with tracheal irritation, trauma, or failure to protect the airway. Although the mammalian larynx and trachea are relatively resilient structures, excessive force will result in damage, perforation, rupture, or irritation of the delicate mucosa. An endotracheal tube must therefore be chosen, maintained, placed, and monitored with care.

- Intubation may stimulate the vagus nerve and cause an increase in parasympathetic tone, particularly in brachycephalic dogs. This in turn may cause bradycardia, hypotension, and cardiac arrhythmias. Occasionally, cardiac arrest may occur, particularly in an animal with preexisting cardiovascular disease. In some cases, anticholinergics may need to be given in the preanesthetic period help to prevent parasympathetic stimulation.
- Some animals are difficult to intubate. Brachycephalic dogs, for example, have a large amount of redundant tissue within the oral cavity that falls over the back of the pharynx when the animal's mouth is opened, obscuring the glottis. To compound this challenge, these animals must be intubated quickly after induction to prevent airway collapse, so the anesthetist must use all means to facilitate intubation. A laryngoscope is helpful in these patients to increase visibility of the oropharynx, to retract the redundant tissue gently away from the glottis, and to avoid airway trauma during intubation.
- Overzealous efforts to intubate may damage the larynx, pharynx, or soft palate. Particular care should be used when intubating cats, which have a narrow glottis that is easily traumatized. Irritation of the larynx during intubation causes laryngospasm, which can occlude the airway if severe.
- Overinflation of the cuff may cause pressure necrosis of the tracheal mucosa. Cats are particularly sensitive to pressure necrosis from endotracheal tubes, and it is sometimes recommended that uncuffed tubes or tubes with low-pressure cuffs are used with this species. Some anesthetists suggest that if tubes with high-pressure cuffs are used, the cuff should be inflated for no longer than 30 minutes before being deflated and moved slightly to a new location in the trachea. Others suggest that more risk to the patient is caused by moving the

BOX 9.5 Complications of Endotracheal Intubation

Cuff Not Inflated or Underinflated
- Inability to create a seal between the cuff and trachea
- Difficulty with or inability in keeping the patient anesthetized
- Aspiration of stomach contents
- Aspiration of foreign material and fluid during a COHAT
- Pollution of the workspace with anesthetic gas

Tube Diameter Too Small
- Inability to create a seal between the cuff and trachea, leading to the same complications as when the cuff is not inflated
- Small tubes more likely to block with mucus
- Increased resistance to breathing with increased respiratory effort

Cuff Overinflated or Tube Diameter Too Large
- Necrosis of the tracheal mucosa
- Possibility of tracheal rupture in extreme situations

Tube Too Long
- If placed past the thoracic inlet, intubation of only one mainstem bronchus, leading to hypoxemia and difficulty in keeping the patient anesthetized
- If extending beyond the mouth, increased mechanical dead space, leading to hypoventilation and hypoxemia

Tube Too Short
- Inability to intubate the patient successfully
- Displacement of the tube from the glottis if the patient's body position is changed

Overzealous Intubation
- Tracheal irritation, leading to tracheitis and postoperative cough
- Trauma or tracheal rupture, resulting in pneumomediastinum and/or pneumothorax

Tube Kinked or Obstructed
- Dyspnea and hypoxemia
- Asphyxia and cardiac arrest, if not corrected

Tube Not Removed Before Return to Consciousness
- Damage to the tube from chewing
- Blockage of the airway
- In extreme situations, a severed portion of the tube can be aspirated or swallowed

Tube Not Cleaned and Disinfected
- Transmission of infectious agents, leading to tracheitis, bronchitis, or pneumonia
- Blockage of the tube with dried mucus or other foreign material

Adapted from Bassert JM, Beal AD, Samples OM: *McCurnin's clinical textbook for veterinary technicians and nurses,* ed 10, St Louis, 2022, Elsevier.

tube through accidental extubation, inadvertent esophageal intubation, or damage to the tracheal mucosa.

- Endotracheal tubes may become obstructed by saliva, mucus, blood, or foreign material such as gauze. This material may also occlude the patient end of the tube after use, making this a hazard for the next patient if the tube is not cleaned properly. Obstruction may also occur if the tube is kinked or twisted or if the end is occluded against the wall of the trachea. If the endotracheal tube is obstructed for any of these reasons, the patient will not receive oxygen, resulting in hypoxemia.
- Intubated animals require careful monitoring during recovery to ensure that the tube is removed when the animal begins to swallow. If the patient regains consciousness with the tube in place, the patient may chew the tube. In fact, patients can chew the tube in half and aspirate the distal portion into the airway. The presence of such a tracheal foreign body is dangerous, requires bronchoscopy to remove, and is difficult to explain to the owner.
- Although endotracheal tubes used in human patients are routinely discarded after a single use, tubes used in veterinary patients are commonly reused. Tubes must therefore be thoroughly disinfected between patients to prevent the spread of infectious diseases such as canine infectious respiratory disease complex ("kennel cough"). Keep in mind that red rubber tubes soaked in a disinfectant solution for too long or in a solution that is too concentrated will become impregnated with the disinfectant. When next used, the disinfectant may irritate the tracheal mucosa. This can result in coughing after anesthesia or may even cause the tracheal mucosa to slough.
- Despite all precautions, some intubated patients will develop minor irritation of the trachea and larynx. Animal owners should be warned that it is not uncommon for animals to cough for 1 to 2 days after anesthesia if an endotracheal tube has been used.

> **TECHNICIAN NOTE** Despite all precautions, some intubated patients will develop minor irritation of the trachea and larynx. Animal owners should be warned that it is not uncommon for animals to cough for 1–2 days after anesthesia if an endotracheal tube has been used.

Given the problems associated with the use of endotracheal tubes and for reasons of convenience, not all animals undergo endotracheal intubation during anesthesia. If an endotracheal tube is not used, anesthesia may be maintained by use of injectable drugs or by delivery of inhalant anesthetic by mask. Both options have significant disadvantages including inability to manually ventilate the patient and increased waste gas pollution if an inhalant anesthetic is used.

Animals sedated or lightly anesthetized with IM or IV agents for the performance of short procedures may not require the use of an endotracheal tube if the animal maintains the ability to swallow throughout anesthesia and can breathe adequately. In the absence of intubation, the patient must be monitored closely for adequate ventilation (normal respiratory rate [RR] and tidal volume [V_T]) and pulse oximetry should be used to monitor oxygen saturation. Also, the anesthetist should frequently assess the patient to be sure there is no indication of airway obstruction (such as fluid sounds in the airway), and that respiratory effort is normal.

With these exceptions, the animal should be intubated for safety reasons if inhalation anesthetics are used for maintenance or if a lengthy procedure is performed with the patient under injectable anesthesia.

PLACEMENT OF SUPRAGLOTTIC AIRWAY DEVICES

An SGAD is an alternative to an endotracheal tube for maintaining an open airway and transferring anesthetic gases directly from the breathing circuit to the lower respiratory tract (see Chapter 4 for a discussion of SGADs). Like endotracheal tubes, SGADs help to increase efficiency of anesthetic gas delivery, reduce exposure of personnel to waste gas, reduce the risk of aspiration of foreign material, decrease anatomic dead space, and support intermittent positive-pressure ventilation. SGADs also reduce the risk of laryngeal or tracheal trauma and are less likely to induce laryngospasm than conventional endotracheal tubes because they are placed in contact with the tissue surrounding the laryngeal opening instead of the laryngeal and tracheal mucosa directly.

The v-gel advanced SGAD (Docsinnovent) is a veterinary species-specific SGAD designed for use in cats, rabbits, and dogs. The v-gel advanced has specially designed features, including (1) a bowl shape that mirrors the anatomic structure of the larynx and pharynx; (2) a large airway channel; (3) an esophageal plug designed to help prevent regurgitation (in the case of the cat and rabbit v-gel) or a secondary gastric channel (in the case of the dog v-gel) through which a gastric tube can be placed to suction bile and other gastric contents; (4) a low dead space connector; and (5) ridges near the machine end to facilitate placement of a tie (see Chapter 4, Fig. 4.10).

The manufacturer states that the v-gel advanced is quick and easy to place and is useful for a wide variety of procedures, including emergency resuscitation and dental work. Detailed information about v-gel advanced may be found on the manufacturer's website at: https://docsinnovent.com/.

Selection of an appropriately sized v-gel advanced device is based on the species of patient (cat, rabbit, or dog) and lean body weight. The manufacturer recommends placing the patient in sternal recumbency during placement. Safe placement and use of this device require knowledge of specific considerations (detailed in the instructions for use) regarding how it is prepared, placed, and monitored. For example, the patient should be preoxygenated prior to insertion and all outer surfaces should be lubricated with water-soluble lubricant. It is placed by advancing it gently along the hard palate with the open airway channel facing ventrally until it drops into position over the larynx. Proper placement of the v-gel can be confirmed by visualization of a normal capnograph tracing. The patient should be in a surgical plane of anesthesia and topical local anesthetic may be placed on the larynx before insertion. After insertion, the v-gel can be displaced if torque or tension is exerted on it. Consequently, care must be taken to support the breathing circuit and to pay close attention to the position of the tie and the patient's head at all times during the procedure.

A wide range of training resources and support is available at https://docsinnovent.com/technical/ to help users learn to prepare, place, and use the v-gel advanced safely and effectively. The end user should review these materials carefully before using this device.

MAINTENANCE OF ANESTHESIA

After anesthetic induction and endotracheal intubation or placement of an SGAD, patients that are in a light plane of anesthesia must be brought into surgical anesthesia. When the patient reaches the desired anesthetic depth, general anesthesia is maintained with injectable anesthetics, inhalant anesthetics, or a combination thereof. General anesthesia is most commonly maintained with inhalant agents delivered via an anesthetic machine. Less frequently, anesthesia is maintained with either IV boluses approximately every 3 to 8 minutes or a CRI of a short-acting agent such as propofol, or with IM protocols. See Protocol 9.6 for maintenance protocols in dogs and cats, and Procedure 9.7 for details regarding anesthetic maintenance.

Maintenance With an Inhalant Agent

To maintain general anesthesia with an inhalant agent, periodic changes in the vaporizer dial setting must be made on the basis of information derived from physical and machine generated monitoring parameters. Frequent and effective monitoring is paramount so that subtle changes in anesthetic depth are detected in time to make adjustments before the anesthetic depth becomes seriously too light or deep, thus risking that the patient will move or become aware, or will be endangered.

In general, if the anesthetic depth is slightly too light or deep, small dial changes are necessary (about 0.5% to 1% increments with isoflurane and sevoflurane). In contrast, if anesthetic depth is significantly light or deep, large dial changes are necessary. For instance, if the patient's anesthetic depth is significantly light (patient exhibits spontaneous movement, swallowing, active reflexes, strong muscle tone), settings of 3% to 5% isoflurane or 4% to 5% sevoflurane and a high oxygen flow rate are generally necessary to bring the patient back into surgical anesthesia. If the patient's anesthetic depth is significantly too deep (e.g., absent reflexes, flaccid jaw tone, central dilated pupils), then the vaporizer should be turned off, the oxygen flow increased, and the patient monitored carefully until signs of decreased depth are evident. Be aware that these are only general guidelines and each case must be handled differently as circumstances warrant.

Maintenance With Repeat IV Boluses of a Short-Acting Injectable Anesthetic

When maintaining anesthesia with repeat IV boluses of a short-acting injectable anesthetic such as propofol or alfaxalone, frequent and effective monitoring is necessary so that the anesthetist has an accurate assessment of the patient's condition and anesthetic depth. Approximately every 3 to 8 minutes, depending on the agent, additional boluses are administered to effect, often in volumes of approximately one-tenth to one-quarter of that required for induction, as needed to maintain depth at an optimal plane. If the anesthetist is distracted during this process, there is a danger that the patient will unexpectedly awaken in the midst of a procedure, endangering itself and hospital staff.

PROTOCOL 9.6 Maintenance Protocols for Physical Status Class P1 and P2 Dogs and Cats

1. **Isoflurane:** Administer isoflurane at 1.5%–2.5%
2. **Sevoflurane:** Administer sevoflurane at 2.5%–4%
3. **Propofol (IV):** Propofol by repeat boluses to effect approximately every 3–5 min or at a rate of 0.1–0.4 mg/kg/min by constant rate infusion
4. **Alfaxalone (IV):** Alfaxalone by repeat boluses to effect approximately every 6–8 min in dogs or every 3–8 min in cats, or at a rate of 0.1–0.15 mg/kg/min in dogs or 0.11–0.18 mg/kg/min in cats by constant rate infusion
5. **Desflurane:** Administer desflurane at 8%–12%

IV, Intravenous.

PROCEDURE 9.7   Anesthetic Maintenance in a Dog or Cat

General anesthesia is maintained with inhalant or injectable agents. As with anesthetic induction, there are subtleties in the way each agent is handled to ensure that the patient is at an optimum anesthetic depth and is safe. The administration of these agents is summarized here.

Maintenance With an Inhalant Agent
- Choose the initial dial setting appropriate to the anesthetic depth following intubation.
- Make periodic changes in the vaporizer dial setting based on monitoring parameters.
- If the anesthetic depth is slightly too light or deep, make small dial changes of approximately 0.5%–1% increments with isoflurane or sevoflurane.
- If the patient's anesthetic depth is significantly light (e.g., the patient exhibits spontaneous movement, swallowing, active reflexes, strong muscle tone), increase the oxygen flow to 50–100 mL/kg body weight per minute and set isoflurane at 3%–5% or sevoflurane at 4%–5% (induction levels) until signs of increased depth are evident.
- If anesthetic depth is significantly too deep (e.g., absent reflexes, flaccid jaw tone, central dilated pupils), then increase the oxygen flow to 50–100 mL/kg body weight per minute, turn off the vaporizer, bag the patient as needed to support ventilation, and monitor the patient carefully until signs of decreased depth are evident. As soon as depth starts to decrease and the patient is safe, resume the anesthetic.

Maintenance With Repeat IV Boluses of Propofol, Alfaxalone, or Another Short-Acting Agent
- Monitor the patient every few minutes.
- Administer additional boluses as needed to effect, typically every 3–8 min.
- The necessary volume for each bolus varies but is often approximately one-tenth to onequarter of that required for induction.
- Maintain the patient at an optimal plane and avoid overdose.

Maintenance With a Constant Rate Infusion of Propofol or Alfaxalone
- Place an intravenous (IV) catheter, attach an administration set, and begin IV fluid administration.
- Calculate the volume of anesthetic needed to last the anticipated length of the procedure.
- Draw this volume into a syringe.
- Place the syringe in a syringe pump and program in the prescribed infusion rate in milliliters or microliters per minute, or in milliliters or microliters per hour (the manual will indicate accepted units).

- Attach the syringe to the port of a winged infusion set primed with anesthetic to be administered.
- Place the needle of the winged infusion set into the injection port of an IV administration set near the catheter.
- After induction and intubation, start the syringe pump at the calculated rate.
- Based on the results of monitoring parameters, make subtle changes in the infusion rate as needed to maintain the patient in surgical anesthesia.

Induction and Maintenance With an Intramuscular Injection
- Calculate the volume to be administered.
- Administer the agent via the intramuscular (IM) route.
- Place the patient in a quiet area for 15–20 min where it can be monitored.
- After peak effect, check the anesthetic depth and start the procedure if depth is adequate.
- If the anesthetic depth is inadequate, give additional drug intramuscularly or intravenously or administer an inhalant agent by mask.

Maintenance With Concurrent Use of an Inhalant Agent and a Supplemental Injectable Agent
- Place an IV catheter, attach an administration set, and begin IV fluid administration.
- Calculate the volume of the supplemental injectable agent needed to last the anticipated length of the procedure.
- Draw this volume into a syringe.
- Place the syringe in a syringe pump and program in the prescribed infusion rate in milliliters or microliters per minute, or in milliliters or microliters per hour (the manual will indicate accepted units).
- Attach the syringe to the port of a winged infusion set or infusion line primed with the supplemental agent to be administered.
- Place the needle of the winged infusion set into the injection port of an IV administration set near the catheter or into a separate vein.
- After induction and intubation, turn on the vaporizer to an appropriate maintenance rate (this will typically be significantly lower than the percent needed when maintaining with an inhalant agent alone).
- Start the syringe pump at the calculated rate.
- Based on the results of monitoring parameters, make subtle changes in the vaporizer setting and/or the infusion rate as needed to maintain the patient in surgical anesthesia.

No matter how attentive the anesthetist is, patients maintained this way tend to have frequent fluctuations in anesthetic depth, which can be problematic. For this reason, this technique is most appropriate for brief procedures. For patients undergoing prolonged procedures, it is preferable to use a CRI of an injectable agent to maintain anesthesia.

Maintenance With a Constant Rate Infusion

To maintain anesthesia with a CRI, before induction and intubation, a calculated volume of anesthetic is drawn into a syringe large enough to accommodate the anticipated amount needed to maintain surgical anesthesia for the duration of the procedure. The syringe is placed in a syringe pump that has been programmed with an infusion rate based on a calculated dose and attached to a winged infusion set, the needle of which is inserted into the injection port of an IV administration set that is closest to the patient. After induction and intubation, the pump is started, causing the agent to be delivered at a constant rate. Based on results of

monitoring parameters, subtle changes are made in the infusion rate as needed to maintain surgical anesthesia. This method of administration is most suited to propofol and alfaxalone, which do not accumulate in body fat stores because they are rapidly metabolized. Although etomidate can also be used to maintain anesthesia, it is rarely used for this purpose in small animal practice.

Administering an anesthetic as a CRI involves math calculations that are different from those used for bolus administration. This is because unlike calculation of a drug bolus, these calculations involve a unit of time. For instance, the rate used for a CRI of both propofol and alfaxalone is usually expressed in mg/kg/min (e.g., in the case of propofol, the recommended CRI dose is between 0.1 and 0.4 mg/kg/min). Syringe pumps may accept infusion rates expressed in volume (mL)/unit time (hours or minutes), dose (mcg or mg)/unit time (hours or minutes), and/or volume/kg/min, and some are programmed to perform the necessary calculations internally when given the CRI dose. For a pump with this capability, the dose for propofol or alfaxalone, expressed in mg/kg/min, is entered into the machine directly, along with the syringe size and brand (e.g., Monoject, Becton Dickinson), the patient weight, and the drug concentration. *(Note that some pumps detect the syringe size automatically when it is loaded into the pump.)*

Even if the calculations are performed internally by the pump, it is prudent for the anesthetist to manually calculate the volume to be given per unit time so that administration of the drug can be periodically checked to make sure that an error has not been made in machine programming and that the drug is being infused at the correct rate. Errors in calculations or pump programming and startup may result in devastating consequences because drugs given this way often have low therapeutic indices and are dangerous if over- or underdosed. Box 9.6 illustrates the calculations and actions required to prepare and administer an IV anesthetic by CRI via a syringe pump.

Maintenance With Concurrent Use of an Inhalant Agent and a Supplemental Injectable Agent

As an alternative to maintenance of general anesthesia with either an inhalant or an injectable agent, inhalant and injectable agents can be used concurrently, sometimes referred to as balanced anesthesia. This technique involves giving periodic small boluses or administering a low dose CRI of a supplemental injectable agent while also using low vaporizer dial settings of an inhalant agent such as isoflurane. The advantage of this technique is that less of each agent is needed to maintain surgical anesthesia and the adverse effects of both the inhalant and injectable drugs are minimized.

Periodic bolus administration of a supplemental injectable agent during maintenance with an inhalant agent may be used on an as-needed basis to meet specific patient needs. For instance, if a patient shows a response to a painful surgical stimulus or wakes prematurely, small doses of an opioid or other appropriate injectable agent can be given intravenously to rapidly deepen the anesthetic plane.

In contrast, administration of one or more supplemental injectable agents by CRI works well as a strategy to minimize the dose-dependent vasodilatation and resulting hypotension that is frequently observed when using an inhalant agent alone, especially when higher dial settings are necessary to maintain surgical anesthesia. This technique involves choosing one or more injectable agents that provide either additional analgesia or sedation. Drugs that are commonly used in this fashion include the opioid agonists fentanyl, hydromorphone, and morphine, the local anesthetic lidocaine, the dissociative ketamine, and the alpha$_2$-agonist dexmedetomidine. See Protocol 9.7 for supplemental CRI protocols used in PS1 and PS2 dogs and cats to provide additional analgesia or sedation.

BOX 9.6 Calculations and Actions Required to Prepare and Administer an Intravenous Anesthetic by Constant Rate Infusion

Formulas Required to Perform Calculations[a]

Step 1: Calculate the patient body weight (**kg**).
Body weight (kg) = Body weight (lb) ÷ 2.2 (lb/kg)

Step 2: Calculate the drug dose per unit time (**mg/min**).
Drug dose per unit time (mg/min) = BW (kg) × prescribed dose (mg/kg/min)

Step 3: Calculate the volume to be administered per unit time (**mL/min**).
Volume per unit time (mL/min) = Drug dose per unit time (mg/min)/drug concentration (mg/mL)

Step 4: Calculate the estimated total volume to be administered over the duration of the procedure (**mL**).
Total volume (mL) = Volume per unit time (mL/min) × duration (min)

Step 5: Determine the appropriate syringe size.
The size needed should be sufficient to accommodate the sum of the following:
1. The estimated total volume needed to last for the duration of the procedure
2. The volume needed to prime the administration line (fill it with the drug prior to attaching it to the IV catheter—often a minimum of 1–2 mL and sometimes significantly more, depending on the length and diameter of the line)
3. Extra to allow for an increased infusion rate in the event the patient needs a higher dose or an increased infusion volume if anesthetized for a longer time than anticipated

Sample Case:
The anesthetist is asked to use a syringe pump to administer a propofol CRI to a dog undergoing surgery to remove a laryngeal mass.

Assumptions
- Signalment: **35-lb**, mixed breed, 3-year-old male canine
- Anticipated duration of anesthetic maintenance: **30 min**
- Prescribed dose of propofol: **0.15 mg/kg/min**
- Drug concentration: **10 mg/mL**

Performing the Calculations:

Step 1: Calculate the body weight (**kg**).
35 lb ÷ 2.2 (lb/kg) = **15.9 kg**

Step 2: Calculate the propofol dose for this patient (**mg/min**).
15.9 kg × 0.15 mg/kg/min = **2.39 mg/min**

Step 3: Calculate the volume of propofol to be administered (**mL/min**).
2.39 mg/min ÷ 10 mg/mL = **0.24 mL/min**

Step 4: Calculate the estimated total volume to be administered over the duration of the procedure (**mL**).
0.24 mL/min × 30 min = **7.2 mL total over 30 min**

Actions
- **Step 5:** Choose appropriate syringe. The minimum amount needed will be 7.2 mL + 2 mL to prime the line, plus extra in the event more is needed. In this case, it would be prudent to choose a **12-mL syringe** to account for these factors.
- **Step 6:** Fill the syringe with propofol.
- **Step 7:** Attach the winged infusion set or infusion set with needleless connector to the syringe and load the syringe into the pump.
- **Step 8:** Prime the line until it is filled with propofol (being careful that there are no bubbles), then insert the needle or needleless connector into an administration set IV port near the catheter.
- **Step 9:** Program the syringe pump as indicated in the operating instructions. Start the infusion after the patient is induced and intubated. The infusion rate can be adjusted throughout the procedure as needed, based on assessment of anesthetic depth. The anesthetist should check the syringe throughout the procedure to be sure that the correct amount of drug is being administered (which in this case is 0.24 mL/min).

[a]Note: For all calculations, units must match (i.e., all figures involving body weight must be converted to kg; all figures involving prescribed drug doses and concentrations must be converted to either mg or mcg; and all figures involving time must be converted to either minutes or hours.

PROTOCOL 9.7 Supplemental Constant Rate Infusion Protocols Used in PS1 and PS2 Dogs and Cats (To Provide Additional Analgesia or Sedation During Anesthetic Maintenance)

1. **Fentanyl (IV by CRI):** Fentanyl 5–10 mcg/kg/h (following a loading dose of 1–2 mcg/kg)
2. **Hydromorphone (IV by CRI):** Hydromorphone 0.01–0.05 mg/kg/h
3. **Morphine (IV by CRI):** Morphine 0.1–0.2 mg/kg/h
4. **Dexmedetomidine (IV by CRI):** Dexmedetomidine 0.5–1.0 mcg/kg/h
5. **Ketamine (IV by CRI):** Ketamine 0.4–0.6 mg/kg/h

Additional Protocol for Dogs only:

1. **Lidocaine (IV by CRI):** Lidocaine 2–3 mg/kg/h (following a loading dose of 2 mg/kg)

Note: Inhalant anesthetic and injectable anesthetic requirements for maintenance of anesthesia are often considerably reduced when using supplemental CRIs.
CRI, Constant rate infusion; *IV,* intravenous.

Supplemental CRIs may be administered in one of two ways: (1) use of a syringe pump to administer the supplemental drug by CRI through an IV catheter dedicated for this purpose; (2) use of a fluid pump to administer a supplemental drug mixed in a bag of IV crystalloid fluids by CRI.

Use of a Syringe Pump to Administer the Supplemental Drug by Constant Rate Infusion Through an Intravenous Catheter Dedicated for This Purpose

This technique allows the IV fluid and IV drug infusion rates to be controlled independently. When using this technique, the supplemental drug can be titrated—that is, the infusion rate can be changed in response to patient need independently of the IV fluid administration rate. Many analgesic drugs (such as fentanyl, morphine, ketamine, and hydromorphone) as well as drugs used to support cardiovascular function and blood pressure (such as dopamine, dobutamine, phenylephrine, or norepinephrine) are best given this way.

When using this technique, a loading dose of the supplemental injectable drug is prepared (i.e., a relatively high dose intended to raise the blood levels rapidly). Next a CRI dose is mixed with a relatively small volume of 0.9% saline or other diluent (*check a formulary for fluid types that are compatible with the drug you are using*) such that administration of **1 mL/h** of the solution results in administration of **1 mcg/kg/h** (if using a drug commonly dosed in mcg/kg/h, such as the potent opioid analgesic fentanyl and the alpha$_2$-agonist dexmedetomidine). Alternatively, the drug can be mixed with the diluent such that administration of **1 mL/h** of the solution delivers **1 mcg/kg/min** (if using drugs commonly dosed in mcg/kg/min, such as ketamine, dobutamine, and lidocaine). Note that in small patients as well as patients prone to fluid overload, such as cats, it may be necessary to mix the drug at a higher concentration such that administration of 1 mL/h of the solution results in administration of 10 mcg/kg/h or 10 mcg/kg/min. Box 9.7 consists of three examples of how to use the process just described to determine the appropriate mixing ratios of drug and diluent for a CRI of a supplemental drug that can be titrated.

BOX 9.7 Determining Appropriate Mixing Ratios for a Constant Rate Infusion of a Supplemental Drug That Can Be Titrated

Example #1: Canine; 2-Year-Old Male Labrador Retriever; Body Weight 86 lb/39.1 kg
Attending Veterinarian's Orders

- Administer a hydromorphone constant rate infusion (CRI) that can be titrated as part of a multimodal intraoperative analgesia protocol
- Prescribed rate of hydromorphone infusion = **30 mcg/kg/h** with a range of 10–50 mcg/kg/h depending on patient need
- Prescribed IV fluid infusion rate = **196 mL/h** (39.1 kg × 5 mL/kg/h) of IV crystalloid fluids *through a separate IV catheter*[a]

Preparing the Infusion:

- The standard approach to this problem would be to prepare a dilution such that administration of **1 mL/h would deliver 1 mcg/kg/h of the drug**
- At this concentration, the fluid infusion rate of **30 mL/h would be needed to deliver the drug at the required rate (30 mcg/kg/h)**—a rate of fluid administration well within the safe range for this patient as long as the IV fluid infusion rate (given through a separate catheter) is decreased by 30 mL/h (from 196 mL/h to 166 mL/h)

Example #2: Feline; 4-Year-Old Female DSH; Body Weight 8.5-lb/3.9 kg
Attending Veterinarian's Orders

- Administer a dobutamine CRI that can be titrated to manage intraoperative hypotension during a surgical procedure
- Prescribed rate of dobutamine infusion = **3 mcg/kg/min** with a range of 2–5 mcg/kg/min, depending on patient need
- Prescribed IV fluid infusion rate = **12 mL/h** (3.9 kg × 3 mL/kg/h) of IV crystalloid fluids *through a separate IV catheter*

Preparing the Infusion

- The standard approach to this problem would be to prepare a dilution such that administration of **1 mL/h would deliver 1 mcg/kg/min of the drug**
- At this concentration, a fluid infusion rate of **3 mL/h would be needed to deliver the drug at the required rate (3 mcg/kg/min)**—a rate of fluid administration well within the safe range for this patient as long as the IV fluid infusion rate (given through a separate catheter) is decreased by 3 mL/h (from 12 to 9 mL/h)

Example #3: Canine; 8-Year-Old Male Terrier Mix; Body Weight 11 lb/5 kg
Attending Veterinarian's Orders

- Administer a lidocaine CRI that can be titrated as part of a multimodal intraoperative analgesia protocol
- Prescribed rate of lidocaine infusion = **50 mcg/kg/min** with a range of 25–80 mcg/kg/min, depending on patient need
- Prescribed IV fluid infusion rate = **25 mL/h** (5 kg × 5 mL/kg/h) of IV crystalloid fluids *through a separate IV catheter*

Preparing the Infusion

- The standard approach to this problem would be to prepare a dilution such that administration of **1 mL/h would deliver 1 mcg/kg/min of the drug**
- At this concentration, an infusion rate of **50 mL/h would be needed to deliver the drug at the required rate (50 mcg/kg/min)**—a rate of fluid administration significantly too high for a patient this size and that may result in fluid overload
- Consequently, for this patient, an infusion should be created such that administration of **1 mL/h would deliver 10 mcg/kg/min and 5 mL/h would be required to deliver 50 mcg/kg/min**. This rate is safe in this patient without the danger of fluid overload as long as the IV fluid infusion rate (given through a separate catheter) is decreased by 5 mL/h (from 25 to 20 mL/h).

[a]Note: When supplemental drugs are known to be compatible with the IV fluids being administered, they can be given through the same catheter as the crystalloid fluids.

This technique for diluting the drug has a few distinct advantages. First, use of a low infusion rate (i.e., often in the range of 1 to 20 mL/h, depending on the drug and the prescribed dose as well as patient body weight) helps to prevent overhydration in the event that the dose of the supplemental drug infusion rate has to be increased. Second, if the infusion rate needs to be increased or decreased, this can easily be done without revising the CRI calculations. For instance, the dose of the drug can be doubled by doubling the infusion rate or halved by halving the infusion rate. Box 9.8 illustrates the calculations and actions required to prepare and administer an IV supplemental drug by CRI that can be easily titrated.

BOX 9.8   Calculations and Actions Required to Prepare and Administer an IV Supplemental Drug by Constant Rate Infusion That Can Be Titrated

Formulas Required to Perform Calculations[a]

Step 1: Calculate the patient body weight (**kg**).
Body weight (kg) = Body weight (lb) ÷ 2.2 (lb/kg)

Step 2: Calculate the loading dose of the prescribed drug (**mL**).
Loading dose (mL) = BW (kg) × prescribed dose (mg/kg or mcg/kg) ÷ drug concentration (mg/mL or mcg/mL)

Step 3: Choose an appropriate syringe size for the constant rate infusion (CRI) solution.
Assume you will prepare a dilution such that administration of **1 mL/h** would deliver a prescribed dose of **1 mcg/kg/h** or **1 mcg/kg/min**, depending on the specific drug used *(or possibly 10 mcg/kg/h or 10 mcg/kg/min for patients at risk for fluid overload)*.

The syringe size needed should be sufficient to accommodate the sum of the following:

1. The estimated total volume needed to last for the duration of the procedure
2. The volume needed to prime the fluid line (fill it with the drug prior to attaching it to the IV catheter—often a minimum of 1–2 mL and sometimes significantly more, depending on the length and diameter of the line)
3. Extra to allow for an increased infusion rate in the event the patient needs a higher dose or an increased infusion volume if anesthetized for a longer time than anticipated.

Step 4: Determine how long the finished solution will last at the prescribed infusion rate (**hours** or **minutes**).
Maximum infusion time (hours or minutes) = syringe size (mL) ÷ infusion rate (mL/h or min)

Step 5: Calculate the CRI drug dose for this patient in **mcg or mg/h** or **mcg or mg/min**.
Drug dose per unit time (mcg or mg/h or mcg or mg/min) = BW (kg) × prescribed dose rate (mcg or mg/kg/h or mcg or mg/kg/min)

Step 6: Calculate the total amount of drug (**mcg or mg**) that will be needed to last for the maximum infusion time (**hours** or **minutes**) *(see step 4)*
Total drug amount (mcg or mg) = Drug dose per unit time (mcg or mg/h or mcg or mg/min) × maximum infusion time (hours or minutes.)

Step 7: Calculate the total volume of the drug needed (**mL**)
Total drug volume (mL) = Total drug amount (mcg or mg) ÷ drug concentration (mcg/mL or mg/mL)

Step 8: Calculate the volume of saline (**mL**) that should be added to the drug to fill the syringe.
Saline volume (mL) = Syringe size (mL) − Total drug volume (mL)

Sample Case:
The anesthetist is asked to administer a fentanyl CRI to a cat undergoing surgery to provide intraoperative analgesia.

Assumptions
- Signalment: **12-lb**, 5-year-old female DSH

- Anticipated duration of anesthetic maintenance: **60 min (1 hr)**
- Prescribed dose of fentanyl: **Loading dose of 1 mcg/kg IV** followed by a **CRI at a rate of 2.5 mcg/kg/h**
- Drug concentration: **0.05 mg/mL (50 mcg/mL)**
- The fentanyl must be diluted with normal saline such that administration of the finished solution at a rate of **1 mL/h will infuse fentanyl at a rate of 1 mcg/kg/h** (thus a rate of 2.5 mL/h will infuse fentanyl at the prescribed CRI rate of 2.5 mcg/kg/h)

Performing the Calculations

Step 1: Calculate the patient body weight in kg.
12 lb ÷ 2.2 (lb/kg) = **5.5 kg**

Step 2: Calculate the loading dose of fentanyl in mL.
5.5 kg × 1 mcg/kg ÷ 50 mcg/mL = **0.11 mL**

Step 3: Choose an appropriate syringe for the CRI solution.
In this case, a filled **12-mL syringe** would be sufficient (2.5 mL [for the estimated 60 min duration of the procedure] + 1- to 2 mL for priming, + a minimum of 3 to 6 mL in case more is needed).

Step 4: Determine how long the finished solution would last at an infusion rate of 2.5 mL/h.
12 mL ÷ 2.5 mL/h = **4.8 hrs**

Step 5: Calculate the CRI dose of fentanyl for this patient in mcg/h.
5.5 kg × 2.5 mcg/kg/h = **13.75 mcg/h**

Step 6: Calculate the amount of fentanyl (mcg) that will be needed to last 4.8 hrs.
13.75 mcg/h × 4.8 hrs = **66 mcg fentanyl needed to last 4.8 hrs**

Step 7: Calculate the volume of fentanyl needed to last 4.8 hrs.
66 mcg fentanyl ÷ 50 mcg/mL = **1.3 mL fentanyl total**

Step 8: Calculate the volume of saline that should be added to the fentanyl to fill the syringe.
12 mL syringe − 1.3 mL fentanyl = **10.7 mL saline**

Actions

Step 9: Draw up **10.7 mL normal saline** in the 12-mL syringe. Add **1.3 mL fentanyl** to the syringe for a total of 12 mL of finished solution.

Step 10: Attach the fluid line to the syringe and load it into the syringe pump.

Step 11: Prime the line until it is filled with the finished solution (being careful that there are no bubbles), and then attach it to a dedicated IV catheter or port.

Step 12: Program the pump as indicated in the operating instructions and start the infusion at a rate of **2.5 mL/h[b]** after the patient has been induced, intubated, and has received the loading dose. The supplemental CRI infusion rate will be adjusted throughout the procedure as needed based on assessment of reaction to painful stimuli and other monitoring parameters. The anesthetist should check the syringe throughout the procedure to be sure that the correct amount of fentanyl is being administered (which in this case is 2.5 mL/h).

---

[a]Note: For all calculations, units must match (i.e., all figures involving body weight must be converted to kg; all figures involving prescribed drug doses and concentrations must be converted to either mg or mcg; and all figures involving time must be converted to either minutes or hours.
[b]Note that the total amount of IV fluids the patient should receive via an IV fluid pump (separate from the CRI) should ideally be decreased by 2.5 mL/h to adjust for this extra fluid load and minimize the risk of overhydration.

Use of a Fluid Pump to Administer a Supplemental Drug Mixed in a Bag of Crystalloid Fluids IV by Constant Rate Infusion

This technique may be used if the practice does not have a syringe pump. The disadvantage of this approach is that the IV fluid infusion rate and the supplemental drug infusion rate cannot be independently adjusted. The appropriate amount of the supplemental drug to add to the bag is calculated based on a prescribed infusion rate and a fixed IV fluid infusion rate must be used throughout the procedure. If the fluid infusion rate or drug infusion rate needs to be changed, the calculations must be revised and a new mixture prepared, or a separate fluid bag should be used to administer the additional fluids required. In most cases, isotonic replacement crystalloid fluids (e.g., 0.9% saline, lactated Ringer solution, Normosol R) can be used for this purpose, but a formulary should be checked to ensure compatibility of the fluids and the drug. Box 9.9 illustrates the calculations and actions required to prepare and administer an IV supplemental drug mixed in a bag of crystalloid fluids by CRI.

When using this method, it is possible to have flexibility to titrate the infusion rate by calculating and preparing the CRI such that it can be administered at a low rate (e.g., 1 or 2 mL/kg/h) through a separate IV catheter dedicated for this purpose. The patient's remaining fluid needs can be met via a second catheter placed in another vein.

Note that various online CRI calculators and smartphone apps (such as Vetcalculators) that perform CRI calculations are available. For example, the International Veterinary Academy of Pain Management (IVAPM) has an online calculator available at https://ivapm.org/professionals/cri-calculator/. This calculator is designed for administration of individual drugs, including commonly used opioids, lidocaine, and ketamine, as well as for administration of multiple drug CRIs. Because of the high risk associated with incorrectly giving drugs by CRI, it is the technician's or nurse's responsibility to check all calculations before administration, regardless of whether the calculations were performed manually or electronically.

BOX 9.9 Calculations and Actions Required to Prepare and Administer a Supplemental Drug Mixed in a Bag of Crystalloid Fluids IV by Constant Rate Infusion

Formulas Required to Perform Calculations[a]

Step 1: Calculate the patient body weight (**kg**).
Body weight (kg) = Body weight (lb) ÷ 2.2 (lb/kg)

Step 2: Calculate the loading dose of the prescribed drug (**mL**).
Loading dose (mL) = BW (kg) × prescribed dose (mg/kg or mcg/kg) ÷ drug concentration (mg/mL or mcg/mL)

Step 3: Determine the IV fluid infusion rate (**mL/h**).
Fluid infusion rate (mL/h) = Patient body weight (kg) × Prescribed fluid infusion rate (mL/kg/h)

Step 4: Determine how long the solution will last at the prescribed infusion rate (**hours**) based on the volume of the fluid bag.
Maximum infusion time (hours) = fluid bag size (mL) ÷ fluid infusion rate (mL/h)

Step 5: Calculate the CRI drug dose for this patient in **mcg or mg/h** or **mcg or mg/min**.
Drug dose per unit time (mcg or mg/h or mcg or mg/min) = BW (kg) × Prescribed dose rate (mcg or mg/kg/h or mcg or mg/kg/min)

Step 6: Calculate the total amount of drug (**mcg or mg**) that will be needed to last the maximum infusion time (**hours**) *(see step 4)*.
Total drug amount (mcg or mg) = Drug dose per unit time (mcg or mg/h or mcg or mg/min) × maximum infusion time (hours)

Step 7: Calculate the total volume of the drug needed (**mL**)
Total drug volume (mL) = Total drug amount (mcg or mg) ÷ drug concentration (mcg/mL or mg/mL)

Sample Case:
The anesthetist is asked to administer a CRI of the analgesic ketamine to a canine patient undergoing orthopedic surgery by adding it to a bag of IV fluids and administering the resulting solution.

Assumptions
- Signalment: **48-lb**, 4-year-old male Spaniel mix
- Anticipated duration of anesthetic maintenance: **90 min (1.5 hrs)**
- Prescribed intraoperative IV fluid infusion rate: **5 mL/kg/h**
- Volume of fluid bag: **1 L (1000 mL)**
- Prescribed dose of ketamine: **Loading dose of 0.4 mg/kg IV** followed by a **CRI at a rate of 0.4 mg/kg/h (0.0067 mg/kg/min)**

- Drug concentration: **(100 mg/mL)**
- The volume of ketamine that will be added to the bag of fluids must be such that administration of the finished solution at a rate of **5 mL/kg/h will infuse ketamine at a rate of 0.4 mg/kg/h**

Performing the Calculations

Step 1: Calculate the patient body weight in kg.
48 lb ÷ 2.2 (lb/kg) = **21.8 kg**

Step 2: Calculate the loading dose of ketamine in mL.
21.8 kg × 0.4 mg/kg ÷ 100 mg/mL = **0.09 mL**

Step 3: Determine the IV fluid infusion rate in mL/h.
21.8 kg × 5 mL/kg/h = **109 mL/h**

Step 4: Determine how long the bag of fluids will last at an infusion rate of 109 mL/h.
1000 mL in bag ÷ 109 mL/h = **9.2 hr**

Step 5: Calculate the CRI dose of ketamine for this patient in mg/h.
21.8 kg × 0.4 mg/kg/h = **8.72 mg/h**

Step 6: Calculate the amount of ketamine (mcg) that will be needed to last 9.2 hrs.
8.72 mg/h × 9.2 hrs = **80.2 mg ketamine needed to last 9.2 hrs**

Step 7: Calculate the volume of ketamine needed to last 9.2 hr.
80.2 mg ketamine ÷ 100 mg/mL = **0.8 mL total**

Actions

Step 8: Remove 0.8 mL of fluid from the 1 L bag of fluids and discard.

Step 9: Draw up **0.8 mL ketamine** and add it to the 1 L bag of fluids.

Step 10: Label the bag with the following:
Drug name (in this case, "**Ketamine**")
Drug concentration/volume (in this case, "**80 mg/1000 mL**" or "**0.08 mg/mL**")
Time and date the bag was prepared
Initials of the person who prepared the solution

Step 11: Program the fluid pump as indicated in the operating instructions. Start the infusion at a rate of **109 mL/h** after the patient has been induced, intubated, and has received the loading dose. In the event that either the fluid administration rate or drug infusion rate needs to be changed, the calculations must be revised and a new mixture prepared.

---

[a]Note: For all calculations, units must match (i.e., all figures involving body weight must be converted to kg; all figures involving prescribed drug doses and concentrations must be converted to either mg or mcg; and all figures involving time must be converted to either minutes or hours.

TECHNICIAN NOTE The International Veterinary Academy of Pain Management (IVAPM) has an online CRI calculator available at https://ivapm.org/professionals/cri-calculator/. Smart phone apps for CRI calculations are also available. Because of the high risk associated with giving drugs by CRI incorrectly, it is the technician's or nurse's responsibility to check all calculations before administration regardless of whether the calculations were performed manually or electronically.

Maintenance With an Intramuscular Injection

Finally, anesthesia can be induced and maintained with a single IM injection. IM injection offers a flexibility that is unmatched by other anesthetic techniques because the anesthetist is able to select from a wide variety of drugs and doses to produce a combination of effects that can be tailored precisely to meet the patient's needs. Although used for many years for sedation, preanesthesia, and even general anesthesia, IM induction has emerged in recent years as an excellent alternative to IV and inhalant anesthesia by providing balanced anesthesia (premedication, induction, maintenance, analgesia, and muscle relaxation) in a single injection. IM protocols generally produce general anesthesia of relatively short duration (only long enough to perform routine procedures such as spays and castrations). This technique is most commonly used in shelter medicine for elective surgeries in cats. In contrast, when used in general small-animal practice, IM protocols are often supplemented with administration of inhalant agents or IV agents during anesthetic maintenance. Only tranquilizers, alpha$_2$-agonists, opioids, dissociatives, anticholinergics, and alfaxalone can be given intramuscularly. In contrast, propofol and etomidate should be given only by the IV route. Protocol 9.8 lists two examples of IM anesthetic protocols used in PS1 and PS2 cats.

TECHNICIAN NOTE Any time an intubated patient is turned over, the endotracheal tube should be temporarily disconnected from the anesthetic circuit. Rolling or twisting the animal while it is still connected to the circuit may cause the endotracheal tube to twist and collapse, resulting in an airway obstruction, or may cause the distal end of the tube to traumatize or lacerate the trachea.

PROTOCOL 9.8 Intramuscular Anesthetic Protocols for PS1 and PS2 Cats

1. **Dexmedetomidine–ketamine–butorphanol (IM):** Dexmedetomidine 0.02–0.03 mg/kg with ketamine 3–5 mg/kg and butorphanol 0.2 mg/kg IM for elective surgeries
2. **"TTDex" (telazol–butorphanol–dexmedetomidine) (IM):** Add 2.5 mL butorphanol (10 mg/mL) and 2.5 mL dexmedetomidine (0.5 mg/mL) to 1 vial of Telazol powder. The final mixture contains 100 mg/tiletamine-zolazepam, 0.25 mg dexmedetomidine, and 5 mg butorphanol/mL of the mixture. Give at a rate of 0.015 mL/kg IM for castration and 0.02 mL/kg IM for ovariohysterectomy.

IM, Intramuscular.

PATIENT POSITIONING, COMFORT, AND SAFETY

During anesthetic induction and maintenance, a number of considerations must be observed to ensure that the patient is not harmed.

- During induction, the animal should be supported as it loses consciousness. Particular care should be taken to be sure that the animal does not strike its head on the table during induction or transfer to surgery.
- After IV induction, as soon as the patient is intubated, remove the needle and syringe to avoid accidental overdose in the event that the syringe plunger is accidentally pushed while the patient is being moved
- Immediately after intubation, place the patient in lateral recumbency, then secure and cuff the tube
- Before preparing the patient for surgery, the anesthetist must ensure that the patient's endotracheal tube is correctly placed (i.e., in the trachea) and that the cuff is functional and inflated. Once the surgical preparation begins, it is difficult to reposition the animal to allow reintubation without compromising aseptic technique.
- Check the endotracheal tube for kinks or bends. An open airway must be maintained at all times (Fig. 9.15).
- Any time an intubated patient is turned over, the endotracheal tube should be temporarily disconnected from the anesthetic circuit. Rolling or twisting the animal while it is still connected to the circuit may cause the endotracheal tube to twist and collapse, resulting in an airway obstruction, or may cause the distal end of the tube to traumatize or lacerate the trachea. This risk is of most concern in feline patients.
- The hoses of the anesthetic machine should be supported so that there is no drag on the endotracheal tube, which could result in tracheal trauma or displacement of the tube. Displacement is of particular concern when using an SGAD.
- The position of the hoses and endotracheal tube should be checked during patient transfer and after repositioning. Hyperflexion of the neck should be avoided because it may lead to endotracheal tube obstruction.

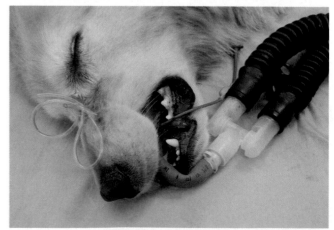

FIG. 9.15 The endotracheal tube is kinked and the airway is blocked because of the position of the breathing tubes in relation to the position of the patient.

- The reservoir bag should be placed so that it is clearly visible at all times
- When positioning the animal on the surgery table, the anesthetist should ensure that the animal assumes as normal a posture as possible. In particular, hyperextension or hyperflexion of the limbs should be avoided because either may result in permanent neurologic injury.
- Heavy drapes or instruments must not compress the chest of a small patient because they may interfere with respiration
- Do not overtighten leg restraint ropes or circulation may be compromised.
- Place the patient on a heat-retaining surface designed for veterinary use such as a warm-water circulating blanket. Do *not* use an electric heating pad, which can burn the patient!
- If one lung is diseased, place the normal side up whenever possible to maximize oxygen exchange.
- Tilting the surgery table so that the patient's head is down gives the surgeon easier access to some abdominal organs, particularly the uterus and ovaries. However, the anesthetist should be aware that more than a 15-degree elevation of the caudal aspect of the body may cause the abdominal organs to compress the diaphragm, which may compromise heart and lung function. Head-down, tilted positions should be avoided entirely in animals with breathing difficulties, especially those with diaphragmatic hernias.
- Artificial tear solution or other corneal lubricant should be instilled into the eyes of an anesthetized patient every 2 to 4 hours unless the patient is undergoing ocular surgery. This is particularly important if an anticholinergic is used. General anesthesia decreases tear secretion for a period of up to 24 hours after anesthesia and some dogs may need periodic application of a corneal lubricant for up to 36 hours after recovery. Cats maintain some tear production throughout anesthesia; however, lubrication is advisable if an anticholinergic or ketamine is given.

> **TECHNICIAN NOTE** Artificial tear solution or other corneal lubricant should be instilled into the eyes of an anesthetized patient every 2–4 hrs. General anesthesia decreases tear secretion for a period of up to 24 hrs after anesthesia, and some dogs may need periodic application of a corneal lubricant for up to 36 hrs after recovery.

ANESTHETIC RECOVERY

The anesthetic recovery period may be defined as the period between the time the anesthetic is discontinued and the time the animal is able to stand and walk without assistance. The length of the recovery period depends on many factors, including the following:

- The length of the anesthetic period. As a general rule, the longer the patient is under anesthesia, the longer the expected recovery.
- The condition of the patient. Lengthy recoveries are seen in animals that have almost any debilitating disease (particularly liver and kidney disease).
- The type of anesthetic given and the route of administration. Lengthy recoveries are more common if an injectable agent is given intramuscularly rather than intravenously.
- The patient's temperature. Hypothermic patients are slow to metabolize and excrete anesthetic drugs.
- The breed of the patient. Certain dog breeds (e.g., Greyhounds, Salukis, Afghan Hounds, Whippets, and Russian Wolfhounds) may be slow to recover from certain anesthetic agents such as propofol.

Anesthetist's Role in the Recovery Period

The anesthetist's intraoperative duties toward the patient does not end until the patient is awake, alert, normothermic, and ambulatory (unless nonambulatory prior to the procedure). On completion of the procedure, the patient should be transferred to a recovery area where it can be monitored. A crash cart, monitoring equipment, materials for intubation, and oxygen should be readily available. The anesthetist must remain vigilant during recovery because this is often one of the most dangerous periods, even for animals that have had no problems during induction or maintenance.

During anesthetic recovery, the anesthetist must fulfill each of the following responsibilities:

- Discontinue administration of all anesthetic agents
- Monitor the patient on a continual basis
- Administer oxygen as necessary
- Administer reversal agents (see Protocol 9.9 for reversal agent protocols in dogs and Protocol 9.10 for reversal agent protocols in cats)
- Maintain a patent airway and extubate the patient at the appropriate time
- Provide general nursing care (reassure the patient, provide patient hygiene, warm the patient, and prevent self-injury)
- Provide adequate analgesia and administer other medications as requested by the veterinarian

Procedure 9.8 shows the sequence of events during the recovery period.

> ### PROTOCOL 9.9   Reversal Agent Protocols for Dogs
>
> 1. **Atipamezole:** Administer IM according to the following dosage guidelines. Give IV only for emergency resuscitation. To reverse the effects of dexmedetomidine, administer atipamezole IM at a 1:10 agonist: antagonist ratio (0.01 mg/kg dexmedetomidine is reversed with 0.1 mg/kg atipamezole). This means that equal volumes of Dexdomitor (0.5 mg/mL) and Antisedan should be administered. The volume of Antisedan needed to reverse the effects of Dexdomitor 0.1 is approximately one-fifth the volume of Dexdomitor 0.1 given.
> 2. **Naloxone:** To reverse the effects of opioids, administer naloxone at a dose of 0.01–0.02 mg/kg IM or by slow IV injection. If renarcotization occurs, additional doses may be needed.
> 3. **Flumazenil:** To reverse the effects of benzodiazepine toxicity, administer flumazenil at a dose of 0.01 mg/kg by slow IV injection. Repeat every hour if needed.
> 4. **Yohimbine:** To reverse the effects of xylazine, administer yohimbine slowly IV at a 10:1 agonist:antagonist ratio (1 mg/kg xylazine is reversed with 0.1 mg/kg yohimbine).

PROTOCOL 9.10   Reversal Agent Protocols for Cats

1. **Atipamezole:** Administer intramuscularly according to the following dosage guidelines. Because of marked side effects, atipamezole should not be given intravenously except when necessary for emergency resuscitation. To reverse the effects of dexmedetomidine, administer atipamezole intramuscularly to cats at a 1:6 agonist:antagonist ratio (0.01 mg/kg dexmedetomidine is reversed with 0.06 mg/kg atipamezole)[c]. Note that the manufacturer recommends a 1:10 agonist:antagonist ratio in cats (the same dose as that used for dogs).
2. **Naloxone:** To reverse the effects of opioids, administer naloxone at a dose of 0.01–0.02 mg/kg intramuscular (IM) or by slow intravenous (IV) injection. If renarcotization occurs, additional doses may be needed.
3. **Flumazenil:** To reverse the effects of benzodiazepine toxicity, administer flumazenil at a dose of 0.01 mg/kg by slow IV injection. Repeat every hour if needed.
4. **Yohimbine:** To reverse the effects of xylazine, administer yohimbine slowly intravenously at a dose of 0.1 mg/kg.

PROCEDURE 9.8   Recovery From General Anesthesia in a Dog or Cat

1. Prepare the patient for recovery, including removal of drapes, any other equipment used for the procedure, and monitoring equipment.
2. Prepare a cage without food, water, a litter pan, or anything else that has the potential to cause injury to the patient during the recovery period.
3. Discontinue the anesthetic but continue administering oxygen at a rate of 50–100 mL/kg/min up to a maximum of 5 L/min for 5 min or until the patient is extubated (whichever comes first).
4. Continue measures to normalize body temperature until it is ≥98°F (36.7°C).
5. Transfer the patient to the recovery area or cage, paying attention to positioning so that an open airway is maintained, and continue monitoring.
6. Deflate the cuff, untie the endotracheal tube, and extubate the patient at the appropriate time. Ensure that the airway is open and the patient is breathing without difficulty.
7. Calm and reassure the patient. Turn the patient every 10–15 min. Take precautions to prevent self-trauma or injury.
8. As soon as it is clear that the patient is recovering normally, ask the attending veterinarian whether continued intravenous (IV) access is needed for ongoing care. When and if ordered by the attending veterinarian, stop fluid administration and remove the IV catheter.
9. Prepare the patient for continued hospitalization or discharge by applying bandages, administering medications, and performing any other procedures ordered by the doctor.
10. When the patient is able to remain in sternal recumbency unsupported, return the patient to the cage (if not already done) and close the cage door securely.
11. Check body temperature as well as vital signs and other indicators of general wellness at least one more time within the first few hours after return to the wards.

TECHNICIAN NOTE During recovery, it is important to monitor carefully. This is often one of the most dangerous periods, even for animals that have had no problems during induction or maintenance.

---

[c]Lemke KA: Anticholinergics and sedatives. In Tranquilli WJ, Thurmon JC, Grimm KA, editors. *Lumb & Jones' veterinary anesthesia and analgesia,* ed 4, Ames, IA, 2007, Blackwell, pp 225–227.

Signs of Recovery

An animal recovering from general anesthesia gradually progresses back through the anesthetic stages and planes. As the animal moves from deep to moderate to light anesthesia, vital signs and reflexes change in predictable ways. The heart rate, respiratory rate, and respiratory volume increase. After assuming a ventromedial position, as is usually the case during surgical anesthesia, the eyeballs move back to a central position. Reflex responses return, and muscle tone strengthens. The animal may shiver, swallow, chew, or attempt to lick. Shortly after swallowing reflexes return, the animal will normally show signs of consciousness, including voluntary movement of the head or limbs and possibly vocalization.

While passing through stage II, some patients may exhibit a variety of alarming signs, including head bobbing, delirium, mydriasis, hyperventilation, head thrashing, and rapid limb paddling, especially if not premedicated. Occasionally, a patient may attempt to stand and fall, or may appear blind and bump into the sides of the cage. Some patients (particularly those recovering from ketamine anesthesia) may chew at their paws or claw their faces. Animals showing these signs of a rough or stormy recovery usually return to normal within a short time, but these signs should not be ignored and steps must be taken to prevent self-trauma or disruption of the surgical wound. Administration of preanesthetic medications before the procedure often prevents or moderates these signs, but additional tranquilization or administration of analgesics during the postoperative period may be necessary in these patients.

TECHNICIAN NOTE During recovery, the patient must be watched continuously at close range because a recovering animal may develop hypoxemia, cardiac arrhythmias, or other complications, yet show no signs that are evident to the casual observer.

Monitoring During Recovery

During recovery, the patient must be watched continuously at close range because a recovering animal may develop hypoxemia, cardiac arrhythmias, or other complications, yet show no signs that are evident to the casual observer. Evaluation from across the room is not acceptable because problems such as vomiting, chewing the tube, and airway occlusion occur with some regularity and must be managed without delay to prevent serious consequences. These problems are discussed in detail in Chapter 13.

To minimize these risks, the patient should be positioned in the cage so that mucous membranes and respiration can be observed. Vital signs should be evaluated at least every 5 minutes. Ideally, the patient should be monitored with a pulse oximeter during the recovery period and a capnograph up until extubation.

Abnormal vital signs or a delayed return to consciousness may indicate a variety of serious conditions that must be treated promptly by the veterinarian, such as shock, hemorrhage, hypoglycemia, or hypothermia. See Box 9.10 for ACVAA monitoring guidelines for the recovery period.

BOX 9.10 American College of Veterinary Anesthesia and Analgesia Monitoring Guidelines for the Recovery Period

The objective of the American College of Veterinary Anesthesia and Analgesia (ACVAA) monitoring guidelines for recovery is "to ensure a safe and comfortable recovery from anesthesia." To accomplish this, the ACVAA makes the following recommendations: "Monitoring in recovery should include at the minimum evaluation of pulse rate and quality, mucous membrane color, respiratory pattern, signs of pain, and temperature."

Note that the 2020 Anesthesia and Monitoring Guidelines also recommend use of a pulse oximeter during the recovery period and capnograph up until extubation.

Oxygen Therapy

As soon as the anesthetic depth decreases sufficiently, most recovering patients begin to shiver. Shivering is a protective response to hypothermia that raises the body temperature. During shivering, contracting muscle tissue converts oxygen and chemical fuel into heat. Consequently, muscle contractions associated with shivering increase oxygen consumption. Oxygen administration during recovery is necessary to meet these needs and to compensate for residual respiratory depression until anesthetic depth decreases.

TECHNICIAN NOTE Recovering patients often consume more oxygen as a result of shivering. Oxygen administration during recovery is necessary to meet these needs.

Oxygen should be administered via the endotracheal tube at a rate of 50 to 100 mL/kg/min (up to a maximum of 5 L/min) for 5 minutes after discontinuation of the anesthetic or until the animal swallows. This route of administration allows exhaled anesthetic gases to be scavenged and gives the anesthetist the ability to bag the patient during recovery to help reinflate collapsed alveoli.

If the patient is at a light depth of anesthesia and must be extubated, oxygen can be administered by mask. Some patients do not tolerate a mask without becoming agitated, however, and may require an alternative means of oxygen delivery. The following options are alternatives to the use of a mask during the postoperative period.

- An oxygen source such as the Y-piece or the fresh gas inlet of a nonrebreathing system can be placed near the nasal openings
- An Elizabethan (E-)collar can be placed around the patient's neck with an oxygen line secured to the inside of the collar. The front of the collar is covered with cellophane, with a small ventilation hole. A flow rate of 1 L/min provides approximately 30% to 40% oxygen.
- Oxygen can be delivered via a nasal catheter. A lubricated soft red rubber catheter (5- to 10-French, depending on the size of the patient) is introduced into the ventral nasal meatus. Intranasal proparacaine or 2% lidocaine can be used to desensitize the nasal tissues to allow insertion. The catheter is advanced to the level of the carnassial teeth and attached to the dorsum of the nose with tissue glue (cyanoacrylate). A

flow rate of 100 to 150 mL/kg provides approximately 30% to 50% oxygen. Alternatively, nasal prongs used in human hospitals may be used. They can be secured to the patient with tissue glue or staples.
- The patient can be placed in an oxygen cage

Note that a patient that is intubated and breathing oxygen from an anesthetic machine receives close to 100% oxygen. This is beneficial for the relatively short duration of most procedures, but prolonged inhalation of high levels of oxygen (e.g., greater than 50% oxygen for more than 24 hours) can be toxic.

Extubation

To prepare the patient for extubation, deflate the cuff by drawing out all the air until the pilot balloon is empty. Untie the tube so that it can be rapidly removed. At all times during recovery, keep the patient's neck in a natural but extended position to protect the airway. Some anesthetists prefer to deflate the cuff and untie the gauze or tubing before signs of arousal are seen so that the tube can be quickly removed when swallowing occurs.

As soon as the patient shows signs of imminent arousal, the endotracheal tube must be removed using a slow, steady motion. In dogs, return of the swallowing reflex is the most appropriate time to remove the tube because this reflex will help protect the animal from pulmonary aspiration if vomiting occurs during recovery. Animals that show voluntary limb, head, or chewing movements are close to consciousness, however, and should be extubated even if swallowing has not been observed. These patients typically swallow on removal of the endotracheal tube.

A notable exception to this general rule is brachycephalic dogs. In these patients, many anesthetists prefer to delay extubation until the patient is able to lift its head unassisted because early extubation may lead to respiratory distress from upper airway obstruction. In these patients, it is wise to prepare by having a laryngoscope, endotracheal tubes (the same size as used during the procedure and one size smaller), and the appropriate dose of a short-acting IV induction agent such as propofol or alfaxalone nearby in case reintubation is necessary.

If a recovering patient shows signs of respiratory distress after extubation, the anesthetist must determine whether this is because of pulmonary disease (in which case oxygen therapy may be needed) or upper airway obstruction. One helpful clue is that upper airway obstruction is often associated with *stridor* (noisy respiration), especially on inspiration. If obstruction is present, the anesthetist should reposition the patient and gently pull the tongue forward. If the obstruction persists, it may be necessary to reinduce and reintubate the patient.

With cats, the endotracheal tube may be removed when signs of impending arousal are observed. These include swallowing, an active palpebral reflex, and voluntary limb, tail, or head movements. Delaying extubation is not advisable with cats because it may predispose the patient to laryngospasm.

> **TECHNICIAN NOTE** After a COHAT, oral surgery, or any other procedure in which blood or other fluids are present in the oral cavity, the patient should be positioned with the nose slightly lower than the neck to allow drainage of secretions, blood, and debris away from the trachea. The cuff may be left partially inflated during removal to sweep out the fluid and prevent it from entering the airways.

> **TECHNICIAN NOTE** A recovering patient should be turned every 10–15 min to prevent pooling of blood in the dependent lung and tissues—a condition called *hypostatic congestion.*

After a COHAT, oral surgery, or any other procedure in which blood or other fluids are present in the oral cavity, the patient should be positioned with the nose slightly lower than the neck to allow drainage of secretions, blood, and debris away from the trachea. The cuff may be left partially inflated during removal to sweep out the fluid and prevent it from entering the airways. After extubation, all animals should be placed in lateral or sternal recumbency with the neck extended. This position helps maintain a patent airway. Occasionally, fluid or mucus may accumulate in the pharynx or trachea and must be removed by suction. The anesthetist should do this before the patient is fully awake to avoid being bitten.

POSTANESTHETIC PERIOD

In the postanesthetic period, patients require general nursing care to ease recovery, ensure their safety, and prepare them for return to the hospital ward. The anesthetist should be sensitive to the fact that the animal has no means of understanding the events that have produced the disorientation, fear, and discomfort that often accompanies the return to consciousness. Quiet, calm handling; reassurance; and attention to the patient's comfort level are therefore essential.

The anesthetist can take several steps to minimize patient discomfort during recovery. All ties restraining the animal to the surgery table should be removed before the animal regains consciousness. The anesthetist should ensure that all accessory procedures, such as bandaging, chest tube placement, and urinary catheterization, have been completed, and that all monitoring equipment probes, cuffs, and electrocardiographic electrodes have been removed. The anesthetist should also be gentle when moving a recovering patient so as not to increase discomfort and pain.

The IV catheter should be left in place until the endotracheal tube has been removed and it is clear that the patient is recovering normally. This provides venous access in the event that the patient's current condition or an unexpected complication necessitates administration of IV drugs or fluids.

Patient recovery may be hastened by gentle stimulation in the form of talking softly to the patient, gently patting or rubbing the chest, turning the patient, or gently moving the endotracheal tube. These actions stimulate breathing and increase the flow of information to the reticular activating system (RAS) of the brain—the area responsible for maintaining consciousness in the awake animal. A lack of stimulation of the RAS may cause drowsiness in the conscious animal. It is therefore speculated that stimulation of this area may help the animal to awaken.

A recovering patient should also be turned every 10 to 15 minutes to prevent pooling of blood in the dependent lung and tissues—a condition called hypostatic congestion. When the intubated patient is turned from one side to another, the breathing circuit must be briefly detached from the endotracheal tube or SGAD, and the head and neck should be turned as a single unit to minimize the risk of tracheal damage by the tube. Although not proven, there may be a risk of causing the stomach to twist if a patient is turned by moving the limbs over the body from one side to the other. For this reason, some anesthetists recommend turning a patient by sliding the limbs under the body instead, especially if the patient is a member of a breed prone to gastric dilatation–volvulus.

Never leave a recovering patient in an open cage or on a table unattended because once spontaneous movement returns, a recovering patient may fall and be injured. Food and water should not be left in the cage during recovery because it is possible for a recovering animal to drown in a water bowl or suffocate in a food bowl. Some patients may be able to drink soon after standing; however, most have little appetite for food for several hours after recovery. Vomiting during the recovery period is not uncommon, but provided that the patient is conscious and has a swallowing reflex, this is seldom dangerous.

Nursing care of hypothermic patients should include the provision of heat. This can be accomplished by a variety of means including warm air or water blankets and incubators. Never use electric heating pads, which have a significant potential to burn a recovering patient. Box 9.11 lists strategies recommended to normalize body temperature. Recovering patients are unable voluntarily to move away from a heat source if it is excessive; therefore the anesthetist must prevent burns by ensuring that the heat source never exceeds 42°C (approximately 107.6°F). Gradual rewarming is preferred to rapid rewarming because the latter may cause dilation of cutaneous vessels, leading to hypotension and afterdrop (worsening of hypothermia due to shunting of cool blood from the extremities to the core).

Analgesics should be administered as requested by the veterinarian, preferably before the onset of pain (see Chapter 8).

BOX 9.11 Acceptable Strategies to Normalize Body Temperature for Recovering Patients[a]

- Provide ample bedding
- Dry the patient's haircoat with a hairdryer on low heat
- Place warm towels over the patient
- Wrap the patient in a forced warm air blanket
- Use an in-line intravenous (IV) fluid warmer
- Place the patient on a circulating warm water blanket
- Avoid excessive oxygen flow rates
- Place the patient in an incubator designed for human babies

[a]Note that heat sources should never exceed 42°C (107.6°F).

If analgesia is adequate, the patient should be able to sleep comfortably and should demonstrate minimal signs of discomfort. A change in the dose or frequency of administration or use of a different or additional agent may be necessary if postoperative pain is not well controlled.

After recovery, the anesthetist must provide ongoing care and prepare the patient for release or continued hospitalization.

Most small-animal patients should be given nothing by mouth for the first hour or two and no food for at least several hours. On discharge, the client should be instructed to reintroduce water gradually after arriving home and to feed a small meal after several hours. Exceptions to these guidelines include very small and neonatal patients, which require reintroduction of water and food more rapidly.

■ KEY POINTS

1. Small-animal patients are restrained and anesthetized with a variety of techniques, but general anesthesia is most commonly selected for many procedures. In many practices, IV, or IM induction followed by maintenance with an inhalant agent is most commonly employed.

2. General anesthesia can be divided into the following periods: preanesthesia, induction, maintenance, and recovery. Traditionally, anesthetic depth during general anesthesia has been described in terms of stages and planes of anesthesia, with the surgical plane of stage III being suitable for most surgical procedures.

3. When a protocol is being selected, great care must be used in calculating drug dosages, oxygen flow rates, and fluid administration rates, and in drawing up and administering anesthetic agents and adjuncts.

4. To anesthetize a patient safely and effectively, the anesthetist must have a clear understanding of the expected sequence of events and dynamics associated with each anesthetic technique.

5. Equipment must be carefully prepared before anesthetic induction- because once induction commences, the anesthetist has little to no time to gather missing equipment.

6. The goal of anesthetic induction is to take the patient from consciousness to stage III anesthesia smoothly and rapidly. This requires finesse, watchfulness, and an ability to make decisions rapidly and act quickly on the basis of patient monitoring parameters.

7. IV induction agents are most often given to effect by using a process called *titration*. When inducing anesthesia by IV injection, in general, the entire calculated dose should not be administered at once.

8. Mask and chamber inductions involve risks of which the anesthetist must be aware to prevent serious complications. Vigilant patient monitoring is required when these methods are used.

9. There are many advantages to endotracheal intubation or SGAD placement that justify these techniques, even in patients anesthetized only with injectable drugs.

10. Successful and safe endotracheal intubation requires careful preparation, excellent technique, and watchfulness for potential complications.

11. General anesthesia can be maintained with inhalant agents, repeat IV boluses of short-acting injectable anesthetics, constant rate infusion, concurrent use of an inhalant agent and a supplemental injectable agent, or IM techniques.

12. Supplemental CRIs are most commonly used to administer analgesic drugs as well as drugs used to support cardiovascular function. CRIs can be administered by use of a syringe pump attached to a dedicated IV catheter or port or by adding the supplemental injectable drug to a bag of IV fluids.

13. Patient positioning, comfort, and safety must be considered during anesthetic maintenance to avoid problems such as traumatic injury, accidental overdose, airway blockage, hypoxemia, circulatory compromise, burns, hypostatic congestion, and corneal drying.

14. The length of the recovery period depends on many factors, including the anesthetic protocol and the patient's condition. Return to consciousness is accompanied by increasing heart and respiratory rates, increased reflex responses, and voluntary movement.

15. During the recovery period, the anesthetist must continue to monitor the patient's vital signs, including temperature, as anesthetic complications commonly occur during this period. It is advisable to administer oxygen for 5 minutes after the anesthetic has been discontinued or until the patient has been extubated.

16. In dogs, extubation should occur when the swallowing reflex returns. In cats, extubation should occur when the patient shows signs of impending arousal, such as voluntary movements, swallowing, or active reflexes.

17. Other duties during recovery include stimulation of the patient, administration of oxygen, provision of postoperative analgesia, and general nursing care.

18. Anesthetic safety is improved through the use of preanesthetic agents, use of the minimum effective dosages, selection of a protocol well suited to the patient, and close monitoring of the patient.

REVIEW QUESTIONS

1. Consider the following scenario: You are performing a procedure on a canine patient that you feel is at an appropriate anesthetic depth. If using sevoflurane in this patient, which of the following settings would be within the usual accepted range of maintenance rates?
   a. 2%
   b. 2 L/min
   c. 3.5%
   d. 4 mL/min
   e. 5%

2. Which of the following statements about how to induce anesthesia in a young, healthy patient using an IV agent such as alfaxalone or propofol is least accurate?
   a. If, after giving the initial amount, the patient is not adequately anesthetized to allow intubation, give the rest of the calculated dose
   b. Draw up the calculated dose, give about one-quarter to one-half first, and give the rest to effect
   c. You must be sure the drug gets in the vein
   d. These agents may be given through an IV administration set injection port

3. Which of the following statements regarding IV induction agents is least accurate?
   a. Ketamine–diazepam takes slightly longer to act and lasts somewhat longer than propofol
   b. When using propofol, give about 25% to 50% of the calculated dose every 30 seconds to effect
   c. Sick, old, or debilitated patients often require significantly lower doses of injectable anesthetics
   d. Propofol is generally given intravenously for anesthetic induction, but it can be given intramuscularly in uncooperative patients

4. Which of the following agents is not an analgesic commonly administered as a CRI to control pain?
   a. Ketamine
   b. Dexmedetomidine
   c. Fentanyl
   d. Propofol

5. Which of the following statements about alfaxalone is least accurate?
   a. It can cause respiratory depression and apnea
   b. It provides good quality analgesia
   c. It causes minimal cardiovascular depression
   d. It can be given IM to cats

6. Which of the following statements concerning endotracheal intubation is false?
   a. Choosing a tube that is too small may result in increased resistance to breathing
   b. Choosing a tube that is too long may result in hypoxemia.
   c. Choosing a tube that is too short may cause increased mechanical dead space
   d. Failure to cuff the tube may result in aspiration of foreign material

7. Which of the following is an indicator that the endotracheal tube has been placed in the esophagus instead of the trachea?
   a. The patient coughs as the tube is placed
   b. The unidirectional valves do not move
   c. The pressure manometer indicates 1 to 3 cm H_2O while the patient is spontaneously breathing
   d. Only one firm structure in the neck is palpated

8. The term atelectasis refers to:
   a. Increased fluid in the alveoli
   b. Hyperinflation of the alveoli
   c. A decrease in blood perfusion around the alveoli
   d. Collapsed alveoli

9. After an anesthetic procedure, when is it best to extubate a dog?
   a. Right after you turn off the vaporizer
   b. About 10 minutes after turning off the vaporizer
   c. When the animal begins to swallow
   d. Right after detaching the breathing circuit

10. Hypostatic congestion may be present at the end of the anesthetic protocol. This term refers to the:
    a. Accumulation of mucus in the trachea
    b. Pooling of blood in the dependent lung
    c. Leakage of fluid into the chest
    d. Pooling of ingesta in one area of the gastrointestinal tract

11. Which of the following protocols would result in the fastest induction time and the best control over anesthetic depth?
    a. IM induction and maintenance
    b. IV induction with a short-acting agent and maintenance with bolus injections of the same
    c. Inhalant induction and maintenance
    d. IV induction with a short-acting agent and maintenance with an inhalant

12. Mask inductions in small-animal patients are:
    a. Easier for the anesthetist than IV inductions
    b. Less likely to cause cardiac arrhythmias and hypotension than IV inductions
    c. An excellent technique for brachycephalic breeds
    d. Possible only with use of inhalant agents with a low solubility coefficient

13. Which of the following techniques are used most often in most general small-animal practices?
    a. General anesthesia and sedation
    b. Sedation and regional techniques
    c. Neuromuscular blockade and neuroleptanalgesia
    d. Regional techniques and general anesthesia

14. An 18-kg adult dog of normal conformation would likely require a _____ endotracheal tube.
    a. 7- to 7.5-mm
    b. 8- to 8.5-mm
    c. 9- to 9.5-mm
    d. 10- to 10.5-mm

The following questions may have more than one correct answer. Select all that apply.

15. An endotracheal tube is used to:
    a. Decrease anatomic dead space
    b. Maintain a patent airway
    c. Protect the patient from aspiration of vomitus
    d. Allow the anesthetist to ventilate the patient

16. Potential problems associated with endotracheal intubation include:
    a. Decreased mechanical dead space
    b. Pressure necrosis of the tracheal mucosa
    c. Intubation of a bronchus
    d. Spread of infectious disease

17. During anesthetic induction and maintenance:
    a. The patient should be supported as it loses consciousness
    b. The patient should be placed on an electric heating pad to prevent hypothermia
    c. If a patient has one diseased lung, it should be positioned with the diseased side down
    d. The anesthetist should avoid any more than a 15-degree elevation of the rear quarters

18. The length of the anesthetic recovery period may be influenced by:
    a. Body temperature
    b. Patient condition
    c. The length of time the patient was under
    d. The breed of the patient

19. Patients may exhibit alarming signs while passing through Stage II anesthesia during recovery. Which of the following are expected signs of passage through this anesthetic stage?
    a. Head bobbing
    b. Mydriasis
    c. Seizures
    d. Rapid limb paddling

20. Which of the following actions is appropriate during anesthetic recovery?
    a. Administer oxygen at a high flow rate for 5 minutes after discontinuation of the anesthetic or until extubation
    b. Leave the cage door open so you can monitor the patient from across the room
    c. Turn the patient about every 10 to 15 minutes
    d. Use warming methods to increase the body temperature

ANSWERS TO CASE PRESENTATION

Case Presentation 9.1

Question #1: There are many possible causes of an inability to keep a patient anesthetized during a general anesthetic event, most of which are factors that affect the delivery of anesthetic to the patient. These factors include (1) inadequate carrier gas flow (caused by an empty oxygen tank, failure to turn on the flowmeter, use of an inadequate flow rate, or disconnection of the ETT from the Y-piece), (2) airway blockage (due to a blocked or kinked ETT or blocked tracheal lumen), (3) leakage in the breathing system or airway (caused by an inadequately inflated ETT cuff or a leak in the anesthetic machine, breathing circuit, or ETT), (4) inadequate uptake of anesthetic (due to respiratory depression, intubation of one bronchus, esophageal intubation, increased dead space, or pulmonary disease), and (5) inadequate anesthetic delivery (due to an empty vaporizer, inadequate dial setting, or vaporizer malfunction).

Question #2: Julia should first rule out possible causes that can be assessed very rapidly (within seconds). This would include the oxygen flow rate, vaporizer setting, vaporizer fill level, and the ETT connection with the breathing circuit. If this very rapid assessment does not reveal a cause, then she may need to call for assistance in case 1) Caesar must be reanesthetized with an injectable agent; 2) steps must be taken to prevent him from chewing the tube; 3) the anesthetic machine must be changed; or 4) or Caesar must be reintubated. As soon as help arrives, she can begin to explore other causes such as esophageal intubation, ETT blockage, inadequate cuff inflation, and misassembly of the anesthetic machine (by disconnecting the machine and performing a rapid leak test). As soon as a cause is discovered, rapid steps should be taken to correct it, and Caesar should be closely monitored until safely reanesthetized and at a stable anesthetic depth.

Outcome of This Case

Julia very rapidly determined that there was 1200 psi oxygen remaining in the tank, the oxygen flow was set at 2.5 L/min, and the vaporizer was half full and was set at 2.5%. She also determined that the ETT was attached to the breathing circuit, the respiratory rate and quality were adequate, and that the machine appeared to be correctly assembled.

After calling for help, Julia attempted to ventilate Caesar manually and noticed that the abdominal wall expanded in response to a breath whereas the chest wall did not, leading Julia to deduce that the tube was improperly placed. Revisualization of the larynx confirmed esophageal intubation, thus explaining Caesar's imminent arousal. With help, she was able to reintubate Caesar. She then cuffed the tube, increased the vaporizer dial setting to 4%, and increased the oxygen flow rate to 4 L/min. Although she had to hold Caesar's mouth closed to prevent him from chewing the tube, his anesthetic depth began to increase within 1 to 2 minutes. At that point, she gradually decreased the vaporizer setting in response to monitoring parameters until he was stable and again in stage III surgical anesthesia. He remained stable, and both the surgical prep and the surgical repair were completed uneventfully.

This case illustrates the importance of carefully checking the ETT for proper placement before commencing any procedure.

SELECTED READINGS

Bednarski RM: Anesthesia management of dogs and cats. In Grimm KA, Tranquilli WJ, Lamont LA, editors: *Essentials of small animal anesthesia and analgesia*, ed 2, Ames, IA, 2011, Wiley-Blackwell, pp 274–299.

Clarke KW, Trim CM, Hall LW: *Veterinary anaesthesia*, ed 11, St. Louis, MO, 2014, Elsevier, pp 405–534.

Grubb T, Sager J, Gaynor JS, et al: 2020 AAHA anesthesia and monitoring guidelines for dogs and cats, *J Am Anim Hosp Assoc* 56(2):59–82, 2020.

Mosing M: General principles of perioperative care. In Duke-Novakovski T, DeVries M, Seymour C, editors: *BSAVA manual of canine and feline anaesthesia and analgesia*, ed 3, Gloucester, UK, 2016, British Small Animal Veterinary Association, pp 13–23.

Muir WW, Hubbell JA, Bednarski RM, Lerche P: *Handbook of veterinary anesthesia*, ed 5, St. Louis, MO, 2013, Elsevier.

Pascoe PJ, Pypendop BH: Comparative anesthesia and analgesia of dogs and cats. In Grimm KA, Lamont LA, Tranquilli SA, et al, editors: *Lumb and Jones' veterinary anesthesia and analgesia*, ed 5, Ames, IA, 2015, John Wiley & Sons, Inc., pp 723–730.

Plumb DC: Plumb's Veterinary Drugs. https://plumbs.com/solutions/plumbs-veterinary-drugs/.

Robertson SA, Gogolski SM, Pascoe P, et al: AAFP feline anesthesia guidelines, *J Feline Med Surg* 20:602–634, 2018.

Steagall P, Robertson S, Taylor P: *Feline anesthesia and pain management*, Ames, IA, 2018, John Wiley & Sons, Inc., pp 1–138.

Equine Anesthesia

OUTLINE

LEARNING OBJECTIVES

When you have completed this chapter, you will be able to:

- Describe anesthetic techniques commonly used in equine practice.
- Explain the special anesthetic challenges resulting from the patient's temperament, large body size, and equine anatomy and physiology.
- List the causes of nasal congestion, atelectasis, neuropathy, and myopathy, and describe strategies to prevent these anesthetic complications.
- Describe the differences between anesthetic protocols and procedures used for field anesthesia and anesthesia in a fully equipped equine hospital.
- Explain the indications for, the advantages of, and risks associated with standing chemical restraint in horses.
- Describe anesthetic induction by intravenous (IV) injection and by inhalation via a nasotracheal tube.
- Prepare an equine patient, anesthetic equipment, and anesthetic agents and adjuncts for general anesthesia.
- Explain cautions and risks associated with each method of anesthetic induction and strategies to maximize patient safety.
- Explain how to do each of the following: (1) select and prepare an endotracheal tube (ETT) for placement; (2) place an ETT in a horse; (3) check for proper ETT placement; (4) inflate the cuff; and (5) extubate a horse during anesthetic recovery.
- Describe maintenance of general anesthesia with an inhalant agent and with IV agents.
- List principles of providing appropriate patient positioning, comfort, and safety during anesthetic maintenance.
- Explain the significance of hypoventilation, hypoxemia, and hypotension in equine patients, as well as prevention and management strategies for these anesthetic complications.
- List factors that affect patient recovery from anesthesia, the signs of recovery, appropriate monitoring during recovery, and oxygen therapy during recovery.
- Describe general nursing care during the postanesthetic period.

KEY TERMS

Atelectasis
Demand valve
Epistaxis
Field anesthesia
Hypotension

Hypoventilation
Hypoxemia
Insufflation
Myopathy
Neuropathy

Partial intravenous anesthesia
Positive inotrope
Standing chemical restraint
Total intravenous anesthesia
Ventilation–perfusion mismatch

INTRODUCTION TO EQUINE ANESTHESIA

The basic principles of anesthesia discussed in Chapter 9 apply to equine anesthesia. Additionally, horses present unique challenges to the anesthetist because of their temperament, size, anatomy, and physiology. The anesthetist should be aware of these concerns before anesthetizing equine patients.

Different breeds of horses and even individuals within the same breed can have varying temperaments, ranging from calm and stoic to excitable and nervous. Also, because horses are flight animals (animals that tend to run away from stressful situations), even a normally calm, stoic horse can become excited in an unfamiliar environment such as a veterinary hospital. An excited horse may behave unpredictably and can cause injury to itself and veterinary personnel. A complete discussion of handling the equine patient is beyond the scope of this chapter; however, it is important to have a good understanding of how to catch, handle, and physically restrain a horse in order to minimize risk to the horse, the anesthetist, and other personnel. An aspect of equine behavior that differs from other species is that horses have an instinctive desire to stand shortly after awakening from anesthesia, which makes any equine anesthetic recovery a relatively high-risk event. Ideally, both induction and recovery from anesthesia should occur in a calm, quiet environment, with subdued lighting, if possible.

The average adult horse weighs 350 to 500 kg and some larger breeds may weigh as much as 1000 kg. This requires use of specialized equipment such as induction and recovery stalls, hoists, and special large-animal surgery tables and anesthetic machines, in addition to small-animal machines and equipment, which are used for patients weighing less than 150 kg (foals, miniature horses). The equine anesthetist must be familiar with the operation of all related equipment in addition to anesthetic machines and monitors.

Anatomic concerns involve the respiratory, gastrointestinal, and musculoskeletal systems. Horses are obligate nasal breathers; thus anything that causes nasal obstruction, such as congestion (which develops when the head is below the withers during general anesthesia) or a horse pressing its nostrils against the recovery stall wall, can quickly lead to respiratory compromise and death without intervention. The large, heavy gastrointestinal tract places pressure on the lungs when horses are placed in dorsal or lateral recumbency, causing atelectasis (collapsed alveoli). Atelectatic lung tissue is not available for gas exchange and therefore horses are prone to hypoxemia under anesthesia. Many anesthetic drugs affect the gastrointestinal tract (anticholinergics, opioids, alpha$_2$-agonists); this must be taken into consideration when selecting protocols because horses are susceptible to developing colic in the perianesthetic period. Some superficial nerves (e.g., the facial nerve) can become damaged (neuropathy) if intraoperative padding is not appropriate or if the halter is inadvertently left on during anesthesia when the horse is positioned in lateral recumbency.

Muscle blood flow must be maintained during anesthesia in order to prevent myopathy, which manifests in recovery as muscle hardness, pain, and weakness and is commonly referred

---

> ## BOX 10.1 Examples of Procedures Commonly Performed Under Sedation or Standing Chemical Restraint
>
> **Sedation**
> - Radiographic studies
> - Ultrasonographic studies
> - Endoscopy
> - Dental floating
> - Minor wound suturing
> - Hoof trimming and shoeing
> - Nasogastric intubation
> - Venipuncture for catheter placement
>
> **Procedures Performed Under Standing Chemical Restraint in Conjunction With Local Nerve Blocks or Epidural Anesthesia**
> - Eye and eyelid surgery
> - Sinus and dental surgery
> - Castration
> - Major wound evaluation and repair
> - Mass removals
> - Rectovaginal fistula repair
> - Laparoscopy
> - Ovariectomy

---

to using the lay term "tying up." Insufficient padding and/or inappropriate positioning of limbs may also lead to myopathy.

Given these challenges it is preferred, if the horse's temperament and surgical approach allow, to perform procedures on lightly or heavily sedated horses. Heavy sedation is often referred to as standing chemical restraint and these terms are used interchangeably. Many diagnostic and surgical procedures can be performed under standing chemical restraint with the addition of local anesthetic nerve blocks (Box 10.1). Horses that are not cooperative after sedation and horses undergoing more complex procedures (e.g., abdominal surgery, arthroscopy) do, however, require general anesthesia. General anesthesia is frequently carried out at farms or stables, and this is referred to as field anesthesia. As the name implies, field anesthesia occurs away from the veterinary hospital in a relatively clean stall or paddock and is appropriate for short procedures (20 to 60 minutes). Procedures that will last longer than 60 minutes, those that are complex, and those involving compromised patients should be performed at a well-equipped veterinary hospital where inhalant anesthetics and oxygen can be administered using an anesthetic machine and anesthetic monitoring is available.

As with small-animal anesthesia, neuromuscular blockers are rarely used in general practice but are sometimes used to provide muscle relaxation for ocular and orthopedic procedures in veterinary schools and referral practices.

PATIENT PREPARATION

The reader is referred to Chapters 2 and 9 for a detailed discussion of the essentials of preparation before anesthesia. See

PROCEDURE 10.1 Preparation for Anesthesia of the Horse

1. Assess, prepare, and weigh the patient. If a large-animal scale is not available, the weight must be estimated, preferably with a weight tape. (See Chapter 2 for a discussion of patient assessment, preparation, and stabilization.)
2. Prepare equipment for and place an IV catheter, which may require intramuscular (IM) sedation in some horses (clippers, local anesthetic, antiseptic scrub, catheters, tape, normal saline, suture material, catheter cap, and/or extension line with three-way stopcock).
3. Rinse the horse's mouth, clean the hooves, and remove or wrap shoes when appropriate.
4. Determine the protocol (anesthetic agents, including dosages, routes, and sequence of administration).
5. Calculate the volume of each agent to give, including fluid administration rates (preanesthetic, induction, maintenance, and analgesic agents).
6. Review oxygen flow rates (see Table 10.1).
7. Prepare equipment required to administer drugs (syringes, needles, agents, reversal agents, emergency cart, controlled substance log).
8. Prepare fluid administration equipment (fluids, administration/extension set, syringe pump, tape, normal saline).
9. Prepare equipment for endotracheal intubation (see Chapter 10, page 349).
10. Prepare monitoring equipment including arterial catheterization materials, anesthesia record, monitors, and probes (see Chapter 6).
11. Assemble and test the anesthetic machine and ventilator.

BOX 10.2 Example of Dosage Calculations for Injectable Drugs

How much ketamine and diazepam should you draw up to induce a 1200-lb Quarter Horse for arthroscopy? The prescribed dose of ketamine is 2.2 mg/kg, and the drug concentration is 100 mg/mL. The prescribed dose of diazepam is 0.05 mg/kg and the drug concentration is 5 mg/mL.

$$\text{Patient body weight (kg)} = \frac{1200 \text{ lb} \times 1 \text{ kg}}{2.2 \text{ lb}} = 545 \text{ kg}$$

$$\text{Volume of ketamine (mL)} = \frac{545 \text{ kg} \times 2.2 \text{ mg/kg}}{100 \text{ mg/mL}} = 12 \text{ mL}$$

$$\text{Volume of diazepam (mL)} = \frac{545 \text{ kg} \times 0.05 \text{ mg/kg}}{5 \text{ mg/mL}} = 5.5 \text{ mL}$$

Procedure 10.1 for additional tasks pertinent to preparation of the equine patient undergoing general anesthesia. Additionally, the anesthetist should be familiar with operation of any other equipment such as surgical tables and hoists that will be used during the anesthetic episode.

SELECTING A PROTOCOL

A suitable protocol takes into account the minimum patient database, the patient's physical status class, and the type and duration of procedure to be performed. Location also plays a role; field anesthesia is most commonly performed using total intravenous anesthesia (TIVA), whereas in a veterinary clinic, the anesthetic protocol may be TIVA or induction with an injectable drug followed by maintenance with an inhalant agent.

Regardless of the protocol, the correct drugs and amounts, as well as oxygen flow rates and fluid administration rates, must be prepared. Chapter 9, Box 9.3 shows the steps required to calculate the dosages of most injectable drugs and Box 10.2 shows an example of drug calculations for a horse. Table 10.1 lists oxygen flow rates used for large-animal patients. Ill, geriatric, pediatric, or otherwise compromised patients (physical status class P3 to P5) require use of modified protocols based on the patient's primary condition. Management of these cases can be quite challenging and requires customization of the anesthetic protocol by the attending veterinarian.

See Chapter 9 for additional information on selecting a protocol and strategies to minimize adverse effects.

SUMMARY OF A GENERAL ANESTHETIC PROCEDURE

The dynamics associated with commonly used protocols in equine anesthesia are very similar to those associated with small-animal protocols (see Chapter 9), with the exception that induction with an intramuscular (IM) agent is not used in clinical practice, although it is used for capture of feral horses.

EQUIPMENT PREPARATION

During a typical anesthetic induction, many events occur in rapid succession. Anesthetic agents are administered, the patient becomes unconscious and recumbent, and the endotracheal tube is placed, secured, and cuffed. The horse is then moved to or hoisted onto the surgery table, the halter is removed, the endotracheal tube connected to the anesthetic machine, and the anesthetic gas vaporizer is adjusted, all within the first few minutes. Because these events follow one another so rapidly, the technician does not have the luxury of leaving the patient in order to locate equipment. For this reason, all equipment must be carefully gathered, checked, and organized before commencing the procedure.

Equine patients weighing more than 150 kg are usually placed on a large-animal anesthetic machine (Fig. 10.1). Large-animal anesthetic machines typically incorporate a ventilator (see Fig. 10.1 D). Both the circle system and the ventilator of the machine should be assembled and checked before use. Smaller horses, ponies, and foals weighing less than 150 kg can be placed on a small-animal anesthetic machine. Hypothermia is uncommon in anesthetized adult horses; however, methods such as forced air warming and warm water circulating blankets can be used for smaller horses and foals. A crash cart containing emergency equipment and drugs should also always be available.

PREMEDICATION OR SEDATION

Premedication refers to the administration of anesthetic agents and adjuncts to calm and prepare the patient for anesthetic

TABLE 10.1   Large-Animal Oxygen Flow Rate Quick Reference Chart

	LARGE-ANIMAL OXYGEN FLOW RATES (L/min)			
Body Weight (kg)	Full Rebreathing (Based on 3–5 mL/kg/min)	Partial Rebreathing During Maintenance (Based on 10 mL/kg/min)	Partial Rebreathing Induction, Recovery, and Changes (Based on 20 mL/kg/min)[a]	Minimal Rebreathing[a,b]
300	1–1.5	3	6	10
450	1.4–2.3	4.5	9	10
600	1.8–3	6	10	10
750	2.3–3.8	7.5	10	10
900	2.7–4.5	9	10	10

[a]Note that flowmeters on large-animal machines are not typically calibrated above 10 L/min.
[b]Minimal rebreathing occurs only when the oxygen flow is greater than or equal to the respiratory minute volume (RMV).

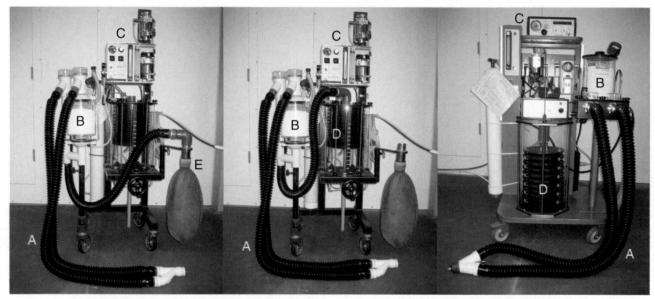

FIG. 10.1 Large-animal anesthetic machines (Drager[a] *left* and *middle*, and Mallard[b] *right*). *A,* Large-animal breathing tubes and Y-piece; *B,* CO_2 absorber canister; *C,* ventilator control panel, flowmeters, and vaporizers; *D,* ventilator bellows and housing; *E,* 35 L reservoir bag. [a]Note that the hose connected to the breathing bag must be moved over to the top of the ventilator housing when switching the Drager to mechanical ventilation. The pop-off valve should then be closed because the ventilator has an internal pop-off valve. [b]Note that because the Mallard has a standing bellows (a bellows that is attached at the bottom- and depresses from the top down during inspiration), it can be used as pictured for spontaneous breathing as well as mechanical ventilation.

induction. Preanesthetic medications are chosen specifically to produce a set of desired effects such as sedation, analgesia, and muscle relaxation. Tranquilizers, alpha₂-agonists, and opioids are commonly used as preanesthetic medications, and are given IM or intravenously (IV). Anticholinergic drugs are not used to premedicate horses because they reduce gastrointestinal motility, which may result in colic. This class of drugs is therefore reserved for treatment of arrhythmias and for cardiopulmonary resuscitation (CPR) in this species.

The preanesthetic procedure in horses differs slightly from that used for small animals. After appropriate patient assessment, the first step is placement of an IV catheter (4 to 6 inches, 14- to 16-gauge), almost always in one of the jugular veins. Some horses object to venipuncture and must be sedated first. Such horses may be premedicated at this time (Box 10.3). Alternatively, a low dose of xylazine (0.2 to 0.5 mg/kg IV) may be

sufficient to achieve catheter placement. Once the horse is cooperative, a small bleb of local anesthetic is administered over the proposed site of catheterization to desensitize the skin.

Following catheterization, the horse's mouth should be washed out with a large syringe (Fig. 10.2) to flush out any feed material. This prevents aspiration of the material during intubation or during recovery following extubation. Some horses may require sedation if they object to having their mouths rinsed. The feet should be cleaned before sedation and the shoes should be removed or wrapped. Just before or immediately after premedication, the horse is positioned in an induction area or placed adjacent to a tilt table. Some breeds generally require higher doses of sedatives than others, for example, Arabians and Thoroughbreds, particularly those in training, whereas draft horses typically require lower doses (see Box 10.3 for preanesthetic/sedative protocols used in horses).

Protocols for Light–Moderate Sedation (for minor procedures such as wound debridement or radiography):

1. **Acepromazine (IV or IM):** Acepromazine: 0.03–0.05 mg/kg IV or IM (not for use in debilitated patients, or in breeding stallions)
2. **Xylazine (IV):** Xylazine: 0.1–0.3 mg/kg IV
3. **Detomidine (IV):** Detomidine: 0.005–0.01 mg/kg IV
4. **Romifidine (IV):** Romifidine: 0.03–0.05 mg/kg IV
5. **Butorphanol (IV):** Butorphanol: 0.02–0.05 mg/kg; can be combined in the same syringe with any one of the sedatives listed above and given IV for additional sedation

Protocols for Premedication or Moderate–Deep Sedation

1. **Xylazine (IV):** Xylazine: 1.1 mg/kg IV
2. **Detomidine (IV):** Detomidine: 0.01–0.02 mg/kg IV
3. **Romifidine (IV):** Romifidine: 0.05–0.1 mg/kg IV
4. **Butorphanol (IV):** Butorphanol: 0.05–0.2 mg/kg IV; can be added to any of the alpha$_2$-agonists listed above to provide neuroleptanalgesia
5. **Morphine (IV):** Morphine: 0.05–0.1 mg/kg IV; can be added to any of the alpha$_2$-agonists listed above to provide neuroleptanalgesia

IM, Intramuscular; *IV,* intravenous.

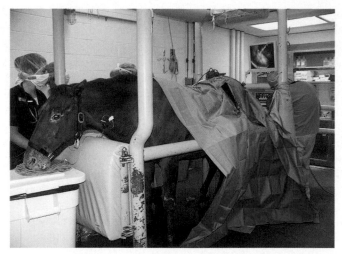

FIG. 10.3 Standing chemical restraint. A sedated horse is standing in the stocks before preparation for a procedure. An assistant should always be present to control the head of the horse.

(For major procedures such as laparoscopy, rectovaginal fistula repair, sinus, eye or dental surgery, note that local anesthetic blocks or opioid epidurals may be required to facilitate some of these procedures.)

1. **Xylazine–butorphanol (IV):** Xylazine 0.5–1.1 mg/kg and butorphanol 0.05–0.1 mg/kg (provides 20–30 min of chemical restraint). Extend sedation with xylazine 0.25–0.5 mg/kg + butorphanol 0.025–0.05 mg/kg as needed.
2. **Detomidine–morphine (IV):** Detomidine 0.02 mg/kg IV and morphine 0.1 mg/kg (provides approximately 60 min of sedation). Administer detomidine 0.01 mg/kg to extend sedation. (Morphine has a longer duration of action than detomidine, therefore does not need to be redosed.)

IV, Intravenous.

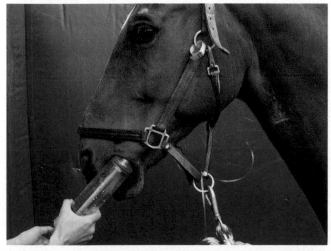

FIG. 10.2 Preparing a horse for general anesthesia. The horse's mouth is flushed with water using a large dosing syringe. The nozzle of the syringe is inserted between the horse's cheek and teeth. This is done on both sides of the mouth to flush out feed material.

Standing Chemical Restraint

Standing chemical restraint is essentially a continuation or extension of sedation. The patient is prepared as if it were having general anesthesia, with placement of an IV catheter and extension set. The patient is usually secured in stocks for the procedure (Fig. 10.3). If the level of sedation required for the procedure is inadequate, additional drugs are given intravenously (see Box 10.4 for standing chemical restraint protocols in horses). The dynamics of standing chemical restraint differ because general anesthesia is not the goal; the horse remains standing. The horse's level of consciousness may change from light to heavy sedation, which can be gauged on the basis of the

horse's level of interest in the environment, head position, and stance. On rare occasions, general anesthesia may be required after or during standing restraint. If a horse becomes excessively sedated; becomes excited and panics falling in the stocks; or if the veterinarian cannot perform the procedure because of inadequate sedation or surgical access, the anesthetist should be prepared to anesthetize the horse under instruction from the attending veterinarian. If the period of standing anesthesia required to perform the procedure is lengthy, the horse may develop nasal congestion, which could lead to respiratory obstruction. To avoid this, the head should be held up in a neutral position. If the horse is placed in stocks, cross-ties can be used for this purpose.

Signs of appropriate sedation before anesthetic induction or for standing restraint include lowering of the head and neck, drooping of the lower lip, reluctance to move, a wide-based stance, and a lack of interest in the surrounding activity. Some horses remain sensitive to sudden loud noises and movements. This can be diminished by ensuring the work area of the induction stall is quiet, by covering the horse's eyes, or by placing cotton in the horse's ears. Moving a horse into position behind a squeeze gate or into stocks may cause brief excitement or loss of sedation. Waiting for a few minutes will usually allow the horse to settle down. It may be necessary to give additional sedative if the horse is not adequately sedated. It is also possible that external stimuli in an environment unfamiliar to the horse may result in the horse becoming excited, even if it initially appeared to be adequately sedated with an alpha₂-agonist. If this occurs, the horse should be given time to calm down (decrease external stimuli, refrain from trying to move the horse into the induction area) before proceeding. In order to help produce a stable plane of anesthetic depth during the maintenance phase, it is essential that a horse is adequately sedated prior to induction. Administration of additional sedative drugs may therefore be required. Once the patient is adequately sedated, anesthetic induction should immediately follow or, as an alternative, these protocols can be used alone to provide sedation for diagnostic and therapeutic procedures.

> **TECHNICIAN NOTE** Remember that a horse can easily become aroused or excited after sedation with an alpha₂-agonist or acepromazine. Covering the horse's eyes with a towel or placing cotton in the horse's ears will decrease visual and auditory stimuli, which may enhance sedation. It is essential that a horse is adequately sedated prior to induction. Administration of additional sedative drugs may therefore be required.

ANESTHETIC INDUCTION

Anesthetic induction is the process by which the horse loses consciousness and enters surgical anesthesia. In addition to the goals set out for induction of small animals in Chapter 9, an additional goal for equine anesthetic induction is to render the horse unconscious as quickly as possible so that its transition from standing to recumbency occurs with minimal risk of injury to the horse or personnel. In healthy horses, induction drugs are therefore given as rapid bolus injections, rather than to effect. Induction is most commonly accomplished by intravenous administration of injectable agents, typically ketamine alone or in combination with other agents. Inhalant induction is reserved for foals that can be nasotracheally intubated while still awake; foals that will tolerate this are typically compromised and will require careful anesthetic management. What follows is a description of specific techniques used to induce a patient. (See Box 10.5 for IV induction protocols in horses and Procedure 10.2 for the sequence of events.)

> **TECHNICIAN NOTE** One of the main goals of anesthetic induction is to render the horse unconscious as quickly as possible so that its transition from standing to lateral recumbency occurs with minimal risk of injury to the horse or personnel. Induction drugs are therefore given as a rapid IV bolus.

Intravenous Induction

Unless it occurs in the field, induction typically occurs in a special induction stall that has padded walls and often a padded floor. Induction may be done without a restraining gate, often

---

BOX 10.5 Intravenous Induction Protocols for Physical Status Class P1 and P2 Horses

1. **Ketamine (IV):** Ketamine 2.2 mg/kg IV
2. **Ketamine–midazolam (IV):** Ketamine 2.2 mg/kg IV and midazolam[a] 0.05–0.1 mg/kg IV mixed in the same syringe, administered as a rapid bolus.
3. **Ketamine–propofol (IV):** Ketamine 2.2 mg/kg IV and propofol 0.5 mg/kg IV either mixed in the same syringe and administered as a rapid bolus, or in separate syringes with ketamine administered as a rapid bolus first, immediately followed by propofol administered as a rapid bolus.
4. **Guaifenesin–ketamine (IV):** Guaifenesin 25–50 mg/kg is administered IV under pressure to effect (horse becomes ataxic and buckles at the carpus joints) followed by ketamine 2.2 mg/kg bolus IV.

[a]Note: An equivalent volume of diazepam can be substituted for midazolam.

IV, Intravenous.

PROCEDURE 10.2 Sequence of Events for Induction With an Intravenous Agent and Maintenance With an Inhalant Agent in a Horse

1. Administer premedications intramuscularly (IM) approximately 20–30 min before or intravenously (IV) approximately 5–10 min before anesthetic induction.
2. If the horse is adequately sedated, administer the induction agent; otherwise, give additional IV sedation before induction.
3. Check the patient's readiness for intubation.
4. Place and secure the endotracheal tube.
5. Inflate the endotracheal tube cuff.
6. Check the patient's vital signs.
7. Hoist, position, and secure the patient for the procedure, with attention to padding of the face and lower limbs if the horse is in lateral recumbency, maintenance of an open airway, unrestricted blood flow, and unrestricted chest excursions. If the patient is placed in lateral recumbency, the dependent forelimb should be extended forward as far as possible, and padding should be placed between the hindlimbs. The forelimbs are usually secured, e.g., using a thin rope.
8. Remove the halter.
9. Turn on the oxygen and attach the endotracheal tube to the breathing circuit.
10. Turn on the inhalant anesthetic to the appropriate level.
11. Determine the patient's anesthetic depth and commence regular monitoring.
12. Attach monitoring devices, including placement of an arterial catheter.
13. Continue to monitor and adjust the anesthetic and oxygen levels as needed until completion of the procedure.

---

termed "free fall," or behind a gate that restrains the horse (Fig. 10.4). Sometimes the induction stall is also used for recovery. In comparison to small animals, where IV induction agents are given to effect, the goal of induction in horses is to take the horse rapidly from standing (sedated) to lateral recumbency (unconscious) so as to minimize excitement, which can lead to the horse injuring itself or personnel. All drugs are thus given as a bolus, with the exception of the muscle relaxant guaifenesin, which is administered rapidly IV to effect by placing it in a pressure bag (Fig. 10.5). Once the horse shows signs of ataxia,

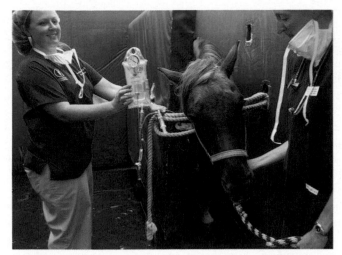

FIG. 10.4 Equine anesthetic induction gate. A premedicated horse is restrained behind a gate before induction. The purpose of the rope (which is looped through a ring in the wall of the induction stall) is to prevent the horse from moving forward during induction and potentially injuring itself or personnel. One person controls the rope and an assistant should always be present to control the head of the horse.

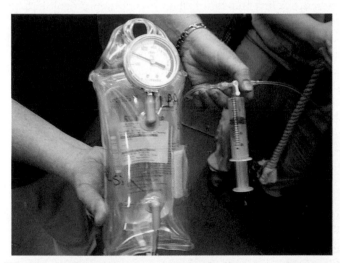

FIG. 10.5 Guaifenesin in a pressure bag. Guaifenesin is administered as a rapid infusion using a pressure bag. Note that the induction drug (in this case, ketamine) is attached to the three-way stopcock so that once the desired level of muscle relaxation has been reached, the horse can be induced.

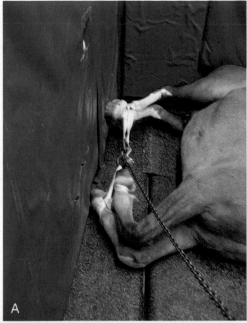

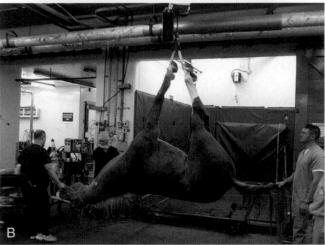

FIG. 10.6 Hoisting a horse after induction. **(A)** Hobbles are placed distal to the fetlock joints of the forelimbs and hindlimbs and attached to the hook of a hoist. **(B)** The horse is hoisted so that a large-animal surgery table can be positioned underneath it. The hoist can then be used to facilitate correct positioning on the table. The anesthetist controls and supports the head, while an assistant controls the tail.

typically bending or buckling of the forelimbs at the carpi and/or fetlocks, the induction agent is given as a bolus. Once the horse has been induced, it is then intubated and the vital signs briefly checked.

In some practices, the floor of the induction stall forms part of the surgery table, but in many the horse must be hoisted onto a table (Fig. 10.6). It is important to understand how the hoist functions so that the horse can be transported safely and any problems can be resolved rapidly.

It is necessary to ensure that muscles and prominent nerves are protected when a horse is placed on a surgical table or surface. The anesthetist should make sure that muscle groups are well supported and do not rest on hard surfaces to prevent myopathy ("tying up"), and that the facial nerve is protected

when placing a horse in lateral recumbency (Fig. 10.7). Horses in lateral recumbency should also have the forelimb closest to the table pulled forward if possible to decrease the pressure placed on it by the chest and opposite limb, and the hindlimbs should be separated by padding so that they are in a neutral position (Fig. 10.8).

> **TECHNICIAN NOTE** It is important to ensure that the horse's muscles and prominent nerves are protected when it is placed on a surgical table or surface. The anesthetist should make sure that muscle groups are well supported and do not rest on hard surfaces during anesthesia in order to help prevent myopathies and neuropathies.

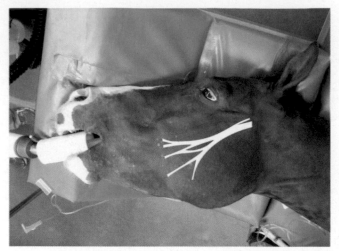

FIG. 10.7 Location of the facial nerve in the laterally recumbent horse. The position of the facial nerve is shown (in *white*) as it runs across the cheek. The halter should be removed when a horse is positioned in lateral recumbency for anesthesia to avoid damaging this nerve and causing facial paralysis.

Agents commonly used to induce general anesthesia in horses by intravenous injection include: (1) ketamine as a bolus injection; (2) a mixture of ketamine and midazolam, ketamine and diazepam, or ketamine and propofol as a bolus injection; and (3) guaifenesin infused under pressure to effect followed by ketamine as a bolus injection.

Following induction with the commonly used IV injectable agents, the duration of surgical anesthesia varies but is usually no more than 10 to 20 minutes. If more than 20 minutes of surgery time is required, anesthesia is maintained with inhalation anesthetics or administration of repeat boluses or a constant rate infusion (CRI) of injectable drugs. Occasionally, horses will be too light to intubate or place on the hoist after the induction dose. If this is the case, a bolus dose of ketamine at 0.4 to 0.5 mg/kg (one-quarter to one-fifth of the induction dose) is given IV. See Procedure 10.3 for IV induction in horses.

Inhalation Induction via Nasotracheal Tube

This technique is limited to use in young foals, particularly those that are sick or those that will tolerate nasotracheal intubation. The anatomy of the horse's nasal passages and nasopharynx is such that an endotracheal tube passed from the nostril into the ventral nasal meatus will emerge in the nasopharynx in a position that favors entry into the larynx. Once the nasotracheal tube has been placed and the cuff inflated, the tube is connected to the breathing system of a small-animal machine. Oxygen and inhalant are then administered. See Box 10.6 for inhalant induction protocols in foals, Procedure 10.4 for the technique, and Fig. 10.9.

This technique has the same risks as mask induction in small animals (see Chapter 9). The nasotracheal tube has the advantage of having few, if any, leaks compared to mask induction; thus induction should be faster and can occur at lower vaporizer settings, causing far less environmental pollution.

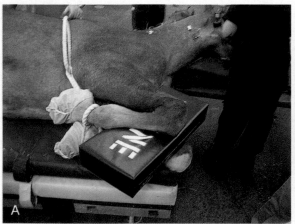

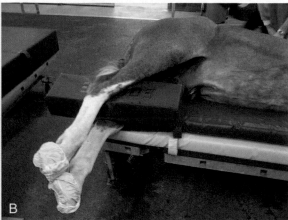

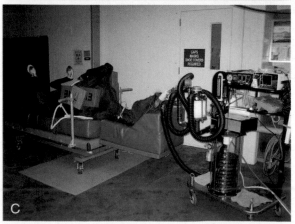

FIG. 10.8 Correct padding of a horse on a surgery table. **(A)** In lateral recumbency, the dependent forelimb is pulled forward before both forelimbs are secured with a rope. **(B)** In lateral recumbency, a pad is placed between the hindlimbs so they remain in a neutral position. **(C)** In dorsal recumbency, the horse's forelimbs are tied and supported with pads. The hindlimbs are not tied and are left in a neutral, flexed position whenever possible. Note the thick foam pad used to support the horse; this prevents muscles of the rump and back from coming into contact with hard surfaces, which could lead to the development of myopathy.

PROCEDURE 10.3 Intravenous Induction in Horses

Induction of horses differs from that of small animals in that the goal is to achieve lateral recumbency without excitement or injury to the horse or personnel. In order to do this, the induction agent is given as a rapid intravenous (IV) bolus to horses in PSC P1 and P2. The only drug that is given to effect in horses during induction (see Procedure 9.3 in Chapter 9) is guaifenesin.

- **Ketamine–midazolam, ketamine–diazepam,** and **ketamine–propofol mixtures**: After checking to make sure that the IV catheter is patent and still in the jugular vein, the entire calculated dose is rapidly injected into the catheter or extension set, then the catheter is flushed using normal saline. Care must be taken to ensure all connections are secure to avoid administering partial doses, which could result in a partially induced and excited horse.
- **Guaifenesin and ketamine**: A bag of guaifenesin with an IV administration set attached is placed in a pressure sleeve, which is inflated up to 300 mmHg pressure. The administration set is connected to the IV catheter or extension set. After checking to make sure that the IV catheter is patent and still in the jugular vein, the guaifenesin is then administered under pressure to effect. Approximately 0.5–1 mL/kg will produce signs of ataxia (buckling at the carpus and fetlock), at which point ketamine is administered as a bolus.

BOX 10.6 Inhalant Induction Protocols for Physical Status Class P1 and P2 Foals

1. **Isoflurane:** Administer isoflurane at 3%–5% via nasotracheal tube[a]
2. **Sevoflurane:** Administer sevoflurane at 4%–6% via nasotracheal tube[a]

[a]Note: lower percentages should be used in sick foals.

PROCEDURE 10.4 Inhalant Induction via Nasotracheal Intubation in Foals

1. In a tractable or sedated foal, place a nasotracheal tube by extending the head and neck and passing a lubricated endotracheal tube through a nostril into the ventral meatus of the nasal cavity. Gently advance the tube into the nasopharynx. As the foal inhales, advance the tube into the larynx.
2. Connect the Y-piece of a rebreathing system to the endotracheal tube.
3. Give 100% oxygen for 2–3 min at 1–3 L/min.
4. Set the anesthetic vaporizer to deliver 0.5% isoflurane or 1% sevoflurane. Sevoflurane is less pungent than isoflurane and therefore better accepted.
5. Gradually increase the concentration of anesthetic by small increments (0.5% every 30 sec for isoflurane and 1% every 30 sec for sevoflurane) until an anesthetic concentration of 3%–5% is reached for isoflurane and 4%–6% for sevoflurane. Use lower maximum concentrations for compromised or very young foals. If the foal struggles, the vaporizer concentration can be increased more rapidly.
6. Monitor the foal carefully for increasing depth of anesthesia and turn the vaporizer to maintenance levels as soon as the patient is in a surgical plane of anesthesia (1.5%–2.5% for isoflurane and 2.5%–4% for sevoflurane).

Foals that require general anesthesia and are amenable to nasotracheal intubation without sedation are often compromised. Care should be taken during inhalant induction in these patients because they may become deep relatively quickly when compared with their healthy counterparts.

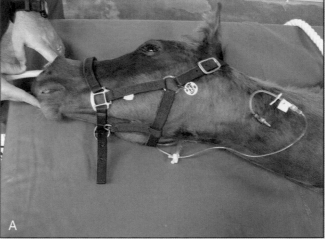
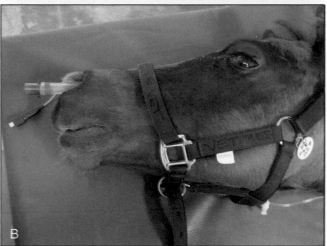

FIG. 10.9 Nasotracheal intubation in a foal. **(A)** In an amenable or sedated foal, the anesthetist directs the tube into the ventral nasal meatus. It is helpful to use the finger of the hand not holding the tube to palpate the ventral meatus as well as to direct the tube ventrally into it. As with orotracheal intubation, the head and neck should be extended. **(B)** Once the tube has been placed in the ventral meatus, it is gently advanced toward and into the larynx. The tube can then be connected to an anesthetic machine for inhalant induction.

ENDOTRACHEAL INTUBATION

Following induction of general anesthesia, an endotracheal tube is usually placed. The advantages of intubation are discussed in Chapters 4 and 9.

Equipment for Endotracheal Intubation

The following equipment is required to perform endotracheal intubation in the horse (Fig. 10.10):
- Appropriately sized endotracheal tubes (at least two of slightly different diameters)
- A mouth gag to hold the jaws apart
- A 60-mL syringe to inflate the cuff
- Gauze sponge to grasp the tongue (if required)

Selecting an Endotracheal Tube

The general principles for selecting an endotracheal tube are discussed in Chapter 9. Adult horses typically require a 22-, 26-,

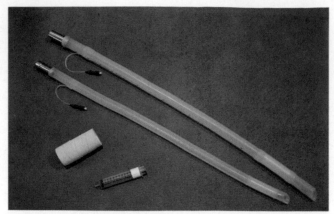

FIG. 10.10 Equipment for intubation of the horse. Appropriately sized endotracheal tubes, mouth gag ("homemade" from polyvinyl chloride [PVC] pipe in this case), and a 60-mL syringe for inflating the cuff.

or 30-mm diameter cuffed tube. Because of the length of the head and neck, intubation of one mainstem bronchus is rarely of concern in horses. Typically, two tube sizes are selected for intubation—the anticipated size and one size smaller. Foals require smaller tubes but rarely smaller than 10 mm diameter. Longer tubes of smaller diameter may be required for successful nasotracheal intubation in foals. Miniature horses also require smaller endotracheal tubes. Endotracheal tubes are further discussed in Chapter 4.

Preparing the Tube

Before using an endotracheal tube, it must be checked for integrity. It should be clean, sanitized, and free of blockages, holes, deterioration, or other damage. The connector must be securely attached and the cuff must inflate and hold pressure after detaching the syringe from the valve. The tube may be lubricated with a small amount of sterile, water-soluble lubricant, although this is not essential for most horses.

Intubation Procedure

Intubation in the horse is performed blindly. This means that the anesthetist does not directly visualize the larynx but instead passes the tube by feel. The oral and oropharyngeal anatomy of the horse makes blind intubation relatively easy. Unlike other species, it is uncommon for the tube to pass into the esophagus.

The horse's head is extended, the tongue is gently pulled to the side of the mouth, and a mouth gag or speculum is placed. Mouth gags can be purchased or "homemade" from polyvinyl chloride (PVC) pipe. The endotracheal tube is passed through the mouth gag, over the base of the tongue, and into the larynx. If the anesthetist meets resistance at the level of the laryngopharynx, the tube should be withdrawn 1 to 2 inches, rotated 90 degrees, and advanced again (Fig. 10.11 and Procedure 10.5).

Advancement of the tube without resistance indicates successful placement in the trachea. Intubation is confirmed by feeling air move when the horse exhales or when an assistant pushes on the thoracic wall. The endotracheal tube is either tied to the mouth speculum or taped to the horse's muzzle.

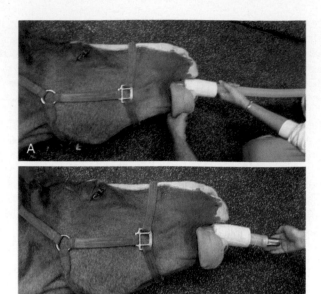

FIG. 10.11 Intubation of the horse. **(A)** The anesthetist advances the endotracheal tube blindly through a speculum in the mouth into the larynx with the horse's head extended. **(B)** The anesthetist feels for movement of air when the horse breathes out to confirm correct placement of the tube in the trachea.

PROCEDURE 10.5 Intubation Procedure for Horses

Horses are generally intubated in lateral recumbency.[a]
1. Place a mouth speculum or mouth gag between the incisors.
2. Grasp the tongue and pull it out of the mouth between the lips and the speculum.
3. Extend the head and neck.
4. Taking care to keep the tube in the center of the oral cavity to avoid laceration of the cuff by the molars, the tube is gently advanced toward, then through, the larynx.
5. If the anesthetist encounters resistance at the level of the larynx, the tube is withdrawn 1–2 inches and rotated 90 degrees before trying to advance it again.
6. Check to ensure the tube is in the trachea by feeling air pass during exhalation or when an assistant presses down on the horse's chest.
7. A small volume of air may be placed in the cuff (20–60 mL) before hoisting the horse.
8. After the horse has been positioned on the surgery table, connect the endotracheal tube to the anesthetic breathing system and allow the horse to breathe 100% oxygen.
9. Check the cuff for leaks.
10. Turn on the anesthetic vaporizer and adjust to the appropriate level.
11. Commence regular monitoring.

[a]Horses can be intubated in sternal recumbency, although this requires the horse to be supported in this position. Sternal intubation is typically reserved for horses that have significant nasogastric reflux due to colic and those with preanesthetic respiratory compromise.

In the event that a tube will not pass into the larynx, changing the angle of the head slightly, changing the angle of the tube slightly, or using a smaller tube usually results in success. If there is any resistance, it is important not to force the tube because this may damage the larynx.

TECHNICIAN NOTE Orotracheal intubation in the horse is performed with the head and neck of the horse extended using a blind technique.

The cuff is inflated as for small-animal intubation (see Chapter 9). Often, it is partially inflated before hoisting or moving the horse into position on the surgery table; then, once the patient is connected to the anesthetic machine, the cuff is checked for proper inflation in the same way as for a small-animal patient.

Nasotracheal intubation may be preferred over orotracheal intubation in horses undergoing some surgeries of the head and neck (e.g., sinus surgery, dental surgery). Nasotracheal intubation is performed by passing a well-lubricated tube one to two sizes smaller than will likely pass orotracheally into the ventral nasal meatus, with the head extended in the same position as for orotracheal intubation. The tube should be passed very gently in order to avoid damaging the nasal mucosa and turbinates, causing epistaxis (nose bleed).

Complications of Intubation

Complications are similar to those in small-animal anesthesia. Additional concerns are:
- Epistaxis may follow nasal intubation.
- Animals with abnormal anatomy (miniature horses, diseases of the oral and nasal cavity, laryngeal paralysis) may be difficult or impossible to intubate. These patients may require endoscopy-assisted intubation, in which an endoscope is passed through the tube and into the larynx, then the tube is threaded off the endoscope. In some cases, placement of an endotracheal tube through a tracheostomy incision may be indicated.

Healthy horses do not regurgitate under anesthesia, so when undergoing intraoral surgery and for reasons of convenience, not all horses are intubated. This is particularly true of field anesthesia. However, when oxygen is available, it is recommended that anesthetized horses are intubated and allowed to breathe oxygen.

MAINTENANCE OF ANESTHESIA

Following anesthetic induction and endotracheal intubation, patients that are in a light plane of anesthesia must be brought into surgical anesthesia. When the patient reaches the desired anesthetic depth, general anesthesia is maintained with injectable anesthetics (using TIVA) and inhalant anesthetics are delivered via an anesthetic machine, or a combination thereof. (See Box 10.7 for maintenance protocols used in horses.)

Maintenance With an Inhalant Agent

Maintenance of anesthesia with an inhalant agent is similar to the technique described for small-animal patients, with the exception that sudden, unexpected movement can occur without any change in signs of anesthetic depth. Owing to the large breathing circuit volume and patient size, responses to changes in inhalant anesthetic and oxygen flow rates generally occur too

---

BOX 10.7 Maintenance Protocols for Physical Status Class P1 and P2 Horses

1. **Isoflurane:** Administer isoflurane at 1.5%–2.5%.
2. **Sevoflurane:** Administer sevoflurane at 2.5%–4%.
3. **Desflurane:** Administer desflurane at 8%–12%.
4. **"Triple drip" (IV by CRI):** Administer at 1.5 mL/kg/h (see Procedure 10.8 for details).
5. **Xylazine + ketamine (IV):** Administer xylazine 0.25 mg/kg IV + ketamine 0.5 mg/kg IV. This is repeated each time the horse becomes light.

CRI, Constant rate infusion; *IV*, intravenous.

slowly to return the patient to surgical anesthesia simply by altering machine settings. A syringe of ketamine is typically drawn up before anesthesia and either attached to a three-way stopcock in the fluid administration line or kept close to the IV port for this purpose. Approximately one-quarter to one-fifth of the IV induction dose is administered to the horse to return it to surgical anesthesia, which corresponds to 0.4 to 0.5 mg/kg ketamine IV as a bolus (Procedure 10.6).

Compared with other species, horses are more likely to develop hypoventilation, hypotension, and hypoxemia during maintenance of anesthesia, particularly when using inhalant agents. In order to monitor blood pressure more accurately and to obtain arterial blood gas values, it is recommended that horses anesthetized with inhalants for procedures lasting more than 1 hour have an arterial catheter placed in a peripheral artery (facial, transverse facial, dorsal metatarsal; Fig. 10.12). Blood gas samples should be taken every 30 to 60 minutes or more frequently if the situation warrants.

TECHNICIAN NOTE Hypoventilation, hypotension, and hypoxemia are common complications in horses anesthetized with inhalant agents.

Hypoventilation is so common in anesthetized horses, particularly those placed in dorsal recumbency, that a ventilator is often used to maintain normal ventilation. See Chapter 7 for a

---

PROCEDURE 10.6 Anesthetic Maintenance With Inhalant Anesthetic in Horses

General anesthesia maintained with inhalant is similar to the procedure described for small animals (see Procedure 9.7).

1. Choose the initial dial setting based on the anesthetic depth following intubation.
2. Set the oxygen flow rate to 8–10 L/min for an adult horse for 10–15 min to wash out the large volume of nitrogen that is present in a horse's lungs. Then, turn the flow rate down to 3–5 L/min for the remainder of the procedure.
3. Make periodic changes in the vaporizer dial setting based on monitoring parameters.
4. If the anesthetic depth is slightly too light or deep, make small dial changes of approximately 0.5%–1% increments with isoflurane and sevoflurane.
5. If the patient is significantly light (exhibiting spontaneous movement, swallowing, active reflexes, strong muscle tone, etc.), administer a bolus of ketamine (0.4–0.5 mg/kg IV). It may also be necessary to increase the oxygen flow to 8–10 L/min and set isoflurane at 3%–4%, or sevoflurane at 4%–6% (induction level).

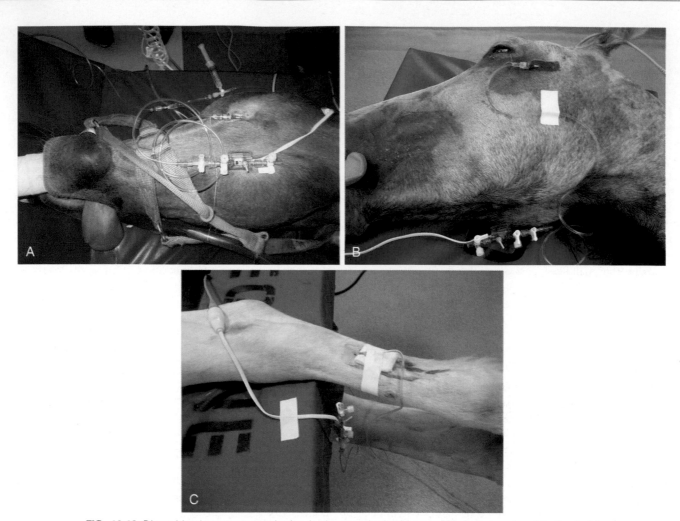

FIG. 10.12 Direct blood pressure monitoring in the anesthetized horse. **(A)** Catheter placed in the facial artery. **(B)** Catheter placed in the transverse facial artery. **(C)** Catheter placed in the dorsal metatarsal artery.

discussion of mechanical ventilation. See Case Presentation 10.1 for an example of management of hypoventilation in the equine patient.

Hypotension (mean arterial blood pressure <70 mmHg) has been shown to contribute to myopathy; therefore treatment with drugs is frequently indicated if increasing the IV fluid rate, decreasing anesthetic depth, and surgical stimulation do not

increase blood pressure. The most common drug used to support blood pressure is the positive inotrope dobutamine (frequently administered via a syringe pump). Dobutamine and many other positive inotropes may cause arrhythmias, so it is important to monitor the electrocardiogram (ECG) closely when starting an infusion. (See Procedure 10.7 for preparation and administration of dobutamine.)

CASE PRESENTATION 10.1 Management of Hypoventilation in the Equine Patient

"Mike" is a healthy, 400-kg 4-year-old Standardbred gelding being anesthetized for arthroscopy of his left carpus. He was sedated with 300 mg xylazine intravenously (IV) and induced with 900 mg ketamine plus 25 mg midazolam IV. Following induction, he underwent orotracheal intubation and was placed on the surgery table in dorsal recumbency. Currently, anesthesia is being maintained with 2% isoflurane delivered in 100% oxygen. His heart rate is 30 beats/min, he is spontaneously breathing with a respiratory rate of 4 breaths/min, his mean arterial blood pressure is 90 mmHg, and he has a strong palpebral reflex with occasional nystagmus.

1) *What is your assessment of Mike at this time?*
2) *What steps, if any, would you like to take at this point?*

TECHNICIAN NOTE Dobutamine, a positive inotrope, is commonly used to treat hypotension in horses. Positive inotropes may cause arrhythmias, so the ECG should be closely monitored during infusion of dobutamine.

Hypoxemia, usually defined as a Pao_2 lower than 80 mmHg, can occur in any horse, regardless of the physical status class. It is more common in horses that are obese, pregnant, or have intestinal torsion, and those that are placed in dorsal recumbency. Hypoxemia has several possible causes, including hypoventilation, ventilation–perfusion mismatch, lung disease, and low cardiac output. Wherever possible, the cause should be investigated and corrected.

PROCEDURE 10.7 How to Prepare and Administer Dobutamine Using a Syringe Pump

1. Draw 56 mL of 0.9% sodium chloride into a 60-mL syringe.
2. Draw 4 mL of dobutamine (15 mg/mL) into the syringe. The concentration of dobutamine is now 60 mg in 60 mL, i.e., 1 mg/mL (or 1000 mcg/mL).
3. Place the syringe in a syringe pump and program in the infusion rate in mL or mcg/min, or in mL or mcg/h (the pump instructions will give accepted units).
4. Typical infusion rates for dobutamine in horses range from 0.5–5 mcg/kg/min, usually starting at the lower end. Administering 1 mcg/kg/min to a 500-kg horse results in an infusion rate of 30 mL/h.
5. Attach the syringe to the port of a primed winged infusion set.
6. Place the needle of the winged infusion set into the injection port of an IV administration set near the catheter.

Maintenance With Intravenous Agents or Total Intravenous Anesthesia

Intravenous maintenance of anesthesia in horses is generally reserved for shorter procedures (less than 1 hour) in healthy patients and for procedures done away from a veterinary clinic ("field anesthesia"). TIVA is generally characterized by higher blood pressure, less respiratory depression, and more active palpebral reflexes than inhalant anesthesia. When used for procedures lasting less than 1 hour, TIVA is associated with recoveries of good quality.

Anesthesia can be extended by administering additional bolus doses of an alpha$_2$-agonist and ketamine. Typically, one-quarter of the amount of each drug used to sedate and induce the horse is administered IV to prolong anesthesia. An alternative method of administering TIVA in horses is to use a combination commonly referred to as "triple drip." As its name suggests, this is a combination of three drugs: guaifenesin, ketamine, and xylazine (or any other alpha$_2$-agonist). Ketamine and xylazine are added to the guaifenesin and infused together to maintain anesthesia (see Procedure 10.8 for preparation and administration of triple drip).

Recently, commercially manufactured guaifenesin has become harder to obtain in the United States. Xylazine and

PROCEDURE 10.8 How to Prepare and Administer "Triple Drip"[a]

1. Add 2.5 mL of xylazine (100 mg/mL) to 500 mL of 5% guaifenesin.
2. Add 5 mL of ketamine (100 mg/mL) to 500 mL of 5% guaifenesin.
3. Each milliliter of "triple drip" contains 0.5 mg xylazine, 1 mg ketamine, and 50 mg guaifenesin.
4. Administer CRI at 1.5 mL/kg/h, which equates to xylazine 0.75 mg/kg/h, ketamine 1.5 mg/kg/h and guaifenesin 75 mg/kg/h IV.
5. Temporarily increase the infusion rate if patient becomes light (movement, rapid nystagmus, swallowing).

[a]Note that there are other ways to formulate "triple drip." Some practices substitute detomidine or romifidine for xylazine, and some will use different final concentrations of drugs. In the latter case, infusion rates will vary.
CRI, Constant rate infusion; IV, intravenous.

ketamine can be placed in a bag of normal saline without guaifenesin and infused at similar rates to triple drip. Alternatively, 25 mg midazolam can be added instead of guaifenesin and the mixture of midazolam, ketamine, and xylazine administered IV to maintain anesthesia.

> **TECHNICIAN NOTE** Maintenance of anesthesia in the field and for procedures of less than 1 hour's duration is typically accomplished using TIVA. An example of a drug combination used for TIVA is a coinfusion of guaifenesin, ketamine, and xylazine, known as "triple drip."

Maintenance With Injectable and Inhalant Agents

As an alternative, inhalant and injectable agents can be used in combination to maintain anesthesia, a technique referred to as partial intravenous anesthesia (PIVA). For instance, triple drip or ketamine and xylazine in saline can be infused at a very slow rate (using a 10 gtt/mL administration set, 1 drop every 5 to 10 seconds is delivered to an adult horse), which will allow a reduction in the amount of inhalant required and will provide muscle relaxation and analgesia. Lidocaine or detomidine infusions are also commonly administered to decrease inhalant requirements and produce analgesia.

PATIENT POSITIONING, COMFORT, AND SAFETY

During anesthetic induction and maintenance, a number of considerations must be observed to ensure that the patient is not harmed. Many of the principles of small-animal anesthesia apply to equine anesthesia (see Chapter 9). In addition, it is important to observe the following:
- Physically control the head to protect the eyes during gate inductions—horses will tend to fall against the wall or the gate, which leaves their eyes vulnerable to corneal injury
- When hoisting horses, ensure that hobbles are correctly applied so that the horse cannot fall from the hoist or be injured by hobble placement
- Ensure correct positioning and padding on the surgery table to prevent neuropathies and myopathies

ANESTHETIC RECOVERY

Horses have a psychologic need to stand up shortly after awakening from anesthesia and this makes recovery particularly dangerous. Some steps can be taken to minimize injury to the horse and anesthetist, but there is a high incidence of complications from anesthetic recovery in horses and clients should be informed of the risks. In veterinary clinics and hospitals, specific padded areas or rooms are dedicated as recovery stalls. In some clinics, the induction stall is also used for recovery. Depending on the facilities and personnel available, horses may be left to recover unassisted after extubation or may have ropes attached to the halter and tail with which personnel can assist the horse as it attempts to stand (Fig. 10.13). Under field conditions, the anesthetist typically restrains the horse by kneeling on

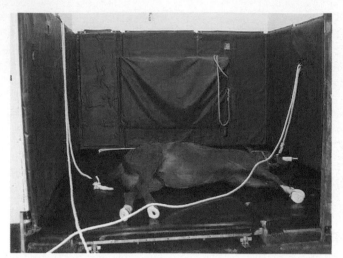

FIG. 10.13 Rope placement for assisted recovery in a horse. One rope is attached to the halter and the other is attached to the tail.

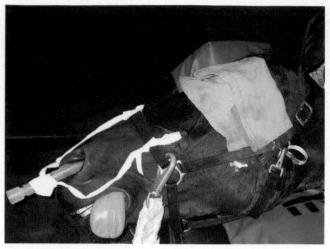

FIG. 10.15 Nasopharyngeal tube placed for recovery. Using the same technique as for nasotracheal tube placement, a nasopharyngeal tube can be placed for recovery and secured to the halter. The tube is gently removed after the horse stands.

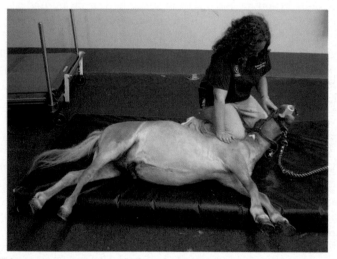

FIG. 10.14 Anesthetist restraining a horse. The anesthetist can restrain a horse by kneeling on the horse's neck and lifting its muzzle slightly off the ground. Once the horse is awake and strong enough to lift the anesthetist off its neck, the anesthetist may leave the recovery area and allow the horse to make an attempt to stand. This technique is useful for horses of any size, in this case, a miniature horse.

its neck until they believe the horse is ready to make a successful attempt to stand (see below for signs of recovery) (Fig. 10.14). Personnel then typically hold the head and tail until the horse is able to stand unassisted.

Preparation for Recovery

Replace the halter. Place a nasopharyngeal tube before movement if nasal congestion or edema is present (Fig. 10.15). Upon completion of the procedure, turn off the inhalant and transfer the horse to a padded recovery stall, where it can be extubated and monitored. Horses are often placed on thick foam or air mattresses, although a padded floor may give enough support. If possible, and particularly if the horse was hypoxemic during anesthesia, provide oxygen support using a demand valve (Fig. 10.16), or insufflation (5 to 10 L/min nasally or through the endotracheal tube) until the horse is extubated or too light

to tolerate an insufflation hose. A demand valve provides oxygen at a very high flow rate (160 to 280 L/min). An assisted breath can be given as follows: 1) remove the endotracheal tube connector from the tube; 2) connect the demand valve to the endotracheal tube of the intubated horse; 3) manually depress the button while observing the chest wall—oxygen should flow into the patient's lungs and expand the chest; 4) once an adequate chest expansion is observed, release the button and disconnect the demand valve from the endotracheal tube to allow complete exhalation. Insufflation involves the passive provision of oxygen: 1) a tube that is able to fit inside the endotracheal tube, nasopharyngeal tube, or nostril is advanced to at least the level of the oropharynx; 2) oxygen flow is set at 10 L/min.

> **TECHNICIAN NOTE** If nasal congestion is present following anesthesia, a nasopharyngeal tube should be placed for recovery.

If the recovery is to be assisted by ropes, a head rope should be attached to the halter and another rope tied to the tail (see Fig. 10.13). See Procedure 10.9 for the sequence of events when preparing a horse for recovery.

Monitoring During Recovery

During recovery, it is ideal to watch the horse on a continual basis so that it can be assisted or sedated if necessary. While the horse is lying quietly, the anesthetist should watch respirations to make sure the horse is breathing normally, take the pulse (from the facial artery) every 5 to 10 minutes, and assess the eye for depth of anesthesia. The anesthetist stays close to the head of the horse in order to monitor the pulse, be ready for extubation, and to physically control the horse if it attempts to stand too soon.

Signs of Recovery

As the patient recovers, it will progress back through the stages and planes of anesthesia. Many horses develop nystagmus

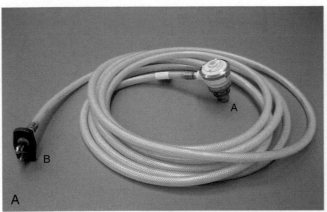
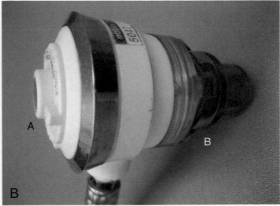
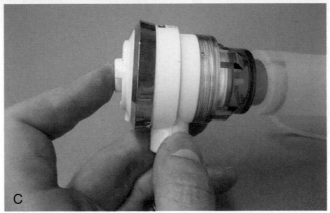

FIG. 10.16 Oxygen demand valve. **(A)** An oxygen demand valve showing *A*, the demand valve and *B*, the quick-release connector, which is inserted into a hospital oxygen supply outlet. **(B)** Close-up view of the demand valve showing *A*, manual button and *B*, connector for endotracheal tube. **(C)** Demand valve connected to endotracheal tube (it is usually easier to remove the endotracheal tube connector before connecting the demand valve to the tube).

during recovery, and rapid nystagmus accompanied by paddling of the limbs generally means that a horse will try to get up too soon and have a rough recovery. In this event, it may be prudent to sedate the horse with 0.1 to 0.2 mg/kg xylazine IV and/or 0.01 to 0.03 mg/kg acepromazine IV. Generally, maintaining control of the head by sitting on the neck or holding the head up off the floor will provide some control over the

horse. However, once the horse is strong enough to lift an anesthetist off its neck, the anesthetist should retreat to a safe distance to observe the remainder of recovery. Other signs that a horse is recovering and may be close to extubation are chewing, swallowing, and purposeful ear, limb, head and neck, or tail movement.

Extubation

To prepare the patient for extubation, deflate the cuff by drawing out all the air until the pilot balloon is empty. Both before and following tube removal, keep the neck in a natural but slightly extended position to protect the airway. Remove the endotracheal tube gently when the swallowing reflex returns, using a slow, steady motion. You may also remove it when signs of imminent arousal are present such as voluntary movement of the limbs or head, movement of the tongue, or chewing. Check to make sure the horse can breathe without obstruction by placing your hand in front of the nostrils and feeling for air flow. Horses can only breathe through their noses and will become distressed and compromised if they are unable to. If a nasopharyngeal tube has not been placed and the nasal passages are or become obstructed, a tube must be placed immediately. In the event that a nasopharyngeal tube does not alleviate the obstruction, a tracheostomy must be performed by the veterinarian, so materials for performing one must be close to the recovery stall at all times.

PROCEDURE 10.9 Recovery From General Anesthesia in the Horse

1. Prepare the patient for recovery, including placement of a nasopharyngeal tube, removal of monitoring equipment, and replacing the halter. Ensure the recovery area has been prepared.
2. Discontinue the anesthetic and transfer the horse to the recovery area, paying attention to positioning, and pull the dependent forelimb forwards.
3. Extubate the patient at the appropriate time and ensure the horse can breathe either through its nostrils or the nasopharyngeal tube without obstruction.
4. Assist the horse until it stands, as directed by the attending veterinarian.
5. Remove the nasopharyngeal tube, if present. Ensure that the horse can breathe through its nostrils.
6. Prepare the patient for continued hospitalization or discharge by applying bandages, administering medications, flushing and securing the IV catheter, and performing any other procedures ordered by the attending veterinarian.

Standing After Regaining Consciousness

The ideal recovery to standing is one where the horse, after it has been extubated, rolls smoothly from lateral to sternal recumbency. After lying in sternal recumbency for several minutes, the horse makes a coordinated, strong attempt to stand and is successful on its first try. Head and tail ropes can be used to assist the horse each time it attempts to stand (Fig. 10.17). A challenging aspect of equine anesthesia is that many horses, particularly those that have been anesthetized for several hours with inhalants, do not have ideal recoveries. With experience, the anesthetist will learn when it is appropriate to provide additional sedation, analgesia, or physical assistance in the recovery stall to minimize injury to the horse. There is, unfortunately, always the possibility that a horse may suffer a catastrophic event during recovery, such as a fractured long bone (femur, tibia, humerus, radius). In such an event, the attending veterinarian should assist the anesthetist in immediately reanesthetizing the horse to assess the situation.

THE POSTANESTHETIC PERIOD

Once the horse is standing and able to walk steadily, it can be returned to its stall. This can be assessed by walking the horse in a circle inside the recovery stall. Once back in its own stall, the horse should be muzzled for 1 to 3 hours but should have free access to water. The horse should also be observed for any

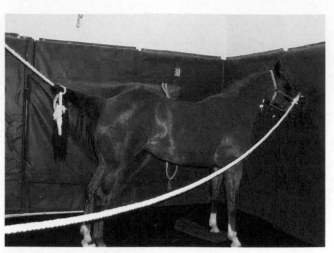

FIG. 10.17 Assisted anesthetic recovery using ropes in the horse. The head and tail ropes are used to guide the horse as it attempts to stand. After the horse has made a successful attempt to stand, it may be necessary to leave the ropes on for several minutes as the horse continues to recover from the effects of anesthesia.

signs of neuropathy (e.g., facial nerve paralysis: drooping eyelid and lip on the affected side; radial nerve paralysis/inability to extend affected forelimb fully), myopathy (hard, swollen muscles; stiff and painful gait), or colic (rolling, kicking at the abdomen) in the postanesthetic period.

■ KEY POINTS

1. Horses present unique challenges to the anesthetist because of their size, physiology, and temperament. Horses also seem to have a psychologic need to stand following anesthesia, making recovery from anesthesia challenging and potentially dangerous to both horse and anesthetist.
2. Horses are susceptible to hypoventilation, nasal congestion, atelectasis, hypoxemia, and hypotension during general anesthesia.
3. Superficial nerves are susceptible to pressure injury, leading to neuropathy, and muscles are prone to injury if blood flow to them is inadequate during anesthesia. Attention must be paid to positioning and padding on the surgery table and in recovery.
4. Standing chemical restraint may be used to perform many surgical and medical procedures in horses instead of general anesthesia, which is fraught with risks to the patient. The head should be supported in a neutral position in a standing sedated horse in order to minimize nasal congestion.
5. A horse should always be appropriately sedated before induction of general anesthesia.
6. General anesthesia is typically induced by rapidly injecting a bolus of IV anesthetic. This provides a smooth transition from standing to lateral recumbency, with minimal risk of injury to the horse and anesthetist.

7. Maintenance of anesthesia in the field and for short procedures (<1-hour duration) is typically accomplished using total intravenous anesthesia (TIVA). An example of a drug combination used for this is a co-infusion of guaifenesin, ketamine, and xylazine, known as "triple drip."
8. Foals that are easily restrained may be nasotracheally intubated after sedation. The nasotracheal tube can then be attached to an anesthetic machine and anesthesia can be induced using an inhalant anesthetic.
9. Intubation in equine patients is a blind procedure, which is facilitated by extending the head and neck.
10. Common problems encountered during maintenance of anesthesia are hypoventilation, hypoxemia, and hypotension. These problems are more common in horses maintained with inhalant anesthetics and those positioned in dorsal recumbency.
11. Recovery is the most challenging part of equine anesthesia. Various strategies can be employed to minimize injury to the horse and personnel; however, it is possible for any horse to have a recovery that is not ideal.
12. Following general anesthesia, horses should be monitored for signs of neuropathy, myopathy, pain, and colic.

REVIEW QUESTIONS

1. Which of the following is true regarding use of standing chemical restraint for performing surgery on a horse?
   a. Horses must be endotracheally intubated for standing chemical restraint
   b. Risk of myopathy or neuropathy is higher with standing chemical restraint
   c. The head must be supported in a normal position to avoid nasal congestion
   d. Hypoxemia is a common complication of standing chemical restraint

2. If a horse becomes excited after it has been premedicated with xylazine IV before general anesthesia, the next step the anesthetist should take is to:
   a. Allow the horse time to calm down before proceeding
   b. Physically restrain the horse using ropes
   c. Induce the horse with acepromazine
   d. Induce the horse with ketamine

3. Appropriate positioning and padding of the horse on the surgery table are essential to prevent:
   a. Hypoxemia and hypotension
   b. Myopathies and neuropathies
   c. Hypoventilation and hypertension
   d. Regurgitation and aspiration

4. What is/are the main reason(s) for including guaifenesin in an induction protocol in horses?
   a. Muscle relaxation
   b. Analgesia
   c. Sedation
   d. All of the above

5. An inhalant induction via nasotracheal tube placement is appropriate for which of the following patients?
   a. A 2-year-old Arabian stallion undergoing arthroscopy
   b. A 25-year-old Thoroughbred mare undergoing sinus surgery
   c. A 3-week-old foal undergoing colic surgery
   d. A 6-month-old foal undergoing umbilical hernia repair

6. Which of the following statements best describes endotracheal intubation in the horse?
   a. Intubation is performed blindly, with the head and neck extended
   b. Intubation can only be performed in lateral recumbency
   c. A laryngoscope is useful for visualization of the larynx
   d. An endoscope is commonly used to facilitate intubation

7. The most common complications in horses during maintenance of anesthesia with inhalant anesthetics are:
   a. Hypoxemia, hypertension, and bradycardia
   b. Hypoxemia, hypotension, and bradycardia
   c. Hypoxemia, hypertension, and hypoventilation
   d. Hypoxemia, hypotension, and hypoventilation

8. Which drug is used to treat hypotension in the anesthetized horse?
   a. Dextrose
   b. Digoxin
   c. Dobutamine
   d. Doxycycline

9. Of all phases of anesthesia, recovery poses the highest risk to the horse and is the phase over which the anesthetist has the least control.
   True
   False

10. A horse has recovered from anesthesia following arthroscopy, and shows the following clinical signs: hard, swollen gluteal muscles; stiff gait; and reluctance to walk. The most likely diagnosis is:
    a. Colic
    b. Myopathy
    c. Neuropathy
    d. Nephropathy

ANSWERS TO CASE PRESENTATION

Case Presentation 10.1

Question #1: Heart rate and blood pressure are within the normal range for an anesthetized horse. Blood pressure may be higher than typically seen in the average anesthetized horse, which may indicate a lighter plane of anesthesia. The respiratory rate is lower than the acceptable range (6 being the minimum), so Mike is most likely hypoventilating, a common occurrence in anesthetized horses, regardless of health status. Anesthetic depth is too light because horses should not have nystagmus and should have a slight palpebral reflex when in a surgical plane of anesthesia.

Question #2: Hypoventilation can be confirmed by obtaining a blood gas and looking at the $Paco_2$ or attaching an end-tidal CO_2 monitor. At a respiratory rate of 4 breaths/min, it is very likely that $Paco_2$ will be elevated. Ventilation should be increased by placing this horse on a mechanical ventilator, if one is available. Respiratory rate should be set at 6 to 8 breaths/min and tidal volume should be 15 mL/kg (i.e., 6 L) per breath. Mike is also too light for surgery at this time based on his eye signs, so the isoflurane concentration should be increased. Placing the horse on a mechanical ventilator will increase anesthetic delivery; therefore a small change on the vaporizer dial to 2.5% is appropriate and Mike should continue to be monitored closely for changes in anesthetic depth, which may warrant further adjustments.

SELECTED READINGS

Clark-Price SC, editor: Topics in equine anesthesia, *Vet Clin North Am Equine Pract* 29(3), 2013.

Muir WW, Hubbell JAE: *Equine anesthesia*, ed 2, St. Louis, 2009, Saunders.

Robertson SA: Sedation and anesthesia of the foal, *Equine Vet Educ* 9:37–44, 1997.

Tranquilli WJ, Thurmon JC, Grimm KA: *Veterinary anesthesia and analgesia*, ed 5, Ames, IA, 2015, Wiley Blackwell.

11

Anesthesia of Ruminants, Camelids, and Swine

OUTLINE

LEARNING OBJECTIVES

When you have completed this chapter, you will be able to:
- Describe the main physiologic and anatomic differences that influence anesthetic management of ruminants, camelids, and swine.
- Explain how to prepare a ruminant, camelid, or porcine patient for anesthesia.
- Select an anesthetic protocol for an ASA PS1 or PS2 adult cow, small ruminant, camelid, or pig.
- Explain how to intubate an adult cow, a small ruminant, a calf or camelid, and a pig.

- Explain the importance of proper positioning of anesthetized ruminants and camelids.
- Explain how to position a ruminant for recovery.
- Explain how to position a camelid for recovery.
- Explain the unique concerns and challenges when anesthetizing pigs.
- Describe the clinical signs of porcine stress syndrome.

KEY TERMS

Bolus
Eructate
Porcine stress syndrome

Regurgitus
Tilt table
TKX

Total injectable anesthesia

RUMINANT ANESTHESIA

The basic principles of anesthesia discussed in Chapter 9 apply to ruminant anesthesia. Ruminants do not pose quite the same challenge to the anesthetist as horses do (see Chapter 10); however, an understanding of their unique digestive physiology is important regarding how it impacts the well-being of the patient under general anesthesia and in recovery. Additionally, ruminants present for general anesthesia less frequently than small animals or horses do, so it takes longer to gain anesthetic experience. There are several reasons for this. Due to their relatively calm nature, ruminants require general anesthesia for relatively few procedures. Many surgeries can be conducted using local or regional anesthetic techniques (see Chapter 7) in conjunction with physical restraint. Consideration must also be given to drug withdrawal times when dealing with animals that produce milk or meat for human consumption. Finally, the administration of general anesthesia to production animals is often uneconomical.

Ruminant patients range in size from a few kilograms (lambs and kids) to over 1000 kg (adult bulls). Thus as with horses, specialized tilt tables, head gates, hoists, and transporters may be required to allow the veterinarian to perform surgery or procedures such as hoof trimming safely without causing injury to the animal or personnel. Equipment suitable for anesthetizing small-animal patients is commonly used for smaller patients (sheep, goats, calves). However, if young cattle >150 kg in body weight and adult cattle are to undergo general anesthesia, the anesthetist must have access to a large-animal anesthetic machine and be familiar with its operation as well as that of related equipment and monitors.

The main anesthetic concerns in ruminants result from their unique digestive anatomy and physiology. Ruminants constantly produce large volumes of saliva compared with other species and this is generally not inhibited by general anesthesia. They are thus prone to aspiration if the airway is not protected. Additionally, regurgitation of rumen contents (known as regurgitus) can occur at any stage of general anesthesia, most commonly during the light or deep planes. Fermentation in the rumen is only slightly decreased by general anesthesia; thus ruminants are predisposed to bloat because they cannot eructate when they are unconscious.

As with small-animal anesthesia, neuromuscular blockers are rarely used in general practice but are sometimes used to provide muscle relaxation for ocular and orthopedic procedures in veterinary schools and referral practices.

Patient Preparation

The reader is referred to Chapters 2 and 9 for a detailed discussion of the essentials of patient preparation before anesthesia. See Procedure 11.1 for additional tasks pertinent to preparation of the ruminant patient undergoing general anesthesia. Additionally, the anesthetist should be familiar with operation of equipment such as surgical tables, transporters, head gates, and hoists that will be used during the anesthetic episode.

It is essential to ensure that ruminants have been adequately fasted before anesthesia. Fasting reduces the size of the rumen and also decreases microbial activity. This in turn decreases gas production prior to and during anesthesia. Normally, ruminants eructate to expel gas from the rumen; however, under anesthesia, this does not happen and can lead to bloating. A bloated rumen can put pressure on the diaphragm and large blood vessels (aorta, caudal vena cava) in the abdomen, resulting in respiratory as well as circulatory compromise. Once an anesthetized ruminant develops severe bloat, it can be very difficult to treat and may lead to death if it goes unnoticed or untreated. Bloat often goes unrecognized when a patient is small and covered by surgical drapes. Clinical signs include development of a distended, tight abdomen; decreased blood pressure; increased heart rate; and decreased ventilation.

Selecting a Protocol

A suitable protocol takes into account the minimum patient database, the patient's physical status class, and the type and duration of procedure to be performed. Regardless of the protocol, the correct drugs and amounts must be prepared. Ill, geriatric, pediatric, or otherwise compromised patients (physical status classes P3 to P5) require use of modified protocols based

---

PROCEDURE 11.1 Preparation for Anesthesia of a Ruminant or Camelid

1. Assess, prepare, and weigh the patient. (See Chapter 2 for a discussion of patient assessment, preparation, and stabilization.)
2. Prepare equipment for and place an intravenous (IV) catheter (clippers, local anesthetic, antiseptic scrub, catheters, tape, normal saline, suture material, catheter cap, and/or extension line with a three-way stopcock). Catheter placement in large or aggressive cattle may require restraint in a chute with a head gate.
3. Determine the protocol (anesthetic agents, including dosages, routes, and sequence of administration).
4. Calculate the volume of each agent to give, including fluid administration rates (preanesthetic, induction, maintenance, and analgesic agents).
5. Review the oxygen flow rates (see Table 10.1 for oxygen flow rates used in large animals and Table 9.2 for oxygen flow rates when using a circle system in small animals).
6. Prepare the equipment required to administer drugs (syringes, needles, agents, reversal agents, emergency cart, controlled substance log).
7. Prepare fluid administration equipment (fluids, administration/extension set, syringe pump, tape, normal saline).
8. Prepare equipment for endotracheal intubation. Have suction equipment assembled and turned on for ruminants and camelids. Remove jewelry and watch, and ensure fingernails are trimmed short for digital intubation of adult cattle.
9. Prepare monitoring equipment, including arterial catheterization materials, anesthesia records, monitors, and probes (see Chapter 6).
10. Assemble and test the anesthetic machine and ventilator.

on the patient's primary condition. Management of these cases can be quite challenging and requires customization of the anesthetic protocol by the attending veterinarian.

See Chapter 9 for additional information on selecting a protocol and strategies to minimize adverse effects.

Summary of a General Anesthetic Procedure

The dynamics associated with commonly used protocols in ruminant anesthesia are very similar to those associated with small-animal protocols (see Chapter 9), with the exception that induction with an intramuscular (IM) agent is not commonly used in clinical practice.

Equipment Preparation

During a typical anesthetic induction, many events occur in rapid succession. Anesthetic agents are administered, the patient becomes unconscious and recumbent, and the endotracheal tube is placed, secured, and cuffed. The patient is then lifted or hoisted onto the surgery table, the endotracheal tube is connected to the anesthetic machine, and the anesthetic gas level is adjusted, all within the first few minutes. Because these events follow one another so rapidly, the technician does not have the luxury of leaving the patient to locate equipment (Fig. 11.1). For this reason, all equipment must be carefully gathered, checked, and organized before commencing the procedure.

Patients weighing more than 150 kg are usually placed on a large-animal anesthetic machine (see Fig. 10.1). Most large-animal anesthetic machines incorporate a ventilator (see Fig. 10.1 D). Both the circle system and the ventilator of the machine should be checked before use. Small ruminants and calves weighing less than 150 kg can be placed on a small-animal anesthetic machine. Hypothermia is uncommon in anesthetized adult cattle; however, devices such as warm air blankets or warm water circulating blankets can be used to maintain body temperature in small ruminants and calves, as in small-animal patients.

Any specialized equipment required for restraining or positioning anesthetized ruminants, such as head gates, transporters, and tilt tables, should be checked. In addition to items from the standard checklist, it is extremely helpful to have suction available for small ruminants to allow feed material, regurgitus, or saliva to be removed from the pharynx during intubation.

A crash cart containing emergency equipment and drugs should also always be available.

Premedication and Sedation

Many ruminants are calm and tractable enough to allow intravenous (IV) catheterization and induction of anesthesia, with minimal or no premedication and only mild restraint. Adult cattle are typically restrained using the head gate of a transporter or chute, or against a tilt table. Premedication is often reserved for patients that are aggressive, excited, or stressed. Although many ruminants do not require sedation before anesthesia, premedication will still provide benefits such as decreased doses of induction and maintenance drugs, muscle relaxation, and analgesia.

> **TECHNICIAN NOTE** Ruminants are very sensitive to xylazine, requiring one-tenth of the dose given to horses.

Anticholinergic drugs are not used to premedicate ruminants because they do not reduce salivation and instead cause the saliva to become thick and ropy. These thicker strands of saliva are more easily aspirated, which can cause airway obstruction. This class of drugs is therefore reserved for treatment of arrhythmias and for cardiopulmonary resuscitation (CPR) in these species. (See Box 11.1 for premedication and sedative drugs and doses in ruminants.)

BOX 11.1 Premedication/Sedative Protocols for Physical Status Class PS1 and PS2 Ruminants and Camelids

Protocols for Light–Moderate Sedation[a]:
1. **Acepromazine (IV):** Acepromazine 0.01–0.03 mg/kg IV (may increase regurgitation)
2. **Xylazine (IV/IM):** Xylazine 0.01–0.05 mg/kg IV or IM (unlikely to cause recumbency)
3. **Detomidine (IV):** Detomidine 0.005–0.02 mg/kg IV

Protocols for Moderate–Deep Sedation (for minor procedures such as radiography or wound assessment) **or for Premedication[b]:**
1. **Acepromazine (IV):** Acepromazine 0.03–0.05 mg/kg IV
2. **Xylazine (IV/IM):** Xylazine 0.05–0.1 mg/kg IV or 0.05–0.2 mg/kg IM (likely to cause recumbency and potentially light anesthesia)
3. **Detomidine (IV):** Detomidine 0.01–0.03 mg/kg IV
4. **Midazolam–Butorphanol (IV):** Midazolam 0.1–0.5 mg/kg and butorphanol 0.1–0.2 mg/kg IV (may produce ataxia, so recommended for small ruminants/camelids or restrained cattle)

[a]Note that ruminants may require no sedation for procedures performed with local anesthetic when the patient is standing.
[b]Note that ruminants and camelids may not require premedication before anesthesia.
IM, Intramuscular; *IV,* intravenous.

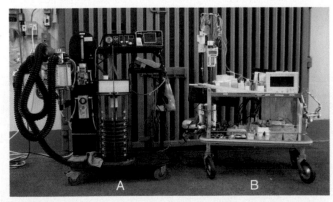

FIG. 11.1 Anesthetic equipment for anesthetizing a large ruminant. **(A)** Large-animal anesthetic machine and ventilator. **(B)** An anesthetic cart with drugs, syringes, endotracheal tubes, a mouth gag for adult cattle, and anesthetic monitor ready for anesthetizing a large ruminant.

TECHNICIAN NOTE Anticholinergics should not be used for premedication of ruminants because they do not decrease salivation and instead make it thick and ropy, increasing the risk of aspiration.

Anesthetic Induction

Anesthetic induction is the process by which an animal loses consciousness and enters surgical anesthesia. Of the goals set out for induction in Chapter 9, it is particularly important to gain control of and protect the airway as quickly as possible in ruminants because they are more likely to regurgitate than other species, which places them at much greater risk for aspiration of rumen contents.

What follows is a description of specific techniques used to induce a patient. (See Box 11.2 for IV induction protocols in ruminants and Procedure 11.2 for the sequence of events for induction with an IV agent and maintenance with an inhalant agent in a ruminant.)

Intravenous Induction

Induction of anesthesia in large cattle may occur in a special induction stall that has padded walls and often a padded floor, in a transporter, or on a tilt table. Smaller ruminants can generally be induced next to the surgery table or, if small or severely compromised, while lying on the surgery table. Although ruminants do not typically become excited during induction of anesthesia, the goals with adult cattle are similar to those with horses: to produce unconsciousness rapidly and to minimize injury to the patient or personnel. Drugs are thus given to the larger ruminants as a rapid bolus, with the exception of double drip (see Box 11.2 and Fig. 11.2), which is administered rapidly IV to effect. Smaller ruminants, particularly those that are compromised, can be given induction drugs to effect as for small-animal patients.

Once the patient is unconscious, it should be kept in sternal recumbency for intubation whenever possible. It is important to be vigilant for regurgitation, which can occur at any point of the anesthetic procedure but occurs most frequently when anesthesia is light or too deep. If regurgitation occurs, the head should immediately be positioned so that the mouth is lower

---

BOX 11.2 Intravenous Induction Protocols for Physical Status Class PS1 and PS2 Ruminants and Camelids

1. **Ketamine–Midazolam (IV):** Ketamine 2.5 mg/kg IV and midazolam[a] 0.12 mg/kg IV mixed in the same syringe. (This is equivalent to 1 mL of the mixture per 20 kg of body weight.) Note the difference from the small-animal dosage. This combination is used most commonly in small ruminants and camelids.
2. **"Double drip" (IV):** "Double drip" IV to effect (approximately 1–2 mL/kg). "Double drip" can be made by adding 500 mg ketamine to a 500 mL bag of 5% guaifenesin. Each milliliter of double drip therefore contains 1 mg ketamine and 50 mg guaifenesin. In smaller patients, draw the correct number of milliliters from the bag in 50- or 60-mL syringes for increased dosing accuracy and give slowly to effect.
3. **Telazol (IV):** Telazol 1–4 mg/kg IV (use a lower dose after premedication with xylazine).
4. **Propofol (IV):** Propofol 2–4 mg/kg IV (for small ruminants/camelids only; not economical for adult cattle).

[a]An equivalent *volume* of diazepam can be substituted for midazolam.

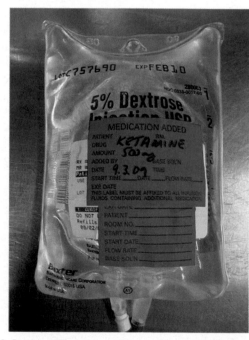

FIG. 11.2 Double drip, using a 500-mL bag of 5% dextrose in water containing 5% guaifenesin to which 5 mL of ketamine has been added. Final concentrations are therefore 1 mg/mL ketamine and 50 mg/mL guaifenesin.

PROCEDURE 11.2 Sequence of Events for Induction With an IV Agent and Maintenance With an Inhalant Agent in a Ruminant or Camelid

1. Administer premedications approximately 20–30 min (intramuscular [IM]) or 5–10 min (intravenous [IV]) before anesthetic induction if this is considered necessary.
2. Administer the induction agent.
3. Check the patient's readiness for intubation.
4. Place and secure the endotracheal tube.
5. Inflate the endotracheal tube cuff.
6. Confirm placement of the endotracheal tube with capnography.
7. Check the patient's vital signs.
8. Hoist or lift (as appropriate), position, and secure the patient for the procedure. It is imperative that the pharynx be positioned higher than the mouth whenever possible.
9. Turn on the oxygen and attach the endotracheal tube to the breathing circuit.
10. Turn on the anesthetic vaporizer to the appropriate level.
11. Determine the patient's anesthetic depth and commence regular monitoring.
12. Attach monitoring devices, including the placement of an arterial catheter.
13. Continue to monitor and adjust the anesthetic and oxygen levels as needed until completion of the procedure.

PROCEDURE 11.3 Intravenous Induction in Adult Cattle

Induction of anesthesia in adult cattle is similar to horses in that the goal is to achieve lateral recumbency without excitement or injury to the patient or personnel. In order to do this, the induction agent is given as a rapid IV bolus to PS1 and PS2 cows. The only induction agent that is given to effect (see Chapter 9) is double drip.

- **Ketamine–midazolam** and **ketamine–diazepam mixtures:** After checking to make sure that the IV catheter is patent and still in the jugular vein, the entire syringe of the calculated dose of drugs is rapidly injected into the catheter or extension set, then the catheter is flushed using heparinized saline.

- **Double drip (guaifenesin 50 mg/mL** and **ketamine 1 mg/mL):** A bag of double drip with an IV administration set attached is placed in a pressure sleeve, which is inflated up to 300 mmHg pressure. The administration set is connected to the IV catheter or extension set. After checking to make sure that the IV catheter is patent and still in the jugular vein, double drip is administered under pressure to effect. Approximately 1–2 mL/kg will produce signs of ataxia (swaying), followed by recumbency. If intubation is not possible, a further 1–2 mL/kg may be administered more slowly or a bolus of ketamine 1 mg/kg IV may be given.

---

than the pharynx, which allows regurgitus to drain out and helps to prevent aspiration.

Once anesthesia has been induced, the patient's vital signs should be briefly checked before intubation. (See Procedure 11.3 for IV induction techniques in adult cattle.)

Endotracheal Intubation

Following the induction of general anesthesia in ruminants, it is ideal to place an endotracheal tube to protect the airway. If intubation is not carried out, the head must be positioned with the poll higher than the mouth. Ruminants being placed in dorsal recumbency for surgery should always be intubated. The advantages of intubation are discussed in Chapters 4 and 9.

Equipment for Endotracheal Intubation

The following equipment is required to perform endotracheal intubation:
- Appropriately sized endotracheal tubes (at least two of slightly different diameters)
- Stylet (small ruminants and calves only)
- A mouth gag to hold the jaws apart (adult cattle only)
- Laryngoscope (small ruminants and calves)
- Gauze sponge to grasp the tongue (if preferred)
- A syringe to inflate the cuff (10 mL for small ruminants and calves or 60 mL for adult cattle)
- Long forceps to remove feed material if present
- Suction to remove liquid regurgitus if present

Selecting an Endotracheal Tube

The general principles for selecting an endotracheal tube are discussed in Chapter 9. Adult cattle typically require a 22-mm, 24-mm, 26-mm, or 30-mm diameter cuffed tube. Two tube sizes are usually selected for intubation—the anticipated size and one size smaller. Small ruminants and calves require smaller tubes.

Endotracheal tubes are further discussed in Chapter 4.

Preparing the Tube

Before using an endotracheal tube, it must be checked for integrity. It should be clean, sanitized, and free of blockages, holes, deterioration, or other damage. The connector must be securely attached and the cuff must inflate and hold pressure after detaching the syringe from the valve. The tube may be lubricated with a small amount of sterile, water-soluble lubricant, although this is not essential for adult cattle.

Intubation Procedure

The procedure for intubation differs between small ruminants and calves, and adult cattle.

Small ruminants and calves. Intubation in these patients is accomplished in a similar way to small-animal patients. The oral opening is small in these patients compared to the distance between the mouth and larynx, so visualization of the airway can be challenging. Additionally, the caudal half of the tongue is thickened, particularly in sheep and goats, which further obstructs the anesthetist's view. Attempting to pass the endotracheal tube alone typically completely obstructs the view, making successful placement extremely challenging and more a matter of luck than skill. Therefore using a narrow stylet that protrudes beyond the patient end of the tube as a guide allows better visualization of the larynx.

With the head extended by an assistant, the anesthetist places a laryngoscope to visualize the larynx. It often helps to grasp the tongue with a gauze sponge and gently pull it forward. The anesthetist then passes the stylet into the airway, taking care not to cause injury to the larynx or trachea. The endotracheal tube can then be passed over the stylet and into the larynx (Fig. 11.3).

The cuff is inflated as for small animal intubation (see Chapter 9).

Adult cattle. Adult cattle are intubated manually using a blind technique (Fig. 11.4 and Procedure 11.4). A speculum or mouth gag is placed, which prevents the cow from closing its mouth (see Fig. 11.4 A). This protects the anesthetist's arm and hand from being injured if the cow should become light enough to chew. The anesthetist then inserts their nondominant hand into the mouth up to the larynx, holding (and protecting) the endotracheal tube in their hand (see Fig. 11.4 B and C). The dominant hand is used to push the tube toward the larynx. Once the anesthetist's fingers are at the level of the larynx, the anesthetist palpates the epiglottis, reflects it forward if necessary, and directs the end of the endotracheal tube into the trachea, while simultaneously advancing it with their dominant hand. Extending the head and neck of the cow, while sometimes challenging due to its weight, is often helpful while passing the tube. Upon successful placement, the endotracheal cuff is inflated. The tube is then secured by tying it to

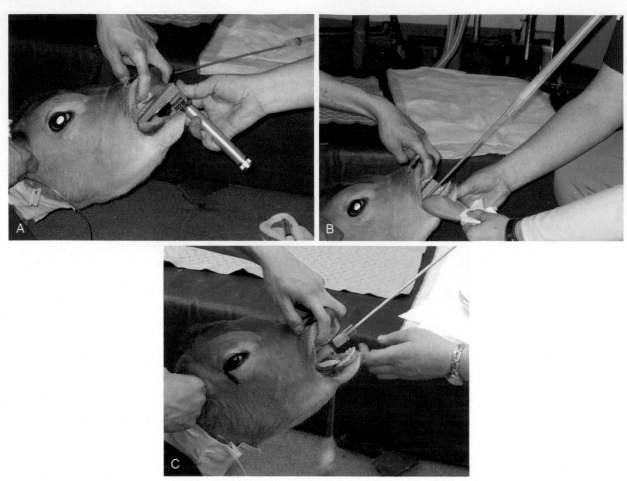

FIG. 11.3 Intubation of a calf. **(A)** Following induction, an assistant holds the patient's head in an extended position. The anesthetist places a laryngoscope and directly visualizes the larynx. The tongues of ruminants, particularly sheep and goats, have a raised area in the caudal portion that makes correct positioning of the laryngoscope more difficult than in small animals. **(B)** A stylet, which is preplaced within and extends beyond the endotracheal tube, is advanced until it is positioned 2 to 5 cm within the larynx. **(C)** The tube is then advanced over the stylet into the trachea. The stylet can then be removed. This technique is also used for intubating sheep, goats, and camelids.

the halter or around the muzzle in a similar manner to that used for a dog.

Maintenance of Anesthesia

Following anesthetic induction and endotracheal intubation, patients that are in a light plane of anesthesia must be brought into a surgical plane of anesthesia. When the patient reaches the desired anesthetic depth, general anesthesia is most commonly maintained with inhalant anesthetics but can also be maintained with total intravenous anesthesia (TIVA). (See Box 11.3 for maintenance protocols in ruminants.)

Maintenance of Anesthesia With Inhalant

Maintenance of anesthesia with inhalants in small ruminants and calves is similar to maintenance in small animals (see Procedure 9.7), whereas maintenance of anesthesia with inhalants in adult cattle is similar to maintenance in horses (see Procedure 10.6). Healthy ruminants typically have relatively few problems during the maintenance phase of anesthe-

sia. Blood pressure is usually well maintained and is often higher than that seen in small animal and equine patients. Ruminants do, however, tend to hypoventilate, and are often observed to breathe rapidly and shallowly, somewhat like a panting dog. This type of breathing pattern may lead to hypoventilation, hypoxemia, and difficulty keeping the patient anesthetized because of inadequate delivery of inhalant anesthetic to the lungs. Patients that demonstrate this breathing pattern should be placed on a ventilator (see Chapter 7).

Most ruminants have accessible arteries in their ears. These are often catheterized so that blood pressure can be monitored directly and blood samples can be taken for blood gas analysis, particularly during long surgical procedures or in compromised patients.

Intravenous Maintenance of Anesthesia

IV maintenance of anesthesia in ruminants is generally reserved for procedures shorter than 20 minutes in healthy, nonintubated patients. If the patient is intubated, the duration of anesthesia

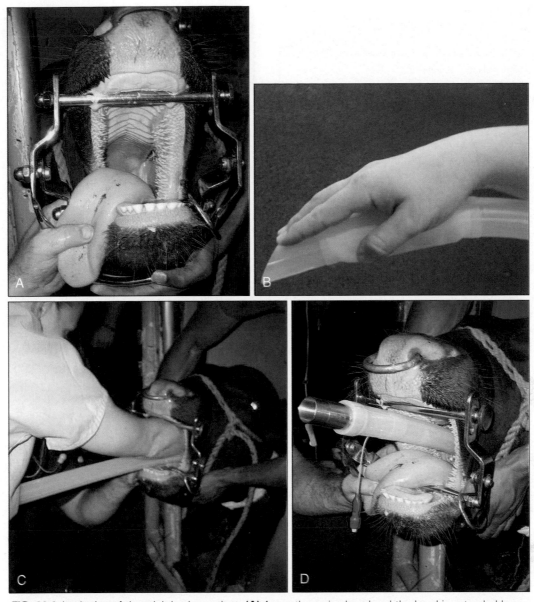

FIG. 11.4 Intubation of the adult bovine patient. **(A)** A mouth gag is placed and the head is extended by an assistant. **(B)** The anesthetist protects the endotracheal tube cuff with the nondominant hand. **(C)** Using the nondominant hand, the anesthetist palpates the larynx with their fingers and directs the endotracheal tube into the larynx while advancing the tube with the dominant hand. **(D)** With the tube in place, the cuff can be inflated and the mouth gag removed.

PROCEDURE 11.4 Intubation Procedure for Adult Cattle

Ruminants are generally intubated while in sternal recumbency.

1. Place a mouth speculum or gag.
2. Grasp the tongue and pull it forward.
3. Extend the head and neck.
4. Hold the tube at the patient end and cover the cuff with the nondominant hand.
5. Holding the tube in this manner, extend the nondominant arm into the mouth and advance to the larynx. Use the dominant hand to assist with advancement of the machine end of the tube.
6. Palpate the epiglottis and laryngeal opening with one or two fingers of the nondominant hand.
7. Pass the tube into the larynx, using the nondominant hand to push the end of the tube into the airway and the dominant hand to advance the tube.

8. Check to ensure the tube is in the trachea by feeling air pass during exhalation or when an assistant presses down on the patient's chest.
9. Place 20–60 mL of air in the cuff before hoisting or positioning the cow.
10. Secure the tube to the halter or to the muzzle.
11. After the cow has been positioned on the surgery table, connect the endotracheal tube to the anesthetic breathing system and allow the patient to breathe 100% oxygen.
12. Check the tube for leaks.
13. Turn on the anesthetic vaporizer and adjust to the appropriate level.
14. Commence regular monitoring as for small ruminants.

can be extended. Double drip is commonly used for this purpose.

Patient Positioning, Comfort, and Safety

During anesthetic induction and maintenance, a number of considerations must be observed to ensure that the patient is not harmed. Many of the principles of small animal anesthesia apply to ruminant anesthesia (see Chapter 9). Additional concerns are:

- All ruminants should be positioned for surgery with the mouth lower than the pharynx to allow drainage of saliva and any regurgitated material from the mouth, preventing buildup in the pharynx, which could lead to aspiration during recovery following extubation.
- Ruminants, even large cattle, are not predisposed to developing myopathy or neuropathy, unlike horses; however, appropriate physical support and padding during anesthesia are prudent (Fig. 11.5).

Anesthetic Recovery

Unlike horses, ruminants generally are content to lie in sternal recumbency following anesthesia. The development of complications from anesthetic recovery is generally limited to the residual effects of bloat. Ruminants rarely develop nasal edema during anesthesia and usually do not require nasal intubation. (See Procedure 11.5 for information regarding anesthetic recovery.)

Preparation for Recovery

Upon completion of the procedure, turn off the inhalant and transfer the patient to a padded recovery stall where it can be extubated and monitored (large cattle), or to a quiet, clean area on the floor (small ruminant). Support or prop the patient in sternal recumbency with the mouth lower than the pharynx. Sternal recumbency allows eructation as the patient regains consciousness, while the head position allows for drainage of saliva and/or regurgitus that may have accumulated in the pharynx and mouth during anesthesia (Fig. 11.6).

Monitoring During Recovery

The patient should be monitored for signs of excessive bloating (a visibly large abdomen that feels tight to the touch). It is common for ruminants to eructate as the depth of anesthesia decreases and eructation often occurs before extubation.

Signs of Recovery

As the patient recovers, it will progress back through the stages and planes of anesthesia. Generally, this is not as dramatic in ruminants as it is in horses, even if the patient did not receive premedication.

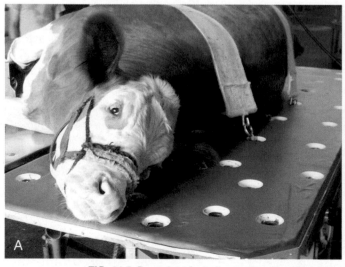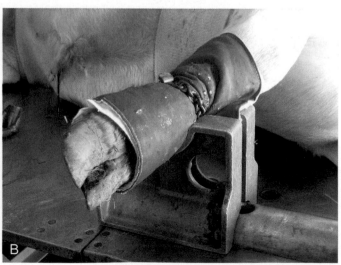

FIG. 11.5 Restraint of a bull on a tilt table. **(A)** A bull is appropriately restrained with two support bands on a tilt table that has a padded surface. The bull's halter is secured by passing a rope through one of the holes and tying it underneath the table. **(B)** Appropriate padding of the bull's distal right forelimb, which is placed in a metal foot support.

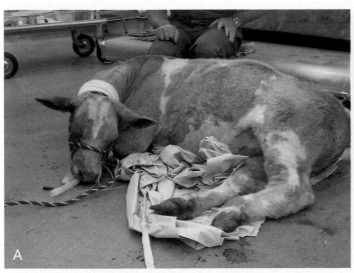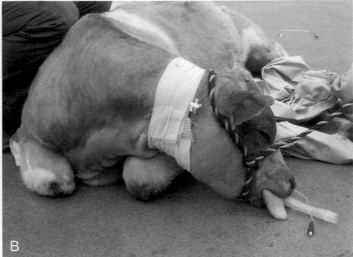

FIG. 11.6 Appropriate positioning of a ruminant for anesthetic recovery. **(A)** This heifer, recovering from anesthesia for umbilical hernia repair, is placed in sternal recumbency and maintained in that position, in this case by an assistant, to allow eructation. The head is positioned so that the pharynx is higher than the mouth, thus allowing drainage of saliva and regurgitus. **(B)** Folding the front limbs underneath the heifer makes it easier to keep her in sternal recumbency.

Extubation

In contrast to the norm for other species, the endotracheal tube cuff should either be kept inflated or only partially deflated in ruminants in order to prevent aspiration of any material that may have become lodged in the pharynx during anesthesia. The anesthetist should wait for strong swallowing movements or coughing before extubation. Both before and after tube removal, keep the neck in a natural but slightly extended position to protect the airway. Remove the endotracheal tube gently using a slow, steady motion. If there is difficulty removing the tube, remove some more air from the cuff and try again.

> **TECHNICIAN NOTE** Ruminants should be placed in sternal recumbency for recovery from anesthesia to allow the patient to eructate. The endotracheal tube cuff should either be kept inflated or only partially deflated to assist the removal of saliva and regurgitus from the laryngopharynx on extubation.

The Postanesthetic Period

Once a ruminant is lying in sternal recumbency without support and is no longer in danger of bloating, it can be left unattended. Many ruminants will lie quietly after anesthesia, only standing some time after the anesthetic period unless they are stimulated to rise. It is not necessary to withhold food or water from ruminants postoperatively unless specifically instructed to do so by the attending veterinarian.

CAMELID ANESTHESIA

Llamas and alpacas, collectively referred to as South American camelids, have become more popular as herd animals in North America over the last few decades and present for anesthesia for a variety of reasons, including orthopedic, abdominal, and dental

surgery. General anesthesia of camelids is very similar to that of small ruminants because they have a similar digestive system. Although camelids are not true ruminants, the first stomach compartment plays a similar role to the rumen. Camelids produce copious saliva even when anesthetized and have the ability to chew cud; thus it is common to find food material in the oral cavity at induction. Unlike ruminants, anesthetized camelids are prone to developing nasal congestion when placed in lateral or dorsal recumbency. Like horses, camelids are obligate nasal breathers and may also develop upper airway obstruction during recovery. Anesthetic management therefore tends to focus on these specific concerns in addition to the general concerns for anesthetizing any veterinary patient (see Chapter 9).

Patient Preparation

Camelids are prepared for anesthesia in the same manner as small ruminants (see Procedure 11.1). IV catheters are commonly placed in the jugular or cephalic veins. The skin on the neck of camelids is typically thicker and much tighter than that of small ruminants. This can make it comparatively more difficult to place an IV catheter in the jugular vein successfully and a little easier to mistake the carotid artery for the jugular vein, resulting in inadvertent carotid puncture. If a hematoma forms as a result of unsuccessful venipuncture of the neck, the tight skin tends to compress it inwards, leading to the possibility that the trachea will be compressed and partially obstructed. In the event that a hematoma develops, it may be prudent to postpone a nonemergency procedure for 24 hours to allow some resolution of the hematoma.

Selecting a Protocol

Camelids are generally easy to handle and the protocols used in small ruminants are recommended (see Boxes 11.1, 11.2, and 11.3). Aggressive camelids may be quite resentful of restraint

> **BOX 11.4**   **Premedication/Sedative Combinations for Aggressive PS1 and PS2 Camelids**
>
> 1. **Xylazine–Butorphanol (IM):** Xylazine 0.2–0.5 mg/kg and butorphanol 0.1–0.2 mg/kg IM
> 2. **Ketamine–Xylazine–Butorphanol (IM):**[a] Ketamine 3–5 mg/kg, xylazine 0.2–0.5 mg/kg, and butorphanol 0.1–0.2 mg/kg mixed in a syringe and administered intramuscularly

[a]This combination may produce general anesthesia in some camelids, allowing short procedures to be performed.
IM, Intramuscular.

for examination or venipuncture and may require alternative sedative protocols (Box 11.4).

Summary of a General Anesthetic Procedure

The general procedure for anesthetizing a camelid is essentially the same as that for small ruminants (see Procedure 11.2), with the following exceptions.

Maintenance of Anesthesia

Camelids tend to maintain ventilation better than ruminants under anesthesia; however, some individuals may require the use of a mechanical ventilator. The heart rate is frequently more variable compared to ruminants. Bradycardia is commonly encountered, and can be treated with glycopyrrolate or atropine.

Patient Positioning, Comfort, and Safety

Care should be taken with the long, flexible neck during induction, positioning, and recovery to prevent injury. The eyes of camelids are large and prominent and should be protected during movement of the patient during induction, positioning, and recovery.

As with ruminants, the head should be positioned to allow drainage of saliva and regurgitus by placing the mouth lower than the pharynx.

Anesthetic Recovery

Camelids should be placed in sternal recumbency for recovery from general anesthesia. The head and neck should be held upright in a normal position to promote venous drainage of any upper airway congestion that may have developed during the procedure (Fig. 11.7). The anesthetist should hold their hand close to but not obstructing the nares after extubation to feel for the passage of air during exhalation (Fig. 11.8). If breathing seems labored after extubation, if stridor is present, or the camelid is breathing with an open mouth, oxygen can be delivered by face mask. If dyspnea develops, a small endotracheal tube can be placed into the ventral meatus of one or both nostrils by gently advancing it toward the nasopharynx until passage of air is felt through the tube when the camelid exhales (Fig. 11.9). If placement of nasopharyngeal tubes does not alleviate the obstruction, the attending veterinarian should be notified immediately. Complete airway obstruction is an emergency and may require reintubation of the trachea or a tracheostomy.

Like ruminants, camelids tend to remain calm and consequently rarely require sedation in the recovery period.

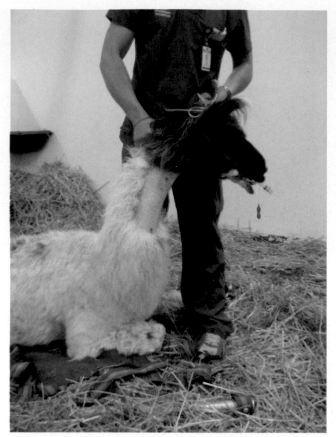

FIG. 11.7 Camelid positioned for recovery from general anesthesia. The camelid is positioned in sternal recumbency. The anesthetist, or an assistant, holds the head and neck upright in a normal, neutral position until the patient is extubated and able to hold up its own neck.

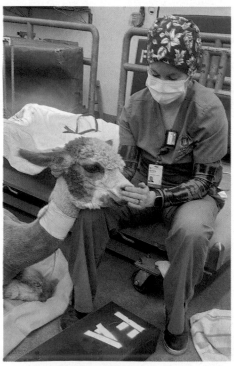

FIG. 11.8 Immediately post extubation, the anesthetist holds her hand in front of the nares to detect adequate flow of air during exhalation.

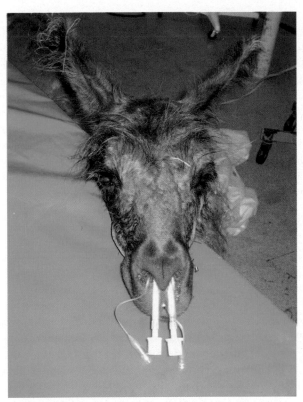

FIG. 11.9 Nasopharyngeal tubes placed bilaterally in a llama that developed dyspnea from upper airway obstruction following dental surgery.

> **TECHNICIAN NOTE** Camelids should be placed in sternal recumbency with the head and neck held upright and supported in a normal, neutral position to promote venous drainage from the head. If upper airway obstruction develops after extubation, nasopharyngeal tubes can be placed. If nasopharyngeal intubation does not relieve the obstruction, the attending veterinarian should be informed immediately.

SWINE ANESTHESIA

Pigs are challenging patients to restrain, sedate, and anesthetize because of unique characteristics of this species that make physical examination, sedation, IV catheterization, and intubation much more difficult than in the species discussed so far.

> **TECHNICIAN NOTE** Pigs are challenging patients to restrain, sedate, and anesthetize because of unique characteristics of this species that make physical examination, sedation, IV catheterization, and intubation difficult.

Patient Preparation

In most swine, physical examination is impossible beyond general observation of the animal, assessment of respiratory rate and character, and detection of obvious problems such as nasal discharge. Conscious pigs typically squeal in protest when restrained, making procedures such as thoracic auscultation impossible. The anesthetist must often rely on patient history to determine health status. Pigs also do not have readily accessible peripheral veins or arteries, making further investigation of cardiovascular status and blood sample collection very difficult or impossible without causing extreme stress to the animal and the handler.

Premedication and Sedation

Sedative drugs are most commonly administered by IM injection in pigs owing to the lack of easily accessible peripheral veins, but the presence of a thick layer of subcutaneous fat makes IM administration of drugs difficult without the use of needles that are at least 1.5 inches long. The most accessible site for IM injection is in the muscles of the neck caudal to the ear and at least 3 to 5 cm lateral to the dorsal midline (Fig. 11.10).

Of the domestic species, swine are generally considered to be the most resistant to sedative drugs, and many protocols for IM sedation, premedication, or total injectable anesthesia include a tranquilizer or sedative, an opioid, and a dissociative. Various combinations of drugs have been used to sedate swine (Box 11.5). Generally, drug combinations that include a dissociative produce more predictable and heavier sedation that in some pigs, may produce anesthesia for short surgical and nonsurgical procedures. A combination that is widely used to produce heavy sedation or anesthesia is Telazol, ketamine, and xylazine, or TKX (Procedure 11.6).

A technique known as "forking" may be useful to calm some friendly pigs prior to injection. A plastic fork (or similar implement, like a back scratcher) is either repeatedly dragged like a comb from the pig's neck toward the hindquarters on either side of the midline, or the fork is used to gently and repetitively prod both sides of the pig's thorax and flanks (Fig. 11.11). Some pigs will not tolerate this, on some it has no effect, and others may become calmer and have a much lesser response to IM injection. Some pigs will even lie down as a result of forking, as seen in videos shared online.

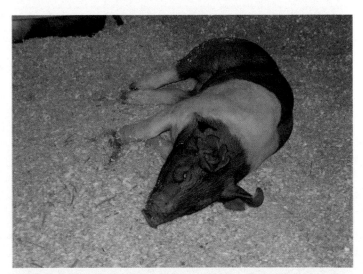

FIG. 11.10 Pig sedated with Telazol, ketamine, and xylazine (TKX). This pig became laterally recumbent 15 minutes after intramuscular (IM) injection of TKX (the blood on the side of the neck marks the site of IM injection).

PROCEDURE 11.6 How to Prepare and Administer Telazol–Ketamine–Xylazine to Swine

1. Reconstitute a bottle of Telazol with 2.5 mL of 100 mg/mL ketamine and 2.5 mL of 100 mg/mL xylazine.
2. The final mixture of Telazol, ketamine, and xylazine (TKX) then contains the following drugs and concentrations:
   - Tiletamine 50 mg/mL
   - Zolazepam 50 mg/mL
   - Ketamine 50 mg/mL
   - Xylazine 50 mg/mL
3. Administer TKX at 1 mL/50 kg by intramuscular (IM) injection up to a maximum of 3 mL.

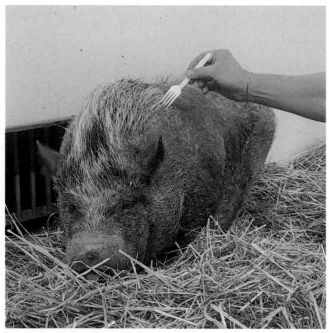

FIG. 11.11 A friendly Vietnamese pot-bellied pig being forked with a plastic fork to calm the patient and facilitate restraint.

Anesthetic Induction

Using a combination of drugs such as TKX will often induce anesthesia in pigs. The eyes of pigs are very small and sunken, and do not provide reliable information about depth of anesthesia. Readiness for intubation is often best assessed by seeing whether the mouth can be opened without resistance. If after TKX the patient is not quite deep enough to intubate, the anesthetist has two options. An IV catheter can be placed in an aural vein (Fig. 11.12) and small increments of an IV induction drug such as ketamine can be administered (i.e., 0.5 to 1.0 mg/kg boluses), or anesthetic depth can be increased by administering an inhalant anesthetic via face mask (Fig. 11.13).

Endotracheal Intubation

Endotracheal intubation of swine is particularly challenging because of poor visibility resulting from the limited extent to which the mouth can be opened, a long soft palate, the relatively narrow dental arcade, and the anatomy of the larynx and proximal trachea. A ventral laryngeal diverticulum is present in the floor of the larynx into which the tube can easily be misdirected, and the laryngotracheal junction is at an angle rather than being straight, as in other domestic species. Finally, the larynx of a pig is sensitive and may spasm when stimulated, making intubation even harder. The novice anesthetist should seek assistance from an experienced person when intubating a pig, as it is easy to damage the larynx by forcing the tube. There are several methods of intubating pigs. The pig may be placed in either sternal or dorsal recumbency. Similarly to small ruminants, a straight stylet is placed within the tube such that several inches of it extend beyond the bevel of the tube. Using a laryngoscope to visualize the airway, the stylet is passed into the larynx, bypassing the diverticulum. The tube can then be gently threaded over the stylet into the trachea. Care must be taken with the stylet to avoid damage to the larynx and trachea (Fig. 11.14). Alternatively, a stylet with a 20- to 30-degree curve in it is placed in the tube, ensuring that it does not extend beyond the end of the tube. The tube is initially inserted into the larynx in the same manner as intubating small animals, i.e., with the convex side of the tube toward the hard palate and the end of the tube pointing "down" toward the ventral neck when placed in the larynx. Once the tube is placed in the larynx, the tube and stylet are then rotated 180 degrees so that the end of the tube now points "up" toward the dorsal neck and advanced into the trachea; this technique bypasses the laryngeal diverticulum. If it is hard to rotate the tube, it may have become lodged in the diverticulum; in this case, withdraw the tube slightly and try again. Patience should be exercised and if the pig becomes light during intubation, further attempts at intubation should be halted until IV or inhalant drugs have been administered and an appropriate depth of anesthesia for intubation is achieved.

Maintenance of Anesthesia

Most pigs can be maintained with an inhalant anesthetic delivered using a small-animal anesthetic machine and rebreathing system. Maintenance of anesthesia is similar to that in small-animal patients (see Chapter 9). In the rare case of very large pigs that

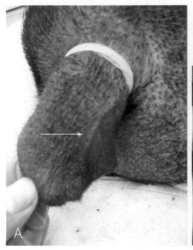
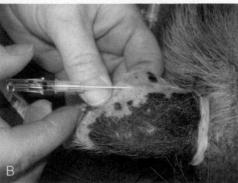
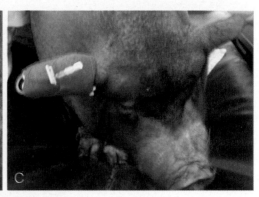

FIG. 11.12 Placement of a catheter in the aural vein of a pig. **(A)** A rubber band placed around the base of the ear acts as a tourniquet, causing the marginal ear vein to distend *(white arrow)*. **(B)** Placement of an intravenous (IV) catheter in the aural vein. Note the blood flashback in the hub of the catheter. Because of the small size of ear veins in pigs, blood does not commonly flow out of the catheter after the stylet is removed. After the catheter has been placed, the rubber band is removed. It is usually easier to cut the rubber band off, taking care not to cut the ear, than to risk dislodging the catheter while moving the rubber band over the catheter and off the ear. **(C)** If required, the catheter can be secured and wrapped to allow for the administration of postoperative intravenous medication.

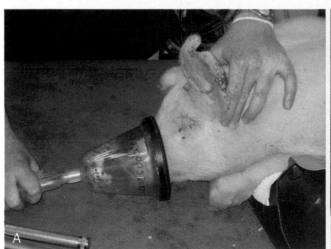
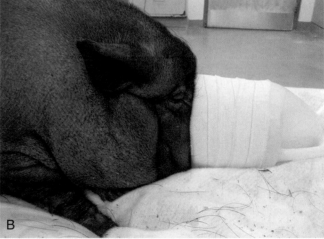

FIG. 11.13 Administering an inhalant anesthetic via a face mask in a pig. **(A)** Use of a clear small-animal face mask for a small pig. **(B)** Use of a homemade face mask for a large pig. In both cases, it is important that the mask fit tightly to avoid pollution of the work area and to ensure that the inhalant anesthetic is not diluted by room air, which will delay induction.

can be intubated with a 16-mm endotracheal tube, a large-animal machine can be used.

Monitoring

Pigs can be challenging to monitor effectively because they have few palpable peripheral arteries, and their cone-shaped legs make the use of blood pressure cuffs, which are designed for the more cylindrical arms of people, difficult. In most pigs, the pulse can be palpated in the ear and on the medial aspect of the carpus. In smaller pigs, the brachial artery may be palpable, a Doppler signal may be obtained from it, and oscillometric cuffs

will often give pressure readings (Fig. 11.15). A Doppler signal is also relatively easy to elicit from the tail artery, which runs along the ventral midline of the tail. Pulse oximeter transmission probes will usually work on the tongue, but can also be placed on other areas such as the snout and ears of pink pigs (Fig. 11.16).

The respiratory system can be monitored by observing the breathing bag and with capnometry as for other species.

Porcine Stress Syndrome

Also known as malignant hyperthermia, porcine stress syndrome has been associated with anesthesia, particularly

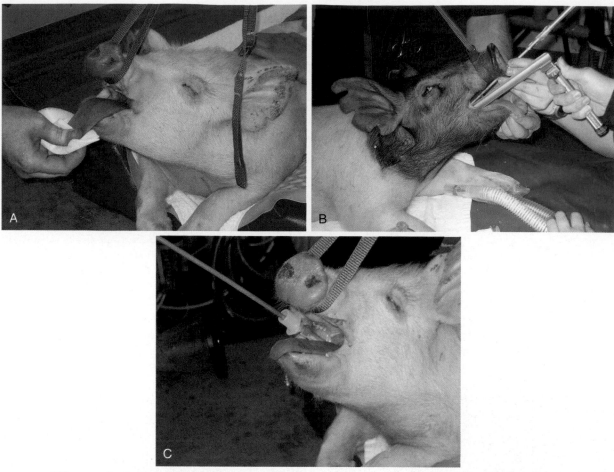

FIG. 11.14 Intubation of a pig. **(A)** Following anesthetic induction, the tongue is gently pulled forward and down, while the upper jaw is pulled upward using a lead. **(B)** Using a laryngoscope to aid visualization, a stylet placed through and beyond the end of an endotracheal tube is advanced into the larynx. **(C)** The tube is advanced over the stylet into the larynx.

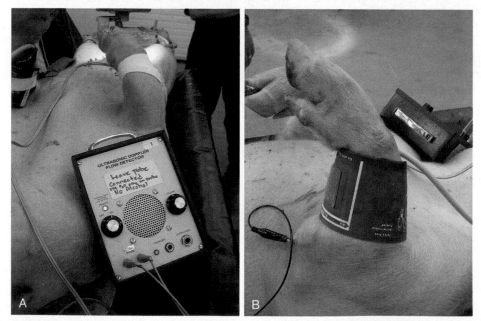

FIG. 11.15 Placement of Doppler probe and oscillometric blood pressure cuff on the forelimb of a small pig. **(A)** Placement of the Doppler probe on the medial aspect of the carpus. **(B)** Placement of an oscillometric blood pressure cuff on the forelimb.

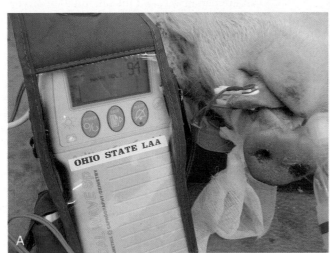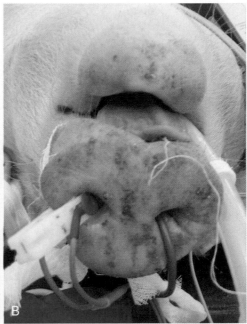

FIG. 11.16 Pulse oximetry probe placement on a pig. **(A)** Placement of a pulse oximetry transmission probe on a pig's tongue. **(B)** Placement of a pulse oximetry transmission probe on a pig's snout. Notice the temperature probe entering the pig's right nostril.

when inhalant anesthetics are used. This metabolic condition is due to a mutation in one of the genes that controls calcium metabolism in the muscle. Symptoms include muscle rigidity, a rapid rise in temperature, hypercapnia, hyperkalemia, and death. Treatment includes immediate termination of all anesthetic drugs, delivery of oxygen at high flow rates, and treatment with the muscle relaxant dantrolene.

Patient Positioning, Comfort, and Safety

Commercial pigs are managed in a similar way to small animals during anesthesia. Vietnamese pot-bellied pigs tend to have fairly lax shoulder and hip joints and should never be picked up by their limbs to adjust position, as this can lead to dislocation of a limb.

Anesthetic Recovery

The general principles applicable to extubation and recovery for small animals apply to pigs, including detection and treatment of hypothermia. Typically, the IV catheter is removed before full awakening, although if a pig is to be hospitalized, it may be prudent to secure the IV catheter for administration of IV medications (see Fig. 11.12 C).

KEY POINTS

1. The main anesthetic concerns in ruminants arise from their unique digestive anatomy and physiology.
2. Ruminants are susceptible to bloat, regurgitation, and hypoventilation when under general anesthesia.
3. Ruminants are generally very tractable; surgery, particularly flank laparotomy, is often accomplished using local anesthesia with or without sedation.
4. Intubation in small ruminants and calves is performed under direct visualization with a laryngoscope, often with the use of a stylet.
5. Intubation of adult cattle is performed manually using a blind technique that involves direct palpation of the larynx.
6. Ruminants should be positioned for surgery as well as during recovery with the mouth lower than the pharynx to allow drainage of saliva and any regurgitated material, thus decreasing the risk of aspiration.

7. Ruminants should be placed in sternal recumbency during anesthetic recovery to allow eructation. The endotracheal tube should be left in place with the cuff partially inflated to minimize the risk of aspirating rumen contents or saliva.
8. Anesthesia of camelids is generally similar to anesthesia of small ruminants.
9. Camelids have very tight-fitting neck skin and consequently, hematomas after venipuncture of the jugular vein or carotid artery may partially obstruct the trachea.
10. Camelids are prone to developing nasal congestion under general anesthesia and should be recovered in sternal recumbency with the head and neck held up in a normal, neutral position to allow venous drainage to occur.
11. Preoperative physical examination of swine is limited to observation.

12. The main anesthetic concerns in swine are an inability to perform blood work, resistance to sedation, paucity of peripheral veins and arteries, and the difficulty of intubation.
13. Pigs are more resistant to sedation than other species. A combination of Telazol, ketamine, and xylazine (TKX) is commonly used to provide heavy sedation or total injectable anesthesia in pigs.
14. After sedation or induction, the ear vein is usually accessible for catheterization in pigs.
15. Intubation of swine is challenging because of poor visualization of the larynx, the unique anatomy of the oral cavity and upper airway, and the potential for laryngospasm.
16. There are few palpable arteries in pigs, making monitoring difficult. Oscillometric blood pressure cuffs may not work well on the cone-shaped limbs of pigs.

REVIEW QUESTIONS

1. Comparing the sensitivity of cattle, horses, and swine to xylazine, which of the following is true?
   a. Cattle are more sensitive than horses, which are more sensitive than swine
   b. Cattle are more sensitive than swine, which are more sensitive than horses
   c. Horses are more sensitive than cattle, which are more sensitive than swine
   d. Swine are more sensitive than cattle, which are more sensitive than horses
2. An anticholinergic is an essential component of premedication in ruminants.
   True
   False
3. "Double drip" contains which two drugs?
   a. Guaifenesin and dobutamine
   b. Guaifenesin and ketamine
   c. Xylazine and ketamine
   d. Acepromazine and ketamine
4. You plan to anesthetize a 1000-kg bull and maintain anesthesia using an inhalant technique. Which of the following statements regarding intubation is correct?
   a. The inhalant can be safely delivered via a face mask
   b. You will need a laryngoscope to visualize the larynx
   c. You will have to intubate the bull manually
   d. All of the above
5. It is common for anesthetized ruminants to hypoventilate.
   True
   False
6. Positioning the head of an anesthetized ruminant with the pharynx higher than the mouth helps to prevent:
   a. Hyperventilation
   b. Hypotension
   c. Aspiration
   d. Hypoxemia
7. Ruminants should be placed in sternal recumbency during recovery to allow them to:
   a. Eructate
   b. Regurgitate
   c. Salivate
   d. Hyperventilate

8. A hematoma that results from unsuccessful jugular catheterization in a camelid may result in which of the following?
   a. Bloat
   b. Excessive blood loss
   c. Nasal congestion
   d. Pressure on the tracheal wall
9. When recovering a camelid after general anesthesia, how should it be positioned?
   a. In lateral recumbency, with the head on the ground
   b. In lateral recumbency, with the head elevated
   c. In sternal recumbency, with the head on the ground
   d. In sternal recumbency, with the head elevated
10. Intubation is made easier in pigs by
   a. The presence of a laryngeal diverticulum
   b. The possibility of laryngospasm
   c. The use of a stylet
   d. The angle of the laryngotracheal junction
11. Which of the following statements regarding porcine anesthesia is TRUE?
   a. Oscillometric blood pressure monitors work well in pigs
   b. All pigs should have complete blood work before anesthesia
   c. Pigs are very sensitive to alpha$_2$-agonists
   d. Intravenous sedation is virtually impossible in healthy pigs
12. Which of the following is NOT a symptom of porcine stress syndrome?
   a. Hypothermia
   b. Hyperthermia
   c. Hyperkalemia
   d. Hypercapnia

SELECTED READINGS

Greene SA: Protocols for anesthesia of cattle, *Vet Clin North Am Food Anim Pract* 19(3):679–693, 2003.

Tranquilli WJ, Thurmon JC, Grimm KA: *Veterinary anesthesia and analgesia*, ed 5, Ames, IA, 2015, Wiley-Blackwell.

12

Rodent and Rabbit Anesthesia

Paul Flecknell

OUTLINE

LEARNING OBJECTIVES

When you have completed this chapter, you will be able to:
- Summarize the common problems that may arise when anesthetizing rodents and rabbits.
- List the preanesthetic and anesthetic agents suitable for use in these species.
- Describe the technique of endotracheal intubation in rabbits.
- Describe the problems that can arise when monitoring anesthesia in rodents and rabbits.
- State aspects of intraoperative care that are of particular importance when anesthetizing rodents and rabbits.
- Describe how to cope with common anesthetic emergencies in rodents and rabbits.
- Describe the most common problems associated with postanesthetic care of rodents and rabbits.
- List the analgesics that can be used in rodents and rabbits.

KEY TERMS

Fluanisone
Intraosseous

Intraperitoneal

Supraglottic airway device

Anesthesia of small mammals (rabbits, guinea pigs, rats, mice, gerbils, and hamsters) is a specialized branch of veterinary anesthesia, but the general principles of good anesthetic practice provide basic guidance. The main difficulties encountered when anesthetizing these animals are due to:

- Lack of familiarity with the species
- Lack of suitable equipment
- A failure to appreciate the poor health status of some patients
- The difficulties of providing supportive care

Once these problems are appreciated, anesthesia of small mammals and other exotic species should be as successful as anesthesia of dogs and cats.

PATIENT EVALUATION

To anesthetize small mammals safely and effectively, it is important to perform a clinical examination and obtain a case history. Although the information required is similar to that needed for more familiar species, many of these small animals are owned by children and accurate information may not always be obtainable. Even when an adult or older child is caring for the animal, it may be difficult to be certain that the animal is eating and drinking normally, because many of these species are fed ad lib.

Remember that the life span of these small mammals is considerably shorter than that of dogs and cats. Geriatric animals present a greater risk when anesthetized; a hamster, for example, will be nearing the end of its natural life when aged only 18 to 24 months. Some basic biologic data are given in Table 12.1.

> **TECHNICIAN NOTE** It is important that the techniques for restraining the different species of small mammals are understood to avoid injury to the patient and handler.

For a physical examination to be performed, any animal must be safely and humanely handled and restrained. Handling is easier if small rodents are brought to the veterinary clinic in a small container, although they should not be left in a cardboard box for long as they can easily gnaw through the container and escape. Rabbits can usually be transported in a small transport box and cat-sized carriers are suitable. Rabbits are a prey species and, because cats are one of their predators, it is not surprising that placing a rabbit in a transport box that has been previously used for cats can be extremely stressful and should therefore be avoided. Similarly, it is advisable to wash your hands and preferably wear a fresh gown or coat before examining and handling these species if you have previously been working with dogs and cats.

Before the animal is handled, it should be observed undisturbed so that its normal behavior and respiratory pattern and rate can be noted.

Handling and Restraint
Mouse

Mice are best picked using your cupped hands, or with a Perspex or cardboard handling tube. They can then either be observed in a clear hard plastic tube (Fig. 12.1) or in your cupped hands while gently restraining them by the base of the tail if needed. To restrain them for administration of injectable anesthetics or other drugs, allow mice to rest on a rough surface (e.g., a towel or the bars of their cage). They can then be grasped by the skin overlying the shoulders and lifted clear. The tail can be gripped between the operator's fingers, as shown in Fig. 12.2. Subcutaneous administration of medication is made into the skin overlying the shoulders and can be carried out single-handedly. An assistant should administer intraperitoneal injections while the operator restrains the animal as shown in Fig. 12.3. Intramuscular (IM) injections are best avoided in mice and other small mammals because of their very small muscle mass. Restraining the mouse by its scruff can interfere with respiration. This causes no problems in healthy animals, but care should be taken if the animal is showing signs of respiratory disease. Young mice can be extremely active and may jump out of their transport box as soon as the lid is removed; handling these agile young animals requires fast reactions.

TABLE 12.1	Biologic Data for Small Mammals					
	Gerbil	**Guinea Pig**	**Hamster**	**Mouse**	**Rabbit**	**Rat**
Adult body weight (g)	85–150	700–1200	85–150	25–40	2000–6000	300–500
Respiratory rate (bpm)	90	50–140	80–135	80–200	40–60	70–115
Heart rate (bpm)	260–300	150–250	250–500	350–600	135–325	250–350
Average adult blood volume (mL) (65–70 mL/kg)	9	60	9	2.5	250	30
PCV (%)	41–52	37–48	36–55	36–49	36–48	38–50
Blood glucose (mg/dL)	54–126	81–108	54–144	63–162	72–144	54–144
Total protein (g/dL)	4.3–12.5	4.6–6.2	5.9–6.5	3.5–7.2	5.4–7.5	5.6–7.6
BUN (mg/dL)	17–27	9–32	10–25	12–28	17.0–23.5	6–23
ALT (IU)	—	25–59	12–36	74–232	35–38	17.5–30
Life span (years)	3–5	4–8	1.5–2	2–2.5	5–10	2–3.5

ALT, Alanine aminotransferase; *BUN,* blood urea nitrogen; *IU,* international units; *PCV,* packed cell volume.

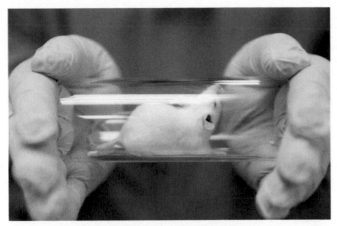

FIG. 12.1 Use of a handling tube to examine a mouse. The animal is encouraged to run into the tube while in its cage or transport box.

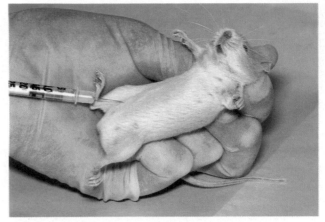

FIG. 12.3 Intraperitoneal injection in a mouse. Intraperitoneal injection is made into one posterior quadrant of the abdomen, along the line of the hindlimb.

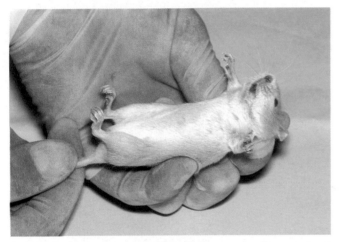

FIG. 12.2 Restraint of a mouse. Mice can be restrained by grasping the skin overlying the shoulders, with the tail held between the operator's fingers.

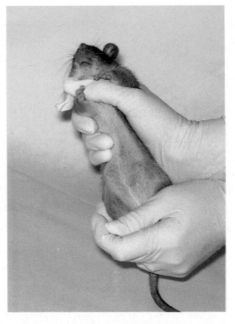

FIG. 12.4 Restraint of a rat. Note that the thumb is positioned below the mandible to prevent biting. The chest is held gently to avoid interfering with respiration.

Rat

Most pet rats are friendly and easy to handle. They should be picked up around the shoulders and lifted clear of the transport box. They can then be allowed to rest on the handler's forearm and be gently restrained by the tail or around the shoulders. If the animal resents handling (which it may if it is in pain, e.g., if it has arthritis), it can be picked up by the base of the tail in the same way as mice are. It can then be placed on a rough surface and grasped around the shoulders. When holding a rat in this way, the operator can avoid being bitten by positioning their thumb under the rat's mandible, as shown in Fig. 12.4. It is important not to grasp the animal's chest too firmly because this can interfere with respiratory movements, causing the animal to panic and struggle. Although subcutaneous (SC) injections can be given into the scruff while also restraining the animal, it is usually easier to obtain the assistance of a colleague. Intraperitoneal injections are given in the same way as in the mouse, but an assistant is needed for this procedure (Fig. 12.5). Assistance is also required for intramuscular injections, which may be given in the quadriceps muscle (Fig. 12.6). Intravenous (IV) administration of anesthetic agents and fluids is also

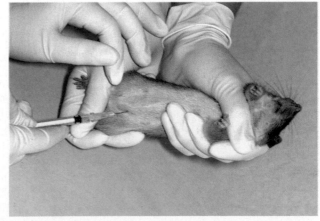

FIG. 12.5 Intraperitoneal injection in the rat. An assistant restrains the rat with one hindlimb extended, while another person injects into one posterior quadrant of the abdomen.

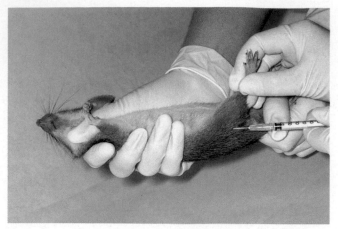

FIG. 12.6 Intramuscular injection in the rat. An assistant restrains the rat, while another person extends and immobilizes one hindlimb and injects into the quadriceps muscle.

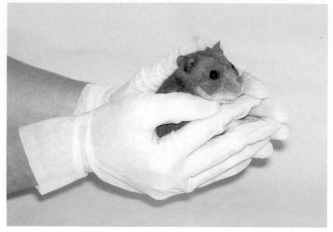

FIG. 12.8 Gentle restraint of a hamster for clinical examination by cupping it in the operator's hands.

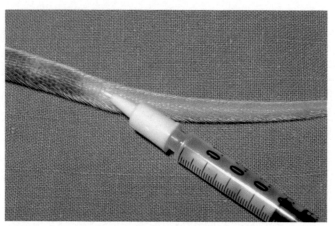

FIG. 12.7 A 24-gauge over-the-needle catheter placed in the lateral tail vein of a rat.

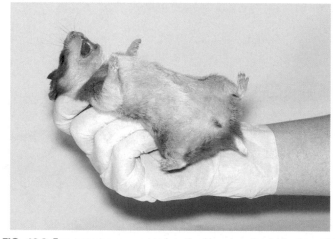

FIG. 12.9 For more secure restraint, the hamster should be immobilized with the operator's hand grasping the skin overlying the back and shoulders firmly.

possible using the lateral tail veins. Although technically difficult, it is no more challenging than venipuncture in other small patients such as puppies and kittens. Rats can be restrained firmly but gently by an assistant by being wrapped in a towel and venipuncture carried out using a 23- to 26-gauge needle. Alternatively, an over-the-needle catheter can be inserted to provide a secure route for administering IV anesthesia or for fluid support (Fig. 12.7).

Hamster

Hamsters vary considerably in their temperament and care should be taken when handling them. This species is normally active at night and asleep during the day and, if necessary, they should be gently awakened before being handled. Most animals can be cupped in the operator's hands, as shown in Fig. 12.8 and an external examination carried out. If it is necessary to immobilize the animal, it should be covered by the operator's hand with the skin overlying the shoulders and back grasped firmly (Fig. 12.9). It is important to grasp sufficient skin; otherwise, the animal can turn in the operator's grasp and may bite. An assistant can make intraperitoneal or subcutaneous injections into

the same sites as in the rat and mouse (Fig. 12.10). Hamsters should not be allowed to run unrestrained on the consulting room table because they appear to lack depth perception and may fall to the floor and injure themselves.

Gerbil

Gerbils are very active and can easily escape from their transport container unless quickly immobilized. Preventing escape is best achieved by the operator covering the animal with a hand and grasping around the animal's shoulders with the thumb positioned under the mandible to prevent biting. With the animal immobilized in this way, an assistant can administer subcutaneous injections into the flank, or intraperitoneal injections can be made in the same site as for other small rodents. Gerbils can also be immobilized by grasping the base of the tail, but the skin of the tail is delicate and easily damaged.

Guinea Pig

On initial examination, a guinea pig may be completely immobile, but when attempts are made to restrain it, the animal can

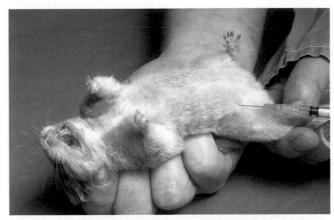

FIG. 12.10 Injection in the hamster. The hamster should be held securely for injections to be carried out by an assistant.

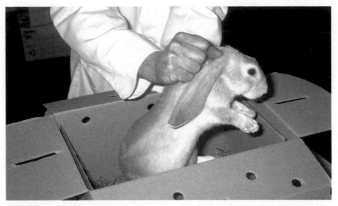

FIG. 12.12 Lifting a rabbit. When lifting a rabbit out of its transport box or cage, the skin overlying the shoulders should be grasped firmly and the abdomen supported. The operator's forearms are used to provide support to the animal's back.

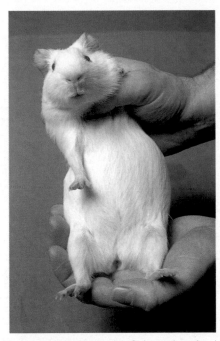

FIG. 12.11 Restraint of a guinea pig. Guinea pigs should be grasped around the shoulders and the hindquarters supported.

become very agitated and run around its transport box at high speed. It should be immobilized by grasping it swiftly and firmly around the shoulders. It can then be lifted clear of the transport container, and the operator's other hand can be used to support its hindquarters (Fig. 12.11). With the animal restrained in this way, an assistant can administer subcutaneous injections into the flank and intramuscular and intraperitoneal injections into the same site as with other rodents. If drugs are to be given by the subcutaneous route, an alternative approach is for the restrainer's hands to be placed on each side of the guinea pig's body to immobilize the animal on the examination table. An assistant can then inject into the skin overlying the shoulders.

Rabbit

Rabbits vary considerably in body weight, ranging from dwarf breeds weighing as little as 400 g up to giant breeds that can

weigh 10 kg. Most domestic rabbits weigh between 2 and 5 kg and are relatively easy to restrain, but care must be taken because they are easily frightened. When attempting to escape, they may kick out with their hind legs. This can injure the person attempting to handle them and may also result in serious injury to the rabbit (e.g., fracture of the lumbar vertebrae). It is therefore important to provide support to the animal's back at all times and never leave the animal unrestrained on the examination table.

Rabbits should be grasped by the skin overlying the shoulders and lifted clear of the transport container. As the rabbit is lifted, the operator's other hand should be positioned under the animal's abdomen to support its body weight, as shown in Fig. 12.12. The rabbit can then be placed on the examination table. The animal should not be released until its feet are in firm contact with the table surface. It can then be restrained by gently holding the skin over the shoulders. Rabbits should never be picked up by the ears because these are delicate structures.

An assistant can make intramuscular injections into the quadriceps or into the lumbar muscles while the operator restrains the animal by placing their hands and arms along each side of its body. IV injection is most easily carried out into the marginal ear veins. The skin of the ears is sensitive and animals will often jerk in response to venipuncture. To avoid a jerk and to prevent discomfort, the skin overlying the vein can be desensitized using a local anesthetic cream (e.g., EMLA, AstraZeneca). The cream is applied thickly over the vein and covered with a waterproof dressing (e.g., plastic food wrap) and a protective adhesive bandage. The cream is left in place for approximately 45 minutes, then removed and the ear wiped clean. This provides full skin thickness anesthesia for at least an hour. This technique is particularly useful when placing over-the-needle catheters. It is important to place the catheter in the marginal vein close to the edge of the ear and not the central artery for administration of anesthetics or blood sampling (Fig. 12.13). As an alternative to the ear veins, the cephalic veins in the forelegs or the lateral saphenous veins in the hindlegs (Figs. 12.14 and 12.15) can be used. These vessels are, however, fragile, and it is easy to produce a hematoma, even when

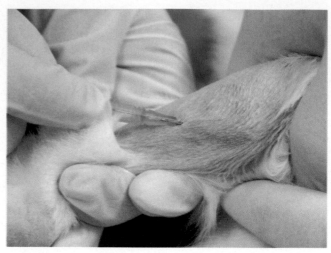

FIG. 12.13 Rabbit ear blood vessels. The marginal ear vein is used for venipuncture and catheter placement for intravenous injection. The central ear artery can be used for direct measurement of arterial pressure but should not be used for blood sampling because of the high risk of hematoma formation.

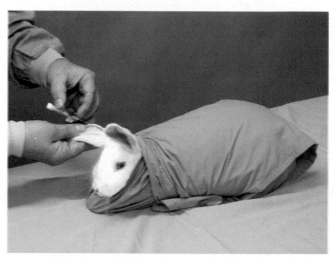

FIG. 12.15 Saphenous vein catheter in a rabbit. The lateral saphenous vein in the hindlimb can also be used for catheter placement or venipuncture. Like the cephalic vein, it is also fragile.

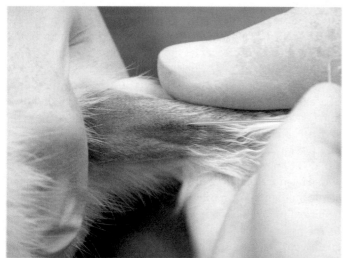

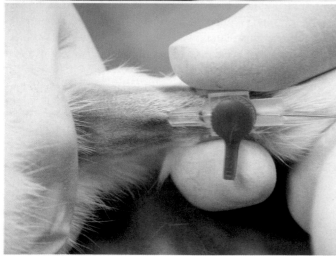

FIG. 12.14 Cephalic vein catheter. The cephalic vein can be used for catheter placement or venipuncture in the rabbit, but the vein is a little more mobile and more fragile than in dogs and cats.

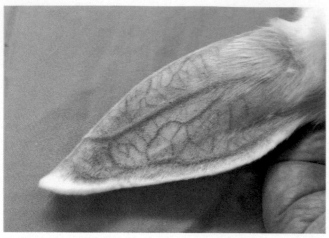

FIG. 12.16 Restraint of a rabbit by wrapping it in a surgical gown.

venipuncture has been carried out successfully at the first attempt.

If an assistant is unavailable, rabbits can be securely restrained by wrapping them in a towel, lab coat, or surgical gown. Provided it is wrapped securely, the animal will remain immobile and it is usually possible to carry out venipuncture successfully in the marginal ear veins, as shown in Fig. 12.16.

> **TECHNICIAN NOTE** The patient should first be observed undisturbed in its transport box. Respiratory rate and character can be noted during observation.

Physical Examination of Small Mammals

The animal should first be observed undisturbed in its transport box if possible and can then be restrained as previously described for more detailed examination. The animal's respiratory rate and pattern can be assessed and its heart rate recorded, either by palpating the heartbeat or by using a stethoscope. Although normal rates are given in Table 12.1, these will rarely be observed in patients because most will show a marked increase in heart and respiratory rates due to the stress of examination. Rabbits, for example, frequently have respiratory rates in excess of 250 breaths/min during routine clinical examination. The type of examination that can be carried out is limited by the size of the species being examined, but in rabbits, it is possible to auscultate and percuss the chest, as in cats.

In all species, the following are of particular importance:
- Discharges from the eyes and nose may indicate the presence of respiratory disease. Rats are commonly seen with a black or reddish-brown discharge around their eyes or nose. This is a buildup of porphyrin secretions which, when wiped with a damp swab, will appear bright red. This can lead owners to report that their animal has been bleeding from its eyes or nose. These secretions are a nonspecific response to stress or illnesses such as chronic respiratory disease.
- Labored or noisy respiration is also indicative of respiratory disease
- Soiling of the perineum can indicate gastrointestinal disturbances
- An unkempt or staring appearance of the coat is a general sign of ill health in small mammals
- Loss of skin tone in response to dehydration is more difficult to detect in small mammals than in the dog and cat. If loss of elasticity is noted, it usually indicates that more than 10% of body weight has been lost as fluid. When small mammals are markedly dehydrated, the eyes become sunken. This is commonly seen in rabbits and small mammals that are anesthetized for treatment of dental disease. Because the disease may have been present for some time, the animal may have had a prolonged period of reduced food and water intake. It is essential that these animals receive supportive fluid therapy before anesthesia.
- Palpation of the regions overlying the spine and pelvis is helpful in assessing body condition. If the prominences of the vertebrae and of the pelvis are easily palpable, it is likely that the animal has lost a considerable amount of body fat.
- It is difficult to examine the mucous membranes in small rodents, but in the rabbit, both the gingiva and conjunctiva can be inspected easily. They should have a normal reddish coloration and the capillary refill time should be under 1 second. As with the dog and cat, abnormal coloration of the mucous membranes may indicate underlying disease.

> **TECHNICIAN NOTE** Dehydration is more difficult to detect in small mammals than in dogs and cats. If loss of skin elasticity is noted, it usually indicates that more than 10% of body weight has been lost as fluid.

Diagnostic Tests

Preanesthetic blood tests are rarely undertaken in small rodents but may be of value in some circumstances (e.g., in rabbits with suspected hepatic lipidosis). Urine samples are easily obtained from small rodents because these species frequently urinate when handled. Diabetes mellitus is relatively common in Chinese hamsters and is also seen occasionally in rabbits and guinea pigs. In these latter species, it is frequently asymptomatic.

Radiography may be required before some surgical procedures. For example, radiography of the skull is helpful in assessing underlying dental problems before flushing the nasolacrimal (tear) ducts to correct an obstruction since blockage may occur secondary to elongation of a maxillary incisor or an abscessed tooth. Radiography is also indicated before removal of a suspected uterine adenocarcinoma in rabbits to identify secondary tumors in the lungs.

PREANESTHETIC PATIENT CARE

> **TECHNICIAN NOTE** There is generally no reason to withhold food or water before anesthesia because small rodents and rabbits do not vomit; the practice may lead to hypoglycemia. Food should be made available until 1–2 hr before anesthesia and immediately following recovery from anesthesia.

Withholding Food Before Anesthesia

Small rodents and rabbits do not vomit and there is generally no reason to withhold food or water before anesthesia. Withholding food from small rodents for prolonged periods can be detrimental because it can predispose to hypoglycemia. Withholding food from rabbits and guinea pigs can also trigger digestive disturbances that can result in enterotoxemia, which may be fatal. One exception to the no-fasting rule is if the planned operation involves the stomach, in which case a 3- to 4-hour fasting period will reduce the volume of digesta.

Successful recovery from an operation and anesthesia in these species is critically dependent on reestablishing a normal feeding pattern. It is therefore strongly recommended that food be available up until 1 to 2 hours before anesthesia and provided again as soon as the animal has recovered. Ask the owner about the animal's favorite foods and provide these during recovery. Although these might not represent a balanced diet, advice can be given later on this. The priority is to encourage the animal to eat. The anesthetist should be aware that many of these animals are nocturnal and will not feed during the day. Postoperative pain and discomfort can also decrease appetite in the period after the operation.

Correction of Preexisting Problems

If animals are in poor condition, every attempt should be made to commence supportive therapy before anesthesia. One common problem is dehydration. Unfortunately, the small body size of these animals makes administration of fluids difficult. In the rabbit, the marginal ear veins and cephalic veins can be used, but in rodents, the small size of the veins does not allow easy IV catheterization, although placement of a catheter in the tail vein of rats is practicable. One alternative is to administer fluids by the subcutaneous or intraperitoneal route, although subcutaneous administration is unlikely to be effective if

TABLE 12.2	Volumes of Fluid for Administration to Adult Small Mammals[a]					
Route	**Gerbil**	**Guinea Pig**	**Hamster**	**Mouse**	**Rabbit**	**Rat**
Intraperitoneal	2–3 mL	20 mL	3 mL	2 mL	50 mL	5 mL
Subcutaneous	1–2 mL	10–20 mL	3 mL	1–2 mL	30–50 mL	5 mL

[a]All fluids should be warmed to body temperature before administration.

dehydration is severe. The intraosseous route can also be used and can be a valuable means of providing prolonged fluid therapy in rabbits, guinea pigs, and rats.

Calculation of fluid volume and administration rates is done according to body weight. Small mammals require higher maintenance rates than dogs and cats (100 mL/kg every 24 hours). All of the types of fluid commonly used in small animal practice can be administered to rodents and rabbits. Suggested volumes for administration are listed in Table 12.2.

PREANESTHETIC AGENTS

> **TECHNICIAN NOTE** Atropine is often relatively ineffective in rabbits because many animals have high levels of atropinase, an enzyme which inactivates atropine. Glycopyrrolate should be used instead.

Although the general principles governing the use of preanesthetic agents (see Chapter 3) apply to small mammals, these agents are less frequently used than in dogs and cats. This is primarily due to the methods of anesthesia that are used in small mammals. Because many anesthetic protocols include a combination of anesthetic agents to be given by subcutaneous, intraperitoneal, or intramuscular injection, there is often little advantage in giving a sedative agent before this. If anesthesia is to be induced in an anesthetic chamber in small rodents, prior sedation is rarely needed.

Preanesthetic agents should also be used in the following circumstances:

- Anticholinergic agents can be used to reduce salivation associated with some anesthetics (e.g., ketamine) and to reduce bronchial secretions, particularly in animals with preexisting respiratory disease. Atropine is frequently used for this purpose, but in rabbits, it is often relatively ineffective because many have high levels of atropinase. It is therefore advisable to use glycopyrrolate in rabbits.
- Opioid analgesics may be given 30 to 45 minutes before induction of anesthesia. This reduces the concentration of volatile anesthetics needed to maintain anesthesia and provides preemptive analgesia (see Chapter 8).
- Sedatives or tranquilizers should be given to rabbits before induction of anesthesia with volatile agents (see detailed discussion later in this section).

All of the agents that are commonly used for preanesthetic medication in dogs and cats can be used in small mammals. Their properties and side effects are very similar, but some vary in their actions. Suggested dose rates and their effects are listed in Table 12.3.

Anticholinergics

Both atropine and glycopyrrolate can be used in small mammals, with the same indications as in dogs and cats. As mentioned earlier, glycopyrrolate is preferred to atropine for use in rabbits because the effect of atropine is less predictable in this species. These agents should not be administered if an alpha$_2$-agonist like dexmedetomidine is to be used as part of the anesthetic regimen.

Phenothiazines

Phenothiazines such as acepromazine can be used to sedate small mammals. When used in rodents, acepromazine will sedate the animal but will not immobilize it. In rabbits, acepromazine has excellent sedative effects and will often provide sufficient restraint for procedures such as radiography.

Benzodiazepines

Both diazepam and midazolam have marked sedative effects in rodents and rabbits, unlike their effects in dogs and cats. They can be administered by intraperitoneal, intramuscular, or IV injection and are often used in combination with other agents to produce balanced anesthesia. Their sedative properties, although pronounced, are not usually sufficient to immobilize an animal for minor procedures such as radiography.

Alpha$_2$-Adrenoreceptor Agonists

Dexmedetomidine, medetomidine, and xylazine can be used to produce sedation with some analgesia in small mammals. At higher dose rates, the effects can be sufficient to immobilize some animals. This effect is most reliable in the rabbit, and dexmedetomidine or medetomidine can be used to provide sedation and restraint for radiography in this species. Vomiting, one side effect of medetomidine and dexmedetomidine (which is often seen in dogs and cats), does not occur in small mammals because these animals do not vomit. The other side effects of these agents, such as hyperglycemia, diuresis, and respiratory and cardiovascular system depression, do occur. A major advantage of these sedatives is that their action can be reversed by administration of specific antagonists. Both yohimbine and atipamezole have been used for this purpose in small mammals. Atipamezole is preferable because it has fewer side effects. It can be given through the subcutaneous, intraperitoneal, intramuscular, or IV routes. Absorption after subcutaneous injection is rapid and the drug generally acts within 5 to 10 minutes. Dose rates of 0.5 to 1 mg/kg are required, depending on the dose of dexmedetomidine that has been administered.

TABLE 12.3   Preanesthetic Agents for Use in Small Mammals

Drug	Species	Doseage	Effect
Acepromazine	Rat, guinea pig	2.5 mg/kg IP or SC	Sedation but still active
	Mouse, hamster, gerbil	3–5 mg/kg IP or SC	
	Rabbit	1 mg/kg SC or IM	Sedation, often immobilized
Acepromazine and butorphanol	Rabbit	0.5 mg/kg + 1 mg/kg IM or SC	Sedation, often immobilized, some analgesia
Atropine	Mouse, hamster, gerbil, rat, guinea pig	0.04 mg/kg SC or IM	Reduced bronchial and salivary secretions, inhibition of vagal responses, ineffective in many rabbits
Diazepam	Mouse, hamster, gerbil, guinea pig	5 mg/kg IP	Sedation
	Rat	2.5 mg/kg IP	
	Rabbit	1–2 mg/kg IM	
Glycopyrrolate	Rabbit	0.01 mg/kg IV or 0.1 mg/kg SC or IM	Reduced bronchial and salivary secretions, inhibition of vagal responses
Innovar Vet (fentanyl/ droperidol)	Rabbit	0.22 mL/kg IM	Sedation and analgesia, often sufficiently immobilized for minor surgical procedures
	Mouse	0.06–0.5 mL/kg IM	
	Hamster	1.5 mL/kg IM	
	Guinea pig	0.4 mL/kg IM	
Hypnorm (fentanyl/ fluanisone)	Mouse, hamster, gerbil, rat, guinea pig	0.5 mL/kg SC or IP	Sedation and analgesia, often sufficiently immobilized for minor surgical procedures
	Rabbit	0.3–0.5 mL/kg SC or IM	
Dexmedetomidine	Mouse, hamster, rat	15–50 mcg/kg SC or IP	Sedation and some analgesia, immobilized at higher dose rates
	Rabbit	50–250 mcg/kg SC or IP	
Midazolam	Mouse, hamster, gerbil, guinea pig	5 mg/kg IP	Sedation
	Rat	2.5 mg/kg IP	
	Rabbit	1–2 mg/kg IM	
Xylazine	Mouse, hamster, rat	5 mg/kg SC or IM	Sedation and some analgesia, immobilized at higher dose rates
	Rabbit	2.5 mg/kg SC or IM	

IM, Intramuscular; *IP,* intraperitoneal; *IV,* intravenous; *SC,* subcutaneous.

Opioids

The use of these agents in the preanesthetic period to provide preemptive analgesia is discussed in Chapter 8. More commonly, opioids are used in small mammals in combination with sedative agents to provide chemical restraint and analgesia for minor procedures such as suturing superficial wounds and draining abscesses. In Europe, a commercially prepared mixture of fentanyl and fluanisone (Hypnorm) is available for this purpose. A mixture of acepromazine and butorphanol is useful when taking blood samples from rabbits because it provides some sedation and analgesia and dilates the ear veins.

GENERAL ANESTHESIA

Induction Techniques and Agents

Although techniques similar to those used for anesthetic induction in dogs and cats can be used in small mammals, practical considerations limit the use of the IV route except in rabbits. A wide range of different anesthetic agents can be used in these species and suggested dose rates are given in Table 12.4. Formulas for anesthetic mixtures used in small mammals are given in Box 12.1. Given the small muscle mass of small rodents, intramuscular administration is best avoided because the relatively

large volumes of anesthetic agents required cause pain on injection and can produce muscle damage.

In rabbits, the subcutaneous or intramuscular routes are often used, but IV injection of short-acting agents provides more controllable induction of anesthesia. For small mammals, intraperitoneal injection is a simple and relatively painless route for induction agents. The intraperitoneal route appears to be less painful than intramuscular injection, although the technique is less familiar. The technique is similar for most small rodents: an assistant extends the right hindlimb and injects the anesthetic into the middle of the right posterior quadrant of the abdomen. This technique avoids the bladder, which lies in the midline just in front of the pelvis. Use of the right side of the abdomen also avoids the cecum, which is large and thin walled in rodents.

Although the technique for intraperitoneal injection is simple to carry out, administration of anesthetics by this route has important practical implications. If an anesthetic is given intravenously, the dose that is administered can be titrated to provide the required effect in that particular animal. It is therefore relatively simple to adjust the dose to account for individual, breed, and strain variation, and overdosing or underdosing is easy to avoid. When anesthetics are given intraperitoneally

TABLE 12.4   Anesthetic and Related Drugs for Use in Small Mammals[a]

Agent	Gerbil	Guinea Pig	Hamster	Mouse	Rabbit	Rat
Atipamezole	1 mg/kg SC, IM, IP, IV	1 mg/kg SC, IM, IP, IV	1 mg/kg SC, IM, IP, IV	1 mg/kg SC, IM, IP, IV	1 mg/kg SC, IM, IP, IV	1 mg/kg SC, IM, IP, IV
Doxapram	5–10 mg/kg IV or IP	5–10 mg/kg IV or IP	5–10 mg/kg IV or IP	5–10 mg/kg IV or IP	5–10 mg/kg IV or IM	5–10 mg/kg IV or IP
Fentanyl/fluanisone and diazepam[b]	0.3 mL/kg IM + 5 mg/kg IP	1.0 mL/kg IM + 2.5 mg/kg IP	1 mL/kg IM + 5 mg/kg IP	0.3 mL/kg IM + 5 mg/kg IP	0.3 mL/kg IM + 2 mg/kg IP or IV	0.3 mL/kg IM + 2.5 mg/kg IP
Fentanyl/fluanisone (Hypnorm) and midazolam[c]	8 mL/kg IP	8 mL/kg IP	4 mL/kg IP	10 mL/kg IP	0.3 mL/kg Hypnorm IM + 2 mg/kg midazolam IP or IV	2.7 mL/kg IP
Ketamine + dexmedetomidine	75 mg/kg 0.25 mg/kg IP	40 mg/kg + 0.25 mg/kg IP	100 mg/kg + 0.125 mg/kg IP	75 mg/kg + 0.5 mg/kg IP	15 mg/kg + 0.125 mg/kg IM	75 mg/kg + 0.25 mg/kg IP
Ketamine + xylazine	50 mg/kg + 2 mg/kg IP	40 mg/kg + 5 mg/kg IP	200 mg/kg + 10 mg/kg IP	80 mg/kg + 10 mg/kg IP	35 mg/kg + 5 mg/kg IM	75 mg/kg + 10 mg/kg IP
Tiletamine and zolazepam[d] (immobilizes, does not usually produce anesthesia)	60 mg/kg IM	40–60 mg/kg IM	50–80 mg/kg IM	80–100 mg/kg IM	5–25 mg/kg IM	20–40 mg/kg IM

[a]Note that there may be considerable variation between strains and these dose rates should be taken as a general guide only.

[b]These drugs cannot be mixed together and must be given separately.

[c]Doses for rodents are given as milliliters of a combination of fentanyl/fluanisone and midazolam, prepared as 2 mL water for injection plus 1 mL of 5 mg/mL midazolam and 1 mL of Hypnorm (Janssen; fentanyl/fluanisone). In rabbits, Hypnorm and midazolam are injected separately, without dilution.

[d]Dosage is combined amount of tiletamine and zolazepam, in the commercial formulation "Telazol".

IM, Intramuscular; *IP*, intraperitoneal; *IV*, intravenous; *SC*, subcutaneous.

BOX 12.1   Formulas for Anesthetic Mixtures for Small Mammals

- Many of these solutions can be stored for a few days if made up carefully and placed in a sterile multidose vial. There is some risk of instability with prolonged storage and this practice is not recommended by the manufacturers.
- If necessary, solutions can be diluted with sterile water for injection or sterile saline to provide an appropriate volume for accurate administration. The appropriate volume for mice is 0.1 mL/10 g (therefore an adult mouse would need 0.2–0.4 mL IP or SC). The appropriate volume for a rat is 0.2 mL/100 g (therefore an adult rat would need 0.5–0.8 mL IP or SC).
- See Tables 12.3 and 12.4 for dosages used in each species

Examples

1. To make a 2-mL mixture of ketamine (75 mg/kg) and dexmedetomidine (0.25 mg/kg) for rats, mix together the following:
   Ketamine (100 mg/mL): 0.75 mL
   Dexmedetomidine (0.5 mg/mL): 0.5 mL
   Sterile saline (0.9%): 0.75 mL
   Administer at 0.2 mL/100 g IP
2. To make up a 5-mL mixture of ketamine (75 mg/kg) and dexmedetomidine (0.5 mg/kg) for mice, mix together the following:
   Ketamine (100 mg/mL): 0.38 mL
   Dexmedetomidine (0.5 mg/mL): 0.5 mL
   Sterile saline (0.9%): 4.12 mL
   Administer at 0.1 mL/10 g IP

IP, Intraperitoneal.

(or by subcutaneous injection), a calculated dose is given and there is no opportunity to adjust it to suit the requirements of the particular animal. As large variations in response to anesthetics have been noted in small rodents, it is advisable to select an anesthetic regimen that has a wide safety margin (preferably one that is completely or partially reversible) if drugs are not being administered intravenously.

A further problem associated with use of the intraperitoneal or subcutaneous route is that relatively high dose rates are required compared with those that are needed when drugs are given intravenously. One consequence is that recovery times tend to be prolonged, which is particularly undesirable in small mammals because of the high risk of hypothermia.

Cyclohexamine Agents

When used alone, ketamine has limited effect in small mammals, even at high doses. In rodents, it barely immobilizes the animal and does not provide sufficient analgesia, even for superficial surgical procedures such as suturing of skin wounds. In rabbits, use of ketamine alone provides restraint, but the degree of analgesia is insufficient for surgery. Ketamine combined with acepromazine and ketamine combined with either diazepam or midazolam produce surgical anesthesia in some rabbits, but these combinations generally produce only light anesthesia in small rodents. Ketamine is most effective when combined with an alpha$_2$-agonist such as dexmedetomidine or xylazine due to the analgesic and muscle relaxant activity of these agents. Ketamine with dexmedetomidine or xylazine produces surgical anesthesia in most rodents and rabbits, but the effects of these agents are less uniform in guinea pigs and some animals may not be at a sufficient depth of anesthesia for an operation to be carried out humanely. As in other species, the dose of dexmedetomidine required is approximately 50% of the medetomidine dose. Because ketamine has limited effects when used alone in small mammals, reversal of dexmedetomidine, medetomidine, or xylazine will considerably reduce the length of the recovery period. However, because the analgesic effects are also reversed, another analgesic should be administered to provide postoperative pain relief.

Tiletamine in combination with zolazepam (Zoletil, Telazol) produces light to medium planes of anesthesia in small rodents. It offers little advantage in comparison with ketamine combined with midazolam or diazepam and it produces less analgesia than ketamine in combination with dexmedetomidine, medetomidine, or xylazine.

Neuroleptanalgesics

As mentioned earlier, the combination of fentanyl/fluanisone provides restraint and analgesia in small mammals. Fentanyl and fluanisone also can be combined with a benzodiazepine to provide surgical anesthesia. The addition of midazolam or diazepam provides muscle relaxation and increases the depth of anesthesia. Recovery can be enhanced by reversal of fentanyl with a mixed agonist/antagonist opioid such as butorphanol or nalbuphine. This reverses the respiratory depression and some of the sedation caused by the fentanyl component of the anesthetic mixture while continuing to provide postoperative analgesia. Although antagonists of benzodiazepines (e.g., flumazenil) can be administered to speed recovery, their duration of action is short and animals may become resedated.

Propofol

Propofol produces short periods of surgical anesthesia in small rodents, but because it is most effective when given by IV injection, it is rarely used in these species. Propofol can be used in rabbits to provide a short period of light anesthesia sufficient for induction of anesthesia, followed by endotracheal intubation and maintenance of anesthesia with inhalant anesthetics. If high doses of propofol are given to rabbits to produce a surgical plane of anesthesia, respiratory depression or respiratory arrest may occur. After induction with a low to moderate dose of propofol, it is safer to increase the depth of anesthesia by administering a low concentration of an inhalational agent (e.g., 0.5% isoflurane). When administering propofol to rabbits, it should be injected slowly (e.g., over 1 to 2 minutes for an induction dose in a 3-kg rabbit). When administered in this way, it rarely causes significant respiratory depression and recovery from anesthesia is smooth and rapid.

Alfaxalone

The steroid anesthetic alfaxalone can be used to induce anesthesia in rabbits when given by IV injection. As with propofol, there is a risk of causing apnea if administration is too rapid. This anesthetic causes minimal cardiovascular depression and recovery following its use is relatively rapid.

Administration by intramuscular injection produces sedation or light anesthesia in rodents. When given intravenously, surgical anesthesia can be produced.

Inhalant Anesthetics

Induction of anesthesia with an inhalant anesthetic agent is probably the safest and most effective means of providing anesthesia in small rodents. Although mask induction is possible, it is usually most convenient to induce anesthesia in an anesthetic chamber. Suitable chambers can be either purchased commercially or constructed from clear plastic containers. The size of the chamber should be such that it can be rapidly filled with anesthetic vapor from the anesthetic machine. This will ensure that the induction of anesthesia is rapid and smooth, with only a brief period of involuntary excitement. Anesthetic vapors are denser than air, so the chamber should be filled from the bottom and excess anesthetic gases removed from the top. A suitable design is shown in Fig. 12.17.

Isoflurane, sevoflurane, and desflurane can all be used safely in small rodents. The concentrations required for induction and maintenance of anesthesia are similar to those used in dogs and cats. Provided the anesthetic chamber is filled rapidly, induction is generally complete in 2 to 3 minutes. Recovery is also rapid, with rodents regaining their righting reflex within 5 to 10 minutes after 20 to 30 minutes of anesthesia. After a further 10 to 15 minutes, they will appear to be fully recovered. As in dogs and cats, induction of anesthesia and recovery are rapid with isoflurane and even more rapid with sevoflurane and desflurane.

Inhalant anesthetics should be delivered with a precision vaporizer. Induction of anesthesia in a chamber in which liquid anesthetic is placed on a gauze pad is extremely dangerous because high concentrations (>20%) of anesthetic vapor are produced.

After induction of anesthesia, the animal can be removed from the chamber and brief (<30 seconds) procedures carried out. For longer procedures, it is usually more convenient to maintain anesthesia by placing a face mask on the animal. Suitable masks can either be purchased commercially or constructed from plastic syringes. Although relatively high gas flow

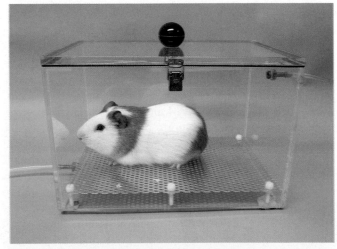

FIG. 12.17 Anesthetic induction chamber suitable for small mammals.

rates should be used to fill anesthetic chambers rapidly, the fresh gas flow rates needed to maintain anesthesia on a face mask are low for small mammals because they are linked to the animal's minute volume. For example, a hamster would typically require less than 100 mL/min. Given that some vaporizers and flowmeters may not perform accurately at very low flows, rates of 200 to 300 mL/min are suggested for use with small rodents. As with dogs and cats, it is important that waste anesthetic gases are scavenged effectively; this is most easily achieved by using a commercial apparatus designed for this purpose.

> **TECHNICIAN NOTE** Rabbits should be premedicated before mask or chamber induction with an inhalant anesthetic in order to avoid violent struggling and prolonged breath holding.

The use of inhalant anesthetics in rabbits can be difficult because these animals frequently hold their breath when exposed to these agents. Breath holding can be prolonged and is sometimes associated with marked bradycardia. If a mask is used, animals appear to resent the procedure and may struggle violently. If placed in an anesthetic chamber, they attempt to avoid inhaling the anesthetic and may make violent attempts to escape. It is therefore preferable to administer preanesthetic medication (e.g., acepromazine, midazolam, or dexmedetomidine) before inducing anesthesia with a face mask. After this medication has taken effect, a mask can be used to administer 100% oxygen for 1 to 2 minutes before introducing the inhalant. The animal may still hold its breath but is unlikely to struggle. If breath holding occurs, the mask should be briefly removed and replaced when the animal commences breathing again. An alternative approach is to administer a short-acting induction agent such as propofol and maintain anesthesia with an inhalation agent.

> **TECHNICIAN NOTE** Due to the ease of control of the depth of anesthesia, the simple and convenient method of induction, and the rapid recovery, inhalation agents are often the anesthesia method of choice in small mammals.

Summary of Recommended Techniques

Inhalation agents are often the anesthesia method of choice in small mammals because of the ease of control of the depth of anesthesia, the simple and convenient method of induction, and the rapid recovery. If injectable anesthetics are preferred, ketamine in combination with dexmedetomidine, medetomidine, or xylazine, or fentanyl and fluanisone with a benzodiazepine, are the combinations of choice. If an injectable anesthetic combination has been administered and the desired depth of anesthesia has not been reached, it is possible to administer an additional drug to deepen anesthesia. However, it is often preferable to deepen anesthesia with a low concentration of an inhalation agent or, alternatively, to provide local analgesia by infiltrating the surgical site with local anesthetic. These techniques are also useful when dealing with high-risk patients. In these circumstances, a low dose of an injectable anesthetic combination can be given to provide a light plane of anesthesia, and inhalation anesthetics or local anesthetics can be used to provide surgical anesthesia. Although local anesthetics are safe to use in small mammals, it is relatively easy to overdose the animal when infiltrating the surgical site. Avoid this by calculating a safe dose in advance, as described on page 394.

Intubation and Maintenance of Anesthesia

The apparatus used to anesthetize small rodents and rabbits is similar to that used in dogs and cats, but the size of the patient limits the suitability of some equipment. Generally, anesthetic gases are delivered with a face mask; however, in rabbits, endotracheal intubation is a relatively simple technique to perform and is recommended as a routine procedure. Endotracheal intubation can be carried out by visualizing the larynx with a laryngoscope and blade created for this purpose (such as a Wisconsin blade) or with a canine otoscope. Alternatively, a blind technique can be used. These procedures are outlined in detail in Procedure 12.1.

Uncuffed endotracheal tubes are preferred. A typical 3-kg rabbit requires a tube with a 3.0 to 3.5 mm diameter. Very small rabbits (<800 g) need tubes with a diameter of <2.5 mm, which can be purchased from specialist suppliers. A rabbit's airway can also be maintained using a supraglottic airway device or laryngeal mask (see Chapter 4). These are simple to use in this species and allow some control of respiration. As an alternative to intubation, a nasal catheter can be passed and positioned in the back of the pharynx. This allows oxygen supplementation during oral surgery but does not enable ventilation to be assisted effectively. Nasal catheters can also be used in small rodents to deliver oxygen or anesthetic gases and should be directed medially and ventrally through the external nares, and inserted about 0.5 cm in a mouse or hamster and 1 cm in a rat or guinea pig (Fig. 12.18). This technique is particularly useful when carrying out dental procedures. Waste anesthetic gases can be removed by placing an extractor tube close to the animal's nose, and the potential problem can be reduced by using appropriately low fresh gas flow rates. The catheter should be connected with tubing directly to the fresh gas outlet of the anesthetic machine because if a reservoir bag or valve is in place, the high resistance of the catheter will result in most of the oxygen supplied being vented through the valve.

When using an anesthetic machine, non rebreathing systems are preferred to rebreathing systems because they offer less resistance and have less equipment dead space. Examples of suitable nonrebreathing systems include the Bain circuit and Ayres T-piece. With smaller rabbits, it is advisable to use low dead space pediatric connectors to attach the endotracheal tube to the breathing circuit. Low dead space T-piece systems designed for use in humans are also useful for rabbits (Fig. 12.19). Fresh gas flow rates are calculated in the same way as for dogs and cats (see Chapter 4, Box 4.5).

Monitoring

Depth of anesthesia. Before a surgical or other painful procedure is started, it is essential to ensure that the animal is at an appropriate depth of anesthesia. The most reliable method in rodents is to assess the pedal withdrawal (discussed in Chapter 6)

PROCEDURE 12.1 Rabbit Endotracheal Intubation

1. Have ready an appropriately sized tube, local anesthetic spray, a laryngoscope or otoscope, and an introducer (Fig. 1). Check that the batteries in the otoscope or laryngoscope are functioning.

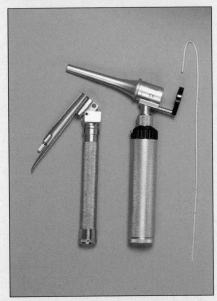

FIG. 1 Apparatus for endotracheal intubation in the rabbit. A laryngoscope *(left)* or otoscope *(center)* is used to visualize the larynx, and an introducer *(right)* is used to guide the endotracheal tube into the airway.

2. Measure from the nares to the thoracic inlet and trim the length of the endotracheal tube if necessary.

3. Anesthetize the animal, ensuring that it has lost the chewing reflex elicited when the mouth is opened. Place the animal on its back and administer oxygen through a face mask for 2 min.

4. Open the mouth and pull the tongue forward into the gap between the incisors and premolars. The incisors are sharp, so take care not to damage the tongue. Insert the blade of the laryngoscope or the otoscope speculum into the gap between the teeth on the opposite side of the mouth and advance it until the end of the soft palate or the larynx is visible. In some animals, the epiglottis will be positioned behind the soft palate, hiding the larynx from view. To expose the larynx, use the introducer to reposition the epiglottis and soft palate (Fig. 2).

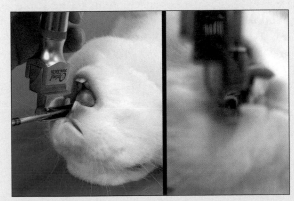

FIG. 2 Endotracheal intubation in a dorsally recumbent rabbit using a laryngoscope (Wisconsin blade) to visualize the larynx. *Left,* Placing the endotracheal tube using an introducer. *Right,* View of the larynx through the laryngoscope blade.

5. Spray the larynx with local anesthetic.

6. Advance the introducer through the larynx into the trachea. If an otoscope is being used, thread the introducer through the speculum, remove the otoscope, and thread the endotracheal tube onto the introducer. If a laryngoscope is being used, the tube and introducer are advanced into the mouth together and then into the larynx and trachea. The introducer is used to guide the endotracheal tube into the trachea and is then withdrawn. Although introducers are commercially available, a dog or cat urinary catheter can be used to stiffen and straighten the endotracheal tube and act as a guide.

7. When a blind intubation technique is used, place the rabbit on its chest and supply oxygen through a face mask for 2 min. Hold the rabbit around the base of the skull and position the rabbit so its head and neck are elevated (Fig. 3). Introduce the endotracheal tube into the gap between the incisors and premolars and slide it on into the pharynx. As it reaches the larynx, some increase in resistance is felt. The tube is then advanced into the larynx and trachea; this is usually accompanied by a slight cough. In some cases, the tube passes into the esophagus and will need to be withdrawn and repositioned. The position of the tube can be monitored by listening at the end of the tube.

If breath sounds can be heard, the tube is in the pharynx or the trachea.

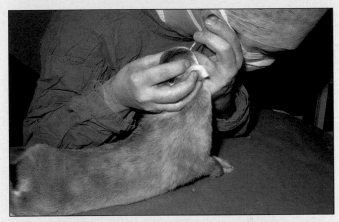

FIG. 3 Rabbit positioned for endotracheal intubation with a blind technique. After successful intubation of the trachea, the operator will hear breath sounds through the tube.

8. Confirm successful placement of the tube by observing condensation in the tube on each expiration, by observing movement of a small piece of tissue paper or a tuft of fur placed at the end of the tube, or by using a capnograph to detect carbon dioxide. After attaching the tube to an anesthetic circuit, auscultate the chest and ensure that both sides are inflated when the reservoir bag is compressed or the expiratory limb of the circuit is occluded.

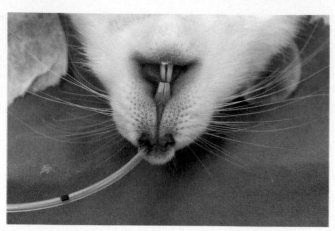

FIG. 12.18 Nasal catheter being used to deliver oxygen to a rat. The catheter is an infant nasogastric feeding tube, but any suitably sized soft catheter can be used.

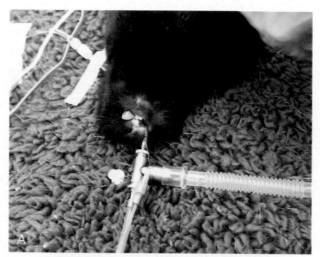

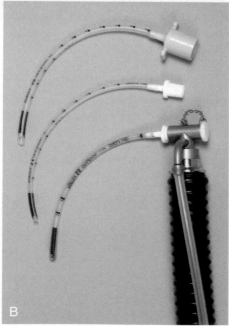

FIG. 12.19 (A) A low dead space pediatric T-piece and endotracheal connector suitable for anesthetic delivery in a rabbit. **(B)** Endotracheal tube connectors. *Top,* Standard connector; *middle,* pediatric connector; *bottom,* pediatric connector and T-piece.

or tail pinch reflex. To assess the tail pinch, the operator firmly pinches the tip of the tail with their fingernails. It is important to pinch hard enough to produce a painful stimulus but not so hard as to damage the tail. If the animal is too lightly anesthetized for surgery, it will flick its tail and may vocalize. The tail pinch response is usually lost at a light to medium plane of anesthesia; this is followed by loss of the pedal withdrawal response at medium to deep planes of anesthesia. Most surgical procedures can be carried out when the pedal withdrawal reflex is absent or barely detectable. In rabbits and guinea pigs, the ear pinch reflex can also be used to measure anesthetic depth.

Ocular reflexes are not as useful in small mammals as in the dog and cat. With most anesthetic regimens, the position of the eye remains fixed in rodents and the palpebral (blink) reflex may still be present at surgical planes of anesthesia. In rabbits, there is considerable variation in the loss of ocular reflexes; however, at deep planes of anesthesia, the eye may rotate and protrude. Because cardiac arrest may occur shortly after the animal reaches such a deep plane of anesthesia, this appearance indicates that supportive measures should be initiated immediately and administration of anesthetic should be reduced or terminated. The eye often remains open during anesthesia and should be protected from drying by applying a suitable lubricating ophthalmic ointment or should be gently taped closed.

> **TECHNICIAN NOTE** Many pieces of monitoring equipment (e.g., blood pressure measuring device, electrocardiogram [ECG], or pulse oximeter) are not designed to function normally within the range of heart rates (often 250–400 beats per minute [bpm]) seen in small mammals.

Heart rate and rhythm. The small size of rodents and rabbits and their rapid heart rates can make it difficult to monitor heart rate and rhythm, and it is usually not possible to palpate a peripheral pulse. Auscultation of the chest wall is possible for rabbits and guinea pigs but difficult with smaller rodents. An esophageal stethoscope can be used for rabbits and the heartbeat can be detected by palpating the chest wall in all species. However, because the heart rate often exceeds 250 bpm in many of these animals, it is not possible to assess the heart rate accurately. Problems can also arise when an electrocardiogram (ECG) is used because many instruments have an upper heart rate limit of 250 or 300 bpm and may also be unable to detect the low amplitude signals generated in small rodents.

Capillary refill time. The small size of rodents usually prevents the use of capillary refill time as an assessment of peripheral perfusion, although it is possible to assess this in rabbits. The color of the mucous membranes can give some indication of problems associated with blood loss, cyanosis, and poor peripheral perfusion. In addition to inspection of the gingiva, the color of light reflected in the eyes can be used to detect cyanosis or pallor caused by blood loss in albino animals.

> **TECHNICIAN NOTE** Loss of 1 mL of blood represents a 15% blood loss in a small mammal weighing 100 g; this puts the patient at risk of hypovolemic circulatory failure.

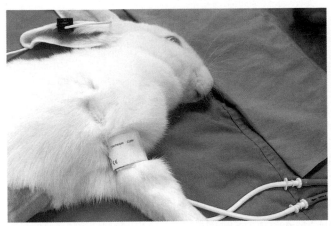

FIG. 12.20 Use of noninvasive blood pressure monitoring in the rabbit. A pulse oximeter probe placed on the pinna is also being used to monitor this animal.

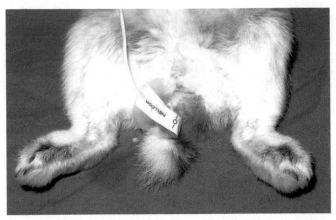

FIG. 12.21 Use of a pulse oximeter in a rabbit, with the probe positioned across the base of the tail.

Blood loss. Because these animals are small, total blood volume is small—approximately 70 mL/kg of body weight. A 100-g hamster will have a total blood volume of only 7 mL. As in dogs and cats, loss of more than 15% of blood volume (approximately 1 mL in this example) can lead to signs of circulatory failure. It is therefore critically important to monitor blood loss by carefully weighing swabs and assessing other losses at the surgical site. Surgical techniques should be adapted to minimize the risk of hemorrhage and any bleeding should be controlled as quickly as possible.

Arterial blood pressure. Blood pressure can be monitored in rabbits using either a catheter placed in the central ear artery or noninvasively using an oscillometric technique. The pressure cuff should be placed either on the forelimb just proximal to the elbow or on the hindlimb proximal to the stifle (Fig. 12.20). The success of this technique depends both on the size of the rabbit and on the particular monitor. As an alternative, a Doppler probe can be placed over a suitable artery and, if combined with the use of a blood pressure cuff and sphygmomanometer, an estimate of arterial pressure can be obtained (see Chapter 6).

Respiratory rate and depth. The pattern and depth of respiration can be monitored by observing the chest movements, although this becomes difficult once surgical drapes have been placed. Because of the small size of these animals, there is usually no reservoir bag in the anesthetic breathing system and respiration cannot be monitored by bag movement. It is helpful to use an electronic monitor but, as with the ECG, the small size of the animal and rapid respiratory rate can make some monitors ineffective.

Although both the pattern and the rate of respiration change during anesthesia, this varies greatly depending on the anesthetic regimen used. Becoming familiar with one or two regularly used regimens allows changes to be interpreted more reliably. In general, once anesthesia has been induced, the respiratory rate decreases markedly, especially because most of these animals will show tachypnea before induction. Typical respiratory rates during anesthesia are 50 to 100 breaths per minute for small rodents and 30 to 60 breaths per minute for rabbits. A reduction to less than 50% of the estimated normal respiratory rate (see Table 12.1) should give cause for concern. As with dogs and cats, it is more common to see gradual changes in rate rather than a sudden

reduction. For this reason, it is helpful to keep a written anesthetic record when assessing the state of the animal during anesthesia.

Pulse Oximetry. Pulse oximeters can be used to monitor both the adequacy of oxygenation and the heart rate, but not all instruments function well in small rodents. The high heart rates may exceed the upper limits of the monitor and the low signal strength may not be detectable. A monitor with an upper limit of at least 350 bpm is needed, and it is useful to have a variety of different probe designs. A reliable signal can usually be obtained by placing the probe across the hind foot in small rodents or across a toe in larger rabbits, but the tail, tongue, and ear are also useful in some animals (Fig. 12.21).

Capnography. Sidestream capnographs can be used to monitor respiratory function in small animals, although the volume of gas sampled may be very large in relation to the animal's tidal volume. Mainstream capnographs introduce too much equipment dead space into the anesthetic breathing system and are not recommended for these species, but lower dead space, human pediatric versions can be used successfully in rabbits.

> **TECHNICIAN NOTE** Because of their small body size, rodents and rabbits have an increased ratio of surface area to body weight, which may lead to rapid cooling during anesthesia. It is therefore critically important to monitor and maintain body temperature during anesthesia and in the postoperative period.

Thermoregulation. It is critically important to monitor and maintain body temperature during anesthesia and in the postoperative period. Because of their small body size, rodents and rabbits have an increased ratio of surface area to body weight, which may lead to rapid cooling during anesthesia. Heat loss can be much more rapid than in dogs and cats. For example, the rectal temperature in a mouse can fall from 5°C to 6°C (9°F to 11°F) within 5 to 10 minutes of induction of anesthesia. The following procedures help avoid hypothermia.

- Monitor rectal temperature using an electronic thermometer rather than a glass clinical thermometer. Glass clinical thermometers can only indicate a minimum temperature of 35°C and the animal may be colder than this when the first measurement is made.

- Adopt good standards of asepsis but keep the area of fur that is shaved at the surgical site to a minimum and use the minimum quantity of skin disinfectant.
- Place the animal on a warming pad as soon as it has lost consciousness and provide additional insulation if needed. Warming pad temperatures should be set to 38°C to 40°C (100.4°F–104°F) for mice and other small mammals.
- Remember that electric heating pads can develop hot spots; using a second thermometer to measure the temperature between the animal and the heat pad can avoid the risk of inadvertent overheating.
- Always warm fluids to body temperature before administration
- Continue measures to prevent heat loss in the recovery period (see the following section).

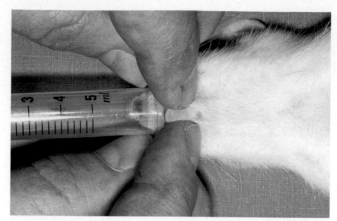

FIG. 12.22 Assisting ventilation in a rat by blowing down the barrel of a syringe placed over the rat's mouth and nose.

POSTOPERATIVE CARE

The provision of appropriate postoperative care is critical to the successful outcome of anesthesia and surgery in small mammals. Supportive measures to maintain body temperature must be continued and a quiet, warm, and secure environment should be provided. Because heat loss can occur relatively rapidly, an appropriate recovery environment should be set up before starting anesthesia and an operation. The animal can then be transferred to the recovery area immediately after the operation is completed. While the animal is immobile and unconscious, an environmental temperature of approximately 35°C (95°F) should be maintained. This can be lowered to 26°C to 28°C (79°F to 81°F) as the animal recovers. Warm and comfortable bedding must be provided. Synthetic sheepskin is ideal, but if this is unavailable, shredded paper or tissues can be used. Sawdust is unsuitable because it tends to crust around the nose, eyes, and mouth. Good-quality hay should be provided to guinea pigs and rabbits once they have recovered their righting reflex. This type of bedding allows the animal to surround itself with insulating material, which provides both warmth and a sense of security and encourages early feeding. Other species of small mammals should also be encouraged to eat soon after recovery and should be given their preferred foods.

Animals should also be provided with water, but care must be taken that they do not spill it because the animal will lose heat rapidly if it becomes wet. The animal may also fail to drink from an unfamiliar water container and, when a case history is obtained before anesthesia, it is important to find out what type of container the animal is accustomed to using. In most circumstances, it is advisable to administer warmed (37°C or 98.6°F) subcutaneous or intraperitoneal dextrose/saline (4% dextrose, 0.15% saline) at the end of the operation to provide some fluid supplementation in the immediate postoperative period.

Postoperative analgesia is discussed on page 391.

ANESTHETIC EMERGENCIES

Respiratory Depression

Changes in the depth and pattern of respiration usually precede respiratory arrest. Careful monitoring of respiratory function will usually allow corrective measures to be taken before an emergency arises. If the animal has been intubated, respiration can be assisted by delivering 100% oxygen from the anesthetic machine with the vaporizer turned off or turned down. As with larger species, it is important to check that the endotracheal tube is properly positioned and has not become obstructed or disconnected from the breathing system. If the animal has not been intubated, respiration can be assisted by extending the head and neck and gently compressing the chest. Attempts to assist ventilation with a face mask are usually unsuccessful. Small rodents normally breathe through the nose and ventilation can be assisted using a small nasal mask. These can be purchased commercially or can be made from the flared end of a Foley urinary catheter. The mask can also be used to deliver anesthetic agents and oxygen using a Y-connector and a small T-piece. Intermittently occluding the end of the T-piece will inflate the lungs. Alternatively, the barrel of a syringe can be placed over the nose and respiration assisted by gently blowing down the barrel (Fig. 12.22). Respiration can also be stimulated by the administration of doxapram, but this drug has a relatively short duration of action (approximately 10 minutes) and repeated doses may be needed. Efforts should be made to determine the cause of the respiratory depression and to initiate corrective measures.

Circulatory Failure

Treatment of circulatory failure and cardiac arrest is similar to that in dogs and cats, but the small size of these animals causes some practical problems. Fluid therapy is difficult because of the small size of the superficial vessels, although it is possible to place over-the-needle catheters in the tail veins of rats and the medial tarsal veins of guinea pigs. In rabbits, IV access is much easier and catheters can be placed in the marginal ear veins or cephalic veins. The jugular vein is relatively mobile in the rabbit and is more difficult to locate and catheterize than in the dog and cat.

Loss of blood can be treated by transfusion from a donor animal. Fortunately, problems of incompatibility are rare on initial transfusion; however, it is likely to be more difficult to locate a suitable donor than when dealing with dogs and cats. As an alternative, a plasma volume expander such as a synthetic colloid can

TABLE 12.5 Dose Rates for Emergency Drugs With Typical Dilutions and Volumes Needed for an Adult Animal[a]

Drug	Concentration in Commercial Preparation	Dilution Instructions	Volume of Diluted Drug for a Typical Adult Animal
Doxapram	20 mg/mL	1 in 10 Not required	Mouse, 0.1 mL; hamster and gerbil, 0.25 mL, SC or IV Rat, 0.1 mL; guinea pig, 0.25 mL, SC or IV
Epinephrine	1 mg/mL	1 in 10	Mouse, 0.03 mL; hamster and gerbil, 0.1 mL; rat, 0.3 mL; guinea pig, 0.7 mL, IV or intracardiac
Lidocaine	20 mg/mL (2%)	1 in 10	Mouse, 0.03 mL; hamster and gerbil, 0.1 mL; rat, 0.3 mL, guinea pig, 0.7 mL, IV or intracardiac
Sodium bicarbonate	1 mEq/mL	Not required	Mouse, 0.03 mL; hamster and gerbil, 0.1 mL; rat, 0.3 mL; guinea pig, 0.7 mL, IV

[a]For rabbits, dose rates are similar to those for dogs and cats.
IV, Intravenous; *mEq,* milliequivalent; *SC,* subcutaneous.

be administered. All of the commonly available products can be administered safely to small mammals, providing that appropriate allowance is made for their smaller circulating volumes. In smaller species in which IV access is not practical, intraperitoneal or subcutaneous administration of warmed electrolyte solutions can slowly replace fluid deficits or blood loss but will be of minimal benefit if rapid hemorrhage is occurring. As discussed earlier, preventing problems by minimizing hemorrhage through meticulous surgical technique is important.

If cardiac arrest occurs, external cardiac massage and emergency drugs such as epinephrine can be used to try to resuscitate the animal (see Chapter 13). One significant problem is the practical difficulty of rapidly calculating drug dose rates when an emergency occurs. It is much simpler to utilize a list of dose rates and volumes, expressed as the dose volumes for a typical adult animal of each species. This will help avoid errors and speed therapy (Table 12.5).

ANALGESIA

As discussed in Chapter 8, the use of analgesics in veterinary practice is now standard practice. Although the vast majority of dogs and cats now receive perioperative analgesia, these drugs are often not used as frequently as they should be in small mammals. This is probably due to a number of factors including poor ability to recognize pain in these small animals and a lack of knowledge of the safety and efficacy of analgesic agents. However, it is critically important to provide postoperative analgesia to these patients because most small mammals will fail to eat or drink if they are experiencing postoperative pain.

Pain Assessment in Small Mammals

Pain assessment in dogs and cats is not always easy, but most veterinarians and veterinary technicians are relatively familiar with the normal behavior of these species. The normal behavior and general appearance of small rodents and rabbits are often less well appreciated, and as a result, the signs associated with pain may be overlooked. In addition, several species of small mammals are nocturnal and may not be active when observed during normal working hours. They may also remain immobile in the presence of an observer if they perceive them as a threat. It is therefore not always easy to use behavior and changes in

posture to assess pain. However, it is important to overcome these difficulties so that pain can be prevented or controlled effectively in these small animals.

As in dogs and cats, an initial assessment of the animal should be made without disturbing the animal. The animal's appearance and posture may be abnormal and it may appear hunched. Its coat may be unkempt and ruffled because of a lack of grooming and the presence of piloerection. Rats may have a blackish discharge around their eyes and nose because of a buildup of secretions from their Harderian glands. It is uncertain whether this buildup of material is due to reduced grooming or whether it is a response to stress, but it is a valuable indicator that the animal is not healthy and may be in pain. While it is being observed, the animal may demonstrate normal inquisitive behavior and explore its environment but, as mentioned earlier, if it remains motionless, this may be because it feels threatened rather than because it is in pain. If the animal has positioned itself in the back of its cage or pen or has hidden in bedding, this can also be a sign of fear but may also be due to pain.

When encouraged to move, the animal may have an abnormal gait or posture and may show uncharacteristic signs of aggression. Rats, mice, and gerbils will usually rear when investigating what has disturbed them, and the absence of this behavior may be due to pain. When handled, rather than attempting to evade capture, animals in pain may be apathetic or may be aggressive and bite the handler. When it is examined, the animal may respond to manipulation or palpation of a painful area by vocalizing or trying to bite. Confusingly, some small mammals such as guinea pigs will also vocalize loudly when not in pain and may respond to any manipulation by tensing their muscles and remaining immobile. Similar immobility can be seen in rabbits. Abdominal pain in rabbits, rats, and mice often produces characteristic behaviors involving contraction of the abdominal muscles, pressing of the abdomen to the floor and, in rabbits and rats, arching of the back. Rats, mice, and rabbits also show characteristic changes in facial expression when in pain. The most easily recognized is tightening of the skin around the orbit (Fig. 12.23). Although sedation can produce similar changes, assessment of facial expression provides a useful additional means of assessing pain in these species.

Rabbits and small mammals may stop eating and drinking when experiencing pain. This can be difficult to detect if food is

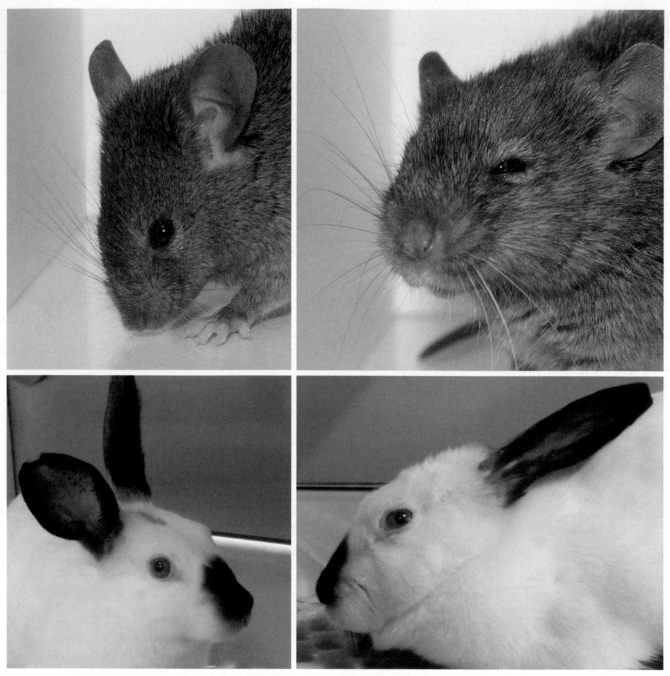

FIG. 12.23 Facial expression in a pain-free mouse *(top left)* and rabbit *(bottom left)*, and a mouse in pain *(top right)* and a rabbit in pain *(bottom right)*. The mouse "pain face" shows tightening of the skin of the orbit, bulging of the cheeks and nose, and flattening of the ears. The rabbit "pain face" shows tightening of the skin of the orbit, and the ears are rotated away from normal position to face towards the hindquarters and have a more tightly folded or curled shape. Contraction of the muscles around the muzzle produces a more angular contour, and the rounded appearance of the cheeks is lost. The nostrils are drawn vertically, giving a more pointed nose with a "V" rather than a "U" shape.

provided ad lib, but the subsequent loss in body weight can easily be monitored. This is one of the easiest ways of following a small mammal's progress after surgery or during treatment of any disease condition. The inappetence caused by pain is a serious problem in small mammals because failure to drink can rapidly lead to significant dehydration, and lack of food intake can predispose to the development of hypoglycemia in small rodents. In rabbits, guinea pigs, and chinchillas, disturbances in

food intake can lead to the development of life-threatening gastrointestinal disturbances.

As experience is gained in observing the normal behavior patterns of small mammals, abnormalities will be detected with greater confidence. Although relatively specific signs of pain such as guarding of an injured area may be seen, many of the signs are relatively nonspecific and can also occur in response to nonpainful conditions. It is therefore important to consider the appearance of the animal in relation to its case history and other clinical findings. Although it is highly desirable to try to assess pain in each individual patient so that appropriate analgesia therapy can be administered, it is not unreasonable to accept that some analgesic treatment will be needed after every surgical procedure.

Analgesic Agents

None of the analgesics that are currently marketed for use in dogs and cats provide any product information regarding use in small mammals. It is worth noting, however, that all of these products were originally tested for safety and efficacy in small rodents. This information provides reassurance that the drugs can be used safely to provide effective pain relief in these species. There is less information available on the use of analgesia in rabbits and guinea pigs, but extensive clinical experience indicates that most analgesics can be used safely in these animals. Suggested dose rates are listed in Table 12.6. The options for pain management are similar to those available in dogs and cats, but the small size of the animal may limit the use of techniques such as epidural administration of drugs or the use of fentanyl patches.

> **TECHNICIAN NOTE** Many opioids (e.g., morphine) have a shorter duration of action in small mammals than in other species. Buprenorphine, with a duration of action of 6–8 hr in small mammals, is preferred.

Opioids

All of the full opioid agonist drugs like morphine that can be used in dogs and cats can also be used in small mammals, but they often have a shorter duration of action in these species. Meperidine lasts for only 30 to 60 minutes in rodents, for example. Buprenorphine, which has a duration of action of approximately 6 to 8 hours in small mammals, is often

preferred. Some authorities question whether partial agonists such as buprenorphine are potent enough to control severe pain; however, clinical experience suggests that this analgesic is effective after most surgical procedures in small rodents and rabbits. Buprenorphine may cause behavioral abnormalities in small rodents (e.g., rats may eat sawdust bedding). However, this side effect appears rare and most animals appear to benefit from the use of buprenorphine after surgery. If other opioid analgesics are to be used, repeated administration is likely to be needed to provide effective pain relief. One useful way to avoid the need for frequent injections of drug is to combine administration of an opioid with the use of a nonsteroidal antiinflammatory drug (NSAID) (see the following section).

Nonsteroidal Antiinflammatory Drugs

NSAIDs (particularly the more potent NSAIDs such as carprofen and meloxicam) can provide very effective pain relief in small mammals. Considerable basic information is available from pharmaceutical companies concerning the safety and efficacy of these analgesics in small rodents. Although there have been no reports of adverse reactions to these drugs in small mammals, it seems advisable to adopt the same precautions as in dogs and cats (see Chapter 8). Prolonged use (more than a few days) should be avoided when possible, although clinical experience suggests that meloxicam can be used for extended periods in rabbits to control dental pain. Due to the risks of renal toxicity, if hypotension is present prior to or is expected to occur during anesthesia, only carprofen or meloxicam should be administered preoperatively. A significant advantage of the use of NSAIDs is that they appear to have a prolonged duration of action in small mammals. A single dose of carprofen or meloxicam may provide analgesia for 12 to 24 hours. Meloxicam has the additional advantage of being available in some countries as a palatable liquid preparation. This makes it easier for owners to continue administration if needed.

TABLE 12.6 Analgesic Agents for Use in Small Mammals[a]

Analgesic	Gerbil	Guinea Pig	Hamster	Mouse	Rabbit	Rat
Buprenorphine	0.1 mg/kg SC	0.05 mg/kg SC	0.1 mg/kg	0.1 mg/kg SC	0.01–0.05 mg/kg SC	0.05 mg/kg SC
Butorphanol	?	2 mg/kg	?	1–5 mg/kg SC	0.1–0.5 mg/kg SC	2 mg/kg SC
Carprofen	5 mg/kg SC	2.5 mg/kg SC daily	5 mg/kg SC	5 mg/kg bid SC or PO	1.5 mg/kg PO daily, 4 mg/kg SC daily	5 mg/kg bid SC or PO
Flunixin	?	?	?	2.5 mg/kg SC bid	1.1 mg/kg SC bid	2.5 mg/kg SC bid
Ketoprofen	?	?	?	?	3 mg/kg IM	5 mg/kg IM
Meloxicam	?	0.1–0.3 mg/kg SC or PO	?	5 mg/kg	0.6 mg/kg SC daily	1 mg/kg SC or PO daily
Meperidine (Pethidine)	?	10–20 mg/kg SC or IM q 2–3 hrs	?	10–20 mg/kg SC or IM q 2–3 hrs	10 mg/kg SC or IM q 2–3 hrs	10–20 mg/kg SC or IM q 2–3 hrs
Morphine	?	2–5 mg/kg SC or IM q 4 hrs	?	2.5 mg/kg SC or IM q 4 hrs	2–5 mg/kg SC or IM q 4 hrs	2.5 mg/kg SC or IM q 4 hrs

[a]Note that these are only suggestions based on clinical experience and the limited published data that are available. Dose rates should be adjusted depending on the clinical response of the animal. A "?" indicates that there is insufficient information to make a firm recommendation of an appropriate dose. Clinical experience suggests the doses used in rats and mice can be administered safely to other rodents.
BID, Twice daily; *IM,* intramuscular; *IV,* intravenous; *PO,* per os; *SC,* subcutaneous.
Data modified from Flecknell PA, Waterman-Pearson AE, editors: *Pain management in animals,* London, 2001, Harcourt International.

Local Anesthetics

Local anesthetics can be used to provide postoperative analgesia. As in dogs and cats, they can be infiltrated around surgical wounds or administered as specific nerve blocks. Although the safety of these agents in small mammals is similar to that in dogs and cats, it is relatively easy to overdose rodents inadvertently because of their small size. Care must be taken to calculate the dose accurately (maximum recommended doses in rodents: lidocaine 10 mg/kg, bupivacaine 4 mg/kg; maximum recommended dose in rabbits: same as for cats, see Chapter 7). Accurate dosing and effective infiltration of the surgical site are made easier if the agents are diluted with saline. It is also advantageous to use a mixture of lidocaine and bupivacaine because lidocaine has a more rapid onset of action and bupivacaine a longer delay before onset with a longer duration. Combining the two agents provides rapid onset and prolonged duration of action. Mixing one part 1% lidocaine, one part 0.5% bupivacaine, and three parts saline produces a solution that contains 2 mg/mL lidocaine and 1 mg/mL bupivacaine. These dilutions are effective at producing local anesthesia. Given that the toxic effects of these agents are additive, this mixture should be used at no more than 0.4 to 0.5 mL/100 g. It is important to note that the duration of action of some local anesthetics may be shorter in rodents than in larger species such as dogs and effective anesthesia may last less than 60 minutes with bupivacaine. Despite this, local anesthetics can provide an effective contribution to the alleviation of immediate postsurgical pain, and contribute to intraoperative analgesia as part of a balanced anesthetic regimen. As mentioned earlier, the application of topical agents such as EMLA cream provides analgesia for venipuncture or the placement of IV catheters.

Chronic Pain

Small mammals have a range of chronic conditions that can cause pain. Rats may have arthritis; guinea pigs, chinchillas, and rabbits may have dental disease; and neoplasia is common in many species. NSAIDs can often be used successfully to control the pain associated with these conditions, although it is necessary to monitor the patient carefully for side effects, especially during long-term use of these agents.

Administration of Analgesics

IV administration of analgesics is difficult in rodents but relatively straightforward in rabbits. Because of the small muscle mass of rodents, subcutaneous administration is preferred. Oral dosing can be difficult and may require firm physical restraint

that can exacerbate pain from surgical wounds. Provided the animal is eating, analgesics can be added to highly palatable food items (e.g., doughnuts for rats and mice). Analgesics for rats or mice can also be incorporated into fruit or gelatin-based food. Commercial flavored jello should be prepared with half the recommended quantity of water and after the mixture has been allowed to cool, a measured quantity of analgesic is added. After the jello has set, it can be cut into cubes of an appropriate weight. The remaining jello should be labeled and stored in a refrigerator, taking note of any legal requirements concerning storage of controlled drugs, and used within the next two days. Commercial gelatin mixed with beef extract may also be used, as may the commercial spread Nutella.

As in dogs and cats, preemptive administration of analgesics may provide more effective pain relief than postoperative use and may reduce the amount of anesthetic required for the surgical procedure. If volatile anesthetics are being used, opioids can be administered safely before the operation and the concentration of anesthetic delivered may be reduced as necessary to maintain a safe level of anesthesia. For example, when buprenorphine is administered preoperatively to rodents, the concentration of isoflurane needed to provide surgical anesthesia can be reduced by approximately 25% to 50%. If injectable agents are used, preemptive analgesia is more difficult because injectable anesthetics are often given as a single dose by the intraperitoneal or subcutaneous routes and cannot be titrated according to their effect in the individual animal. The commonly used opioids will potentiate the actions of injectable anesthetic agents and therefore their preoperative administration could lead to inadvertent anesthetic overdose. Because of the limited information available concerning the degree of interaction between injectable anesthetics and opioids in small rodents, it is safer in this case to administer opioid analgesics at the end of an operation, as the depth of anesthesia is becoming lighter.

Not all NSAIDs can be used safely preoperatively because of potential adverse effects such as renal hypotension and prolonged bleeding times. Carprofen and meloxicam apparently can both be safely used for preemptive analgesia.

Although the use of analgesic drugs remains the most important technique for reducing postoperative pain, pain medication must be integrated into the overall plan for perioperative care. Animals must be provided with a postoperative recovery area appropriate to their particular needs. For example, it is stressful for a small mammal to recover in the same room as its predators (e.g., cats), and the resulting change in their behavior pattern could mask signs of pain.

REVIEW QUESTIONS

1. Glycopyrrolate should be used instead of atropine in rabbits because:
   a. Atropine is highly toxic in rabbits
   b. Many rabbits have high levels of atropinase, so atropine is relatively ineffective
   c. Rabbits are unable to metabolize atropine
   d. Atropine causes marked bradycardia in rabbits

2. Pulse oximeters can be used in small mammals, but they may not be reliable because:
   a. The heart rate of the animal may exceed the upper range of the instrument
   b. The hemoglobin absorption characteristics are different in rodents from those in dogs and cats
   c. Pulse oximeters do not function on animals that have dark fur
   d. Small rodents have a rapid respiratory rate

3. The position of the eye cannot be used to assess the depth of anesthesia in rodents because:
   a. The eye is too small to assess its position accurately
   b. The position of the eye does not change during anesthesia
   c. The eye rotates downwards at very light planes of anesthesia
   d. The eyelids remain closed throughout anesthesia
4. An advantage of using dexmedetomidine combined with ketamine for anesthesia of rodents and rabbits is that:
   a. It is readily absorbed from body fat
   b. It can be given by mouth to produce anesthesia
   c. It promotes gut motility and so reduces the occurrence of postoperative inappetence
   d. It can be partially reversed using atipamezole, allowing faster recovery
5. An adult mouse weighing 40 g will have a blood volume of approximately:
   a. 10 mL
   b. 3 mL
   c. 50 mL
   d. 0.2 mL
6. When fluids such as lactated Ringer solution are given to small mammals, they should be:
   a. Used at about 4°C so that they are rapidly absorbed
   b. Administered orally because it is not possible to use any other route
   c. Warmed to body temperature before administration to avoid causing hypothermia
   d. Only given postoperatively to avoid overloading the circulation
7. Anesthetic breathing systems for use with small rabbits should:
   a. Only be constructed of plastic components because rabbits are allergic to latex
   b. Have low equipment dead space
   c. Have high equipment dead space
   d. Always include a soda lime canister to prevent rebreathing of CO_2

8. When small rodents are anesthetized with injectable anesthetics:
   a. It is not necessary to administer oxygen because most anesthetics stimulate respiration
   b. Oxygen should be administered because most anesthetics depress respiration
   c. A small amount of carbon dioxide should be included in the fresh gas mixture to stimulate respiration
   d. Nitrous oxide should always be used; otherwise the depth of anesthesia will be insufficient for surgery
9. Postoperative analgesia should be given to rodents and rabbits to alleviate pain, but:
   a. NSAIDs cannot be used because they cause gastric ulceration at normal therapeutic doses in these species
   b. Opioids (narcotics) cause severe respiratory depression and so must never be used
   c. Opioids must be given with care if a neuroleptanalgesic mixture has been used for anesthesia
   d. Local anesthetics cannot be used because they produce cardiac arrest even at low doses in these species
10. If postoperative pain is not alleviated in rabbits, then:
    a. Animals will not eat or drink normally
    b. Animals recover much faster from anesthesia
    c. Rabbits will spend a great deal of time grooming themselves
    d. Porphyrin staining will appear around their eyes

SELECTED READINGS

Flecknell PA: *Laboratory animal anesthesia*, ed 4, London, 2016, Elsevier.

Flecknell P: Analgesics in small mammals, *Vet Clin North Am Exot Anim Pract* 21(1):83–103, 2018.

Anesthetic Problems and Emergencies

LEARNING OBJECTIVES

When you have completed this chapter, you will be able to:

- List the most common reasons that anesthetic emergencies occur, including problems arising from increased patient risk, human error, equipment failure, and the adverse effects of anesthetic agents.
- Explain how anesthesia of pediatric and geriatric patients differs from anesthesia of healthy adult dogs and cats.
- Describe the problems involved in anesthetizing each of the following: obese animals; brachycephalic dogs; sighthounds; patients affected by trauma or cardiovascular, respiratory, hepatic, or renal disease; and patients undergoing a cesarean section.
- Describe the role of the veterinary technician or nurse in responding to anesthetic emergencies.

- List common causes of and responses to the following anesthetic problems: inadequate anesthetic depth, excessive anesthetic depth, pale mucous membranes, prolonged capillary refill time, and hypotension.
- List common causes of and responses to the following anesthetic problems: cyanosis and dyspnea, tachypnea, apnea, respiratory arrest, abnormalities in cardiac rate and rhythm, and cardiac arrest.
- Explain the principles of cardiopulmonary resuscitation as recommended in the RECOVER Guidelines, including basic life support and advanced life support.
- List the most common problems that may arise in the recovery period and the appropriate action that can be taken to prevent or treat these problems.

KEY TERMS

Advanced life support (ALS)
Agonal
Basic life support (BLS)
Brachycephalic obstructive airway
  syndrome (BOAS)
Cardiac pump theory
Functional residual volume

Manual resuscitator bag
Opisthotonus
Physiologic anemia
Pleural effusion
Pneumothorax
Postarrest care (PAC)
Pulmonary contusions

RECOVER Initiative
Return of spontaneous circulation
  (ROSC)
Sequestration
Stertor
Thoracic pump theory
Thoracocentesis

The authors and the publisher wish to acknowledge the contribution of K. Wayne Hollingshead, whose original work served as the foundation for this chapter.

General anesthesia poses relatively little risk to most patients when performed by capable personnel using an anesthetic protocol appropriate for the animal. Emergencies are uncommon and the overwhelming majority of patients recover from anesthesia with no lasting ill effects. Consequently, after successfully anesthetizing hundreds of patients, it is easy for the technician or nurse to become complacent. However, it is vitally important that the anesthetist remember that every anesthetic procedure has the potential to cause complications leading to temporary or permanent impairment or, in extreme cases, death of the patient. In fact, the incidence of complications is significant. For example, an American study of 3239 cases found the incidence of anesthetic complications to be 12% in dogs and 10.5% in cats.[a] Therefore the anesthetist must remain watchful for problems that may arise in even the most routine anesthetic procedure.

A number of scientific studies have been conducted over the past seven decades to determine rates of anesthetic deaths in veterinary patients. Although results of these studies vary, most reveal a death rate that is well under 1% for healthy animals and approximately 1% to 4% in animals with preexisting disease, with

a significant decrease in the anesthetic death rate over the past several decades and a slightly higher rate for cats than for dogs.[b]

For example, a study at Colorado State University in the 1950s reported an overall mortality rate of 1.08% in dogs and 1.79% in cats, whereas a study at the same institution almost 40 years later reported an overall rate of 0.43% in dogs and 0.35% in cats. From 2002 to 2004, a study of over 170,000 dogs and cats anesthetized in practices in the United Kingdom revealed an overall mortality rate of 0.17% in dogs and 0.24% in cats. The rates in healthy dogs and cats (ASA physical status 1 and 2 patients) in this study were 0.05% and 0.11%, respectively. In contrast, the rates in sick dogs and cats (ASA physical status 3, 4, and 5 patients) were 1.33% and 1.4%, respectively.

Most anesthetic deaths are due to complications involving the cardiovascular and respiratory systems, thus emphasizing the importance of monitoring these organ systems closely during any anesthetic event. A large proportion of deaths typically occur during anesthetic maintenance, but in many of the mortality studies, the highest number occurred during the postoperative period—a time during an anesthetic event when there is a tendency for anesthetists to let their guard down. This underscores the importance of remaining vigilant during this critical period.

---

[a]Gaynor JS, Dunlop CI, Wagner AE, et al: Complications and mortality associated with anesthesia in dogs and cats. *J Am Anim Hosp Assoc* 35(1):13–17, 1999.

[b]Brodbelt DC, Flaherty D, Pettifer GR: Anesthetic risk and informed consent. In Grimm KA, Lamont LA, Tranquilli WJ, et al: *Veterinary anesthesia and analgesia*, ed 5, Ames, IA, 2015, John Wiley and Sons, Inc, pp 11–22.

This chapter is divided into three parts. The first part describes reasons that anesthetic problems and emergencies arise and includes strategies to prevent them from occurring. In the second part, the challenges associated with the management of patients that have increased anesthetic risk (because of age, body conformation, breed-related issues, or because of preexisting conditions or the nature of the procedure being done) will be discussed. The focus of the third and final part is the causes of and responses to common problems and emergencies ranging from minor (such as maintaining appropriate anesthetic depth) to major (including respiratory arrest and cardiac arrest).

WHY ANESTHETIC PROBLEMS AND EMERGENCIES ARISE

Although an awareness of the correct response to anesthetic problems or emergencies is essential, it is just as important to understand why they arise and how they may be prevented. Most anesthetic problems and emergencies are caused by (1) human error, (2) equipment-related issues, (3) adverse effects of anesthetic agents, and (4) increased patient risk.

Human Error

Human error is a contributing cause of some anesthetic emergencies and deaths. This is partly because the complexity and risk inherent in the practice of anesthesia demand that the technician or nurse have an array of knowledge, skills, and behaviors, including command of a wide range of equipment, well-developed observational and decision-making skills, and constant vigilance. When working under these circumstances, even the best-prepared professional may make an error from time to time, especially when distracted, tired, or in a hurry. Human errors commonly encountered in veterinary practice typically involve:

- Inadequate training
- Lack of familiarity with the anesthetic machine or anesthetic agents
- Failure to adequately prepare the patient
- Drug calculation and administration errors
- Errors caused by fatigue, haste, or inattention

> **TECHNICIAN NOTE**
> Human error is one of the reasons for anesthetic emergencies. Human errors typically involve the following:
> - Inadequate training
> - Lack of familiarity with the anesthetic machine or anesthetic agents
> - Failure to adequately prepare the patient
> - Drug calculation and administration errors
> - Errors caused by fatigue, haste, or inattention

Inadequate Training

It is the responsibility of the veterinarian, and in some states or provinces a requirement of the veterinary association, to ensure that personnel are sufficiently trained and knowledgeable to competently perform all required procedures. Although unskilled personnel working under a veterinarian's direct supervision may assist with some aspects of an anesthetic procedure, skilled tasks, such as calculation and administration of anesthetics and monitoring of anesthetized patients, must be assigned only to personnel (veterinarians or technicians or nurses) who have sufficient training and knowledge, the experience to recognize abnormalities and danger signals, and the ability to respond appropriately.

Lack of Familiarity With the Anesthetic Machine or Anesthetic Agents

The practice of anesthesia is constantly changing as new technologies and anesthetic agents are introduced into the workplace. Consequently, the technician or nurse is constantly faced with the task of keeping up with advancements. Feeling a high level of comfort with a new piece of equipment or a new drug requires opportunities to use it in situations in which the technician or nurse has adequate time to devote their full attention to the mastery of its use. A failure to do this can result in drug under- or overdoses, or complications related to malfunction or incorrect use of equipment. Reading owner's manuals for new equipment and package inserts for new drugs, taking the time to attend in-house training sessions, and acquiring experience under the guidance of someone who is experienced are ways to help develop this comfort level so that the patient can be cared for in a safe and effective manner.

Failure to Adequately Prepare the Patient

Every patient scheduled for anesthesia should have a complete physical examination and a thorough history should be obtained. In practice, this does not always happen. Animals are sometimes dropped off at the veterinary clinic by owners who are in a hurry and reluctant to stop and answer questions. Animals may be brought in by neighbors or friends of the owner, or by other persons unfamiliar with the animal's history. The receptionist or other person admitting the animal to the hospital may fail to ask important questions or may not transmit the information to the anesthetist or veterinarian. The physical examination is sometimes cursory or omitted entirely. The net result is that significant information may be overlooked. For example, the anesthetist may be unaware that a patient has not been fasted or that an animal scheduled for surgery is dehydrated as a result of vomiting and diarrhea. An anesthetic protocol that is safe for a healthy patient may be inappropriate for such a patient and consequently, an anesthetic complication or even death of the patient could result. It is the technician's or nurse's responsibility to ensure that these important aspects of patient preparation are addressed. (See Chapter 2 for a detailed discussion of patient preparation.)

Drug Calculation and Administration Errors

Many anesthetic agents have a narrow margin of safety. Thus dosage calculation or administration errors may have serious or even fatal consequences and may arise from any of the following:

- Failure to weigh the patient and calculate an accurate dose.
- Mathematical errors (particularly decimal errors, which can result in an error of 10 times or even 100 times in the amount of drug given).
- Use of the wrong medication (e.g., calculating a dose of atropine and drawing up acepromazine instead).

- Use of the wrong concentration of a medication. This is a common problem with drugs that are available in different concentrations (e.g., atropine, xylazine, and dexmedetomidine). Obviously, the concentration used in calculating the dose must be the same as that drawn up into the syringe for the amount administered to be correct.
- Administration of anesthetics by the incorrect route (e.g., administration of an IM dose of ketamine by the intravenous [IV] route).
- Confusion between syringes drawn up for two different patients. This involves either a failure to label the syringes or a failure to read the labels correctly.

Errors Caused by Fatigue, Haste, or Inattention

The veterinary technician or nurse anesthetist may be called on to restrain patients for examination or procedures, answer the phone, perform diagnostic tests, discharge animals, clean soiled cages, and carry out other similar tasks. This can lead to a feeling of being pressured and fatigued, especially at the end of a busy day. A technician or nurse who is feeling rushed or tired is more likely to make mistakes, such as perivascular injection of an IV drug or inserting an endotracheal tube (ETT) into the esophagus. Awareness of one's feelings and mood is important so that action can be taken to prevent such mistakes, such as requesting help or taking a break when appropriate.

Inattention may also cause the technician or nurse to make mistakes or may lead to complications due to a failure to recognize danger signals. It is obviously better for the patient—and prudent for the anesthetist—to detect and address anesthetic problems early rather than late. For example, when anesthetic depth is excessive, an animal may show a warning sign, such as a gradually decreasing blood pressure or respiratory rate, at which point the anesthetist should respond to bring the patient back into an appropriate plane. Therefore a high level of vigilance is needed at all times to ensure that the patient is not in trouble. A brief check of the vital signs and physical indicators of depth typically takes less than 1 minute and can prevent such errors.

Equipment-Related Issues

Anesthetic machines, monitors, and associated equipment are complex and require regular maintenance. Working with this equipment requires attention to detail during setup, operation, and maintenance. Failure to use equipment correctly can and often does lead to mild to serious complications; for instance, failure to open the adjustable pressure limiting (APL) valve after checking the machine for leaks, failure to check the oxygen supply, failure to refill an empty vaporizer, or failure to reattach the keyed fitting to the outlet port of the vaporizer after using a nonrebreathing system. Thus the importance of a preanesthetic check of the anesthetic machine, as described in Chapter 4, cannot be overemphasized. These and other equipment-related issues are discussed in the next section.

Misassembly of the Anesthetic Machine

Misassembly of the anesthetic machine is an error that usually results from inattention when preparing a machine for use but is more likely when using a machine that the anesthetist is not familiar with. To prevent misassembly, it is essential that the person handling the anesthetic machine be familiar with every connection, hose, dial, and component. Before using an unfamiliar machine, the anesthetist should take a few minutes to examine it carefully for the location of the controls and to understand the direction and path of gas flow within the machine. Every time a connection, such as a Bain circuit, is added or removed, the anesthetist must trace the flow of gas, ensuring that the correct pattern of flow is maintained and that all connections are secure. After assembling a machine, a low-pressure leak test should be performed on the machine. This will reveal any errors in assembly. Failure to do so can result in the patient not receiving oxygen and anesthetic gases, or rebreathing expired carbon dioxide (CO_2).

> **TECHNICIAN NOTE**
> After assembling a machine, a low-pressure leak test should be performed. This will reveal any errors in assembly. Failure to do so can result in the patient not receiving oxygen and anesthetic gases, or rebreathing expired CO_2.

CO_2 Absorbent Exhaustion

Patients on a rebreathing system rely on the CO_2 absorbent to remove expired CO_2 from the circuit, preventing inhalation of excessive levels of this toxic gas. If CO_2 is not removed from the circuit due to exhaustion of the absorbent, the patient will experience hypercapnia (elevated blood CO_2). This problem usually results from a failure to change the absorbent on a regular basis (e.g., after 6 to 8 hours of use; after 30 days; or when the granules change color—whichever comes first). Signs of hypercapnia resulting from exhausted absorbent include tachypnea (rapid respiratory rate), tachycardia, cardiac arrhythmias, and increased baseline and $ETco_2$ levels on a capnograph tracing. If this complication is suspected, the patient should be placed on an alternative anesthetic machine until the problem can be corrected. If an alternative machine is not available, the oxygen flow rate may be increased to a level that approximates the patient's respiratory minute volume (200 mL/kg/min) or, if this is not possible, the patient should be permitted to breathe room air until the absorbent can be changed. To prevent this problem, the date that the absorbent was last changed should be written on a label or piece of tape affixed to the canister, the number of hours that the absorbent has been in use should be logged on a card attached to the machine, and the absorbent should be checked for color change at the end of every procedure.

> **TECHNICIAN NOTE**
> To prevent CO_2 absorbent exhaustion:
> - Write the date that the absorbent was last changed on a label or piece of tape affixed to the canister and change absorbent at least every 30 days.
> - Log the number of hours that the absorbent has been in use on a card attached to the machine and replace it after 6–8 h of use.
> - Check the absorbent for color change at the end of every procedure and replace it when no more than 33%–50% has changed color.

Failure of the Oxygen Supply

Failure to deliver oxygen to the patient is one of the most serious and yet one of the most easily preventable mistakes that an anesthetist can make. This error results from a failure to turn the tank or the flowmeter on, or a failure to change an empty tank. Before starting an anesthetic procedure, the anesthetist must ensure that the primary oxygen supply contains sufficient oxygen for the duration of the surgery. A secondary supply (usually a size E compressed gas cylinder) should be attached to the machine and checked to make sure that it is full and in working order. (For information on calculating the amount of oxygen present in a tank, refer to Chapter 4, page 126.) During the procedure, the oxygen tank pressure should be checked frequently and the flowmeter should be checked every 5 minutes. The anesthetist must ensure that either oxygen or room air is continuously provided to the patient. At the end of a procedure, the patient should be disconnected from the machine before the oxygen flow meter is turned off.

It is important to be able to recognize when the machine is no longer delivering oxygen to the patient. If the oxygen flow meter reads zero, the patient is not receiving any oxygen, regardless of the oxygen tank pressure. Occasionally, when the oxygen tank is nearly empty, the oxygen tank pressure gauge may read zero, but the flow meter may indicate that some oxygen is still being delivered. In this situation, even though the tank still contains a small amount of oxygen, loss of oxygen pressure is imminent and the tank must be changed immediately.

The anesthetist must be aware of the proper response when oxygen delivery to the patient is stopped, whether because of machine malfunction or an empty tank. If the oxygen flow stops (i.e., the flow meter reads zero despite the efforts of the anesthetist to establish flow), the anesthetist should immediately disconnect the hoses from the ETT, which allows the patient to breathe room air until oxygen delivery can be reestablished. It is important for the anesthetist to understand that having oxygen flowing is even more critical when a patient is connected to a nonrebreathing anesthetic circuit, as cessation of oxygen flow immediately halts the flow of fresh gas to the patient. As the fresh gas flow is responsible for moving exhaled CO_2 away from the patient, the absence of oxygen flowing will result in immediate hypercarbia and hypoxemia, which will lead to patient death within minutes if not addressed by disconnecting the patient from the breathing system or restoring oxygen flow. For comparison, when oxygen stops flowing when a patient is connected to a rebreathing anesthetic circuit, there is some oxygen still available for a few minutes from the reservoir bag and, assuming the circuit and absorber granules are functioning correctly, the one-way movement of gases will prevent CO_2 buildup near the patient from occurring in those few minutes. Once the reservoir bag is empty (i.e., the bag is flat), hypercarbia and hypoxemia will occur, making identification and correction of the lack of oxygen flow critical.

> **TECHNICIAN NOTE**
> To prevent failure of oxygen delivery:
> - Be sure that the primary tank has sufficient oxygen and that a full secondary tank is available.
> - Be sure the oxygen tank and flowmeter are turned on.
> - Check the oxygen supply frequently and the flowmeter every 5 min during any anesthetic procedure.

Endotracheal Tube Problems

ETTs are a critical component of the anesthetic delivery system and are subject to many problems. ETTs may become blocked during anesthesia, cutting off the flow of anesthetic vapor and oxygen to the patient. Blockages may be the result of twisting or kinking of the tube; accumulation of material such as blood, mucus, or saliva within the tube; or inappropriate positioning of the tube (as may occur when the neck is flexed). The ETT should be premeasured from the incisor teeth to the mid-neck and advanced no further than the position of the carina. If the tube is accidentally advanced into a bronchus, the patient may become hypoxic and hypercapnic and may be difficult to keep asleep as only one lung will receive anesthetic gas and oxygen.

ETT blockage (if complete) results in a cessation of oxygen flow to the patient and retention of CO_2. The patient may become dyspneic and may develop cardiac arrhythmias. Eventually, if the problem is not identified and resolved, respiratory arrest will occur. The anesthetist usually becomes aware of ETT blockage by observing an exaggerated breathing pattern or by noting that the reservoir bag no longer inflates and deflates with the patient's respirations. If a problem is suspected, the anesthetist should quickly check the ETT function in two ways:

1. Attempt to bag the patient and observe if the chest rises. If the ETT is blocked, no chest movement will be seen and there will be considerable resistance to the passage of air into the patient.
2. If capnometry is being used, examine the capnogram while attempting to deliver a breath to the patient. If no waveform or a truncated waveform (shark fin appearance) is detected, then complete or partial blockage may be present. In this case, the tube should be removed and another ETT or mask used to deliver oxygen to the patient. If blood, mucus, or similar material is causing the obstruction, suction with a 20-mL syringe and a feeding tube cut to the length of the ETT may be helpful.

> **TECHNICIAN NOTE**
> To prevent ETT blockage:
> - Premeasure the tube prior to placement to ensure it is an appropriate length.
> - Prior to intubation, check the tube for damage, kinks, and blockage with dried mucus or other foreign material.
> - After intubating and positioning the patient, check to be sure the tube is not twisted or kinked.
> - Frequently check that the tube is patent (by watching for movement of the bag and/or unidirectional valves). Accumulation of material such as blood, mucus, or saliva within the tube can block the tube.
> - Frequently check that the neck is not excessively flexed.

Vaporizer Problems

Each vaporizer is designed for a specific agent. A potentially disastrous problem can arise if the wrong anesthetic is put into a vaporizer. Each anesthetic liquid has its own vapor pressure (the amount of anesthetic that vaporizes at 20°C), and anesthetic vaporizers are calibrated on the basis of a particular anesthetic with a unique vapor pressure being used in the vaporizer. If an anesthetic is put into the incorrect vaporizer, it is possible that a higher or lower concentration than that indicated on the dial will be delivered because the anesthetic has a different vapor pressure than the anesthetic for which the vaporizer was designed. This leads to the patient's anesthetic depth becoming unexpectedly deep or light. Other problems involving vaporizers are as follows:

- Vaporizers should not be overfilled. If too much anesthetic is put into the vaporizer, it should be drained until the fluid level is at or below the indicator line and checked for proper output.
- Vaporizers should not be tipped. Tipping may lead to leakage of anesthetic into the oxygen bypass channel, resulting in higher concentrations of anesthetic reaching the patient and therefore potential overdose. Any machine that is tipped should be removed from service until it can be checked for proper operation.
- Occasionally, a vaporizer dial may stick or become jammed. If the dial cannot be adjusted, the patient should be transferred to another machine.
- Anesthetic machines equipped with two or more vaporizers in a series should be monitored carefully to ensure that both vaporizers are not turned on at the same time.

TECHNICIAN NOTE
- Never overfill or tip a vaporizer.
- If using two or more vaporizers in series, use only one at a time.
- Anesthetic vaporizers should be serviced regularly.

Adjustable Pressure Limiting Valve Problems

Occasionally, an anesthetist inadvertently leaves the APL valve in a closed position when using partial rebreathing flow rates with a rebreathing system or when using a nonrebreathing system. In this situation, pressure within the breathing circuit will rapidly rise. This is because the oxygen flow rate used with these systems is greater than the patient's oxygen requirement. This can also happen when using full rebreathing flow rates with a rebreathing system in the event that the oxygen flow rate has inadvertently been set higher than the metabolic oxygen consumption (approximately 5 to 10 mL/kg/min). In either situation, as pressure rises in the circuit, the reservoir bag will expand, as will the patient's lungs. This prevents exhalation and also decreases the venous return to the heart. This in turn decreases cardiac output, causes blood pressure to fall rapidly, and will lead to death within a short time unless recognized and corrected. If left unrecognized, pneumothorax and pneumomediastinum can also occur as intrathoracic pressure increases.

To detect the problem at an early stage, the anesthetist should adjust the APL valve immediately after performing a low-pressure system leak test at the beginning of the day, and should frequently monitor the reservoir bag size during each procedure and attempt to maintain it at no more than two-thirds full of gas at the end of a patient expiration. Additionally, the pressure gauge should always read less than 5 cm H_2O during spontaneous breathing. The reservoir bag size is controlled

by changing the oxygen flow rate or by opening and closing the APL valve.

TECHNICIAN NOTE
If the APL valve is closed and the oxygen flow rate is greater than the patient's oxygen requirement, pressure within the circuit and the patient's lungs and thoracic cavity will rapidly rise. This prevents exhalation and decreases venous return to the heart, which decreases cardiac output and will lead to death within a short time unless recognized and corrected immediately.

Adverse Effects of Anesthetic Agents

As discussed in Chapter 3, each anesthetic agent and adjunct has the potential to harm a patient and, in some cases, cause death. Several strategies are used to reduce this potential:

- The anesthetic protocol must be chosen to reflect the specific needs of the patient. For example, acepromazine is a poor preanesthetic for patients with low blood pressure because this agent may cause vasodilation, further decreasing the blood pressure. Alpha$_2$-agonists such as dexmedetomidine may cause dangerous cardiovascular or respiratory depression in patients with disease of these body systems. Animals that are fearful or excited may have increased levels of epinephrine circulating throughout their bodies. In these patients, mask or chamber induction may precipitate severe hypotension and cardiac arrhythmias. In each case, the veterinarian might choose to use an alternative agent.
- The anesthetist must be familiar with the side effects and contraindications associated with each of the preanesthetic and general anesthetic agents used in the hospital. For example, the anesthetist who administers an alpha$_2$-agonist should be aware of its potential to cause bradycardia, cardiac arrhythmias, vomiting, bloating, and respiratory depression.
- Multidrug use to achieve balanced anesthesia can be safer than anesthesia with a single drug provided that the doses of the individual drugs are appropriately reduced. For example, the concentration of isoflurane needed to anesthetize an animal is significantly reduced if the animal is premedicated with dexmedetomidine and butorphanol compared with an animal that is not premedicated. If the same isoflurane concentration were used in both situations, the patient could be at risk for anesthetic gas overdose.

A detailed description of the pharmacology and physiologic effects of preanesthetic and general anesthetic agents is given in Chapter 3.

ANESTHESIA OF HIGH-RISK PATIENTS

Patients at higher risk for complications include neonates and geriatric animals, brachycephalic dogs, sighthounds, and obese animals. Cesarean delivery of puppies or kittens also places unique demands on the anesthetist because the response of both the dam and the offspring to anesthetic agents must be considered. Animals that have experienced recent trauma may be presented for emergency surgery, and the anesthetist must be prepared to deal with shock, respiratory difficulties, cardiac arrhythmias, and other serious challenges in these patients. Animals with cardiac problems such as heartworm disease or congestive heart failure may require anesthesia for diagnostic or therapeutic procedures. Similarly, animals may require anesthesia despite the presence of hepatic or renal disease. Although a detailed discussion of the anesthetic challenges posed by these and other factors is beyond the scope of this text, it is desirable that the technician or nurse be familiar with some of the special considerations when anesthetizing these animals. These are summarized in Table 13.1.

Neonatal and Pediatric Patients

The neonatal and pediatric periods in the small animal patient encompass the first 6 weeks and 12 weeks (3 months) of life,

TABLE 13.1	Patient Factors That Increase Anesthetic Risk	
Patient Factor	**Anesthetic Problems Encountered**	**Strategies Used to Decrease Risk**
Pediatric patients	• Increased risk of hypothermia, dehydration, overhydration, hypoxemia, hypotension, hypoventilation, and hypoglycemia • Inefficient metabolism and excretion of drugs • Difficult intubation and IV catheterization	• Minimize heat loss • Avoid prolonged fasting and do not withhold water • Consider IV 5% dextrose in isotonic crystalloids using an infusion pump or volume control chamber • Weigh the patient accurately and dilute injectable drugs if necessary • Reduce anesthetic doses • Inhalant agents preferred to injectable agents • Minimize dead space
Geriatric patients	• Reduced organ function • Poor response to stress • Serious illness not uncommon • Increased susceptibility to hypothermia, hypotension, respiratory depression, and overhydration	• Carefully assess and stabilize the patient prior to procedure • Use premedications to minimize adverse effects of general anesthetics • Reduce anesthetic doses by 30%–50% • Allow longer time for response to drugs • Administer fluids at reduced rate • Keep patient warm
Obese animals	• Accurate dosing difficult • May have respiratory difficulties • May exhibit rapid, shallow respirations	• Determine dose according to ideal weigh • Preoxygenate • Induce rapidly • Assist ventilation if necessary • Delay extubation • Observe closely in recovery period
Brachycephalic dogs	• Conformational tendency toward airway obstruction • Abnormally high parasympathetic tone • Small trachea in comparison with physical body size	• Include anticholinergic in anesthetic protocol • Preoxygenate • Rapid induction using IV agents • Place endotracheal tube (ETT) quickly and efficiently; may need a smaller diameter tube • Delay extubation • Observe closely during recovery period
Sighthounds	• Increased sensitivity to barbiturates	• Use alternative agent
Cardiovascular disease	• Circulation is compromised • Pulmonary edema common • Increased tendency to develop arrhythmias, tachycardia, and overhydration	• Identify specific disease process through careful patient assessment and stabilize as needed • Minimize stress and restrain gently • Customize anesthetic protocol for each patient • Monitor carefully for changes in cardiopulmonary function • Preoxygenate for 5 min before induction • Avoid agents that depress myocardial contractility, increase cardiac work, or cause arrhythmias • Avoid overhydration • Titrate drug dosages
Respiratory disease	• Poor oxygenation of tissues • Patient may be anxious and difficult to restrain	• Stabilize prior to induction • Preoxygenate but avoid stress and unnecessary handling • Induce with injectable agents • Intubate rapidly and control ventilation if necessary • Be prepared to perform tracheostomy • Check airway frequently and avoid compressing chest • Monitor Spo_2 and end-tidal CO_2 • Monitor closely during recovery
Hepatic disease	• Delayed metabolism of anesthetic agents • Decreased synthesis of blood clotting factors • May be hypoproteinemic • Dehydration common; may be anemic and/or icteric	• Base protocol on results of preanesthetic blood work and other tests • May reduce dosages of, or omit preanesthetic medication • Inhalation agents preferred over injectable agents • Expect prolonged recovery • Reversible agents are preferred

TABLE 13.1 **Patient Factors That Increase Anesthetic Risk—cont'd**

Patient Factor	Anesthetic Problems Encountered	Strategies Used to Decrease Risk
Renal disease	• Electrolyte imbalances common, including hyperkalemia and metabolic acidosis • Dehydration usually present • Delayed excretion of anesthetic agents	• Withhold water for 1 h or less • Rehydrate before surgery • Obtain renal function test results and electrolyte values, and address abnormalities • Administer intraoperative IV fluids at appropriate rates • Reduce doses of anesthetic agents • Monitor blood pressure and manage hypotension promptly
Cesarean section	Dam: • Increased workload to heart • Respiration may be compromised • Increased risk of vomiting or regurgitation • Increased risk of hypotension and hemorrhage Offspring: • Anesthetic agents cross placenta and may reduce respiratory and cardiovascular function • Hypoxemia and hypercapnia secondary to respiratory depression	Dam: • Administer IV fluids • Clip, prep, and establish IV access before induction • Preoxygenate • Use lowest effective dose of general anesthetic • Induce IV and intubate quickly • Consider epidural analgesia combined with neuroleptanalgesia • Monitor for vomiting during recovery Offspring: • Clear airway with bulb syringe • Use reversal agents under the tongue to stimulate breathing • Administer oxygen by face mask • Administer atropine for bradycardia
Trauma patients	• Respiratory distress common • Cardiac arrhythmias common for 72 h after incident • Shock and hemorrhage common • Internal injuries often present	• Thorough physical examination necessary to check for concurrent injuries • Obtain thoracic radiographs and electrocardiogram • Stabilize before anesthesia • Preoxygenate

respectively. Small animals during the neonatal and pediatric periods are generally considered to be at increased risk when anesthetized compared with mature animals. Therefore when working with these patients, the anesthetist must be aware of special considerations during the preanesthetic, anesthetic, and recovery periods.

Factors That Put Neonatal and Pediatric Patients at Increased Risk

Compared with adult animals, neonatal and pediatric patients are less able to respond to physiological stresses, such as changes in fluid balance and blood glucose level. Liver function is not fully mature in these patients, resulting in decreased metabolism and excretion of many drugs. Kidney function is also not fully developed in these patients, and the ability to alter the body's fluid balance by increasing or decreasing urine output in the face of over- or underhydration is limited. In addition, immaturity of the cardiovascular and respiratory systems makes these patients more susceptible to adverse effects associated with anesthesia such as bradycardia, hypotension, hypoventilation, and hypoxemia. Their small body size predisposes these patients to hypothermia, fluid loss, and drug overdose, and their higher metabolic rate increases oxygen needs when compared with larger patients. These susceptibilities to anesthetic complications necessitate changes in the way these patients are managed.

Management of Fluid and Blood Glucose Balance

Hypoglycemia and dehydration may occur in pediatric patients after even a short period of fasting. Consequently, water should not

be withheld from these patients preoperatively, and patients under 8 weeks old should be fasted for ≤1 to 2 hours or sometimes not at all. To prevent hypoglycemia during surgery, isotonic crystalloid solutions with 5% dextrose added can be used in place of plain isotonic crystalloids such as normal saline, lactated Ringer, or Normosol M. This can be formulated by removing 100 mL of fluid from a 1-L bag of fluids and adding an equivalent volume of 50% dextrose. Alternatively, blood glucose can be measured every 30 to 60 minutes and the administered fluid type changed accordingly.

Fluid administration must be sufficient to maintain hydration because these patients have a decreased ability to respond to fluid deficits; but should not exceed recommended rates (see Chapter 2 for a discussion of these rates) unless shock or dehydration is present because these animals are prone to overhydration if fluid administration is rapid. Consequently, it is important to calculate and monitor fluid administration rates carefully. Ideally, a fluid infusion pump or syringe pump should be used to ensure that fluids are given to these patients at an appropriate rate. In the event that neither is available, the use of a microdrip administration set with a delivery rate of 60 drops/mL is essential in these patients, and a *burette (see Fig. 2.7)* is helpful in preventing inadvertent excessive fluid administration.

Drug Protocols for Neonatal and Pediatric Patients

A variety of injectable drugs including opioids, benzodiazepines, anticholinergics, propofol, and alfaxalone can be used for premedication and anesthetic induction of pediatric patients as long as care is taken to ensure accurate dosing and appropriate use. What follows is a list of precautions that apply to the use of injectable agents:

- For the calculation of drug doses, an accurate weight must be obtained because small inaccuracies will result in significant dosing errors in small patients. For animals weighing less than 5 kg, a pediatric or gram scale is more accurate than a conventional scale and should be used.
- Some injectable agents may require dilution because otherwise, the dose may be too small to measure or administer accurately.
- The dose of injectable anesthetics given to pediatric animals is often one-half to two-thirds of the dose given to mature animals because very young animals have less plasma protein binding of drugs and lack an efficient mechanism to metabolize drugs within the liver. Thus injectable anesthetic agents that have high protein binding (e.g., propofol, ketamine, and etomidate) may have an exaggerated effect, and agents that are metabolized by the liver (e.g., benzodiazepines and opioids) or excreted by the kidneys (e.g., ketamine in the cat) may have a prolonged effect in puppies or kittens less than 8 weeks of age and must be used with care. When selecting agents, preference should be given to reversible drugs.

> **TECHNICIAN NOTE**
> For the calculation of drug doses, an accurate weight must be obtained because small inaccuracies will result in significant dosing errors in small patients. For animals weighing less than 5 kg, a pediatric or gram scale is more accurate than a conventional scale and should be used.

Inhalant agents are commonly used in these patients for both anesthetic induction and maintenance because these drugs are absorbed and eliminated via the respiratory tract and patient recovery tends to be rapid. Inhalants are also easier to administer in some cases because they do not require venous access. It is important to be aware, however, that mask and chamber induction have been shown to be associated with higher mortality rates when compared with injectable drugs, so great care must be taken if these techniques are used. Also, the vaporizer setting must be minimized and the patient closely monitored to avoid the hypotension, hypoventilation, and hypothermia that often accompany the use of these agents.

Other Considerations in Pediatric and Neonatal Patients

Pediatric patients are more at risk for hypothermia, hypotension, and hypoxemia than adult animals because of anatomic and physiologic differences associated with their small body size, such as their proportionally large body surface area. The small body size also makes certain anesthetic procedures such as intubation and IV catheterization more challenging in pediatric patients. The larynx may be difficult to see and the use of a laryngoscope may be required. To minimize dead space and the resulting hypoxemia, it is often necessary to shorten an ETT to an appropriate length by (1) measuring the distance between the nose and the thoracic inlet, (2) removing the ETT connector, (3) cutting the patient end to length, and (4) reattaching the connector to the cut end to avoid bronchial intubation.

Apart from obvious differences in size, the monitoring of pediatric patients is similar to that of adults, although monitoring parameters may have different normal values. For instance, pediatric and neonatal patients tend to have higher heart rates and respiratory rates and slightly lower blood pressure than adult animals. The anesthetist should be particularly watchful for bradycardia, which is associated with poor cardiac output in anesthetized animals under 4 weeks of age because neonates depend much more on heart rate than contractility to maintain cardiac output. Alpha$_2$-agonists may cause significant bradycardia and should be avoided in these patients. Anticholinergics may be helpful in preventing and treating low heart rates when given during the preoperative and intraoperative periods, respectively. Pediatric patients are prone to hypothermia because of their lack of subcutaneous fat, their relatively large body surface area, their reduced ability to shiver, and immature thermoregulatory responses. Particular care should be taken to avoid heat loss during surgery. This is accomplished through the use of circulating warm water blankets or forced air warming blankets such as the Bair Hugger Animal Health Blanket by 3M. It is also essential to make sure that all air is removed from IV lines to avoid the risk of air embolism.

> **TECHNICIAN NOTE**
> Pediatric animals are more prone to dehydration or overhydration, hypoglycemia, hypothermia, hypotension, and hypoxemia than are adult animals.

Geriatric Patients

A geriatric patient is one that has reached 75% of the average life expectancy for that species and breed. Aging is associated with a number of important physiologic changes that put geriatric patients at increased risk during general anesthesia. Therefore the anesthetist must make alterations in anesthetic management to minimize the effects of these changes.

Factors That Put Geriatric Patients at Increased Risk

In geriatric patients, the function of critical organs such as the heart, lungs, kidneys, and liver is often reduced in comparison with the healthy, young adult patient. Geriatric animals have less functional reserve than do younger animals and a relatively poor response to stress. Consequently, they are often less able to maintain an adequate state of hydration than younger patients and are less able to tolerate hypotension. In addition, geriatric animals are more likely to be afflicted with serious disorders such as diabetes mellitus, congestive heart failure, and chronic renal disease, all of which change the way they respond to anesthetic drugs. Because of these factors, including the high incidence of health problems in these animals, acquisition of a thorough history, careful physical assessment, diagnostic testing, and patient stabilization are even more important than for nongeriatric patients.

Geriatric animals typically have reduced anesthetic requirements. Consequently, doses of anesthetic agents are typically decreased by one-quarter to one-half when compared with doses for healthy young patients, although some patients may require even less. Response to drugs can be slower; consequently, the technician or nurse should allow more time for IV injections to take effect, and recovery from anesthesia may be prolonged partly because of decreased renal and hepatic function (and hence decreased ability to excrete drugs). Geriatric patients also have a tendency to develop hypothermia because they have a reduced ability to regulate body temperature.

Drug Protocols for Geriatric Patients

Changes in organ function and physiology typical with aging make geriatric patients more susceptible to adverse effects caused by general anesthetics, such as hypotension and respiratory depression. Therefore steps should be taken to reduce the amount of general anesthetic needed to produce the desired effects. One of the best ways of doing this is to provide effective sedation and analgesia prior to anesthetic induction. This reduces anxiety, stress, and most importantly, the amount of anesthetic required to induce as well as to maintain anesthesia. Use of local and regional anesthetic techniques such as nerve blocks and epidural anesthesia (see Chapter 7) will also help to minimize the amount of general anesthetic needed.

For geriatric patients, the short-acting agents propofol and alfaxalone are generally good choices for anesthetic induction, as are ketamine and midazolam or ketamine and diazepam mixtures given intravenously, and etomidate is a good choice for induction of patients with moderate to severe cardiovascular disease. Mask induction with isoflurane or sevoflurane is not recommended routinely owing to the increased risk of mortality when using this method but, if used, should be preceded by premedication and accompanied by vigilant anesthetic monitoring. Inhalant agents are often used for anesthetic maintenance, however, because the anesthetic depth can be changed relatively rapidly when the need arises.

> **TECHNICIAN NOTE**
> Geriatric animals often have lower anesthetic requirements, decreased ability to respond to stress, longer recoveries, less tolerance for hypotension and overhydration, and decreased organ function when compared with younger adult animals.

Other Considerations in Geriatric Patients

The use of IV fluids during general anesthesia is generally advocated in geriatric patients because they have less tolerance to hypotension and often have reduced kidney function. Geriatric animals are, however, also at increased risk for developing overhydration, so IV fluids should be given with care. Owing to the increased tendency to become hypothermic compared with younger adult animals, steps should be taken to conserve body heat by using techniques similar to those used in pediatric patients.

Obese Animals

According to the Association for Pet Obesity Prevention (http://www.petobesityprevention.org), in 2018, over 50% of cats and dogs in the United States were either overweight or obese. Overweight and obese patients have a higher percentage of body fat than patients of normal body weight. Because

the blood supply to fat is relatively poor, anesthetics are not efficiently distributed to fat stores. Obese patients therefore require lower doses of drugs on a per kilogram basis than do nonobese patients. It is advisable to decrease the dose of preanesthetic and anesthetic agents so that the dose is determined according to a weight halfway between the normal breed weight and the actual weight.

Obese animals also may have some degree of respiratory difficulty, further complicating the anesthetic process. Dogs and cats that show respiratory difficulties should receive oxygen by face mask for 5 minutes before induction. They may also require the use of induction techniques similar to those used in brachycephalic dogs and may require ventilatory support during the maintenance of anesthesia (see Chapter 7).

Obese dogs and toy breeds often exhibit rapid, shallow respirations during anesthesia. This breathing pattern may result in hypercapnia and/or difficulty in keeping the patient at an adequate depth of anesthesia. The anesthetist who observes persistent rapid and shallow respirations should assume control over respiration by providing intermittent manual ventilation (commonly known as bagging the patient) with oxygen and inhalant anesthetic once every 5 seconds until increased anesthetic depth and slower respirations are observed. The anesthetist can also slow down the respiratory rate by administering opioids such as hydromorphone, especially if the elevated rate is a result of pain from surgical stimulation, although occasionally opioids may cause panting.

> **TECHNICIAN NOTE**
> As compared with animals with normal body conformation, obese animals:
> * Require lower drug dosages on a per-kilogram basis
> * Have decreased respiratory function
> * Often require respiratory support

Brachycephalic Dogs

Technicians or nurses are often called on to anesthetize brachycephalic dogs such as the English Bulldog, Pug, Boston Terrier, and Pekingese. These patients are at higher risk primarily owing to anatomic abnormalities that increase their susceptibility to airway obstruction.

Factors That Put Brachycephalic Patients at Increased Risk

Because of their body conformation, particularly as it relates to the skull and upper airway, these animals may have one or more anatomic characteristics that impede air exchange, including stenotic nares (very small nasal openings), an elongated soft palate, everted laryngeal saccules, and a small-diameter trachea compared with nonbrachycephalic breeds. Together, these characteristics form the brachycephalic obstructive airway syndrome (BOAS). Additionally, the tissue in the laryngopharynx is often thick and fleshy, further hampering breathing. Any anesthetic agent that depresses respiration or reduces muscle tone in the pharyngeal and laryngeal area, including many of the commonly used sedatives, tranquilizers and opioids, may cause partial airway obstruction in these animals due to the collapse of the tissues of and adjacent to the airway. This may lead to respiratory distress which, in cases of severe or complete obstruction, may be fatal, particularly if the animal is not intubated and an open airway cannot be maintained. These problems may be further exacerbated in animals undergoing surgery to correct conformation defects of the brachycephalic syndrome in the pharyngeal region (e.g., soft palate resection) because postoperative swelling or hemorrhage may occur, increasing the risk of respiratory difficulty.

In addition to respiratory problems, many brachycephalic animals have abnormally high parasympathetic tone, which may cause bradycardia, especially during endotracheal intubation and manipulation of the head and neck. The use of atropine or glycopyrrolate in these patients is helpful to stabilize the heart rate prior to intubation.

Drug Protocols for Brachycephalic Dogs

The induction period is of particularly high risk for brachycephalic dogs. If possible, the anesthetist should preoxygenate brachycephalic patients for 5 minutes before anesthetic induction. This is done by gently restraining the animal and administering oxygen through a face mask. This procedure helps to maintain adequate blood oxygen levels and gives the animal an extra margin of safety during the induction period that follows. Care should always be taken not to press the edges of the mask into the eyes. Induction should be performed rapidly in order to gain control over the airway and for this reason, IV induction agents are generally preferred over mask induction. Agents that are rapidly metabolized (e.g., propofol, alfaxalone, and ketamine–midazolam or ketamine–diazepam) are preferred. The patient must be adequately anesthetized to allow rapid and efficient intubation. Difficulties may be encountered because of the large amount of redundant tissue in the pharynx. This reduces the visibility of the laryngeal opening, and the use of a laryngoscope is essential in these patients. The anesthetist may also find that the ETT that fits the trachea is smaller than expected, considering the size and weight of the dog.

Anesthesia usually can be maintained safely through the use of an inhalation anesthetic. When the patient is intubated, breathing during anesthesia may, in fact, be superior to that of the normal awake brachycephalic patient.

Management During the Recovery Period

After surgery, the brachycephalic patient should be observed closely until it is extubated and breathing well. Vigilance is necessary well into the recovery period because patients may develop airway obstruction even after attempting to stand. The ETT should be left in place as long as possible because the animal will maintain an open airway as long as the tube is in place. Oxygen can also be delivered until the patient is extubated. Once the ETT has been removed, the animal's head and neck should be extended and the animal should be watched closely for dyspnea and cyanosis. If dyspnea is seen, the mouth can be kept open with a mouth gag and the tongue pulled forward. Administration of oxygen by mask or even reinduction (with ketamine–midazolam, propofol, or other IV induction agent) and reintubation may occasionally be necessary. It is advisable to have supplemental oxygen and supplies for reintubation

(i.e., a laryngoscope, new ETT [the same size or one size smaller than the original], and the appropriate dose of an induction agent) readily available in the recovery area in case severe dyspnea occurs after extubation.

Excitement and stress should be minimized as much as possible in the recovery period, especially if airway surgery was carried out. Some patients may require mild tranquilization or the use of opioid analgesics to reduce the rapid respirations that can worsen laryngeal swelling. Steroidal antiinflammatory medications are also helpful in some patients to decrease airway swelling.

Brachycephalic cats (e.g., Persians) do not typically have elongated soft palates or redundant soft tissue affecting their airways; thus management of these patients is not usually as challenging as it is when anesthetizing brachycephalic dogs.

> **TECHNICIAN NOTE**
> Brachycephalic dogs pose special challenges for the anesthetist, including an increased risk of airway obstruction, hypoxemia, and bradycardia, especially during induction and recovery.

Sighthounds

Several canine breeds (including the greyhound, saluki, Afghan hound, whippet, and Russian wolfhound) show increased sensitivity to some anesthetic agents, particularly thiobarbiturates such as thiopental sodium. The reason for this increased sensitivity is not entirely understood but likely involves inefficient hepatic metabolism. Fortunately, thiobarbiturates have been replaced by commonly used induction agents (including midazolam or diazepam and ketamine, propofol, and alfaxalone), which are appropriate alternatives in these animals.

Cardiovascular Disease

Cardiovascular disease involves a variety of abnormalities, including changes in heart rate and rhythm, reduced cardiac output, fluid buildup in the lungs or abdomen, and altered blood flow. These changes are due to an equally wide variety of causes, including congenital abnormalities, heart muscle injury, valvular disease, and obstruction to blood flow, each of which requires anesthetic management tailored to the individual's circumstances. Regardless of the specific situation, there are general principles concerning the way these patients must be handled that will be emphasized in the following paragraphs.

Management of Patients With Cardiovascular Disease

Careful preanesthetic physical examination with a focus on the cardiovascular system (including evaluation of heart rate, rhythm, heart sounds and synchrony with the pulse, mucous membrane color, and capillary refill time) as well as diagnostic testing (e.g. blood work, thoracic radiographs, cardiac ultrasound, and electrocardiography) can help define many cardiac abnormalities prior to anesthetic induction and alert the veterinary anesthetist to potential problems that may occur during an anesthetic procedure.

Several other practices should be observed to increase the likelihood of a successful outcome in these patients. For example, stress must be minimized and affected animals should be gently restrained. Dehydration and hypovolemia should be managed with appropriate fluid therapy. Patients with potentially dangerous abnormalities associated with their disease such as arrhythmias or pulmonary edema should be stabilized prior to anesthetic induction. Oxygen should be administered via mask for at least 5 minutes prior to anesthetic induction to maximize oxygenation as long as the patient tolerates it without undue stress or struggling.

During an anesthetic event, many common adverse effects of general anesthesia such as hypoxemia, hypercapnia, hypothermia, and vagal stimulation may exacerbate cardiac dysfunction. Therefore recognition and prompt resolution of these abnormalities through careful monitoring and treatment is especially important in these patients.

Drug Protocols for Patients With Cardiovascular Disease

When choosing a protocol for patients with cardiovascular disease, agents must be selected that help to maintain cardiac output and tissue perfusion. Although the specific drug choices vary according to the nature of the heart disease, opioid agonists such as hydromorphone or fentanyl, with or without a benzodiazepine, are often a good choice for sedating patients because both drug classes cause minimal cardiovascular depression and bradycardia can generally be controlled with anticholinergics if necessary. Alpha$_2$-agonists and dissociatives should generally be avoided in these patients because of the adverse cardiovascular effects associated with the use of these agents. A very low dose of acepromazine may be helpful in patients with ventricular arrhythmias to prevent exacerbation and since acepromazine reduces afterload, cardiac output may be improved.

The drugs best suited for anesthetic induction of these patients include alfaxalone, propofol, and etomidate, with or without an opioid agonist. Etomidate is an especially good choice because it minimally depresses cardiac function and does not cause arrhythmias; however, its side effects should always be considered. Alfaxalone has fewer adverse cardiovascular effects than propofol and may be a good choice as long as the speed of injection and volume administered are minimized. Propofol, if used, should be given using a low-dose technique (often combined with an opioid agonist) and should be given slowly to avoid the vasodilation, hypotension, and decreased cardiac conduction that often accompany rapid administration or use of higher doses.

Surgical anesthesia can be maintained with a CRI of opioids, propofol, or alfaxalone, with or without an inhalant agent. Regardless of the technique used, great care must be used to titrate carefully the volume of drug administered so that the minimal amount is used to achieve the desired results.

TECHNICIAN NOTE

Regardless of the techniques used for anesthetic induction and maintenance in patients with cardiovascular disease, great care must be used to titrate carefully the volume of drug administered so that the minimal amount is used to achieve the desired results.

Other Considerations in Patients With Cardiovascular Disease

When anesthetizing animals with cardiovascular problems, the anesthetist should be aware of the increased risk of overhydration through excessive or rapid administration of IV fluids. The recommended intraoperative fluid administration rates (5 mL/kg/h in dogs and 3 mL/kg/h in cats) may be excessive in patients with heart disease. Therefore it is advisable to use lower administration rates (in the range of 1 to 3 mL/kg/h) in these patients. These patients should also be monitored at frequent intervals for signs of volume overload and pulmonary edema such as increased lung sounds, increased respiratory rate, and ocular or nasal discharge. Central venous pressure monitoring, if available, may be helpful for the detection of overhydration.

In some of these patients, the anesthetist may need to support cardiovascular function during general anesthesia by administering drugs that increase the strength of cardiac muscle contraction (e.g., dopamine or dobutamine), improve vascular tone (e.g., norepinephrine), or antiarrhythmic drugs (e.g., lidocaine) given by constant rate infusion (CRI).

Respiratory Disease

As with cardiovascular disease, respiratory disease encompasses a variety of disorders with diverse causes. These disorders may be divided according to whether they affect the upper respiratory system (the nares, nasal cavity, nasopharynx, and larynx) or the lower respiratory system (the trachea, bronchi, and lungs). Upper airway disease usually involves some degree of airway obstruction and may be caused by a variety of disease conditions including BOAS, laryngeal paralysis, foreign bodies, and masses. Lower airway disease may be caused by, among other things, pleural effusion (i.e., free fluid present in the chest cavity), diaphragmatic hernia, pneumothorax, pulmonary contusions resulting from trauma, pneumonia, and pulmonary edema. Regardless of the cause, poor oxygenation is often present in these animals, and many show signs of tachypnea, dyspnea, and cyanosis.

Management of Patients With Respiratory Disease

If possible, anesthesia should be delayed until respiratory function has improved, but if anesthesia is required each patient must be carefully assessed and managed in a way appropriate to its specific condition. Regardless, as with cardiovascular disease, there are commonalities in the way patients with respiratory disease are managed that will be emphasized in the paragraphs that follow.

As previously mentioned, it is important to evaluate the patient thoroughly with a physical exam, blood work, thoracic radiographs, and other diagnostics appropriate to the case as ordered by the attending veterinarian. Blood gas analysis and measurement of electrolytes are two specific assays that are often necessary to guide effective management of these patients.

During preanesthetic assessment, great care must be taken to use minimal restraint, minimize stress, and do nothing to compromise the patient's ability to breathe, such as forcibly placing the patient in dorsal or lateral recumbency unless absolutely necessary, and then only when approved by the attending veterinarian and when preceded by preoxygenation. This is truly a circumstance in which less is more, meaning that the less often and more gently the patient is handled, the better. Never place pressure on a dyspneic patient's chest or neck and always allow them to assume the most comfortable position to breathe, which in many cases is sternal recumbency. Light sedation may be far more useful than physical restraint and is often safer for the patient.

After assessment but before anesthetic induction, most of these patients require supplemental oxygen via oxygen cage, mask, nasal cannula, flow-by, or other method as part of an attempt to stabilize them as much as possible before proceeding. This helps to optimize their condition before subjecting them to the additional stressors associated with anesthesia.

Drug Protocols for Patients With Respiratory Disease

When choosing anesthetic premedications and agents, care must be given to selecting agents that will not compromise the patient's ability to breathe or that will exacerbate respiratory depression. Sedatives must be used with great caution because some, such as the alpha$_2$-agonists, can cause significant respiratory depression, worsen hypercarbia and hypoxemia, and cause upper airway muscle relaxation, which may lead to the collapse of the airway, especially in patients with upper airway obstruction. They also may produce vomiting, especially when administered with opioid agonists. For these reasons, agents such as opioid partial agonists, benzodiazepines, and low-dose acepromazine may be better choices for these patients.

With respiratory disease patients, establishing and maintaining an open airway is of greatest importance; consequently, extreme care should be taken to prepare any and all equipment that may be necessary to secure an airway and support ventilation before anesthesia is induced. Depending on the patient's condition, this may require endotracheal intubation or, especially in patients with severe upper airway disease, may require tracheostomy in the event that an ETT cannot be placed. Arrangements should be made to provide manual or mechanical ventilation in these patients because they often require ventilatory support in order to maintain blood oxygen levels and prevent CO_2 buildup. A pulse oximeter and capnograph should also be made ready to monitor these patients as soon as they are induced.

> **TECHNICIAN NOTE**
> With respiratory disease patients, establishing and maintaining an open airway is of greatest importance; consequently, extreme care should be taken to prepare any and all equipment that may be necessary to secure an airway and support ventilation before anesthesia is induced, including having suction available.

Anesthesia may be induced with a variety of agents but should be done with an agent that allows the airway to be rapidly secured, such as propofol or alfaxalone. Both ketamine and propofol are known to result in bronchodilation, and this may be an advantage in patients with lower respiratory tract disease.

Maintenance may be accomplished with isoflurane or sevoflurane, or with a CRI of a short-acting IV agent such as propofol or alfaxalone, especially if an ETT cannot be placed or if surgery is being performed on the upper respiratory tract.

Other Considerations in Patients With Respiratory Disease

Patients with respiratory disease are at high risk of developing complications during the postanesthetic period, especially if their disease cannot be corrected (e.g., an inoperable laryngeal mass). These patients will then require special care during the recovery period and beyond.

In patients with upper airway disease, debris, blood, and fluid must be carefully removed from the mouth, nasal cavity, and/or oropharynx by suction and/or swabbing. The ETT should not be removed until the patient has a strong swallowing reflex and anesthetic depth is light enough to allow it to reject the tube. The anesthetist must be prepared to reintubate the patient in the event that the airway does not remain open or the patient is unable to ventilate adequately on its own. After extubation, many patients will require oxygen therapy until such time as they are able to maintain adequate oxygenation.

Patients that have a perceived or real decrease in PCV (hematocrit) or oxygen saturation of hemoglobin below 95% should be preoxygenated for a minimum of 5 minutes before anesthesia is induced. This will ensure saturated oxygen levels within the vascular system and the tissues, thus reducing the chance of arrhythmias or hypoxemic events.

> **TECHNICIAN NOTE**
> With respiratory disease patients, great care must be taken to use minimal restraint, minimize stress, protect the airway, and do nothing to compromise the patient's ability to breathe during all periods of anesthesia.

Hepatic Disease

Animals with liver disease are subject to increased anesthetic risk because of the central role the organ plays in drug metabolism, synthesis of blood clotting factors and other serum proteins, and carbohydrate metabolism. Some animals with liver disease are hypoproteinemic, which may lead to increased potency of agents that are highly protein bound, such as ketamine, propofol, and etomidate, and low blood pressure as a result of decreased oncotic pressure. Patients with chronic liver failure are also commonly dehydrated, thin, and icteric, and may be anemic. Patients with severe liver disease may also have hepatic encephalopathy, a disorder caused by increased levels of ammonium and a variety of other physiologic changes that alter the response to anesthetic agents. In addition, blood glucose, which may be low, should be checked prior to anesthesia and supplemented during anesthesia if needed.

Drug Protocols for Patients With Hepatic Disease

Because of the complexity of the metabolic changes that accompany liver disease, drug protocols must be tailored to each patient after considering the results of blood work and other diagnostics. Analgesic agents that can be reversed are preferred for pain control. Preanesthetic medication should be given in reduced dosages or omitted from the protocol because most of these agents require hepatic metabolism before they can be excreted. Acepromazine may have long-lasting effects in patients with compromised hepatic function and benzodiazepines, although reversible, may worsen the signs of hepatic encephalopathy. The use of ketamine and midazolam should also be avoided owing to the potential prolongation of effects. Induction of anesthesia can be performed using short-acting IV induction agents. Maintenance of anesthesia is best achieved using inhalants, which require little to no hepatic function for elimination.

> **TECHNICIAN NOTE**
> Patients with hepatic disease have a decreased ability to metabolize anesthetic drugs. Therefore drugs that are metabolized by the liver (such as acepromazine and the benzodiazepines) should be given in reduced dosages or omitted. Short-acting induction drugs, drugs that are reversible, and those that require minimal hepatic metabolism (such as isoflurane and sevoflurane) should be used.

Renal Disease

The kidneys are the organs most involved in maintaining the volume and electrolyte composition of body fluids. This helps explain why animals with renal disease are often dehydrated and may have severe electrolyte and acid–base imbalances, including hyperkalemia and metabolic acidosis. General anesthesia may be particularly hazardous for these patients because renal blood flow is decreased during anesthesia and renal function may be further compromised, particularly if the animal is hypotensive. The use of injectable nonsteroidal antiinflammatory agents during anesthesia may reduce renal perfusion even further.

Management of Patients With Renal Disease

Tests such as urine specific gravity, blood urea nitrogen (BUN), creatinine, and symmetric dimethylarginine (SDMA) should be used to assess renal function prior to anesthesia.

Preoperative water deprivation is not advisable in patients with renal disease because dehydration can occur rapidly after the withdrawal of oral fluids. Water should be offered up to 1 hour before premedication. Fluid deficits should be corrected before surgery and electrolyte problems should be identified and addressed. Administration of IV fluids is often continued throughout the anesthetic and postanesthetic periods in a patient with chronic renal disease until the animal is fully hydrated and able to drink unassisted. Patients in acute renal failure that are anuric should be given no fluids or fluids at vastly reduced rates.

It is important to maintain adequate renal perfusion in patients with kidney disease by keeping mean arterial blood pressure above 60 to 70 mmHg (systolic pressure above 80 to 90 mmHg) in order to avoid further compromise to kidney function. It may be necessary to use vasoactive agents (norepinephrine) or positive inotropes (dobutamine, dopamine) to maintain appropriate blood pressure.

Patients with chronic renal disease may also be anemic; if a procedure is likely to result in significant intraoperative blood loss, a blood transfusion prior to or during anesthesia may be necessary.

Patients with urinary tract obstruction (e.g., male cats and goats with urethral obstructions) are often compromised when they present to the veterinary clinic. Many of these animals are depressed, dehydrated, uremic, acidotic, and hyperkalemic. The vast majority of patients presenting with urinary obstruction are not anesthetic emergencies as they can be stabilized by performing cystocentesis, placing urethrostomy or cystostomy tubes under sedation or local anesthesia, and addressing electrolyte disturbances.

Hyperkalemic animals are at particular risk of cardiac arrest, and therefore obtaining electrolyte values should be part of the preanesthetic workup if urinary obstruction is suspected. Bradycardia is suggestive of hyperkalemia and is often present if plasma potassium levels exceed 6 mEq/L. Electrocardiography may reveal additional changes indicative of high potassium levels (small or absent P waves, widened QRS complexes, and tall, tented T waves). Hyperkalemic patients with cardiac rhythm changes require prompt treatment with one of several drug protocols, for example, insulin and dextrose or sodium bicarbonate. Calcium gluconate administration may be necessary in severe cases as, while it does not lower potassium, it is cardioprotective.

Drug Protocols for Patients With Renal Disease

Many injectable preanesthetic and anesthetic agents and their metabolites are eliminated from the body by renal excretion. For this reason, animals with compromised renal function may show prolonged recovery after anesthesia if conventional doses are used. It is prudent to reduce doses of anesthetic drugs (including acepromazine, dexmedetomidine, midazolam, and ketamine) in these patients if possible and use inhalants for anesthetic maintenance. Ketamine is excreted unchanged in the urine in some species; thus consideration should be given to using other short-acting IV induction agents like propofol or alfaxalone.

> **TECHNICIAN NOTE**
> Patients with renal disease are especially susceptible to dehydration, overhydration, hypotension, and electrolyte imbalances. Therefore the anesthetist must support and maintain normal hydration and electrolyte levels prior to and throughout the anesthetic event.

Cesarean Section

The parturient patient faces unique risks that must be dealt with by the veterinary team. These risks include the following:
- Aspiration of vomitus if the patient has not been fasted (in the case of an emergency cesarean section) or if the patient regurgitates intra- or postoperatively
- Inadequate ventilation because of pressure exerted on the diaphragm by the gravid uterus, potentially resulting in hypoxemia and hypercarbia
- Increased cardiac workload because of advanced pregnancy
- Physiologic anemia because of increased plasma volume without a corresponding increase in the number of red

blood cells (this is accentuated as the number of fetuses increases)

- Increased risk of hypotension due to pressure on the large vessels exerted by the gravid uterus
- Decreased anesthetic requirements because of the effect of progesterone and its metabolites on gamma-aminobutyric acid (GABA) receptors, increasing the risk of overdose
- Compromise or death of newborns because of drug-induced respiratory depression or prolonged anesthesia
- Increased risk of hemorrhage intra- or postoperatively

Methods used to manage each of these risks are discussed in detail in the sections that follow.

Management of Cesarean Section Patients

Throughout a cesarean section (frequently abbreviated to c-section), steps must be taken to minimize the time that the dam is under anesthesia. For instance, if possible, clipping and surgical site preparation as well as IV catheterization should be performed prior to induction. Whether the patient is awake or anesthetized, it is advisable that preparation be performed with the patient held upright (smaller animals), or gently restrained in lateral recumbency rather than in dorsal recumbency because the latter position may cause the heavy uterus to compress the vena cava, decreasing venous return to the heart (Fig. 13.1).

Hemorrhage from the uterus is a common complication of cesarean surgery and even nonhemorrhaging patients have an increased risk of shock. Therefore IV fluid therapy is essential for all patients undergoing a c-section and must be individually tailored to meet each patient's needs.

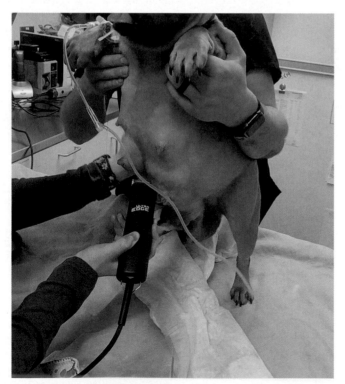

FIG. 13.1 Performing surgical preparation for cesarean section prior to anesthetic induction with the patient in an upright position.

In a patient in the advanced stages of pregnancy, the stomach empties more slowly and the dam is more likely to eat small meals frequently, increasing the likelihood that the stomach may not be empty at the time of surgery. The anesthetist should be prepared for regurgitation during the induction period and an induction agent should be used that allows for rapid control of the airway. Therefore mask induction is not advisable for animals undergoing a c-section.

The distended uterus of the parturient patient causes lung capacity, functional residual volume, and tidal volume (V_T) to decrease. In the parturient patient, there is also an increased demand for oxygen. Consequently, preoxygenation prior to induction is important to reduce the risk of oxygen desaturation.

Neonate vigor is correlated to oxygenation of fetuses in the uterus; therefore the anesthetist should strive to maintain adequate oxygenation and blood pressure to assure oxygen delivery to the uterus during anesthesia.

Drug Protocols for Cesarean Section Patients

Essentially, all anesthetic drugs administered to the pregnant patient (with the exception of neuromuscular blocking agents and local anesthetics) will readily cross the placenta and affect the neonates. Although it is essential that the dam receive enough anesthetic to provide adequate immobilization and analgesia, it is advisable to use minimal doses of any agents that may depress respiration in the neonates.

Various anesthetic techniques are used for c-sections, depending on the preference of the veterinarian:

- Opioids may be given as premedication; however, they are more commonly given after the neonates have been delivered to avoid respiratory depression. Preference should be given to using reversible agents to provide analgesia, sedation, or neuroleptanalgesia, because they may be reversed in both the dam and the neonates with naloxone.
- Use of benzodiazepines should be avoided because they are poorly metabolized by neonates.
- Induction with IV injectable agents and maintenance with inhalant anesthetics is a commonly used protocol for c-sections. The injectable agents propofol, alfaxalone, and ketamine may be used for induction. Inhalants are best used for maintenance as the ability of neonates to metabolize injectable drugs is limited. Isoflurane can be used; however, the low blood gas solubility of sevoflurane offers the advantage of more rapid elimination of inhalant. Regardless of the agents chosen, all drugs should be given at the lowest dose needed to avoid unnecessarily depressing respiratory drive of the neonates. Because of the dam's increased sensitivity to medications, the dose of inhalant anesthetic required is often reduced by up to 40%.
- A local anesthetic line block can be performed along the incision site after the dam is induced and prepped.
- Epidural analgesia combined with a tranquilizer or neuroleptanalgesia is an alternative to general anesthesia because this technique, once mastered, provides effective anesthesia with minimal depression of the dam or the neonates. If the technique is used, IV fluids and oxygen should be administered and blood pressure should be monitored.

> **TECHNICIAN NOTE**
> The anesthetic concerns for patients undergoing cesarean section are as follows:
> - Vomiting and aspiration
> - Hypoxemia and hypercarbia
> - Hypotension
> - Hemorrhage intra- or postoperatively
> - Acid-base imbalances or cardiac arrhythmias
> - Compromise or death of neonates due to respiratory depression

Other Considerations for Cesarean Section Patients

Hypotension is also a potential problem for the cesarean patient. It is important that large-bore catheters be used, and in some situations, such as dogs over 20 kg, it may be advantageous to have two catheters in place to ensure that rapid volume infusion is possible. Drugs known to cause hypotension, such as alpha$_2$-agonists and acepromazine, should generally be avoided.

Because of physiologic anemia, the dam's ability to carry sufficient oxygen to vital tissues is decreased. Oxygen delivery may be further compromised by hypotension, as noted earlier. Preoxygenation lessens these effects and reduces the risk of hypoxemia and anaerobic glycolysis, either of which can result in arrhythmias or acid–base imbalances.

During the postanesthetic period, the veterinary technician or nurse should ensure that the dam has a good swallowing reflex before extubation is performed. The patient should be placed in a sternal position to reduce the risk of any aspiration of vomitus. If the patient does vomit after extubation, the patient must immediately have its head lowered below the rest of the body and suction of the oropharynx should commence immediately. Once the oropharyngeal area is clear, the patient should be placed back in sternal recumbency and may require a short period of oxygenation. The patient should be monitored for the next 24 to 48 hours for aspiration pneumonia (signs of which include pyrexia, dyspnea, hyperpnea, and depression).

Puppies or kittens delivered by cesarean section often show signs of reduced respiratory and cardiovascular function when first delivered. If respiration appears inadequate or if cyanosis is present, oxygen should be administered by face mask. If necessary, the newborn animal can be intubated with a 16- or 18-gauge IV catheter and gently bagged with oxygen every 5 seconds. Fluid may be aspirated from the mouth and nose with an eyedropper or bulb syringe. If bradycardia is present, a drop of dilute atropine (0.25 mg/mL) can be administered under the tongue or injected into the tongue. Gentle cardiac massage and oxygen may also be helpful.

The newborns should be allowed to nurse as soon as the mother appears to be recovered from anesthesia (or, with supervision, during the recovery period). The dam may be disoriented and should be closely watched to ensure the safety of the newborn puppies or kittens. Anesthetic agents excreted in the milk appear to have little effect on nursing or viability of the neonates and so postoperative analgesics such as butorphanol or buprenorphine may be used to provide pain relief for the dam. Low-dose acepromazine may be useful to calm an agitated or disoriented dam in recovery.

Management of Trauma Patients

Animals that have recently undergone trauma, such as being hit by a car, may have problems affecting multiple body systems that greatly increase anesthetic risk. Respiratory difficulties are common and may be the result of pneumothorax, pulmonary contusions, hemorrhage, or diaphragmatic hernia. Any one of these injuries decreases the V_T of the patient and therefore can cause a decrease in oxygenation. Lack of adequate oxygen exchange will cause hypoxemia, which will lead to myocardial hypoxia and therefore arrhythmias, acid–base imbalances, and cell death. Increased CO_2 levels caused by lack of proper ventilation will also lead to acid–base imbalances and arrhythmias. Loss of blood or **sequestration** of fluid will result in hypotension, which must be corrected before anesthesia. Fluid sequestration can result from such situations as burns, in which serum (fluid) oozes from the blood vascular system into the burn site. Anemia may also be present in the traumatized patient as a result of loss of blood directly or sequestration of blood into the trauma site. It has been shown in human medicine that a pelvic fracture can sequester as much as 40% of the circulating blood volume due to severe bleeding into the area around the fracture.

Very few trauma patients require anesthesia immediately after an accident and as a general rule, it is wise to stabilize these animals before anesthesia. Delaying anesthesia offers two advantages: (1) it allows time for a thorough workup to assess the extent of the injuries, and (2) it provides some time to stabilize the animal's condition, which reduces anesthetic risk. The patient should be closely monitored for signs of dyspnea, cardiac arrhythmias, or altered mentation. It is advisable to obtain thoracic radiographs and an electrocardiogram before anesthesia for repair of internal injuries (such as fractures) resulting from trauma. Studies have shown that one-third of patients with traumatic forelimb, hindlimb, or pelvic injuries have concurrent thoracic injuries that could jeopardize their safety under anesthesia. It is obviously advisable to identify and treat a disorder such as pneumothorax before anesthetizing an animal for the repair of a fractured femur. Fortunately, many thoracic injuries improve with cage rest and, if anesthesia can be delayed for 24 to 72 hours after the traumatic incident, the anesthetist usually encounters fewer problems.

> **TECHNICIAN NOTE**
> Very few trauma patients require anesthesia immediately and as a general rule, it is wise to stabilize these animals before anesthesia. Delaying anesthesia offers two advantages: (1) it allows time for a thorough workup to assess the extent of the injuries, and (2) it provides some time to stabilize the animal's condition, which reduces anesthetic risk.

Management of the Patient With Diaphragmatic Hernia

Repair of a diaphragmatic hernia is an example of a surgical procedure requiring anesthesia of an animal in respiratory distress as a result of trauma. When preparing to anesthetize these patients, as with all patients showing signs of dyspnea, it is advisable to preoxygenate for 5 to 10 minutes before surgery.

Patients with diaphragmatic hernias are further compromised because they have a vastly reduced ability to compensate during periods of apnea owing to the fact that the lungs have a greatly decreased functional residual volume; that is, the lungs tend to be much more collapsed at the end of expiration than in an animal with an intact diaphragm. Head-down positions should be avoided before and during the early stages of anesthesia (induction and surgical preparation) because they may result in further movement of abdominal contents into the thorax. If possible, an induction method that allows rapid intubation (i.e., the use of an injectable agent) is preferred over mask induction. After induction, some patients may show signs of respiratory depression and even respiratory arrest, and the anesthetist must be prepared to intubate rapidly and assist or control ventilation. Ventilatory assistance must be provided by manually bagging the patient, or a ventilator may be used. If necessary, the animal can be held up in a vertical position in an attempt to decrease pressure on the lungs from abdominal organs within the chest. It is useful to have a member of the surgical team present at induction as in extreme situations where respiratory compromise occurs, it may be necessary to open the abdomen surgically and remove abdominal organs from the chest. The animal should be closely observed at all times for cyanosis. Pulse oximetry, capnography, and arterial blood gas determination are helpful aids for assessing ventilation. Blood gas (and blood chemistry) values can be obtained with point-of-care analyzers such as the Heska element POC analyzer and the Abaxis Vetscan i-STAT 1 hand-held analyzer (Fig. 13.2).

These patients require close observation during the recovery period. Administration of oxygen may be necessary if signs of respiratory distress are seen. Pneumothorax is usually present after chest surgery and should be the primary differential for respiratory compromise after surgery in which the chest cavity is open to room air. Therefore thoracocentesis or evacuation of air via a chest tube should be a priority.

COMMON ANESTHETIC PROBLEMS AND EMERGENCIES

Despite every precaution, the veterinary technician or nurse is likely to encounter anesthetic problems and emergencies throughout the course of their career. The nature of the technician or nurse's response may mean the difference between life and death for the anesthetized patient.

Role of the Veterinary Technician or Nurse in Emergency Care

Ideally, response to anesthetic problems and emergencies is a team effort involving the veterinarian, technician or nurse, and other hospital staff. Normally, the veterinarian acts as the team leader, directing the staff in emergency response. However, the veterinarian is often performing a surgery or other procedure on the patient when an anesthetic emergency arises and therefore may be unable to respond effectively without assistance. At times such as this, the technician or nurse must be prepared to take an active role in resuscitating the patient and must not rely solely on the veterinarian. Constant communication between the veterinarian and the technician or nurse is obviously important under these circumstances.

In the interest of preparing for just such a contingency, it is a good idea to conduct periodic dress rehearsals, or mock resuscitations in which all staff members participate. Everyone in the hospital should be familiar with the location of ETTs, the crash cart, and IV fluids. Procedures such as warming towels in a clothes dryer, preparing warm water blankets, and preparing syringes and needles can be readily taught to hospital staff. Once the staff has mastered these skills, the veterinarian and technician or nurse can be free to perform more demanding tasks.

Occasionally, an emergency arises when the veterinarian is absent from the hospital or unavailable to assist. For example, seizures or other complications may occur during the postoperative period after regular business hours. Most provincial and state regulations allow the technician or nurse to undertake emergency care if the veterinarian is absent. To protect the veterinarian and technician or nurse from liability, however, it is advisable to discuss in advance the procedures that the veterinarian will authorize the technician or nurse to do in an emergency. In addition, it is helpful to have written instructions available in the form of an emergency protocol authorized by the veterinarian.

It cannot be assumed that every anesthetic emergency should be treated in the same way. For example, the veterinarian and animal owner may elect not to resuscitate a severely ill or debilitated animal that undergoes cardiac arrest during anesthesia. Cost considerations may influence treatment in some cases, because emergency care is labor intensive and treatment costs may be considerable. Most veterinarians, however, will not stop to consider the cost if the emergency arises during a routine surgery, such as a spay, and will do everything possible to revive the animal.

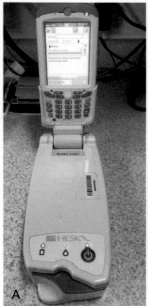
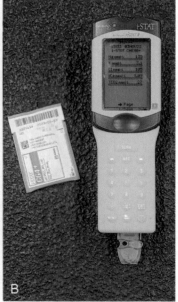

FIG. 13.2 Two point-of-care analyzers used for blood gases and blood chemistries. **(A)** Heska element POC analyzer. **(B)** Abaxis Vetscan i-STAT 1 analyzer. Note that proprietary cartridges (shown to the left of the Abaxis i-STAT), which are analyzer-specific, must be purchased separately. (A, Courtesy of Stacey Reiling, CVT, VTS (Anesthesia/Analgesia), CVPP. B, Courtesy Zoetis; https://www.zoetisus.com/.)

PROCEDURE 13.1 Responding to an Emergency

1. As soon as an anesthetic emergency is identified, the technician or nurse should take a few seconds to think before doing anything. After consulting with the veterinarian, the technician or nurse should mentally list the most important things to be done and undertake them in order of priority.
2. Every veterinary practice should have a well-stocked crash cart for use in emergency situations within the hospital. A list of supplies that may be useful in a crash cart is given in Appendix C.
3. Emergency drugs are listed in Fig. 13.9 and Table 13.2. Doses for emergency drugs should be posted or listed on a laminated page and kept with the crash cart. Emergency drugs kept in the crash cart should be periodically checked to ensure that they have not expired. In particular, epinephrine has a short shelf life and should not be used if a brown discoloration is present; some formulations of epinephrine must be refrigerated.
4. Above all, the technician or nurse should do no harm. In an emergency, it is easy to panic and do things that are not only unnecessary but also potentially harmful to the animal. Sometimes the best course of action is to watch, monitor, and assess.
5. After an anesthetic emergency, the technician or nurse, veterinarian, and hospital staff should discuss the reasons why the emergency arose and determine what could be done to prevent the same thing from happening again. The adequacy of the resuscitation efforts should be analyzed and if a problem exists, it should be addressed.

When responding to an emergency, the technician or nurse should bear in mind the principles of emergency care listed in Procedure 13.1.

Emergency Situations That May Arise During Anesthesia

Although anesthetic emergencies are by their nature unpredictable, certain problems occur with some frequency. The following situations will be addressed in detail:
- Animals that will not stay anesthetized
- Animals that are too deeply anesthetized
- Pale mucous membranes
- Prolonged capillary refill time
- Hypotension
- Dyspnea and/or cyanosis
- Tachypnea
- Abnormalities in cardiac rate and rhythm
- Apnea
- Respiratory arrest
- Cardiac arrest

TECHNICIAN NOTE

Emergencies during anesthesia include the following:
- Inadequate or excessive anesthetic depth
- Pale mucous membranes or prolonged capillary refill time
- Hypotension
- Dyspnea and/or cyanosis
- Tachypnea
- Abnormalities in cardiac rate and rhythm
- Apnea
- Respiratory arrest
- Cardiac arrest

Animals That Will Not Stay Anesthetized

Occasionally, the anesthetist will have difficulty in maintaining a patient at sufficient anesthetic depth despite the use of appropriate techniques to maintain anesthesia. The veterinarian often will become aware of this problem because of patient movement in response to surgical stimulation and will typically call for immediate assistance if a technician or nurse is not present in the room. Inadequate depth may be due to any of the following causes:
- An inadequate vaporizer setting.
- A vaporizer that is inadequately filled with liquid anesthetic.
- A blocked, misplaced, or disconnected ETT.
- An ETT that is too small or is inadequately cuffed.
- Apnea or inadequate tidal volume. Apnea most commonly occurs after induction with an IV agent (e.g. propofol, alfaxalone) and will be apparent immediately after intubation when the animal is connected to the anesthetic machine. Apnea may lead to arousal from anesthesia because adequate quantities of vaporized anesthetic will not enter the lungs or the bloodstream. Inadequate tidal volume may occur secondary to rapid, shallow breathing that is commonly seen in toy dogs and obese animals, and may be associated with insufficient anesthetic depth.
- Misassembly or leakage of the anesthetic machine. This may be due to a failure to set it up correctly, leaks in the system, or inadvertent disconnection of hoses.
- Inadequate oxygen flow. When anesthetic depth is inadequate, a flow of 50 to 100 mL/kg/min should be used for a rebreathing system. Regardless of patient size, for most precision vaporizers, a minimum flow rate of at least 500 mL/min is necessary for accurate delivery of anesthetic. Very high oxygen flow rates or excessive use of the oxygen flush valve may also result in inadequate output.
- Malfunction or incorrect calibration of the vaporizer.

After rapidly checking monitoring parameters, if depth does indeed appear inadequate, the anesthetist should take the actions outlined in Procedure 13.2.

Animals That Are Too Deeply Anesthetized

An animal that is too deeply anesthetized will usually show the following signs:
- A respiratory rate of 6 breaths/min or fewer; shallow respirations, or exaggerated respiratory movements
- Pale or cyanotic mucous membranes
- Capillary refill time greater than 2 seconds
- Bradycardia
- Weak pulse
- Hypotension (systolic blood pressure less than 80 to 90 mmHg or mean blood pressure less than 60 to 70 mmHg)
- Cardiac arrhythmias
- Cold extremities; body temperature is often less than 35°C (95°F)
- Absent reflexes, including palpebral and corneal reflexes
- Flaccid muscle tone
- Dilated pupils; absent pupillary light reflex

The anesthetist must use judgment when interpreting monitoring parameters because the presence of one or two of these

PROCEDURE 13.2 Responding to Inadequate Anesthetic Depth

- Check that the vaporizer setting is appropriate and adjust it accordingly.
- Check that the vaporizer contains an adequate amount of liquid anesthetic and fill it if necessary.
- Confirm that the endotracheal tube (ETT) is not blocked, is in the trachea, and that the breathing circuit is attached. This can be easily determined by checking whether the reservoir bag expands and contracts as the animal breathes. Other techniques used to determine the location and patency of the endotracheal tube include palpation of the neck and compression of the reservoir bag to see if the chest expands in response.
- Check that air is not leaking around the endotracheal tube. Air leakage can be detected by closing the adjustable pressure limiting (APL) valve, inflating the reservoir bag, and gently pressing on the bag while listening for the sound of air escaping from the animal's mouth. A soft hiss caused by escaping air is acceptable at a pressure manometer reading of just over 18–20 cm H2O. Leakage at lower pressure indicates that either the endotracheal tube is too small or the cuff is not sufficiently inflated. If this is the case, the cuff can be further inflated or the tube can be replaced with a larger tube if necessary.
- Check that the patient is breathing and that chest excursions are adequate. Patients with apnea or decreased tidal volume may require assisted or controlled manual ventilation (with the vaporizer on).
- Confirm that the anesthetic machine is correctly assembled and is not leaking, and correct any deficiencies immediately or switch the patient to another machine.
- Check that oxygen flow is adequate. For most precision vaporizers, a minimum flow rate of at least 500 mL/min is necessary for accurate delivery of anesthetic. Very high oxygen flow rates or excessive use of the oxygen flush valve may also result in unpredictable vaporization of anesthetic.
- Recheck the patient's monitoring parameters. Exaggerated respiratory movements may indicate abdominal breathing resulting from excessive anesthetic depth or agonal breaths resulting from impending or actual cardiopulmonary arrest.
- If none of the previously listed causes is identified, switch the patient to another machine and have the machine and vaporizer checked by a professional service technician for proper operation and recalibration. It may also be necessary to take one of several actions such as administering an analgesic or switching to a different anesthetic in order to achieve the desired anesthetic depth.

PROCEDURE 13.3 Responding to Excessive Anesthetic Depth

1. After concluding that the anesthetic depth is excessive, the anesthetist should immediately decrease the vaporizer setting (to zero if necessary) and inform the veterinarian.
2. If the veterinarian decides that the animal's condition has deteriorated so that resuscitation efforts are warranted, the anesthetist should begin to ventilate the animal with pure oxygen. (This assumes that the patient is intubated and is being maintained with an inhalant agent. If an injectable agent is being used to maintain the patient, intubation and oxygen delivery by means of an anesthetic machine should be initiated immediately.)
3. To ventilate the patient, the adjustable pressure limiting (APL) valve is closed, the reservoir bag is filled with oxygen, and the bag is gently squeezed until the animal's chest rises slightly. The APL valve is then opened immediately after giving a breath. This procedure should be repeated every 5 s until the animal shows signs of recovery (such as increased heart rate, stronger pulse, and improved mucous membrane color and refill).
4. The use of IV fluids, external heat, and drugs such as specific reversing agents (such as yohimbine, atipamezole, naloxone, or flumazenil) may also expedite recovery.
5. Occasionally the anesthetist may be unsure of whether a patient's anesthetic depth is excessive. If the veterinarian is not immediately available to assess the patient's condition, it is safest to assume that anesthesia is too deep and to decrease the vaporizer setting while observing the animal carefully for signs of arousal.

TECHNICIAN NOTE
Excessive anesthetic depth may be caused by:
- Anesthetic overdose
- Preexisting disease such as shock or anemia
- Hypothermia

Pale Mucous Membranes

Pale mucous membranes may arise from several causes. Some patients have preexisting anemia secondary to diseases such as hemolytic anemia, bleeding disorders, neoplasia, chronic renal disease, or feline leukemia. In other cases, blood loss may have occurred during surgery. Some anesthetic agents (particularly inhalation agents, propofol, and acepromazine) cause vasodilation and decrease blood pressure, which may result in poor perfusion of capillary beds and pale mucous membranes in some animals due to hypotension. Peripheral vasoconstriction caused by some drugs, such as alpha2-agonists or catecholamines (epinephrine), can also decrease tissue perfusion, resulting in pale mucous membranes. Hypothermia or pain can also reduce blood supply to the tissues and can cause pale mucous membranes.

If pale mucous membranes are observed during surgery, follow Procedure 13.4.

TECHNICIAN NOTE
Pale mucous membranes may be caused by:
- Anemia
- Blood loss
- Hypotension
- Peripheral vasoconstriction
- Hypothermia
- Pain

signs may not indicate excessive depth provided the other parameters are normal. In addition, vital signs are affected by factors other than anesthetic depth such as body temperature, blood volume, and the anesthetics and adjuncts used (e.g., alpha2-agonists may decrease heart rate, blood pressure, and respiratory rate). Consequently, the more parameters that the anesthetist considers, the more accurate the depth assessment is likely to be.

There are several reasons why anesthetic depth may be excessive. Some cases may involve an anesthetic overdose (use of a vaporizer setting that is too high for the patient or administration of too much injectable anesthetic). Occasionally, the animal may have a preexisting problem such as shock or anemia that increases susceptibility to anesthetic overdose. Hypothermia is also a predisposing factor for excessive depth. In the event that a patient's anesthetic depth is excessive, refer to Procedure 13.3.

PROCEDURE 13.4 Treating a Patient with Pale Mucous Membranes

1. The anesthetist should ascertain the animal's anesthetic depth and monitor vital signs including heart rate, respiration, pulse strength, and capillary refill time.
2. The anesthetist should rule out possible causes including hypothermia, hypotension, drug reactions, blood loss, and pain.
3. The attending veterinarian should be consulted because it may be necessary to administer pain medications or other drugs or to initiate treatments such as patient warming, IV fluid therapy, or a blood transfusion to stabilize the patient's condition.

PROCEDURE 13.5 Treating Prolonged Capillary Refill Time

1. The anesthetist who observes a prolonged capillary refill time should immediately check the animal's pulse and blood pressure reading (if available). A mean arterial pressure of less than 60–70 mmHg or a systolic pressure of less than 80–90 mmHg indicates hypotension and poor perfusion.
2. If blood pressure readings are not available, the anesthetist can roughly estimate the systolic pressure by palpating a peripheral pulse. As a general rule, the absence of a palpable pulse at the metatarsal artery indicates a systolic pressure under 60 mmHg, and the absence of a palpable pulse at the femoral artery indicates a systolic pressure under 40 mmHg.
3. If pulse pressure is reduced, the anesthetist should closely observe the animal for other signs of shock, including hypothermia and tachycardia. As circulation to the extremities deteriorates, peripheral temperature decreases. The heart may respond to the fall in blood pressure by increasing the rate and force of contraction, although this effect may not be present in deep anesthesia.

PROCEDURE 13.6 Treatment of Hypotension

1. Anesthetic depth should be reduced, if possible.
2. The use of anesthetic drugs that cause vasodilation (acepromazine, propofol, and inhalant agents) should be minimized.
3. Pain control should be optimized with injectable analgesics such as the opioid agonists. This may allow the dose of inhalant anesthetic to be decreased.
4. Crystalloid fluids should be administered at rates of 3–10 mL/kg rapidly in dogs and large animals and 3–5 mL/kg rapidly in cats. In the short term, it may be necessary to give fluid boluses of up to 20–40 mL/kg, with 50% given over 15 min for dogs (approximately 1 mL/kg/min) and 10–20 mL/kg, with 50% given over 15 min for cats (approximately 0.5 mL/kg/min) to help improve blood pressure quickly.
5. If blood pressure cannot be maintained, colloids may be given in concert with crystalloids. Doses for colloids are approximately 5 mL/kg over 15–20 min in dogs, and 2.5–3 mL/kg over 15–20 min in cats, with additional boluses if needed.
6. If drugs are required to stabilize blood pressure, the veterinarian may choose one or more of various medications such as dopamine (5–12 mcg/kg/min) if the heart rate is low or dobutamine (1–5 mcg/kg/min) for the patient with normal heart rate but decreased blood pressure.
7. The patient must be kept warm through the use of supplemental heat in the form of warm towels, circulating warm water blankets, warm air blankets, or similar devices.

TECHNICIAN NOTE
Prolonged CRT indicates poor tissue perfusion and is most often associated with hypotension.
Hypotension may be caused by:
- Blood loss or dehydration
- Excessive anesthetic depth
- Some anesthetics (e.g., acepromazine, propofol, alfaxalone, inhalant agents)
- Preexisting conditions
- Heart disease/arrhythmias

Prolonged Capillary Refill Time or Hypotension

The observation of a capillary refill time greater than 2 seconds suggests that blood pressure is inadequate to perfuse peripheral tissues. The presence of hypotension should be suspected in any animal with a slow capillary refill time. Hypotension was the most common anesthetic complication found in one study of dogs and cats.[c] Hypotension may be present before the induction of anesthesia, as in the case of animals undergoing emergency surgery after trauma. Hypotension or shock also may develop secondary to blood loss during surgery or may occur in patients with heart disease or arrhythmias, or patients that are at a very deep plane of anesthesia. Acepromazine, propofol, alfaxalone, and the inhalant agents may also cause hypotension, which can be more severe and last longer in hypovolemic patients. Follow Procedure 13.5 if a prolonged capillary refill time is noted. If hypotension is confirmed, the attending veterinarian should be informed and treatment should commence as ordered (Procedure 13.6).

Dyspnea and/or Cyanosis

Dyspnea or cyanosis noted during any anesthetic event should be immediately brought to the veterinarian's attention. The presence of dyspnea indicates that the animal is unable to obtain sufficient oxygen or adequately remove CO_2 with normal respiratory movements. Cyanosis indicates that tissue oxygenation is inadequate. Dyspnea and cyanosis are often seen together and, if not managed quickly, may be followed by respiratory arrest, in which respiratory efforts cease and the amount of oxygen available to the tissues rapidly declines.

The most common sources of respiratory distress during anesthesia are as follows:
- The animal is unable to obtain oxygen from the anesthetic machine because the oxygen supply has run out, the flowmeter has been turned off, or the anesthetic circuit or ETT is blocked.
- The animal is unable to breathe normally because of airway obstruction or respiratory pathology. Causes of airway obstruction include ETT blockage, excessive flexion of the head and neck, laryngospasm, bronchoconstriction, aspiration of stomach contents after vomiting or regurgitation, and BOAS.

[c]Gaynor JS, Dunlop CI, Wagner AE, et al: Complications and mortality associated with anesthesia in dogs and cats. *J Am Anim Hosp Assoc* 35(1):13–17, 1999.

Common causes of respiratory pathology include pneumothorax, pulmonary edema, diaphragmatic hernia, and pleural effusion.

- Use of heavy surgical drapes or constricting bandages also may impair normal respiration.
- The animal may be too deeply anesthetized to the point that respiration and other vital functions are adversely affected.

Dyspnea and cyanosis are life-threatening and should be addressed as discussed in Procedure 13.7.

TECHNICIAN NOTE

Causes of dyspnea and/or cyanosis include:
- Failure of oxygen delivery
- Airway blockage
- Respiratory disease
- Excessive pressure on the chest cavity by drapes, bandages, or other objects
- Excessive anesthetic depth

PROCEDURE 13.7 Treating Dyspnea and/or Cyanosis

1. The anesthetist must first ensure that oxygen is being delivered to the patient. If the oxygen tank has run out, the patient must be disconnected from the machine until another oxygen source can be secured. If the endotracheal tube is blocked, it must be removed and replaced. Endotracheal tube blockage can be suspected when giving the patient a manual breath does not cause the chest to rise and considerable resistance is felt when squeezing the reservoir bag. If a partial or total obstruction has occurred, capnography will show a truncated waveform (shark fin shape) or absent waveform, respectively. If in doubt, it is better to err on the side of caution and replace the tube.
2. Once oxygen flow has been established, the vaporizer should be turned off and the animal should be bagged with 100% oxygen. If the anesthetic machine is temporarily unavailable, a manual resuscitator bag, for example, an Ambu bag (see Fig. 13.3) can be used to deliver room air to the patient. While initiating bagging, the anesthetist should observe the chest for movement. If the chest does not rise when the animal is bagged, the endotracheal tube or airway may be blocked and the blockage must be relieved. If the chest does rise when the reservoir bag is squeezed, oxygen is being delivered to the lungs and bagging should be continued until the mucous membrane color improves or pulse oximeter readings rise to 95%. It is best to watch the anterior thorax for chest movement in the area of the heart so as not to be misled by passive movement of the chest caused by distention of the stomach associated with a misplaced endotracheal tube.
3. On rare occasions, dyspnea and cyanosis may be secondary to complete airway obstruction. If intubation is not possible under these circumstances, the veterinarian may elect to perform an emergency tracheostomy (a surgical incision between the tracheal rings to allow the insertion of a breathing tube). Alternatively, a 14-gauge IV catheter can be placed through the cricothyroid membrane and into the trachea. The catheter is connected to the barrel of a 3-mL syringe, which is in turn attached to the patient connector of an anesthetic machine for oxygen delivery.
4. Administration of IV fluids or emergency drugs such as doxapram may be helpful in reviving patients experiencing respiratory depression or arrest.
5. It is important that the anesthetist observe the patient closely during resuscitative efforts to ensure that cardiac arrest does not occur. If no pulse or heartbeat can be detected, chest compressions should be initiated in conjunction with continued bagging (see page 421).
6. If necessary, supplemental oxygen should be continued into the recovery period, using a mask, oxygen cage, or intranasal insufflation.

Tachypnea

Tachypnea, that is, a respiratory rate that is higher than normal, must be differentiated from dyspnea, in which respiratory distress is present. Tachypnea may arise at any time during anesthesia and may be disconcerting to the anesthetist. Common causes of tachypnea are hypoxemia, hypercarbia, and inadequate anesthetic depth, in which case it is often accompanied by tachycardia and spontaneous movement. Tachypnea is also seen in obese patients and in hyperthermic patients, including animals with malignant hyperthermia. It is not unusual to see a slight increase in respiratory rate with surgical stimulation; however, if surgery results in tachypnea, it is most likely that anesthetic depth is inadequate for the degree of pain the procedure is causing.

If tachypnea is seen, follow Procedure 13.8.

TECHNICIAN NOTE

Causes of tachypnea include:
- Inadequate anesthetic depth
- Surgical stimulation or perception of pain
- Hypoxemia
- Hypercapnia
- Hyperthermia
- Obesity

Abnormalities in Cardiac Rate and Rhythm

Tachycardia, bradycardia, and cardiac arrhythmias are commonly seen in anesthetized patients.

Tachycardia is present if the heart rate during stage III anesthesia is greater than 140 beats per minute (bpm) for a large dog, 160 bpm for a small dog, 200 for a cat, 60 for a horse, or 100 for a cow. It may result from the administration of drugs such as anticholinergics (e.g., atropine), dissociatives (e.g., ketamine), or catecholamines (e.g., epinephrine, dopamine). Tachycardia may also be a preexisting condition in animals with hyperthyroidism, shock, congestive heart failure, and other conditions. The presence of hypoxemia and/or hypercarbia will also cause tachycardia. An elevation in heart rate is also a common response to surgical stimulation, although it does not necessarily indicate insufficient anesthetic depth unless accompanied by rapid respiration, spontaneous movement, or active reflexes. If the elevation

---

PROCEDURE 13.8 Treating Tachypnea

1. The anesthetist should assess the anesthetic depth and check the CO_2 absorber granules or the capnogram, if available, to ensure that hypercapnia is not present.
2. If anesthetic depth is inadequate, increase anesthetic administration to bring the patient into an appropriate plane. If anesthetic depth, body temperature, and vital signs appear to be within acceptable limits, the anesthetist should refrain from changing the vaporizer setting because the condition will usually correct itself within 1–2 min.
3. If tachypnea arises as a result of surgical stimulation and the perception of pain, IV injection of an analgesic such as methadone, hydromorphone, or fentanyl may be helpful.
4. Obese patients are prone to tachypnea, which may result in inefficient ventilation. It may be necessary to assist or control ventilation in these patients.

in heart rate is sustained and no other causes for tachycardia can be found, the attending veterinarian may decide that administration of pain medication intraoperatively is necessary.

Not all cases of tachycardia require treatment (e.g., those in patients with otherwise normal cardiac function), but the anesthetist should notify the veterinarian before assuming that tachycardia is not significant. It is also important to check the vaporizer setting and anesthetic depth and adjust them if necessary.

TECHNICIAN NOTE

Causes of tachycardia include:
- Drug effects (e.g., anticholinergics, dissociatives, catecholamines)
- Preexisting conditions
- Inadequate anesthetic depth
- Surgical stimulation
- Hypoxemia
- Hypercarbia
- Pain

Bradycardia can be defined as a heart rate less than 60 to 70 bpm in a dog, less than 100 bpm in a cat, less than 25 bpm in a horse, or less than 40 bpm in a cow. Bradycardia may be secondary to the administration of alpha$_2$-agonists or opioids, particularly if anticholinergics were not administered preoperatively. Bradycardia also may result from increased activity of the vagus nerve in response to endotracheal intubation, manipulation of the head and neck, ocular surgery, or handling of the viscera by the surgeon. Bradycardia may also occur if the animal is very deeply anesthetized and when seen in this context, it is a warning that respiratory and cardiac arrest may be imminent. Other causes of bradycardia include hypertension, hyperkalemia, hypothermia, and hypoxia.

Not all cases of bradycardia require treatment. If capillary refill, pulse oximeter readings, blood pressure, and pulse strength appear normal, tissue perfusion may be adequate and treatment may be unnecessary. The veterinarian should be consulted and should direct treatment. If anesthetic depth is excessive, the vaporizer setting should be adjusted, and bagging with 100% oxygen (empty the breathing bag into the scavenging system and refill it with pure oxygen) may be helpful. Bradycardia as a result of the administration of drugs or because of excessive vagal stimulation may be treated with anticholinergics, reversal agents, or a change in the anesthetic protocol. See Case Presentation 13.1 for an example of responding to a change in cardiac rate and rhythm.

TECHNICIAN NOTE

Causes of bradycardia include:
- Drug effects (e.g., alpha$_2$-agonists or opioids)
- Preexisting conditions
- Vagal stimulation associated with endotracheal intubation or manipulation of the head and neck
- Vagal stimulation associated with ocular surgery or manipulation of viscera
- Excessive anesthetic depth
- Hypertension or hyperkalemia
- Hypothermia or hypoxia

CASE PRESENTATION 13.1 Responding to Changes in Cardiac Rate and Rhythm

Ariel, a 3-year-old, female, 4.0-kg, physical status class PS1, domestic short-hair (DSH) cat, was anesthetized in preparation for a minor surgical procedure. She was premedicated with 0.005 mg/kg dexmedetomidine and 0.05 mg/kg hydromorphone intramuscularly (IM) 15 min before anesthetic induction and was induced with 5 mg/kg propofol intravenously (IV) to effect. She was intubated and connected to a modified Jackson–Rees nonrebreathing circuit and placed on isoflurane delivered in 100% oxygen. At the time of intubation, she was in light Stage III anesthesia and after receiving 3% isoflurane for a brief period of time, she was found to be in surgical anesthesia and her vital signs stabilized. At this point, the isoflurane was turned down to 1.5% and an esophageal stethoscope was placed to monitor the heart rate, which at that time was approximately 140 bpm.

During surgical preparation, vital signs remained stable, with the exception of the heart rate, which gradually decreased to approximately 95 bpm. At this point, the attending veterinarian was informed. Ariel was found to be at an appropriate anesthetic depth and other vital signs were normal. The veterinarian postulated that the change in heart rate might have been secondary to the preanesthetic medications, both of which are known to cause bradycardia. She therefore ordered administration of the reversal agents atipamezole and naloxone at standard doses. After 5 more minutes, the heart rate had not improved and, in fact, had decreased slightly to approximately 90 bpm.

1. *What are three possible causes of the bradycardia seen in this patient?*
2. *What steps would you take to identify the cause?*
3. *What actions would you take to maximize the likelihood of a successful outcome?*

The term *cardiac arrhythmia* (or *cardiac dysrhythmia*) refers to any one of a number of electrocardiographic abnormalities, including pulse deficits, also known as dropped beats, ventricular premature contractions (VPCs) arising spontaneously from individual heart muscle cells, and sustained episodes of tachycardia or bradycardia. These abnormalities are most easily detected through the use of an electrocardiogram (ECG) and are often suspected from direct auscultation or from hearing irregularities on a Doppler monitor. The alert technician or nurse also may note that a pulse deficit is present in animals with some types of arrhythmias.

Cardiac arrhythmias commonly arise in animals given arrhythmogenic drugs such as anticholinergics, alpha$_2$-agonists, and catecholamines (such as epinephrine). Such arrhythmias are often of short duration and well tolerated in young, healthy patients but may be a significant problem in animals with preexisting heart disease and in geriatric patients. Arrhythmias are particularly common during induction and light anesthesia. They may also be the result of respiratory depression, hypoxemia, and subsequent hypoxia of the heart muscle. Other causes of cardiac arrhythmias include preexisting heart disease, electrolyte and acid–base disturbances, gastric volvulus, splenic disease, thoracic surgery, endotracheal intubation, and hypercapnia. Hypercapnia may arise from poor anesthetic technique, including exhaustion of the CO_2 absorber crystals or inadequate oxygen flow rates.

PROCEDURE 13.9 Treatment of Cardiac Arrhythmias

1. Continuous electrocardiographic monitoring should commence to track the status of the arrhythmia.
2. The anesthetist should rule out inadequate oxygen flow or CO_2 accumulation within the circuit by using a pulse oximeter and capnograph if available.
3. Ventilation should be increased by periodic intermittent manual ventilation or use of a ventilator.
4. In some cases, antiarrhythmic drugs such as atropine or lidocaine (without epinephrine) may be administered on the veterinarian's orders.

Cardiac arrhythmias should be treated in consultation with the veterinarian (Procedure 13.9).

TECHNICIAN NOTE

Causes of cardiac arrhythmias include:
- Drug effects (e.g., anticholinergics, alpha₂-agonists, and catecholamines)
- Anesthetic induction and light anesthesia
- Hypoxia or hypercapnia
- Preexisting conditions (e.g., gastric volvulus, splenic disease, heart disease, electrolyte, and acid–base disturbances)
- Thoracic surgery and endotracheal intubation

Apnea

Apnea is a temporary cessation of breathing secondary to anesthetic administration, hyperventilation, and a variety of other causes. For instance, respiratory efforts may temporarily cease after the IV injection of propofol, alfaxalone, and other respiratory depressants. It may occur after anesthetic induction by IV injection, mask, or chamber in response to exaggerated breathing that sometimes accompanies light anesthesia and endotracheal intubation. It may also occur secondary to overzealous manual ventilation that has caused blood CO_2 levels to be too low to stimulate respiration. It is temporary and is not usually accompanied by other abnormal vital signs.

Apnea resulting from drug administration or manual ventilation generally should be treated in the same way. First, the anesthetist should closely monitor vital signs and other monitoring parameters, particularly heart rate, mucous membrane color, oxygen saturation, and end-tidal CO_2. If the heartbeat is regular, the heart rate is greater than the minimum acceptable rate (see Table 6.4), the pulse is strong, mucous membranes are pink, oxygen saturation is greater than 95%, and end-tidal CO_2 is normal, the patient does not usually require immediate treatment. In fact, periodic manual ventilation, especially in patients with low end-tidal CO_2 levels, may prolong the period of apnea by decreasing levels further. For this reason, patients should be ventilated only if end-tidal CO_2 readings are over 55 to 60 mmHg.

However, during periods of apnea, occasional breaths of oxygen (1 every 30 to 60 seconds) can be delivered to the patient to prevent hypoxia. If spontaneous respiration does not resume within 1 to 2 minutes, the veterinarian should be consulted, as it may be advisable to increase the rate at which manual ventilation is provided. See Procedure 13.10 for treatment of apnea.

PROCEDURE 13.10 Treatment of Apnea

1. Apnea is a common effect following induction of anesthesia with the IV agents propofol and alfaxalone, and may also occur after induction with other intravenous (IV) drugs, but can occur at other times during the anesthetic procedure.
2. The anesthetist should briefly check to make sure that the patient is intubated and that the endotracheal tube is patent and correctly placed in the trachea.
3. The anesthetist should then make sure the patient's other vital signs (heart rate, blood pressure, mucus membrane color and refill time, and oxygen saturation) are acceptable. If one or more of the parameters is not in the expected range for the anesthetized patient, follow the steps in Procedure 13.11.
4. Breathe for the patient by manually bagging once every 30–60 s. If the patient seems to be inadequately anesthetized, maintain or increase the vaporizer setting. If the patient seems adequately anesthetized, maintain or slightly decrease the vaporizer setting. Bagging should be continued until the patient starts to breathe spontaneously.
5. Monitor the patient's end-tidal CO_2 if a monitor is available. If the end-tidal CO_2 is in or below the normal range, reduce the rate and/or depth of manual breaths. If the end-tidal CO_2 is higher than 55–60 mmHg, then ventilate more frequently or deliver larger tidal volumes.
6. If the patient's depth of anesthesia and other signs are stable but regular breathing does not resume after 15 min of bagging, consult the attending veterinarian to determine whether the patient should be placed on a mechanical ventilator.

TECHNICIAN NOTE

Apnea may be caused by:
- Drug effects (e.g., propofol, alfaxalone)
- Hyperventilation that may accompany anesthetic induction, intubation, and light planes of anesthesia
- Overzealous manual ventilation

Respiratory Arrest

Respiratory arrest is the total cessation of breathing. It may occur after a period of prolonged apnea or may be caused by anesthetic overdose, cessation of oxygen flow, and preexisting respiratory disease such as pneumothorax or diaphragmatic hernia. Breathing is controlled by the central nervous system; thus diseases of the CNS, such as brain tumors or meningitis, may also cause respiratory arrest. It is often accompanied by other abnormal vital signs. Consequently, respiratory arrest and apnea are distinguished primarily by seriousness, causes, and accompanying signs. Respiratory arrest is a common precursor to cardiac arrest and is therefore potentially fatal. Affected animals may show warning signs such as a slowing respiratory rate, dyspnea, and/or cyanosis before respiratory arrest occurs. Other vital signs, such as heart rate, capillary refill time, pulse strength, and pupil size, are often abnormal. Pulse oximetry values rapidly fall below 90%. The treatment of respiratory arrest involves the steps shown in Procedure 13.11.

The primary cause of respiratory arrest must be corrected if possible. Periodic, intermittent manual ventilation should be initiated and should continue until the heart rate, mucous membrane color, and pulse oximeter values have been restored to

PROCEDURE 13.11 Treatment of Respiratory Arrest

1. Inform the veterinarian.
2. If the patient is not intubated, an endotracheal tube should be immediately inserted and the patient connected to an anesthetic machine delivering 100% oxygen.
3. Check the heart rate to ensure that cardiac arrest has not occurred.
4. Turn off the anesthetic vaporizer.
5. Ensure oxygen flow is adequate by checking the tank pressure gauge and flowmeter.
6. Ensure the airway is not obstructed by bagging the patient and observing that the chest rises when squeezing the bag (during inspiration).
7. Bag the patient with oxygen at a rate of once every 3–5 s. Continue bagging until vital signs improve (particularly mucous membrane color, heart rate, and pulse oximeter readings).
8. The veterinarian may advise that reversal agents, doxapram, or other drugs be given.
9. Ensure that the patient is kept warm.

normal. Once this is achieved, the anesthetist should discontinue bagging for 15 to 30 seconds and closely observe the patient for respiratory efforts. If none are seen, bagging should resume. It is important not to ventilate excessively, as this can drive CO_2 to low levels, which will eliminate respiratory drive and, if CO_2 is decreased below 25 mmHg, will cause vasoconstriction, leading to cerebral hypoxia. On occasion, the anesthetist may be faced with a patient in respiratory arrest when no anesthetic machine is available. It is possible to substitute a manual resuscitator bag (Fig. 13.3) or even institute mouth-to-ETT or mouth-to-snout resuscitation in these cases.

> **TECHNICIAN NOTE**
> Respiratory arrest may be caused by:
> * Prolonged apnea
> * Anesthetic overdose
> * Cessation of oxygen flow
> * Preexisting respiratory disease such as pneumothorax or diaphragmatic hernia
> * Central nervous system diseases such as brain tumors or meningitis

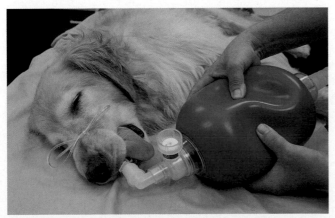

FIG. 13.3 Use of a manual resuscitator bag (Ambu bag) to deliver room air to an intubated patient.

Cardiac Arrest

Cardiac arrest is a cessation of the circulation of oxygenated blood to the tissues due to the failure of the heart to pump effectively. Cardiac arrest usually follows abnormal electrical activity through the cardiac conduction system, which arises from a variety of causes including drug reactions, hypoxia of the heart muscle, disease conditions such as gastric dilatation–volvulus, heart muscle trauma, and anesthetic overdose. Owing to the cardiac depressive effects of many anesthetic agents and adjuncts as well as the hypoxemia, hypotension, and hypoventilation that often accompany the administration of anesthetics, cardiac arrest may occur at any time during general anesthesia and may be preceded by or may follow respiratory arrest. In most cases, the anesthetist receives some warning that arrest is imminent in the form of a short period in which cyanosis, dyspnea or respiratory arrest, and prolonged capillary refill are evident, often accompanied by an arrhythmia. If cardiac arrest appears imminent, the anesthetist should immediately alert the veterinarian and the hospital staff while continuing to monitor the heart rate directly by auscultation or palpation of the chest and the heart rhythm through the use of an ECG. A patient experiencing cardiac arrest rapidly develops the following signs:

* No heartbeat can be auscultated or palpated and normal P waves and QRS complexes are absent from the ECG tracing.
* There is no palpable arterial pulse and blood pressure readings (if available) are ≤25 mmHg.
* Mucous membranes are gray or cyanotic and capillary refill may be prolonged.
* Pupils are widely dilated with no response to light and corneal reflex is absent.
* Respiration is absent except for intermittent, abrupt gasps (agonal breaths).

> **TECHNICIAN NOTE**
> Cardiac arrest may be caused by:
> * Respiratory arrest
> * Drug reactions
> * Hypoxia of the heart muscle
> * Disease conditions such as gastric dilatation–volvulus and heart muscle trauma
> * Anesthetic overdose

Cardiopulmonary Arrest

As previously mentioned, cardiac arrest and respiratory arrest often closely follow one another, with either cardiac failure or respiratory failure occurring first. Once arrest occurs, permanent brain damage is highly likely to occur if oxygen delivery to the brain is not reestablished within approximately 5 minutes by either cardiopulmonary resuscitation (CPR) or restoration of cardiac function. Therefore coordinated action by all hospital staff members is essential to reverse cardiopulmonary arrest.

Cardiopulmonary Resuscitation in Veterinary Species

Until very recently, there was significant controversy regarding the most effective way to perform CPR in veterinary species.

This is because traditionally accepted veterinary CPR guidelines (such as the ABCs of CPR) have primarily been based on the accepted principles of human CPR (which—although often applicable—are not necessarily as effective in animals as they are in people) and the opinions of veterinary clinicians, which differ even among experts in the field of emergency and critical care.

In 2011, a comprehensive study called the "Reassessment Campaign on Veterinary Resuscitation (RECOVER)" was initiated to examine long-held assumptions regarding CPR in a systematic manner by reviewing the available scientific literature on the topic with input from members of the American College of Emergency and Critical Care (ACECC) and the American College of Veterinary Anesthesia and Analgesia (ACVAA). The objective of the **RECOVER initiative** was to develop guidelines based on scientific research. *(See Box 13.1 for a brief summary of the RECOVER initiative.)* The release of the results of this study in 2012 marked the first time that veterinary professionals have had evidence-based guidelines to use when performing CPR on veterinary species.

The RECOVER Clinical Guidelines differ significantly in a number of important ways from the traditional approach to CPR. Therefore it is essential that all veterinary personnel, even those who are experienced, are familiar with and trained to follow these guidelines, which are the basis for the principles of CPR as presented in this chapter.

Terminology of Cardiopulmonary Resuscitation

Before discussing the RECOVER guidelines, it is important that the reader be familiar with some terms and abbreviations that relate to CPR. The foundation of effective CPR is basic life support (BLS), which consists of the recognition that the patient is in cardiopulmonary arrest, and then the application of heart compressions and manual ventilation with the goal of oxygenating the tissues. Advanced life support (ALS) closely follows the initiation of BLS and involves monitoring the patient, as well as administration of drugs, fluid therapy, and electrical defibrillation, if indicated. Successful CPR results in return of spontaneous circulation (ROSC), which is the return of effective tissue perfusion with oxygenated blood, and finally, **postarrest care (PAC)** must follow to minimize permanent effects and maximize the likelihood of recovery and discharge from the hospital. The RECOVER guidelines address each of these aspects of CPR. Table 13.2 lists recommended doses of drugs that may be used in the postarrest period.

Preparation for Cardiopulmonary Resuscitation

The statistics regarding the success of CPR are far from ideal. Several studies suggest that fewer than 6% of veterinary patients are discharged from the hospital following cardiopulmonary arrest (CPA).[d] These percentages are considerably better for animals that suffer CPA during an anesthetic event, primarily because these cases are usually caught very early and CPR is often initiated without delay. Therefore the actions taken during CPR must be coordinated, rapid, and effective in order to maximize the likelihood of successful resuscitation efforts.

All personnel involved must be prepared in every way for an event of CPA well before it happens. This means that equipment must be available in the immediate area and must be functioning,

---

> ### BOX 13.1   The "Reassessment Campaign on Veterinary Resuscitation (RECOVER)"
>
> - A comprehensive study conducted between 2011 and 2012 by Dr. Daniel Fletcher and Dr. Manuel Boller to examine long-held assumptions regarding cardiopulmonary resuscitation (CPR) in a systematic manner.
> - The objectives of this study were:
>   1. To facilitate an evidence-based review of the current literature on veterinary CPR
>   2. To derive a draft set of clinical guidelines for veterinary CPR based on review of the evidence
>   3. To collate and incorporate feedback from the veterinary community at large and develop a set of consensus CPR guidelines
>   4. To disseminate these consensus, evidence-based, veterinary CPR guidelines widely
> - In 2012, the results of this study were published in the *Journal of Veterinary Emergency and Critical Care*, Special Issue: Reassessment Campaign on Veterinary Resuscitation: Evidence and Knowledge Gap Analysis on Veterinary CPR Volume 22, Issue s1, June 2012. The guidelines may be found under "Part 7: Clinical Guidelines" on pages S102–S131 of this issue.
> - As of the time of this writing, a review of the RECOVER Initiative is available at http://www.acvecc-recover.org/, and the Special RECOVER issue is available at https://recoverinitiative.org/cpr-guidelines/current-recover-guideline/. It is likely that the RECOVER guidelines will be reviewed and updated by the time this text is published. We recommend checking the RECOVER Initiative website periodically for updates.

---

[d]Fletcher DJ, Boller M, Brainard BM: RECOVER evidence and knowledge gap analysis on veterinary CPR. *J Vet Emerg Crit Care* 22(S1):S5, 2012.

TABLE 13.2   Drugs Used During the Postarrest Period in Cats and Dogs

Drug	Dose for IV Use	Indications for Use/Mode of Action
Midazolam or diazepam	0.2–1 mg/kg	Treatment of seizures
Dobutamine	1–20 mcg/kg/min infusion in 5% dextrose	Treatment of hypotension by increasing the force of myocardial contractions
Dopamine	5–15 mcg/kg/min infusion in lactated Ringer solution	Treatment of hypotension by increasing the force of myocardial contractions and the heart rate (doses above 10 mcg/kg/min will increase systemic vascular resistance via alpha$_1$ effects)
Doxapram	1–4 mg/kg	Respiratory and central nervous system stimulant
Mannitol (25%)	0.5 g/kg IV/IO over 15–20 min	Osmotic diuretic used to treat cerebral edema
Norepinephrine	0.05–0.1 mcg/kg/min infusion	A vasoconstrictor used for postarrest hypotension due to vasodilation
Vasopressin	0.5–5.0 mU/kg/min infusion	Increases rate and force of cardiac contractions, increases systemic vascular resistance

drugs and drug dosage charts must be available and easily accessible, and personnel must be trained and ready to act quickly.

In addition, CPR is very challenging to perform effectively alone, although it may be performed by one person if circumstances require it. Consequently, a team with three to five members is helpful, provided that all members of the team are well trained and have participated in simulations, have clearly defined roles, and a team leader is identified. Clear communication among team members is essential so that orders are promptly followed, team members act in a coordinated fashion, and actions are effective. Although the optimal team size is unknown, there is evidence that excessively large teams may in fact decrease the effectiveness of CPR.

> **TECHNICIAN NOTE**
>
> The response to CPR is considerably better for animals that suffer CPA during an anesthetic event, primarily because these cases are usually caught very early and CPR is often initiated without delay. The actions taken during CPR must be coordinated, rapid, and effective.

As shown in the RECOVER CPR Algorithm (Fig. 13.4), the initial tasks that must be divided among the team are

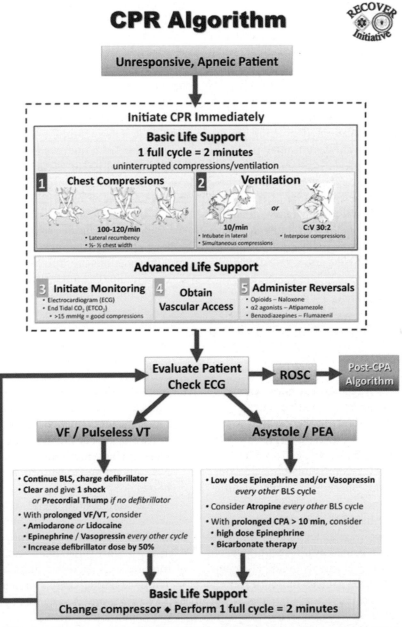

FIG. 13.4 Cardiopulmonary resuscitation *(CPR)* algorithm. Note that the first five steps of CPR (numbered 1 through 5) are summarized in the box outlined with the dashed lines at the top of the page. The first two steps (1. Chest Compressions and 2. Ventilation) constitute basic life support, and the remaining three steps (3. Initiate Monitoring, 4. Obtain Vascular Access, and 5. Administer Reversals) are part of advanced life support. The lower half of the page shows the steps associated with assessment of the cardiac rhythm and therapies intended to normalize the cardiac rhythm. (From RECOVER evidence and knowledge gap analysis on veterinary CPR. Part 7: Clinical guidelines, *J Vet Emerg Crit Care* 22(S1):S102–S131, 2012.)

(1) application of chest compressions, (2) endotracheal intubation and manual ventilation, (3) initiation of ECG and end-tidal CO_2 monitoring, (4) placement of an IV catheter, and (5) administration of reversal agents if opioids or sedatives have been given.

After these actions have been taken, additional steps are followed to identify the heart rhythm and restore the normal heart rhythm by administering drugs or performing electrical defibrillation. If ROSC is achieved, a post-cardiac arrest protocol is followed to optimize blood oxygen and CO_2 levels, oxygen delivery, blood pressure, and brain function. The steps of CPR are detailed below.

Basic Life Support

In any patient that is apneic and nonresponsive, the first step of BLS is to confirm that the animal has arrested, as evidenced by the absence of an audible heartbeat, apical pulse, and peripheral pulse. This initial assessment should be performed quickly (ideally over no more than 5 to 10 seconds). At that point, chest compressions should be initiated, closely followed by endotracheal intubation and manual ventilation. If you are unsure whether or not the patient is in CPA, chest compressions should be instituted immediately and the patient reevaluated by other personnel (if present) as the chest compressions are performed.

If an anesthetized patient is confirmed to be in cardiac arrest, any anesthetic drugs being delivered (inhalants, infusions) should be turned off immediately. The oxygen flow rate can be increased and the reservoir bag emptied and refilled with the oxygen flush valve to quickly decrease the anesthetic concentration in the breathing system.

> **TECHNICIAN NOTE**
> If you are unsure whether or not the patient is in CPA, chest compressions should be instituted immediately and the patient reevaluated by other personnel (if present) as the chest compressions are performed.

Step #1 of cardiopulmonary resuscitation: Chest compressions. High-quality chest compressions should be initiated immediately because they have been shown to be the single most important factor in successful ROSC. Chest compressions are effective when they result in forward blood flow. To understand the reasons behind the RECOVER recommendations, the compressor must understand the two commonly accepted theories regarding how forward blood flow is generated during CPR and how one may exploit each mechanism when providing chest compressions. The cardiac pump theory states that blood flow to the tissues and back to the lungs is caused by direct compression of the ventricles between the ribs (for patients in lateral recumbency) or the sternum and spine (for patients in dorsal recumbency). In contrast, the thoracic pump theory postulates that blood flow to the tissues results from compression of the aorta resulting from increased intrathoracic pressure, which in turn is caused by compression of the chest wall by the hands of the compressor; blood flow back into the thorax and to the lungs is thought to result from negative intrathoracic pressure that occurs during recoil of the chest wall between compressions. It is further thought that in most patients, blood flow is likely to result from

both mechanisms to some extent, with one or the other predominating depending on the size and chest conformation of the patient. For instance, small dogs and cats often have chest walls that are easier to compress, so blood flow can likely be maximized by employing the cardiac pump theory (by compressing the chest wall in a lateral direction directly over the heart using one or both hands). The cardiac pump theory may also predominate in keel-chested breeds, such as the sighthounds, because their chests are narrow side to side and so can be compressed directly over the heart in this direction, and in barrel-chested breeds, such as the English Bulldog, because their chests are often wider than they are deep and so can be compressed over the sternum while in dorsal recumbency. In contrast, the size and stiffness of the chest wall in most other medium- to giant breed dogs renders direct compression of the heart wall very difficult to achieve. Thus the thoracic pump theory is probably more easily employed by applying compressions over the widest portion of the chest wall in a lateral direction in these patients.

In view of these considerations, the RECOVER guidelines recommend that most patients be placed on their right or left side with the feet away from the person applying the compressions. A two-handed technique over the widest part of the chest should be used at a rate of 100 to 120 bpm (Fig. 13.5A). The American Heart Association recommends compressing to the beat of the disco song "Stayin' Alive" by the Bee Gees to achieve this rate. The chest should be compressed by one-third to one-half of its width and the chest wall should be allowed to reexpand completely between compressions (a phenomenon known as full elastic recoil). These recommendations are intended to maximize blood flow by the thoracic pump. The following variations may be considered:

- Two-handed compression directly over the heart in a lateral direction may be considered in keel-chested breeds (such as sighthounds) (see Fig. 13.5 B).
- Two-handed compression on the sternum directly over the heart (while in dorsal recumbency) may be considered in barrel-chested breeds (such as English Bulldogs) (see Fig. 13.5 C)
- A one-handed-technique directly over the heart may be considered in small dogs and cats (Fig 13.6 A)
- As an alternative, a two-handed-technique directly over the heart may be considered in larger cats and small dogs with relatively low chest wall compliance (see Fig. 13.6 B).
- *Note*: Attempting to perform compressions in adult cattle and horses does not produce effective circulation. CPR is limited to drug administration and ventilation in these patients.

When done correctly, especially on medium- to giant breed dogs, chest compressions require an extraordinary amount of energy to perform effectively. Studies indicate that the efficiency of compressions decreases significantly after only 2 minutes or so. For this reason, it is recommended that compressors switch over every 2 minutes. (See Box 13.2 for a summary of Step #1 of Cardiopulmonary Resuscitation: Chest Compressions.)

> **TECHNICIAN NOTE**
> As recommended by the American Heart Association, CPR chest compressions should be timed to the beat of the disco song "Stayin' Alive" by the Bee Gees to achieve the recommended rate of 100–120 bpm.

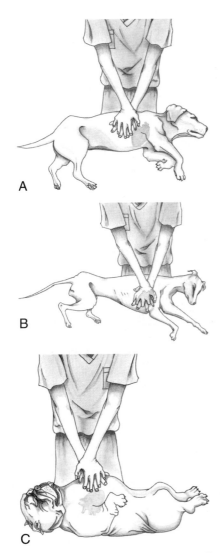

FIG. 13.5 (A) Chest compression technique for medium, large, and giant breed dogs. (B) Alternative chest compression technique for keel-chested breeds. (C) Alternative chest compression technique for barrel-chested breeds.(From RECOVER evidence and knowledge gap analysis on veterinary CPR. Part 7: Clinical guidelines, *J Vet Emerg Crit Care* 22(S1), S102–S131, 2012.)

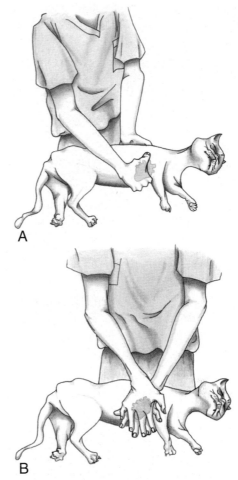

FIG. 13.6 (A) One-handed chest compression technique for small dogs and cats less than 10 kg in body weight that have a relatively compliant chest wall. When using this technique, one hand is wrapped around the sternum directly over the heart. (B) Alternative compression technique for larger cats and small dogs that have a relatively low chest wall compliance. This technique may also be used if the compressor is fatigued. When using this technique, both hands are placed directly over the heart. (From RECOVER evidence and knowledge gap analysis on veterinary CPR. Part 7: Clinical guidelines, *J Vet Emerg Crit Care* 22(S1):S102–S131, 2012.)

Interposed abdominal compressions. Interposed abdominal compressions are felt to maximize blood flow during CPR by increasing return of blood to the heart from the abdomen. To perform this technique, a rescuer should apply pressure to the abdominal cavity with the flat of the hand during the recoil phase of each chest compression (Fig. 13.7). Thus chest compressions and interposed abdominal compressions are applied in a seesaw fashion. This technique is challenging to perform without interrupting chest compressions and so should be used by personnel who have been trained and who have practiced this technique.

Step #2 of cardiopulmonary resuscitation: Intubation and ventilation. As soon as chest compressions are initiated, the patient should be given ventilatory support. This has been found to be especially important in patients with CPA of noncardiac origin (patients that arrest from choking, anesthetic-related CPA, and so on). If working alone, or if endotracheal

---

BOX 13.2   Step #1 of Cardiopulmonary Resuscitation: Chest Compressions

- Start chest compressions immediately after identification of CPA.
- Perform compressions in uninterrupted 2-min cycles.
- Place most patients in lateral recumbency (right or left) with the feet away from you. (Dorsal recumbency may be considered for brachycephalic breeds.)
- Use a two-handed technique over the widest portion of the chest cavity. (A one-handed technique directly over the heart may be considered for small dogs and cats. Compression directly over the heart in a lateral direction may be considered for keel-chested breeds. Compression directly over the heart on the sternum [while in dorsal recumbency] may be considered for barrel-chested breeds.)
- Compress the chest at a rate of 100–120 per minute.
- Compress the chest by one-third to one-half its width.
- Allow full elastic recoil between compressions.

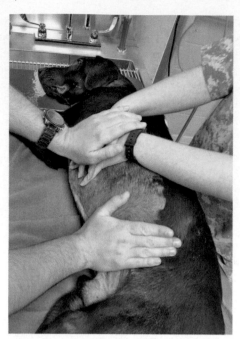

FIG. 13.7 Interposed abdominal compressions. (From Bassert JM, Thomas JA: *McCurnin's clinical textbook for veterinary technicians*, ed 8, St. Louis, MO, 2014, Elsevier.)

intubation is not feasible, mouth-to-snout breaths may be given by pausing briefly after 30 chest compressions to deliver 2 quick breaths, and then immediately resuming chest compressions (Fig. 13.8). These breaths are delivered by holding the patient's mouth closed, placing your lips around the patient's nares, and blowing until the chest wall is expanded as with a normal breath. If multiple rescuers are present, intubation should be performed with the patient in lateral recumbency, and ventilation with 100% oxygen should be initiated at a rate of 10 breaths/min and a tidal volume of 10 mL/kg while another rescuer compresses the chest. Breaths and chest compressions should be delivered simultaneously (compressions should NOT be stopped when breaths are given). In addition, the anesthetist must ensure that the patient's chest rises slightly during bagging, indicating that the airway is not blocked and the tube is not placed in the esophagus.

Ventilation with room air is a reasonable alternative if oxygen is not available and, in fact, prevents over-oxygenation, which may be damaging to pulmonary tissues, especially over a long period of time. However, the use of 100% oxygen is recommended in the RECOVER guidelines unless arterial blood gas monitoring is used to monitor blood oxygen levels. (See Box 13.3 for a summary of Step #2 of Cardiopulmonary Resuscitation: Intubation and Ventilation.)

TECHNICIAN NOTE
During basic life support, breaths and chest compressions should be delivered simultaneously (compressions should NOT be stopped when breaths are given).

Advanced Life Support

As soon as chest compressions and ventilation have been implemented, the following steps of ALS should be initiated: (3) ECG

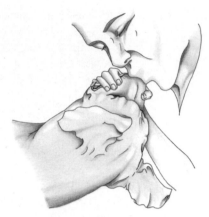

FIG. 13.8 Mouth-to-snout breathing technique. (From RECOVER evidence and knowledge gap analysis on veterinary CPR. Part 7: Clinical guidelines, *J Vet Emerg Crit Care* 22(S1):S102–S131, 2012.)

BOX 13.3 Step #2 of Cardiopulmonary Resuscitation: Intubation and Ventilation

- If multiple rescuers are present:
  1. Intubate the patient while in lateral recumbency without interrupting chest compressions.
  2. Provide breaths of 100% oxygen (if available) with a reservoir bag of an anesthetic machine or a manual resuscitator bag (e.g., Ambu bag) at a rate of 10 breaths/min, a tidal volume of approximately 10 mL/kg, and a short inspiratory time.
- If alone or intubation is not feasible:
  1. After every 30 chest compressions, provide 2 quick breaths using mouth-to-snout ventilation (hold the patient's mouth closed, create a seal with your lips around the patient's nares, and blow until the chest rises as with a normal breath).
  2. The compression to breath ratio should be 30:2.

BOX 13.4 Steps #3, #4, and #5 of Cardiopulmonary Resuscitation: Monitoring, IV Catheterization, and Administration of Reversal Agents

- Attach electrocardiogram (ECG) electrodes and commence ECG monitoring to assess the cardiac rhythm and guide treatment. Use physiologic saline or ECG gel to wet the electrodes.
- Commence end-tidal CO_2 monitoring to assess the effectiveness of chest compressions. An end-tidal CO_2 level of >15 mmHg during the exhalation phase of manual ventilation indicates adequate forward movement of blood.
- Place an intravenous (IV) catheter in a peripheral vein (if not already present) and administer drugs and fluids as directed by the attending veterinarian. If IV access cannot be obtained, the intraosseous route may be used or selected drugs (epinephrine, vasopressin, and atropine) may be given by the intratracheal route via a urinary catheter.
- If the patient has received reversible sedatives or anesthetics (alpha$_2$-agonists, opioids, or benzodiazepines), administer appropriate reversal agents.

and end-tidal CO_2 monitoring, (4) obtaining vascular access, and (5) administration of reversal agents. (See Box 13.4 for a summary of these procedures.)

Step #3: Electrocardiogram and end-tidal CO_2 monitoring. Placement of ECG electrodes is recommended to give the CPR team information regarding the underlying cardiac rhythm of the patient. Compressions should not be halted in order to place leads. It is imperative that alcohol *not* be used to wet electrode–patient contacts if a defibrillator is available, as it could result in an explosion if defibrillation is attempted. Physiologic saline or ECG gel should be used instead.

In addition to ECG monitoring, a capnograph should be used to monitor the quality of chest compressions. In an animal that has arrested, the end-tidal CO_2 will be zero or close to zero because the CO_2 that is produced at the tissue level is not transported to the lungs; thus little to no CO_2 is detected in exhaled air. Forward movement of blood produced by effective chest compressions will transport CO_2 to the lungs in sufficient quantities to be detected. Therefore an end-tidal CO_2 level >15 mmHg during the exhalation phase of manual ventilation is considered to indicate adequate forward movement of blood. If this level is not reached, the method of compression should be adjusted by changing the rate or intensity, by repositioning the patient, or by assigning the compression task to another rescuer.

Step #4: Obtaining vascular access. As soon as feasible, an IV catheter should be placed in a peripheral vein for administration of fluids and emergency drugs, such as those used to normalize the heart rhythm. If attempts to access a vein are unsuccessful, the intraosseous (IO) route can be used as an alternative. This is more likely to be necessary in exotic animal species, small patients, and pediatric patients because these patients have smaller veins that are more difficult to catheterize, especially during CPA.

If IV or IO access is difficult, drugs may be given by injection into the base of the tongue or by intratracheal administration.

Epinephrine, vasopressin, and atropine may be given by the intratracheal route. Although the optimal dose for intratracheal administration is not known, many sources recommend twice the IV dose. The drug should be diluted with saline or sterile water and administered by means of a urinary catheter passed through the ETT to the level of the tracheal bifurcation or beyond.

Intracardiac injections should be avoided if possible because injections by this route require the interruption of chest compressions and have some potential to damage the myocardium or lacerate coronary blood vessels. As a last resort, drugs may be injected into the left ventricle.

Step #5: Administration of reversal agents. If the patient has received sedative or anesthetic drugs prior to arrest for which reversal agents are available (alpha$_2$-agonists, opioids, or benzodiazepines), the appropriate reversal agent(s) should be administered according to the CPR Emergency Drugs and Doses (Fig. 13.9).

> **TECHNICIAN NOTE**
>
> When performing CPR, an end-tidal CO_2 level greater than 15 mmHg during the exhalation phase of manual ventilation is considered indicative of adequate forward movement of blood.

Additional steps of advanced life support. After each 2-minute cycle of BLS, compressions should be briefly paused, during which compressors should be changed, the patient should be evaluated for ROSC, and the ECG tracing should be evaluated for a rhythm diagnosis. This information will be used to determine

CPR Emergency Drugs and Doses

	DRUG	DOSE	Weight (kg) 2.5 / Weight (lb) 5 / ml	5 / 10 / ml	10 / 20 / ml	15 / 30 / ml	20 / 40 / ml	25 / 50 / ml	30 / 60 / ml	35 / 70 / ml	40 / 80 / ml	45 / 90 / ml	50 / 100 / ml
Arrest	Epi Low (1:1000; 1mg/ml) every other BLS cycle x3	0.01 mg/kg	0.03	0.05	0.1	0.15	0.2	0.25	0.3	0.35	0.4	0.45	0.5
	Epi High (1:1000; 1 mg/ml) for prolonged CPR	0.1 mg/kg	0.25	0.5	1	1.5	2	2.5	3	3.5	4	4.5	5
	Vasopressin (20 U/ml)	0.8 U/kg	0.1	0.2	0.4	0.6	0.8	1	1.2	1.4	1.6	1.8	2
	Atropine (0.54 mg/ml)	0.04 mg/kg	0.2	0.4	0.8	1.1	1.5	1.9	2.2	2.6	3	3.3	3.7
Anti-Arrhyth	Amiodarone (50 mg/ml)	5 mg/kg	0.25	0.5	1	1.5	2	2.5	3	3.5	4	4.5	5
	Lidocaine (20 mg/ml)	2 mg/kg	0.25	0.5	1	1.5	2	2.5	3	3.5	4	4.5	5
Reversal	Naloxone (0.4 mg/ml)	0.04 mg/kg	0.25	0.5	1	1.5	2	2.5	3	3.5	4	4.5	5
	Flumazenil (0.1 mg/ml)	0.01 mg/kg	0.25	0.5	1	1.5	2	2.5	3	3.5	4	4.5	5
	Atipamezole (5 mg/ml)	100 µg/kg	0.06	0.1	0.2	0.3	0.4	0.5	0.6	0.7	0.8	0.9	1
Defib	External Defib (J)	4-6 J/kg	10	20	40	60	80	100	120	140	160	180	200
	Internal Defib (J)	0.5-1 J/kg	2	3	5	8	10	15	15	20	20	20	25

FIG. 13.9 Cardiopulmonary resuscitation *(CPR)* emergency drugs and doses. *Anti-arrhyth,* antiarrhythmic drugs; *Defib,* electrical defibrillation; *Epi,* epinephrine. (From RECOVER evidence and knowledge gap analysis on veterinary CPR. Part 7: Clinical guidelines, *J Vet Emerg Crit Care* 22(S1):S102–S131, 2012.)

what steps need to be taken to normalize the heart rhythm. These therapies may include administration of vasopressors, vagolytics, and antiarrhythmic drugs, as well as electrical defibrillation. General anesthesia decreases sympathetic tone; thus administration of vagolytics such as atropine is often prudent in anesthetized patients that have arrested.

Evaluation for return of spontaneous circulation. ROSC is confirmed by the detection of a spontaneous pulse in a peripheral artery (such as the femoral artery). Other signs that support ROSC include the presence of normal complexes on the ECG tracing, the presence of audible heart sounds on auscultation, or the presence of increasing end-tidal CO_2 concentrations on a capnogram.

At any point that ROSC is confirmed, chest compressions should be discontinued and post cardiac arrest care should be instituted (see page 429). Note that bagging must be maintained until spontaneous breathing is established, which may require up to several hours. The anesthetist should periodically check the capillary refill time, mucous membrane color, and heart rate, and should discontinue bagging only if these vital signs appear normal. If mucous membrane color deteriorates or if spontaneous respiration does not occur within 1 minute after bagging has been discontinued, bagging should be resumed.

Evaluation of the electrocardiogram tracing for a rhythm diagnosis. When evaluating the ECG tracing of a patient in CPA, one of four rhythms is commonly observed:

- Asystole (no electrical activity, or flatline): On an electrocardiogram, this rhythm appears as a flat baseline with no visible waveforms or complexes, and the heart is not beating (Fig. 13.10).

- Pulseless electrical activity (PEA): A normal or nearly normal ECG tracing is evident, but this organized electrical activity does not produce any cardiac contractions (Fig. 13.11). Patients with this rhythm have no pulse and no heart muscle contractions and therefore no forward movement of blood. PEA (also known as electromechanical dissociation [EMD]) is the hardest rhythm to treat.
- Ventricular fibrillation (VF): This is a pattern of chaotic and disorganized electrical activity that appears as coarse vertical zigzag lines that do not resemble normal complexes (Fig. 13.12). When viewed directly, the heart muscle writhes and has the appearance of a bag of worms.
- Pulseless ventricular tachycardia (VT): This rhythm is a continuous series of wide and bizarre QRS complexes that occur very close together (ventricular premature complexes or VPCs) in a patient that has no palpable pulse (Fig. 13.13). In patients with this rhythm, forward blood flow is inadequate to maintain blood pressure or tissue perfusion.

TECHNICIAN NOTE

The four most common cardiac rhythms associated with CPA are:
- Asystole
- PEA
- VF
- Pulseless VT

Normalizing the heart rhythm. Appropriate therapy depends on the ECG diagnosis. Asystole and PEA are most likely to respond to BLS and administration of vasopressor drugs (epinephrine or vasopressin). In contrast, VF and pulseless VT

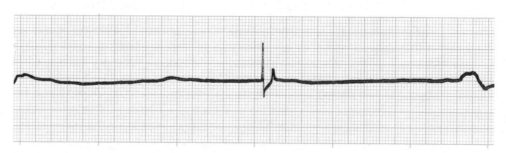

FIG. 13.10 This electrocardiogram (ECG) is from an arrested animal in asystole (flatline). A single escape complex is present near the middle. (From Bassert JM, McCurnin DM: *McCurnin's clinical textbook for veterinary technicians*, ed 7, St. Louis, MO, 2010, Elsevier.)

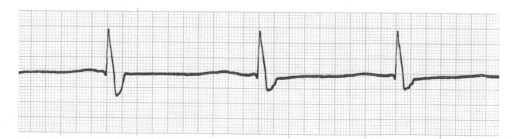

FIG. 13.11 This electrocardiogram (ECG) pattern, accompanied by lack of palpable pulses, is called *pulseless electrical activity,* or *electromechanical dissociation.* Note that at first glance, the QRS complexes resemble normal complexes, but closer evaluation reveals notable differences including wide complexes, prolonged R-R intervals, an absence of P waves, and an absence of normal T waves.

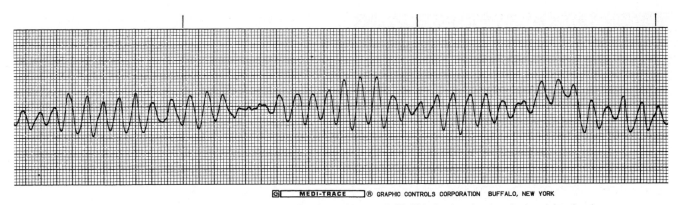

FIG. 13.12 Ventricular fibrillation (dog—lead II; 50 mm/s; 1 cm/mV). This is chaotic electrical activity that is not associated with organized contraction of the heart muscle. (From Birchard SJ, Sherding RG: *Saunders manual of small animal practice*, ed 3, St Louis, MO, 2006, Elsevier.)

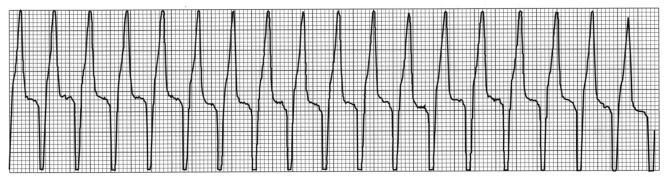

FIG. 13.13 Pulseless ventricular tachycardia (dog—lead II; 25 mm/s; 1.6 cm/mV). This is a series of wide, bizarre QRS complexes followed by T waves.

are most likely to respond to BLS and electrical defibrillation (Procedure 13.12). In all cases, the veterinarian, if present, should authorize the type, dosage, and route of the drugs to be administered, and the use of a defibrillator should be authorized and directly supervised by a veterinarian.

Treatment of asystole or pulseless electrical activity. Asystole and PEA may be treated with low-dose epinephrine and/or vasopressin. Atropine may also be considered if a high parasympathetic tone is suspected. In the event that either of these rhythms persists for longer than 10 minutes, high-dose epinephrine and bicarbonate therapy may be considered. Discussion of each of these drugs follows.

VASOPRESSOR DRUGS. Vasopressors are drugs that increase the tone of the peripheral vessels. This redirects blood to vital organs such as the brain and heart. The two drugs that fall in this category are epinephrine and vasopressin.

Epinephrine. Epinephrine is a powerful sympathetic nervous system stimulant (adrenergic agonist) that increases peripheral vascular tone (by binding to alpha$_1$ receptors) and increases the strength of heart contractions as well as the heart rate (by binding to beta$_1$ receptors). Adverse effects include increasing the heart muscle's oxygen demand, which may result in heart damage owing to the decreased oxygen levels associated with CPA, and tachyarrhythmias. For many decades, it has been the drug most commonly used for the initial treatment of cardiac arrest. It is one of the first-line drugs used to treat asystole and PEA.

Epinephrine may be administered using one of two dosages that differ by a factor of 10. Under the RECOVER guidelines, the low dose (0.1 mL/10 kg body weight IV) is recommended every other 2-minute BLS cycle unless there has been no ROSC for over 10 minutes, in which case the high dose (1.0 mL/10 kg body weight IV) may be considered. Epinephrine is supplied in a concentration of 1:1000 (1 mg/mL). Consequently, when using the low-dose protocol, cats, small dogs, medium dogs, and large dogs receive approximately 0.05, 0.1, 0.2, and 0.3 mL, respectively. When using the high-dose protocol, the volume given is increased by a factor of 10 (*see Fig. 13.9*).

Vasopressin. Vasopressin works in a different way than epinephrine to increase vascular resistance (by binding to V1 receptors). Vasopressin may be used in place of epinephrine or alternated with doses of epinephrine to treat asystole or PEA. The recommended dose is 0.4 mL/10 kg. Like epinephrine, vasopressin is administered every other 2-minute BLS cycle. At the time of this writing, vasopressin is very expensive, costing over $100 per vial and consequently, its use may be cost prohibitive.

ATROPINE. Atropine is a parasympathetic nervous system blocker (anticholinergic) that is used to prevent and treat bradycardia secondary to high parasympathetic tone. Therefore it may be beneficial in animals with asystole or PEA associated with high parasympathetic tone. Atropine is frequently indicated with anesthesia-related cardiac arrest and can be administered by IV every 15 to 20 minutes.

PROCEDURE 13.12 Defibrillation

1. Chest compressions should be carried out for at least 2 min before defibrillation and should be continued at all times unless the patient is being actively defibrillated.
2. The defibrillator should be turned on. Many modern defibrillators require use of the defibrillator's ECG component in order to function correctly.
3. An assistant sets the appropriate amount of joules as directed by the veterinarian. Typically, the first shock uses the lowest setting for the size of the patient.

RECOVER Guidelines for Defibrillation:
External defibrillation: monophasic: 4–6 J/kg; biphasic: 2–4 J/kg
Internal defibrillation: 0.5–1.0 J/kg
If the abnormal rhythm is prolonged, consider increasing the dose by 50%.

4. If external defibrillation is being used, the paddles are coated with conducting gel. If the thorax is open, sterilized internal paddles should be opened using sterile technique, taken by the person performing internal cardiac massage, then soaked with sterile saline. The assistant will have to connect the internal paddles to the defibrillator.
5. The operator then places the external paddles firmly against the skin over the heart according to the directions on the paddles (RECOVER guidelines recommend placing them on opposite sides of the thorax over the costochondral junction); internal paddles are placed on either side of the heart.
6. The defibrillator either makes a "Ready" sound or shows that it is ready on a light-emitting diode (LED) display.
7. The operator clearly announces the word "Clear!" to warn other personnel that an electrical shock is about to be delivered, and that they should stand away from the patient and the table or surface on which the patient is lying.
8. The operator then discharges the paddles by simultaneously depressing the buttons on both handles.
9. Unless there is immediate ROSC, chest compressions should continue for 2 min while the defibrillator recharges.

SODIUM BICARBONATE. Sodium bicarbonate is an alkalinizing agent that is sometimes recommended when CPA has lasted more than 10 minutes to reverse the metabolic acidosis that often accompanies CPA.

Treatment of ventricular fibrillation or pulseless ventricular tachycardia. VF and pulseless VT should be treated with electrical defibrillation. In the event that either of these rhythms persists for longer than 10 minutes, the antiarrhythmic drugs amiodarone or lidocaine may be considered as well as epinephrine or vasopressin, as described in the previous section. Discussion of each of these therapies follows.

ELECTRICAL DEFIBRILLATION. A defibrillator is a device used to perform electrical defibrillation (a procedure used to shock the heart back into a normal sinus rhythm). It has two paddles that are placed on the chest wall (external defibrillation) or directly on the heart (internal defibrillation). When activated, electricity flows from one paddle to the other paddle through the patient's body.

Defibrillators are classified as monophasic or biphasic. In a monophasic defibrillator, current flows only in one direction, whereas in a biphasic defibrillator, it flows in both directions in rapid succession. RECOVER guidelines recommend that use of a biphasic defibrillator is ideal to minimize the setting needed and consequently the potential injury to the heart muscle.

When using a defibrillator, attention to safety is of paramount importance because the operator as well as other rescuers are at risk of electric shock if any part of their skin is contacting the patient, the table top, or any other conductive material (such as any fluids or defibrillator paste or gel) when the defibrillator is activated. Thus great care must be taken to use examination gloves when operating the unit to ensure that any such contact is avoided and to warn other personnel of the intent to deliver a shock by clearly and firmly saying "Clear" prior to activation. Details regarding the use of a defibrillator may be found in Procedure 13.12.

> **TECHNICIAN NOTE**
> When performing electrical defibrillation, attention to safety is of paramount importance because the operator as well as other rescuers are at risk of electric shock if any part of their skin is contacting the patient, the table top, or any other conductive material (such as any fluids or defibrillator paste or gel) when the defibrillator is activated.

ANTIARRHYTHMICS. Antiarrhythmics are a large class of drugs used to treat abnormal heart rhythms. Amiodarone and lidocaine are the two main drugs in this class used to treat patients with VF or pulseless VT that is resistant to electrical defibrillation.

Amiodarone. Amiodarone is an antiarrhythmic that works by a variety of mechanisms including blocking the movement of various cations across cell membranes. It may be administered IV at a dose of 1 mL/10 kg body weight when electrical defibrillation fails to restore a normal cardiac rhythm.

Lidocaine. Lidocaine is a local anesthetic with antiarrhythmic properties that is used to treat ventricular tachycardia. In the context of CPR, lidocaine 2% is given at a dose of 1 mL/10 kg body weight IV to treat nonresponsive VF or pulseless VT when amiodarone is not available.

Other strategies for CPA. During CPR, several other drugs may be indicated for specific purposes, such as potassium to treat hypokalemia, calcium to treat hypocalcemia, and magnesium to treat torsades de pointes (an arrhythmia that may lead to VF). IV fluids are recommended for patients with hypovolemia (low blood volume) but not in those with euvolemia or hypervolemia (normal or excessive blood volume, respectively), as they may adversely affect blood flow to the heart and brain in these patients and may cause pulmonary edema.

Open-chest cardiopulmonary resuscitation. If external chest compressions are not effective, internal chest compressions may be attempted. In the case of dogs weighing over 20 kg, some authorities suggest that internal compressions (also known as open-chest CPR) should be initiated immediately after cardiac arrest is identified because investigators have shown that external chest compression in dogs weighing more than 20 kg results in less than 30% of normal cardiac output, whereas internal massage results in outputs of up to 70% of normal. Open-chest CPR may also be indicated in patients with some thoracic disorders in which closed-chest CPR is unlikely to generate significant forward blood flow, such as tension pneumothorax, pericardial effusion, or diaphragmatic hernia.

Significant resources and training are needed to perform open-chest CPR. Furthermore, during the time it takes to open the chest surgically, compressions must be halted, which will prolong the period during which tissues are not being perfused. Consequently, there is understandable reluctance on the part of many veterinarians, technicians, and nurses to enter the chest to perform internal massage; however, controlled studies have demonstrated that the success rate for resuscitation of large dogs is much greater if internal cardiac massage is performed.

To perform open-chest CPR, the lateral thorax is quickly clipped and rinsed with alcohol, a self-adhering sterile drape is applied to the prepared area, and a scalpel is used to make a skin incision between the seventh and eighth ribs. The incision is extended through the muscle until the chest cavity is encountered. Care should be taken to avoid incising lung tissue, which lies immediately below the pleura. The operator's hand is inserted between the ribs (the use of a retractor may be necessary to separate the ribs adequately). The heart is grasped and gentle but firm pressure is applied to the ventricles at a rate of 100 times per minute. If resuscitation efforts are successful, a palpable heartbeat may return within seconds or minutes. Surgical closure and antibiotic therapy are essential after reestablishment of cardiac function by internal compression.

In the case of a patient that arrests during abdominal surgery, it is faster to enter the chest and perform direct compressions via an incision in the diaphragm, which will be performed by the attending veterinarian.

Aftercare

After ROSC, intensive monitoring of cardiovascular and respiratory function as well as an assessment of brain function are required to guide treatment and watch for the recurrence of CPA. This is because it is very common for patients to experience another cardiac arrest within 24 hours of successful ROSC. Monitoring may include blood pressure (indirect or direct), blood gases, pulse oximetry, continuous ECG, and capnography. Decisions regarding treatment with fluids and infusions are often made on a minute-to-minute basis as patient status changes rapidly in one direction or the other. In an ideal situation, cardiovascular, ventilatory, and neurologic status will improve, infusions will be decreased and finally discontinued, and the patient will be discharged.

Specific post-cardiac arrest care is complex and beyond the scope of this chapter. It focuses on optimization of blood oxygen and CO_2 levels with carefully controlled ventilation and oxygen supplementation, optimization of blood pressure with drug therapy, and IV fluid therapy, as well as protection against brain injury. The RECOVER guidelines contain a detailed discussion of these therapies (see Box 13.5 for a summary of these therapies).

Unfortunately, many patients that sustain cardiac arrest cannot be successfully revived. Even in those patients whose cardiac function is reestablished, conditions such as pulmonary edema and cerebral edema (manifested as seizures, failure to return to consciousness, and temporary or permanent neurologic damage) may occur, leading to recurrent CPA and

ultimately to death. This is the reason that only a small percentage of patients with CPA survive and are discharged from the hospital.

Problems That May Arise in the Recovery Period
Regurgitation and Vomiting

Regurgitation is a passive phenomenon that may occur at any point during an anesthetic event, including deep anesthesia. In a regurgitating animal, stomach contents exit through the cardiac sphincter, move up the esophagus and enter the pharynx, nasopharynx, and oral cavity. Once in the pharynx, stomach contents may be aspirated into the respiratory tract. Regurgitation is most common in ruminants and animals placed in a head-down position during surgery because this causes increased pressure on the stomach. Unlike vomiting, regurgitation is not accompanied by retching or other outward signs, and in fact, the only sign apparent to the anesthetist may be a small amount of fluid draining from the animal's mouth or nose. Treatment of regurgitation involves immediate intubation (if a cuffed ETT is not already present) and removal of as much regurgitated material as possible through suction.

> **TECHNICIAN NOTE**
>
> Treatment of regurgitation involves immediate intubation (if a cuffed ETT is not already present) and removal of as much regurgitated material as possible through suction.

Vomiting during the perianesthetic period is a relatively common phenomenon, particularly in brachycephalic dogs. Unlike regurgitation, vomiting is an active phenomenon often accompanied by retching. Vomiting usually occurs as the animal is losing consciousness during induction or as it is returning to consciousness during anesthetic recovery. Vomiting is potentially most dangerous if the animal is unconscious and the airway is not protected with an ETT. In this situation, the vomitus may easily be aspirated into the trachea. Aspiration of vomitus may cause immediate signs of dyspnea and cyanosis as

---

> **BOX 13.5 Therapies Used in Postcardiac Arrest Care**
>
> - Carefully controlled oxygen therapy to ensure adequate oxygen delivery to tissues, but to avoid overoxygenation, which may injure tissues.
> - Carefully controlled ventilation to normalize blood CO_2 levels, which may cause decreased blood flow to the brain if too low or increased intracranial pressure if too high. Controlled ventilation can also decrease cardiac output if excessive or lead to pulmonary atelectasis and hypoxemia if inadequate.
> - IV fluid therapy to optimize arterial blood pressure and central venous pressure.
> - Use of vasopressors (drugs that increase vascular tone such as norepinephrine, vasopressin, and dopamine) and positive inotropes (drugs that increase the strength of heart muscle contractions such as dopamine and dobutamine) to support blood pressure.
> - Control of body temperature to protect organ function.
> - Treatment of cerebral edema with osmotic agents including mannitol and hypertonic saline.

a result of airway obstruction and bronchospasm. If the patient survives this episode, signs of aspiration pneumonia (including fever, increased respiratory rate, and increased lung sounds) may appear over the next 24 to 48 hours.

It is imperative therefore that the anesthetist prevents the accumulation of vomitus within the oral cavity of the unconscious patient and the subsequent aspiration of the material into the air passages. To do this, an ETT should be inserted immediately if time and level of consciousness of the patient allow. If this cannot be achieved, the animal's head should immediately be placed at a lower level than the rest of its body (e.g., over the edge of the surgery table). This helps prevent the passive flow of liquid material into the trachea. When the vomiting stops, it may be necessary to clean the oral cavity, using suction if available. If respiratory arrest occurs because of airway blockage, the animal should be intubated and bagged with oxygen.

Fortunately, most vomiting episodes occur after the animal has regained consciousness and the ability to swallow. It is not usually necessary to intubate conscious animals during a vomiting episode; however, the anesthetist should ensure that the head is kept extended and as low as possible until the pharynx is clear of stomach contents.

Unconscious animals have a lower risk of aspiration if a cuffed ETT has been placed before a regurgitation episode. It is for this reason that the ETT is customarily left in place until the patient regains the swallowing reflex and is close to consciousness. If regurgitation is seen in an unconscious animal that has a cuffed ETT in place, the anesthetist should ensure that the cuff of the tube is inflated and position the animal's head lower than the rest of its body to prevent accumulation of stomach contents within the oral cavity.

Occasionally, an animal may regurgitate after esophageal intubation. If this occurs, the tube should be left in place to direct the contents away from the pharynx. Another ETT should be placed in the trachea, if possible, while the first tube is still in place.

From time to time, the technician or nurse may be called on to anesthetize an animal that has not been fasted before induction. These patients may be at risk of vomiting and/or regurgitation during induction, maintenance, and recovery. The anesthetist can help avoid problems by ensuring that protocols are used that allow rapid control of the airway. For this reason, an injectable agent is preferred over masking in these patients. A cuffed ETT of the appropriate diameter is essential to create an effective seal between the tube and the trachea. Applying lubricant to the cuff improves the effectiveness of the seal. If possible, head-down positions should be avoided during surgery to prevent excessive pressure on the stomach. The anesthetist should also ensure that suction is readily available in case of regurgitation or vomiting. Premedication with an antiemetic drug such as maropitant may be helpful in these cases. See Box 13.6 for strategies to prevent and respond to regurgitation and vomiting.

Seizures and Emergence Delirium in the Postanesthetic Period

Seizures are occasionally seen in animals recovering from anesthesia. Seizures may be caused by the administration of ketamine,

> **BOX 13.6 Strategies to Prevent and Respond to Regurgitation and Vomiting**
>
> To prevent regurgitation and vomiting:
> - Fast the patient appropriately prior to any anesthetic event.
> - Ensure that the patient is efficiently induced and intubated.
> - Always use a cuffed endotracheal tube of adequate diameter.
> - Keep the head slightly elevated during anesthesia.
> - Leave the endotracheal tube in place until the patient regains the swallowing reflex and is close to regaining consciousness.
>
> If an anesthetized patient regurgitates:
> - Place an endotracheal tube if possible.
> - If intubation is not possible, immediately place the head at a lower level than the rest of its body (e.g., over the edge of the surgery table).
> - If the patient is already intubated, ensure that the cuff of the tube is inflated and position the animal's head lower than the rest of its body.
> - When the regurgitation stops, clean the oral cavity using suction if available.
> - If respiratory arrest occurs because of airway blockage, the obstruction should be removed and the animal should be intubated and bagged with oxygen.

by diagnostic procedures such as myelography, or by medical disorders such as epilepsy or hypoglycemia.

It is important that the anesthetist differentiate between seizures and emergence delirium during recovery. Emergence delirium can occur in any patient, although it may be more commonly seen in patients that have not been given preanesthetic medications, and most often appears as spontaneous paddling of the limbs and occasionally as vocalization. Usually, treatment is unnecessary other than the calm reassurance of the patient; however, sedatives can be helpful, especially if the patient did not receive a sedative in the preanesthetic period. Occasionally, excitement or dysphoria may be seen after the administration of high doses of opioids to animals that have not been tranquilized (particularly cats). Treatment with low doses of naloxone to partially reverse the opioid or a tranquilizer to reduce the dysphoric effects may be helpful in these animals. Excitement is rarely observed in animals that receive opioids for moderate or severe pain.

In contrast, seizures appear as spontaneous twitching or uncontrolled movements of the head, neck, and limbs and are often triggered by a stimulus such as sound or touch. Animals given ketamine may show stiff forelimbs, opisthotonus, and exaggerated responses to touch or noise.

Animals experiencing emergence delirium or having seizures in the postoperative period should be brought to the veterinarian's attention. Elimination of stimuli such as light, sound, and touch may be adequate to resolve the episode. Adequate postoperative analgesia should be provided. If seizures are present, many animals respond well to administration of midazolam or diazepam IV (0.2 mg/kg), rectal diazepam at a dose of 0.2 to 0.4 mg/kg, or intranasal midazolam at 0.2 mg/kg. Lorazepam is another benzodiazepine used to manage seizures and can be given IV at 0.02 to 0.03 mg/kg. If benzodiazepines are not effective or are unavailable, the animal may be reanesthetized with propofol in sufficient quantity to induce sedation and eliminate seizures.

Animals manifesting seizures or emergence delirium during recovery require surveillance and nursing care to prevent self-injury. If the patient is still intubated, it is important to either hold the mouth closed so that the patient does not bite through the ETT or, if it is safe to do so, extubate the patient.

All animals experiencing seizures should be monitored for hyperthermia and cyanosis. Hyperthermia can be treated by the application of cool, wet towels. Cyanosis should be treated by the administration of oxygen by face mask or by ETT (if unconscious). See Box 13.7 for strategies to respond to postanesthetic seizures and emergence delirium.

Dyspnea During the Recovery Period

Dyspnea resulting from upper airway obstruction is the most common cause of death in the postanesthetic period. Dyspnea in cats is usually caused by laryngospasm or laryngeal edema, whereas dyspnea in dogs is most commonly associated with breed-related (e.g., brachycephalic) airway obstruction.

Laryngospasm is a condition in which the cartilages in the laryngeal area become so tightly closed that air is unable to enter the trachea. This condition commonly arises in cats because of this species' extremely active laryngeal reflex. In some recovering cats, the removal of the ETT initiates reflex closure of the airway. This reflex is normally useful to the cat in that it prevents the aspiration of food or water into the larynx in the conscious animal; however, in the unconscious animal, it may well result in complete airway blockage. Laryngeal edema may result from repeated attempts to intubate during light anesthesia. Clinically, this resembles laryngospasm.

Cats undergoing laryngospasm or laryngeal edema may breathe with an audible stertor or wheeze. They typically show exaggerated thoracic movements, gasping, and upward movement of the head during inspiration. If conscious, the animal usually appears anxious or excited. Laryngospasm must be

BOX 13.7 Strategies to Respond to Postanesthetic Seizures and Emergence Delirium

First, differentiate between seizures and emergence delirium.
- Emergence delirium most often appears as spontaneous paddling of the limbs and occasionally as vocalization.
  1. Usually, treatment is unnecessary, other than the calm reassurance of the patient as it returns to being fully conscious.
  2. Administer tranquilizers, sedatives, or reversal agents as ordered by the attending veterinarian.
- Seizures appear as spontaneous twitching or uncontrolled movements of the head, neck, and limbs, and are often triggered by a stimulus such as sound or touch.
  1. Inform the attending veterinarian.
  2. Eliminate stimuli such as light, sound, and touch.
  3. Provide adequate postoperative analgesia.
  4. Administer antiepileptic drugs as ordered.
  5. Monitor the patient for hyperthermia and cyanosis and provide nursing care to prevent self-injury.
  6. Hyperthermia can be treated by the application of cool, wet towels.
  7. Cyanosis should be treated by the administration of oxygen by face mask or by endotracheal tube (if unconscious).

differentiated from growling, which is common in cats recovering from anesthesia. In the case of growling, the noises are particularly evident on expiration, whereas in laryngospasm, the respiration is labored and the noise is most evident during inspiration.

If a cat shows signs of laryngospasm during recovery from anesthesia, the anesthetist should check the mucous membrane color and pulse oximeter readings (if available). If the cat's mucous membranes appear pink and the oxygen saturation (Sao_2) is greater than 90%, the obstruction is likely partial rather than complete. In this case, the situation may resolve without treatment, although administration of oxygen by face mask may be necessary, provided it does not stress the cat. It may be helpful to extend the neck and hold the tongue rostrally if possible. If cyanosis is present or Sao_2 readings are less than 90%, and the cat is losing consciousness—and if these signs are not alleviated by the administration of oxygen by face mask—the animal must be reintubated. If intubation is impossible, the veterinarian may elect to perform a tracheotomy to reestablish airflow. Once an airway has been reestablished, the animal should be given IV corticosteroids to reduce airway swelling and the larynx reassessed after 20 to 30 minutes. The cat can be extubated once the vocal cords appear less rounded and swollen. Nasal oxygen can be administered after extubation.

Laryngospasm is easier to prevent than to treat. When cats are being anesthetized, a gentle intubation technique is essential to avoid unnecessary laryngeal trauma. The anesthetist should also make sure that the patient is at an adequate depth of anesthetic prior to intubation.

Dyspnea in brachycephalic breeds of dogs usually occurs because the airway is obstructed by the soft palate or by other redundant tissue in the pharynx. However, in any patient, there are many other potential causes of upper airway obstruction, including foreign objects such as blood clots, gauze sponges, or even extracted teeth. Animals that have undergone surgery of the pharynx or larynx often undergo postoperative tissue swelling that may lead to airway obstruction.

Regardless of the cause, airway obstruction will usually not become evident until after the ETT has been removed. Strategies to prevent and treat postoperative dyspnea in brachycephalic dogs are outlined on page 406.

A conscious patient that requires supplemental oxygen during the recovery period can have it administered by one of four routes: face mask, nasal cannula, E-collar, or oxygen cage or tent. As a general rule, the flow rate should be at least 100 mL/kg/min. If possible, oxygen being delivered to an awake animal should be humidified (e.g., by directing the flow of oxygen through a bottle of distilled water before delivery to the patient). See Box 13.8 for strategies to respond to dyspnea during the recovery period.

Prolonged Recovery From Anesthesia

Animals experiencing prolonged recovery from anesthesia should be examined by the veterinarian. There are many possible reasons why a patient may be slow to recover, including impaired renal or hepatic function, hypothermia, low blood glucose, breed variation (particularly sighthounds), or the presence of a disorder such as shock or hemorrhage. Excessive anesthetic depth or prolonged

---

BOX 13.8 Strategies to Respond to Dyspnea During the Recovery Period

Cats with laryngospasm/laryngeal edema:

Check the mucous membrane color and pulse oximeter readings (if available).

- If the cat's mucous membranes appear pink and the SpO_2 is greater than 90%:
  1. Administer oxygen by face mask, provided it does not stress the cat.
  2. Extend the neck and hold the tongue rostrally (forward).
- If cyanosis is present or SpO_2 readings are less than 90% and the cat is losing consciousness—and if these signs are not alleviated by the administration of oxygen by face mask:
  1. Place an endotracheal tube.
  2. If intubation is impossible, the veterinarian may elect to perform a tracheotomy to reestablish airflow.
  3. Administer drugs and other treatments as ordered by the attending veterinarian.

Strategies to prevent and treat postoperative dyspnea in brachycephalic dogs are outlined on page 406.

PROCEDURE 13.13 Expediting Recovery from Anesthesia

1. The patient should be placed in a location where frequent observation is possible. If possible, emergency and monitoring equipment and oxygen should be available in the immediate area.
2. It is often helpful to administer IV fluids to support circulation and hasten renal and hepatic elimination of anesthetics. The recommended rate of fluid administration for most intensive care patients is 3–5 mL/kg/h.
3. Good nursing care is important. The patient should be turned frequently and kept warm. If the patient's temperature is less than 37°C, active warming procedures should be instituted, including the use of reflective blankets, circulating warm water blankets, warm air blankets, or warm towels.
4. The animal must be periodically monitored for vital signs, reflexes, and urine production (which should be at least 1 mL/kg/h).
5. Reversal agents are used occasionally to hasten anesthetic recovery. However, the anesthetist whose patients consistently demonstrate slow recoveries should not rely on pharmacologic solutions to solve what may be a problem of technique. The anesthetist should reexamine the anesthetic protocol and consult with the veterinarian to determine whether more appropriate agents or means of administration should be used. It is important to ensure that animals are not maintained at excessively deep levels of anesthesia for routine procedures.

---

anesthesia may also result in delayed recovery. Use of certain agents (e.g., intramuscular [IM] ketamine) may be associated with prolonged recovery, even in healthy animals. In the cat, it is known that hypothermia in itself can cause a significant delay in recovery, even if all other organs are functioning properly.

Recovery may be hastened in several ways (Procedure 13.13).

KEY POINTS

1. Although anesthetic emergencies are relatively uncommon, they are serious and often life-threatening. In contrast, complications are not usually serious but occur relatively frequently. Therefore the technician or nurse must be able to anticipate and respond to both in an efficient and knowledgeable fashion.

2. Human error may result in anesthetic problems. Such errors include the failure to obtain an adequate history or perform a physical examination, lack of training, errors related to a lack of familiarity with the anesthetic machine or drugs used, the incorrect administration of drugs, and errors related to fatigue, inattentiveness, or distraction.

3. Examples of equipment-related issues include CO_2 absorber exhaustion, failure to deliver sufficient oxygen to the patient, misassembly of the anesthetic machine, problems with the vaporizer or APL valve, or ETT problems.

4. Anesthetic agents may cause problems during anesthesia and the anesthetic protocol must be chosen to reflect the special needs of each patient. The anesthetist must be familiar with the adverse effects associated with the use of each agent in the anesthetic protocol.

5. Some patients are at increased risk of anesthetic complications because of preexisting factors such as old age, organ failure, recent trauma, or breed-related conformation.

6. Geriatric patients have less reserve than younger patients and have reduced anesthetic requirements. Pediatric patients also require reduced doses of injectable agents and are prone to hypothermia and hypoglycemia.

7. Brachycephalic dogs have anatomic characteristics that make respiration difficult, particularly during the recovery period. Preoxygenation before induction, rapid induction and intubation, and close monitoring during recovery are essential.

8. Obese animals should receive anesthetic doses according to a body weight halfway between the normal breed weight and the actual weight.

9. Pregnant animals presenting for cesarean section are at increased anesthetic risk. Various anesthetic techniques (including epidural anesthesia, balanced anesthesia, and neuroleptanalgesia) are often used as alternatives to using an inhalant as the sole anesthetic in these patients. Almost all anesthetic agents may cause depression of fetal respiration and/or circulation, and the use of reversal agents may be advisable.

10. If possible, patients that have undergone recent trauma should be stabilized and thoroughly evaluated before anesthesia.

11. Animals with cardiovascular or respiratory disease may require special anesthetic techniques such as preoxygenation and manual control of ventilation.

12. Hepatic or renal disease may delay the excretion of injectable agents and prolonged recovery times may be seen.

13. Emergency care is ideally a team effort involving all hospital personnel. It is helpful to have preauthorized emergency protocols and periodic dress rehearsals.

14. It may be difficult to maintain adequate anesthetic depth in some patients. Incorrect placement of the ETT, incorrect

vaporizer setting, inadequate ETT size, and many other factors may contribute to this problem.

15. Excessive anesthetic depth may result from excessive administration of anesthetic agents or from preexisting patient problems. It may be necessary to bag the patient with 100% oxygen to achieve a lighter plane of anesthesia.

16. Pale mucous membranes may be the result of anemia, hemorrhage, or poor perfusion. Prolonged capillary refill time suggests that hypotension (or, if severe, shock) is present.

17. Cyanosis is a critical emergency and arises because of insufficient delivery of oxygen to the tissues. It may result from a machine problem, airway or ETT blockage, or respiratory difficulties resulting from excessive depth, pneumothorax, or respiratory disease. Oxygen delivery to the patient must be reestablished via a mask, intubation, or tracheostomy.

18. Abnormalities in cardiac rate and rhythm may result from the administration of anesthetic agents, electrolyte abnormalities, hypercapnia, hypoxia, and many other factors.

19. Respiratory arrest that is accompanied by cyanosis and/or bradycardia is an emergency and must be treated by ventilation with 100% oxygen.

20. Cardiac arrest should be treated according to the RECOVER guidelines. The first five steps are (1) initiation of high-quality chest compressions, (2) intubation and ventilation, (3) ECG and end-tidal CO_2 monitoring, (4) obtaining vascular access, and (5) administration of reversal agents.

21. Regurgitation and/or vomiting may be dangerous in the anesthetized animal because of the risk of airway obstruction and aspiration pneumonia.

22. Postanesthesia seizures may be treated by eliminating external stimuli and administering antiepileptic drugs.

23. Dyspnea during the recovery period caused by laryngospasm, laryngeal edema, brachycephalic obstructive airway syndrome, or any other cause of upper airway obstruction may be treated by administration of oxygen by mask, reintubation of the patient, or tracheostomy.

24. Animals experiencing prolonged recovery from anesthesia require close observation and nursing care. An effort should be made to determine the reason for delayed arousal.

REVIEW QUESTIONS

1. When an animal scheduled for a surgical procedure is brought in by a neighbor who is in a hurry, the best thing to do is:
   a. Instruct the receptionist to have the neighbor sign the consent form
   b. Ask the neighbor to take the animal back home
   c. Ask the neighbor some quick questions about the animal
   d. Have the neighbor sign the consent form and ensure that the owner is called before the procedure is initiated

2. In preparation for an anesthetic procedure, you have drawn up a syringe of alfaxalone and an identical syringe of saline. You are then called to the examination room to assist the veterinarian. About 10 minutes later, you return to prepare the animal for induction. With the IV catheter in place, you are just about to inject some saline into the animal when you realize that you are not sure whether the syringe contains saline. The best thing to do would be to:
   a. Inject a small amount of the solution and see what effect it has
   b. Discard both syringes and start over
   c. Ask the person who was holding the animal which syringe had saline in it
   d. Discard both syringes, label some new syringes, and start over

3. You are about to use the anesthetic machine and notice that although the flowmeter is working, the pressure gauge on the oxygen tank reads close to zero. The best thing to do would be to:
   a. Assume that the pressure gauge may be faulty and wait and see whether the flowmeter stops working
   b. Change the oxygen tank
   c. Call the repair person to have the pressure gauge checked
   d. Use low-flow anesthesia techniques and ignore the pressure gauge reading

4. While monitoring a patient on an anesthetic machine, you realize that the oxygen tank has become empty. The best thing to do would be to:
   a. Disconnect the patient from the circuit, put on a new oxygen tank, and then reconnect the patient to the circuit
   b. Remove the circuit from the patient to allow it to breathe room air for the remainder of the procedure
   c. Resuscitate the patient with a manual resuscitator bag, for example, an Ambu bag
   d. Switch to an injectable anesthetic

5. If the APL valve is inadvertently left shut, it will:
   a. Stop the oxygen from entering the breathing circuit
   b. Convert the circuit to low-flow anesthesia
   c. Cause a significant rise of pressure within the circuit
   d. Cause the unidirectional valves to malfunction

6. You look at the oxygen tank and note that 1000 psi of pressure is left in the tank, but the flowmeter now reads zero and you cannot obtain a flow by twisting the knobs. The best thing to do would be to assume:
   a. The oxygen tank pressure gauge is malfunctioning and you need to recheck the flowmeter
   b. The oxygen pressure is adequate and the flowmeter is simply not registering the flow
   c. The animal is not getting oxygen and you need to remove the animal from the circuit until a new machine is found or the problem is corrected

7. A geriatric patient is considered to be one that:
   a. Is greater than 10 years old
   b. Is greater than 15 years old
   c. Has reached 50% of its life expectancy
   d. Has reached 75% of its life expectancy

8. Brain damage is highly likely to occur when there is inadequate oxygenation of the tissues for longer than ___ minutes.
   a. 3
   b. 5
   c. 7
   d. 9
9. When a technician or nurse is performing CPR alone, the ratio of chest compressions to ventilation should be:
   a. 5:1
   b. 10:1
   c. 20:2
   d. 30:2
10. When performing CPR, chest compressions should be discontinued:
    a. When providing breaths
    b. If you are unsure whether or not the patient has arrested
    c. After 10 minutes of CPR if there is no response
    d. Briefly between every 2-minute cycle
11. Respiratory arrest is always fatal.
    True
    False

    For the following questions, more than one answer may be correct.
12. One may suspect that the endotracheal tube is malfunctioning even if it is in the trachea because:
    a. Compression of the reservoir bag does not result in the raising of the chest
    b. The animal is dyspneic
    c. The animal cannot be kept at an adequate plane of anesthesia
    d. The reservoir bag is not moving or is moving very little
13. One may suspect that the APL valve has been closed or that it is malfunctioning if the:
    a. Reservoir bag is distended with air
    b. Patient has difficulty exhaling
    c. Patient wakes up
    d. Flow rate starts to drop
14. Administration of IV fluids at a rate of 5 mL/kg/h during an anesthetic procedure may result in overhydration in the:
    a. Patient with cardiac disease
    b. Obese patient
    c. Feline patient
    d. Brachycephalic patient
15. Brachycephalic dogs may be at increased anesthetic risk because of their:
    a. Physical size
    b. Excess tissue around the oropharynx

c. Increased vagal tone
d. Small trachea in comparison with their physical body size
16. To decrease the anesthetic risk associated with a brachycephalic dog, the anesthetist may elect to:
    a. Use atropine as part of the anesthetic protocol
    b. Preoxygenate the animal before giving any anesthetic
    c. Use an injectable anesthetic to hasten induction rather than masking
    d. Intubate immediately after induction
17. Animals that undergo cesarean section are at increased risk during anesthesia because of:
    a. Decreased respiratory function
    b. Increased chance of aspiration of vomitus
    c. Increased chance of hemorrhage
    d. Increased workload of the heart
18. Anesthetic agents or drugs that one may want to avoid in the animal with cardiovascular disease include:
    a. Ketamine
    b. Isoflurane
    c. Xylazine
    d. Opioids
19. An inadequate plane of anesthesia may be the result of:
    a. An oxygen flow rate that is too low
    b. An incorrect vaporizer setting
    c. Incorrect placement of the endotracheal tube
    d. Use of an anesthetic with a low MAC
20. Tachypnea may result from:
    a. Increased levels of arterial oxygen
    b. Increased levels of arterial CO_2
    c. The use of ketamine
    d. An inadequate plane of anesthesia
21. When a patient's blood pressure drops, the veterinarian may ask the technician or nurse to infuse a colloid. Which of the following is not a colloid?
    a. Hetastarch
    b. Hypertonic saline
    c. Dextran
    d. Plasma
22. Laryngospasm is more common in the dog than in the cat.
    True False
23. Bradycardia can always be treated with an anticholinergic.
    True False
24. Pulseless ventricular tachycardia in the dog is initially treated with:
    a. Lidocaine
    b. Atropine
    c. Defibrillation
    d. Vasopressin

ANSWERS TO CASE PRESENTATIONS

Case Presentation 13.1

Question #1: Bradycardia is often secondary to certain anesthetic agents known to cause this adverse effect, including the opioids and the alpha$_2$-agonists, as was suspected to be the case with Ariel. Other causes include (1) preexisting conditions, (2) excessive anesthetic depth, (3) vagal stimulation due to endotracheal intubation, manipulation of the viscera, or ocular surgery, (4) hypothermia, (5) certain electrolyte disorders, (6) hypertension, and (7) hypoxia.

Question #2: Ariel's anesthetic depth was appropriate, so this cause could be ruled out. It would be prudent to confirm that no known preexisting conditions were present by reviewing the history and performing a rapid assessment. In this patient, vagal stimulation was unlikely because she was not undergoing ocular or abdominal surgery. Rapid assessment of body temperature, blood pressure, and oxygen saturation would be appropriate next steps.

Question #3: Although nothing was occurring to prompt suspicion of an impending emergency, it would be prudent to monitor this patient continuously until a cause of the bradycardia could be identified and corrected. Rapid and effective action to take the steps outlined in the answer to question #2 would be most important. Then, once the cause had been identified, appropriate action could be taken.

Outcome of This Case

Ariel was not known to have any preexisting systemic disorders that would be expected to cause bradycardia. Anesthesia depth was confirmed to be appropriate.

At 37°C, body temperature was decreased as expected for this point in the procedure and mean arterial blood pressure as measured with an oscillometric blood pressure monitor was low normal (63 mmHg). Oxygen saturation (Spo$_2$) was 91% as measured by a lingual probe. Slightly low Spo$_2$ levels are, more often than not, an artifact of probe placement, so this in itself was not of concern unless attempts to reposition the probe continued to yield an Spo$_2$ value less than 95%.

The technician made multiple attempts to rule out probe placement artifact by rewetting the tongue, changing the probe location, orientation, and pressure on the tongue. Despite these attempts, the oxygen saturation remained below 95%, prompting

a suspicion of a failure in oxygen supply to the patient, exchange in the alveoli, or delivery to the tissues.

Adequate oxygen supply and an appropriate flow rate was confirmed (1.5 L/min). The technician observed movement of the bag in response to respiration, although the tidal volume appeared to be low. Periodic manual ventilation was initiated, but the Sao$_2$ did not appreciably improve and chest excursions during bagging did not reflect the amount of pressure applied.

At this point, the veterinarian ordered that the ETT be removed and replaced. A clean 4.0 mm internal diameter (ID) tube was placed, the oxygen flow was increased to 2 L/min, and Ariel was bagged every 15 seconds. The Sao$_2$ increased to 97% almost immediately, and within 5 minutes, the heart rate had returned to approximately 110 bpm. Upon close inspection, the patient end of the original ETT was found to be partially plugged with a large amount of thick, clear mucus.

Ariel's physical parameters continued to improve throughout anesthetic recovery and she recovered without further incident.

This case illustrates bradycardia that was most likely secondary to tissue hypoxia, emphasizing the importance of knowing the causes of abnormal monitoring parameters and being persistent in identifying the reason for any abnormalities observed. This case also illustrates the importance of checking the airway for patency on a regular basis during any anesthetic procedure, particularly in feline patients, because they are especially prone to airway blockage due to their smaller diameter airway. In this case, because the blockage was not complete, it was very difficult to detect and would have been missed were the patient not monitored with care and vigilance. If the technician and veterinarian had not persevered in correcting the cause of this abnormality, respiratory and cardiac arrest would possibly have occurred.

SELECTED READINGS

Arnell K, Hill S, Hart J, Richter K: Postanesthesia regurgitation in a dog, *J Am Anim Hosp Assoc* 49(1):58–63, 2013.

Baetge CL, Matthews NS: Geriatric anesthesia and analgesia, *Vet Clin North Am Small Anim Pract* 42(4):643–653, 2012.

Battaglia AM: *Small animal emergency and critical care for veterinary technicians*, ed 4, St. Louis, MO, 2020, Elsevier.

Brodbelt DC: Perioperative mortality in small animal anaesthesia, *Vet J* 182(2):152–161, 2009.

Brodbelt DC, Flaherty D, Pettifer GR: Anesthetic risk and informed consent. In Grimm KA, Lamont LA, Tranquilli WJ, et al: *Veterinary anesthesia and analgesia*, ed 5, Ames, IA, 2015, John Wiley and Sons, Inc, pp 11–22.

Burns PM: Top 5 considerations for anesthesia of a geriatric patient, *Clin Brief* 71–75, 2015.

Carroll G: *Small animal anesthesia and analgesia*, Ames, IA, 2008, Wiley-Blackwell.

Clarke KW, Hall LW: A survey of anaesthesia in small animal practice: AVA/BSAVA report, *J Assoc Vet Anaesth* 17:4–10, 1990.

Clark-Price S: Anesthesia tips for the obese patient, *Clin Brief* 43–45, 2010.

Cumming K, Wetmore L: Top 5 emergencies requiring anesthesia, *Clin Brief* 13–16, 2014.

Dodman NH, Lamb LA: Survey of small animal anesthetic practice in Vermont, *J Am Anim Hosp Assoc* 28:439–445, 1992.

Dyson DH, Mathews K: Recommendations for intensive care management in small animals following anaesthesia, *VCOT* 5: 66–70, 1992.

Dyson DH, Maxie MG: Morbidity and mortality associated with anesthetic management in small animal veterinary practice in Ontario, *J Am Anim Hosp Assoc* 34(4):325–335, 1998.

Egger CM: Detection and correction of hypoxia during anesthesia, *Clin Brief* 55–59, 2008.

Fletcher DJ, Boller M, Brainard BM: RECOVER evidence and knowledge gap analysis on veterinary CPR. Part 7: clinical guidelines, *J Vet Emerg Crit Care* 22(S1):S102–S131, 2012.

Gaynor JS, Dunlop CI, Wagner AE, et al: Complications and mortality associated with anesthesia in dogs and cats, *J Am Anim Hosp Assoc* 35(1):13–17, 1999.

Grimm KA, Tranquilli WJ: *Essentials of small animal anesthesia and analgesia*, ed 2, Ames, IA, 2011, Wiley-Blackwell.

Grubb TL, Perez Jimenez TE, Pettifer GR: Neonatal and pediatric patients. In Grimm KA, Lamont LA, Tranquilli WJ, et al., editors: *Veterinary anesthesia and analgesia*, ed 5, Ames, IA, John Wiley and Sons, Inc, pp 983–987.

Johnson RA, Snyder LBC, Schroeder CA: *Canine and feline anesthesia and co-exisiting disease*, ed 2, Hoboken, NJ, 2022, John Wiley and Sons, Inc.

Krein S, Wetmore L: Breed-specific anesthesia, *Clin Brief* 17–20, 2012.

Mama K, Rezende M: Anesthesia for patients with renal disease, *Clin Brief* 41–44, 2015.

Mama K, Rezende M: Anesthesia in hepatic disease, *Clin Brief* 65–67, 2015.

Mathews K: *Veterinary emergency and critical care manual*, New York, 2017, Lifelearn.

Miller J, Gannon K: Perioperative management of brachycephalic dogs, *Clin Brief* 54–59, 2015.

Onclin KJ, Verstegen JP: Cesarean section in the dog, *Clin Brief* 72–78, 2008.

Schmiedt CW, Bjorling DE: Repairing diaphragmatic hernia, *Clin Brief* 73–76, 2006.

Seymour C, Duke-Novakovski T: *BSAVA manual of canine and feline anaesthesia and analgesia*, Gloucester, UK, 2016, British Small Animal Veterinary Association.

Sinnott VB, Java M, King LG: Care following successful cardiopulmonary cerebral resuscitation, *Clin Brief* 48–50, 2009.

Weil AB, Ko JC: Anesthetic considerations for specific diseases. In Ko JC, editor: *Small animal anesthesia and pain management*, 2nd edition, Boca Raton, FL, 2019, CRC Press, pp 185–209.

Weil AB, Ko JC: Anesthetic emergencies and cardiopulmonary resuscitation. In Ko JC, editor: *Small animal anesthesia and pain management*, 2nd edition, Boca Raton, FL, 2019, CRC Press, pp 305–316

Welsh E: *Anaesthesia for veterinary nurses*, Oxford, UK, 2009, Blackwell.

Wilson DV, Shih AC: Anesthetic emergencies and resuscitation. In Grimm KA, Lamont LA, Tranquilli WJ, et al., editors: *Veterinary anesthesia and analgesia*, ed 5, Ames, IA, John Wiley and Sons, Inc., pp 114–129.

Procedure for Operation of a Full Rebreathing System

A full rebreathing system (also called a *complete, closed,* or *total rebreathing system*) is one in which the flow of oxygen is very low, providing only the volume necessary to meet the patient's metabolic needs. When using this system, the adjustable pressure limiting (APL) valve may be kept nearly, or in some cases, completely closed.[a] This system is used most often when anesthetizing large animal patients to conserve gas (see Chapter 10, Table 10.1 for appropriate oxygen flow rates when using a full rebreathing system).

If a full rebreathing system is used, the anesthetist should take the following steps to ensure patient safety:

- When using a full rebreathing system, the oxygen flow rate is low, so any loss of oxygen or its dilution by room air may be detrimental. Therefore, the APL valve may be set nearly or in some cases, completely closed, to prevent oxygen escape. If the APL valve is kept closed, it is essential that the anesthetist monitors the pressure in the breathing system.
- Check the machine for leaks before use. If leaks are present, oxygen may escape from the circuit and room air may leak into and dilute the oxygen in the circuit.
- Induction is the most challenging period of anesthesia when using a low oxygen flow rate because it takes significantly longer to increase anesthetic depth. This is because oxygen and other anesthetic gases within the circuit are diluted with exhaled nitrogen and vaporized anesthetic gases are delivered to the patient at a slower rate when oxygen flow is very low. Therefore, the reservoir bag should be emptied and refilled with oxygen two to three times during the first 15 minutes of anesthesia and every 30 minutes thereafter to help prevent patient hypoxemia and to eliminate nitrogen (N_2) (a process known as *denitrogenization*). Alternatively, the anesthetist may provide 5 to 10 minutes of high oxygen flow (200 mL/kg/min) at the start of anesthesia, until the patient reaches a surgical plane of anesthesia. The APL valve should be open when high flow rates are used. This flushes room air and exhaled nitrogen out of the system and replaces it with oxygen. Thereafter, much lower flow rates (5 to 10 mL/kg/min for small animals and 3 to 5 mL/kg/min for large animals) can be used, and the APL valve can be nearly or in some cases completely, closed. This amount of oxygen will meet the metabolic oxygen requirements of the anesthetized patient.

- Closely monitor the reservoir bag. If (1) there is a leak in the system; (2) the APL valve is too far open; (3) the negative pressure (vacuum) associated with an active scavenging system is excessive; or (4) the flow rate of oxygen is inadequate, the bag will not remain inflated. On the other hand, if (1) the APL valve is closed and the fresh gas flow exceeds the patient's demand for oxygen and anesthetic (which can occur if the patient is too deeply anesthetized, the patient is too cold, or any other factor reduces the patient's demand for oxygen); or (2) there is a blockage in the scavenging system, the bag will become distended. In this case, after the patient has been checked and it is apparent that no other problems exist, either the oxygen flow rate should be reduced or the APL valve should be opened. In any case, it is always wise to leave the APL valve at least slightly open during low-flow anesthesia, in case pressure in the circuit rises and excess gas must be vented.
- It may be difficult to change the patient's anesthetic depth quickly when using low oxygen flow rates. If a rapid change in anesthetic depth is required, the vaporizer setting should be changed and the breathing system converted to a partial rebreathing system by increasing the oxygen flow rate and opening the APL valve. If low oxygen flow rates are maintained, changes in the vaporizer setting may not affect the concentration of anesthetic in the circuit for many minutes.
- When a precision out-of-circuit vaporizer is used, the vaporizer setting required during the maintenance period will often be well above the setting normally used to maintain surgical anesthesia with a partial rebreathing system, at least until a state of equilibrium is reached (in which the concentration of anesthetic in the brain and blood is equal to the concentration of anesthetic in the circuit). In a full rebreathing system, this may take a considerable period of time to occur, owing to the low gas flow rate (see Chapter 4, Box 4.4 for a discussion of time constants).
- The low oxygen flow rates used in a full rebreathing system may be inadequate for accurate delivery of anesthetic by some vaporizers and full rebreathing systems should not be used at all with certain vaporizers. Therefore, the owner's manual should be consulted for minimum recommended oxygen flow rates, and to be sure that the vaporizer may safely be used in this manner. Also, it is important to be aware that the anesthetic concentration indicated by the dial may be inaccurate at lower oxygen flow rates.
- The low oxygen flow rates appropriate for a full rebreathing system are unsafe for use with a Bain coaxial circuit or other non-rebreathing system and must therefore never be used for this purpose, as this will lead to rebreathing of CO_2 and hypoxemia.

[a]Note that some clinicians recommend keeping the APL valve open when operating a full rebreathing system. This is because anesthetic gases are not vented from an open APL valve until pressure in the breathing circuit reaches 1 to 3 cm H_2O (assuming the APL valve and scavenging system are functioning properly).

American College of Veterinary Anesthesia and Analgesia Monitoring Guidelines Update, 2009

This document may be accessed online at http://acvaa.org under "Veterinarians," "Guidelines and Position Statement Documents," and then "Small Animal Monitoring Guidelines."

RECOMMENDATIONS FOR MONITORING ANESTHETIZED VETERINARY PATIENTS

Position Statement

The American College of Veterinary Anesthesiologists (ACVA) has revised the set of guidelines for anesthetic monitoring that were originally developed in 1994 and published in 1995.[a] Since then, many factors have caused a shift in the benchmark used to measure a successful anesthetic outcome, moving from the lack of anesthetic mortality toward decreased anesthetic morbidity.

This shift toward minimizing anesthetic morbidity has been facilitated by more objective definition and earlier detection of pathophysiologic conditions such as hypotension, hypoxemia, and severe hypercapnia. This has resulted from the incorporation of newer monitoring modalities by skilled, attentive personnel during anesthesia.

The ACVA recognizes that it is possible to adequately monitor and manage anesthetized patients without specialized equipment and that some of these modalities may be impractical in certain clinical settings. Furthermore, the ACVA does not suggest that using any or all the modalities will ensure any specific patient outcome or that failure to use them will result in poor outcome.

However, as the standard of veterinary care advances and client expectations expand, revised guidelines are necessary to reflect the importance of vigilant monitoring. The goal of the ACVA guidelines is to improve the level of anesthesia care for veterinary patients. Frequent and continuous monitoring and recording of vital signs in the perianesthetic period by trained personnel, and the intelligent use of various monitors are requirements for advancing the quality of anesthesia care of veterinary patients.

Circulation
Objective

To ensure adequate circulatory function.

Methods

1. Palpation of peripheral pulse to determine rate, rhythm and quality, and evaluation of mucous membrane (MM) color and capillary refill time (CRT).
2. Auscultation of heartbeat (stethoscope, esophageal stethoscope, or other audible heart monitor). Continuous (audible heart or pulse monitor) or intermittent monitoring of the heart rate and rhythm.
3. Pulse oximetry to determine the % hemoglobin saturation.
4. Electrocardiogram (ECG) continuous display for detection of arrhythmias.
5. Blood pressure:
   a. Noninvasive (indirect): oscillometric method or Doppler ultrasonic flow detector
   b. Invasive (direct): arterial catheter connected to an aneroid manometer or to a transducer and oscilloscope.

Recommendations

Continuous awareness of heart rate and rhythm during anesthesia, along with gross assessment of peripheral perfusion (pulse quality, MM color, and CRT) are mandatory. Arterial blood pressure and ECG should also be monitored. There may be some situations where these may be temporarily impractical (e.g., movement of an anesthetized patient to a different area of the hospital).

Oxygenation
Objective

To ensure adequate oxygenation of the patient's arterial blood.

Methods

1. Pulse oximetry (noninvasive estimation of hemoglobin saturation).
2. Arterial blood gas analysis for oxygen partial pressure (Pa_{O_2}).

Recommendations

Assessment of oxygenation should be done whenever possible by pulse oximetry, with blood gas analysis being employed when necessary for more critically ill patients.

Ventilation
Objective

To ensure that the patient's ventilation is adequately maintained.

[a]JAVMA 206(7):936–937, 1995.

Methods

1. Observation of thoracic wall movement or observation of breathing bag movement when thoracic wall movement cannot be assessed.
2. Auscultation of breath sounds with an external stethoscope, an esophageal stethoscope, or an audible respiratory monitor.
3. Capnography (end-expired CO_2 measurement).
4. Arterial blood gas analysis for carbon dioxide partial pressure ($Paco_2$).
5. Respirometry (tidal volume measurement).

Recommendations

Qualitative assessment of ventilation is essential as outlined in either 1 or 2 above, and capnography is recommended, with blood gas analysis as necessary.

Temperature
Objective

To ensure that patients do not encounter serious deviations from normal body temperature.

Methods

1. Rectal thermometer for intermittent measurement.
2. Rectal or esophageal temperature probe for continuous measurement.

Recommendations

Temperature should be measured periodically during anesthesia and recovery and if possible, checked within a few hours after return to the wards.

Neuromuscular Blockade
Objective

To assess the intensity of and recovery from neuromuscular blockade.

Methods

1. Hand-held peripheral nerve stimulator.
2. Spirometer.

Recommendations

For any patient in which neuromuscular blockade is used, it is essential to control ventilation, monitor closely for signs of awareness, and be certain of recovery of blockade prior to anesthesia recovery. Recovery of neuromuscular function may be assumed if the evoked response (twitch and/or tetanic fade) to a nerve stimulus, and respiratory tidal volume as measured with a spirometer, return to at least 70% of preblockade status. End-tidal CO_2 may also be used as an indication of adequate ventilation in spontaneously ventilating patients.

Recordkeeping
Objectives

1. To maintain a legal record of significant events related to the anesthetic period.
2. To enhance recognition of significant trends or unusual values for physiologic parameters and allow assessment of the response to intervention.

Recommendations

1. Record all drugs administered to each patient in the perianesthetic period and in early recovery, noting the dose, time, and route of administration, as well as any adverse reaction to a drug or drug combination.
2. Record monitored variables on a regular basis (minimum every 5 to 10 minutes) during anesthesia. The minimum variables that should be recorded are heart rate and respiratory rate, as well as oxygenation status and blood pressure if these were monitored.
3. Record heart rate, respiratory rate, and temperature in the early recovery phase.
4. Any untoward events or unusual circumstances should be recorded for legal reasons and for reference should the patient require anesthesia in the future.

Recovery Period
Objective

To ensure a safe and comfortable recovery from anesthesia.

Methods

1. Observation of respiratory pattern.
2. Observation of MM color and CRT.
3. Palpation of pulse rate and quality.
4. Measurement of body temperature, with appropriate warming or cooling methods applied if indicated.
5. Observation of any behavior that indicates pain, with appropriate pharmaceutical intervention as necessary.
6. Other measurements as indicated by patient's medical status, for example, blood glucose, pulse oximetry, packed cell volume (PCV), total protein (TP), blood gases, etc.

Recommendations

Monitoring in recovery should include *at the minimum* evaluation of pulse rate and quality, MM color, respiratory pattern, signs of pain, and temperature.

Personnel
Objective

To ensure that a responsible individual is aware of the patient's status at all times during anesthesia and recovery, and is prepared either to intervene when indicated or to alert the veterinarian in charge about changes in the patient's condition.

Recommendations

1. Ideally, a veterinarian, technician, or other responsible person should remain with the patient continuously and be dedicated to that patient only.
2. If this is not possible, a reliable and knowledgeable person should check the patient's status on a regular basis (at least every 5 minutes) during anesthesia and recovery.
3. A responsible person may be present in the same room, although not necessarily solely occupied with the anesthetized

patient (for instance, the surgeon may also be responsible for overseeing anesthesia).

4. In either 2 or 3 above, audible heart and respiratory monitors must be available.

5. A responsible person, solely dedicated to managing and caring for the anesthetized patient during anesthesia, remains with the patient continuously until the end of the anesthetic period:
   a. Recommended for all patients assessed as American Society of Anesthesiologists (ASA) status III, IV, or V.
   b. Recommended for horses anesthetized with inhalation anesthetics and/or horses anesthetized for longer than 45 minutes.

Sedation Without General Anesthesia

Sedation is a state characterized by central depression accompanied by drowsiness during which the patient is generally unaware of its surroundings but responsive to noxious manipulation.[b]

[b]Thurmon JC, Short CE: History and overview of veterinary anesthesia. In Tranquilli WJ, Thurmon JC, Grimm KA, editors: *Lumb & Jones' veterinary anesthesia and analgesia*, ed 4, Ames, IA, 2007, Blackwell Publishing, p 5.

If a sedated patient is sufficiently obtunded to lose control of protective airway reflexes, it should be monitored as under general anesthesia.

Objective
To ensure adequate oxygenation and hemodynamic stability in the obtunded patient.

Methods
1. Palpation of pulse rate, rhythm, and quality.
2. Observation of MM color and CRT.
3. Observation of respiratory rate and pattern.
4. Auscultation.
5. Pulse oximetry.
6. Oxygen supplementation.

Recommendations
Intermittent monitoring of basic respiratory and cardiovascular parameters in the heavily sedated animal should be routine. Supplemental oxygen, an endotracheal tube, and materials for IV catheterization should always be readily available. Particular attention should be paid to brachycephalic breeds that are particularly at risk for airway obstruction under heavy sedation.

Equipment and Drugs for Use in an Emergency Crash Cart

The following list of equipment and supplies for an emergency crash cart may be altered depending on the veterinarian's preference and the needs of the practice. The cart must be well organized, with locations of items labeled, and regularly checked and restocked. The items listed below are typical for a small animal crash cart and can be readily adapted for small ruminants, pigs, camelids, and foals.

Personal Protective Equipment
- Examination gloves (small/medium/large)
- Eye protection (goggles or face shield)

Airway Supplies
- Endotracheal (ET) tubes (internal diameter [ID] 3 to 11 mm; whole sizes only)
- Stylet for small and large ET tubes
- Laryngoscope with charged batteries
- Laryngoscope blades (small, medium, and large)
- ET tube ties
- Cuffing syringe (3 mL for cats and 6 to 12 mL for dogs)
- 3 × 3 gauze sponges (quantity—at least 20)
- Mouth gags (1 small and 1 large)
- Anesthetic masks (small, medium, and large)
- Suction tube and tip

Oxygen Source and Means of Providing Ventilation
- E-tank filled to at least 500 psi (with pressure-reducing valve, flow control, tubing, and fitting compatible with manual resuscitator bag)
- Manual resuscitator bag (e.g., Ambu bag). *(Note that an anesthetic machine outfitted with a reservoir bag can be used in place of a manual resuscitator bag.)*

Equipment Required for Intravenous Access and Administration of Drugs
- Needles: 18 to 25 gauge
- Syringes: 1 to 60 mL
- Over-the-needle catheters, 24 to 18 gauge
- Winged infusion sets
- Normal saline flush (250 mL bottle)
- T-ports; intravenous (IV) catheter plugs with injection port
- 1" and ½" porous tape
- 2" elastic gauze bandage
- 2" cohesive bandage
- Bone marrow biopsy needle for intraosseous (IO) access
- 3.5-, 5-, 8-, and 10-French red rubber catheters (to deliver drugs intratracheally via the ET tube)
- #10 and #15 scalpel blades (for venous cutdown)

Emergency Drugs
- Laminated dosage chart

Vasopressors
- Epinephrine (1 mg/mL [1:1000])
- Vasopressin (20 U/mL)

Antiarrhythmics
- Atropine (0.54 mg/mL)
- Lidocaine (20 mg/mL [2%])
- Amiodarone (50 mg/mL)

Reversal Agents
- Naloxone (0.4 mg/mL)
- Atipamezole (5 mg/mL)
- Flumazenil (0.1 mg/mL)

Intravenous Fluid Therapy
- Lactated Ringer's solution; Normosol-R; or other isotonic, polyionic crystalloid solution
- 0.9% saline
- VetStarch colloid
- Macrodrip IV administration sets
- Fluid pump
- Syringe pump
- Pressure infusion bag

Monitoring Equipment
- Electrocardiogram (ECG) monitor, power cord, electrodes, and electrode gel
- Pulse oximeter, lingual probe, and charger
- Capnograph, sampling spacer and tube (for sidestream sampling), adult and pediatric sensor chambers (for mainstream sampling), and charger

Defibrillator
- Defibrillator paddles (internal and external)
- Conducting gel (for external paddles)
- Sterile saline (for internal paddles)

Miscellaneous Supplies
- Surgical gloves sizes 6½ to 8 (at least 2 of each size)
- Sterile pack containing:
  - #3 scalpel blade handle
  - Tissue thumb forceps
  - Curved Mayo scissors
  - Hemostatic forceps
  - Needle holders
  - #10 and #11 surgical blades
  - Army–Navy retractors (quantity 2)
  - 2-0 and 0 PDS (polydioxanone) suture
  - 2-0 and 0 nylon suture
  - Sterile towel

- Chlorhexidine scrub/sponges
- Alcohol rinse/sponges
- Sponge forceps or Allis tissue forceps
- Sterile water-soluble lubricant
- Sterile swabs (1 package)
- Sterile 3 × 3 gauze sponges (minimum 2 packs of 20)
- Tongue depressors
- Trocar catheter chest tube
- 18-French red rubber catheter (for chest tube)
- 12-French red rubber catheter
- Umbilical tape
- Penrose drain

Miscellaneous Emergency Medications (Not Routinely Used for Cardiopulmonary Resuscitation)
- Calcium gluconate (essential cation nutrient)
- Dexamethasone (glucocorticoid)
- Dextrose 50% (glucose-elevating agent)
- Diphenhydramine (H_1 antihistamine)
- Dobutamine (beta-adrenergic inotrope)
- Dopamine (adrenergic/dopaminergic inotrope)
- Furosemide (loop diuretic)
- Midazolam or diazepam (benzodiazepine tranquilizer)
- Norepinephrine (adrenergic vasopressor)
- Potassium chloride (electrolyte)
- Sodium bicarbonate (alkalinizer)

Note: A list of emergency drug doses should be posted or included in the cart.

Standard Volumes, Weights, Measures, and Equivalents

METRIC SYSTEM

Prefixes

"kilo"	*means*	One thousand
"milli"	*means*	One thousandth
"micro"	*means*	One thousandth of one thousandth, or one millionth

Weight to Volume Equivalents

1 gram (g) = the weight of 1 cubic centimeter (cc) of water at 4 degrees centigrade (°C)

Volume Equivalents

1 cc	=	1 milliliter (mL)
1000 mL *or* cc	=	1 liter (L)
1 mL *or* cc	=	0.001 L
1 deciliter (dL)	=	100 mL

Weight Equivalents

1000 microgram (mcg)	=	1 milligram (mg)
1 mcg	=	0.001 mg
1000 mg	=	1 g
1 mg	=	0.001 g
1 million mcg	=	1 g
1000 g	=	1 kilogram (kg)
1 g	=	0.001 kg

Solution Equivalents

1 part in 10 (1:10)	=	10% (1 mL contains 100 mg)
1 part in 100 (1:100)	=	1% (1 mL contains 10 mg)
1 part in 500 (1:500)	=	0.20% (1 mL contains 2 mg)
1 part in 1000 (1:1000)	=	0.10% (1 mL contains 1 mg)
1 part in 5000 (1:5000)	=	0.02% (1 mL contains 0.2 mg)
1 part in 10,000 (1:10,000)	=	0.01% (1 mL contains 0.1 mg)

The number of milligrams in 1 mL of any solution of known percentage strength is obtained by moving the decimal one place to the right. For example, a 1% solution contains 10 mg/mL.

By definition, a percent solution contains the specified weight (in grams) of the solute in 100 mL of total solution. For example, a 5% dextrose and water solution contain 5 g of dextrose dissolved in each 100 mL of water (or 50 mg/mL).

Metric to Household Equivalents

Weight

1 kg	=	2.2 avoirdupois or imperial pounds (lb)
1 oz (0.0625 lb)	=	28.4 g (~0.03 kg)
1 lb (16 ounces [oz])	=	453.6 g (0.454 kg)

Volume

1 L	=	1.06 U.S. quarts	=	33.8 fluid ounces
1 U.S. pint	=	473.2 mL		
1 quart	=	946.4 mL		

Length

1 meter (m)	=	39.37 inches (in)		
1 in	=	$^1/_{12}$ feet (ft)	=	2.54 centimeters (cm)

Pressure Equivalents

Pressure

1 lb/in² (psi)	=	51.7 millimeters (mm) of mercury (Hg)	=	70.3 cm of water (H_2O)
1 mmHg	=	1.36 cm H_2O		
1 cm H_2O	=	0.736 mmHg		
1 atmosphere	=	760 mmHg	= 14.7 psi =	100 kilopascals (kPa)

CONVERSION TABLES

Note: The conversions in each table are calculated using the rounded conversion factors noted and are therefore approximate. All conversions except for gas pressures in kPa and body weights over 100 kg are rounded to one decimal place.

Conversion Table for a Pressure Manometer (cm H_2O to mmHg)

PRESSURE (mmHg) = PRESSURE (cm H_2O)/1.36			
cm H_2O	mmHg	cm H_2O	mmHg
1	0.7	25	18.4
2	1.5	30	22.1
3	2.2	35	25.7
4	2.9	40	29.4
5	3.7	45	33.1
6	4.4	50	36.8
7	5.1	55	40.4
8	5.9	60	44.1
9	6.6	70	51.5
10	7.4	80	58.8
15	11.0	90	66.2
20	14.7	100	73.5

Conversion Table for Endotracheal Tube and Catheter Internal Diameter (French to mm)

INTERNAL DIAMETER (FRENCH) = INTERNAL DIAMETER (mm) × 3					
French	mm	French	mm	French	Mm
1	0.3	9	3.0	40	13.3
1.5	0.5	10	3.3	45	15.0
2	0.7	12	4.0	50	16.7
2.5	0.8	14	4.7	55	18.3
3	1.0	16	5.3	60	20.0
3.5	1.2	18	6.0	65	21.7
4	1.3	20	6.7	70	23.3
4.5	1.5	22	7.3	75	25.0
5	1.7	24	8.0	80	26.7
5.5	1.8	26	8.7	85	28.3
6	2.0	28	9.3	90	30.0
7	2.3	30	10.0	95	31.7
8	2.7	35	11.7	100	33.3

Conversion Table for Gas Pressure in a Compressed Gas Cylinder (psi to kPa)

PRESSURE (kPa) = PRESSURE (psi) × 6.895			
Psi	kPa	Psi	kPa
1	7	500	3,448
5	34	600	4,137
10	69	700	4,827
15	103	800	5,516
20	138	900	6,206
30	207	1,000	6,895
40	276	1,100	7,585
50	345	1,500	10,343
100	690	2,000	13,790
200	1,379	2,200	15,169
300	2,069	2,500	17,238
400	2,758	3,000	20,685

Conversion Table for Body Temperature (°F to °C)

FAHRENHEIT TO CENTIGRADE: °C = (°F − 32) × 5/9					
CENTIGRADE TO FAHRENHEIT: °F = (°C × 9/5) + 32					
°F	°C	°F	°C	°F	°C
32	0.0	92	33.3	102	38.9
68	20.0	93	33.9	103	39.4
84	28.9	94	34.4	104	40.0
85	29.4	95	35.0	105	40.6
86	30.0	96	35.6	106	41.1
87	30.6	97	36.1	107	41.7
88	31.1	98	36.7	108	42.2
89	31.7	99	37.2	109	42.8
90	32.2	100	37.8	110	43.3
91	32.8	101	38.3	212	100.0

Conversion Table for Body Weight (lb to kg)

\multicolumn{12}{c}{BODY WEIGHT (kg) = BODY WEIGHT (lb)/2.2}

lb	kg	lb	kg	lb	kg	lb	kg	lb	kg	lb	kg
1	0.5	11	5.0	22	10.0	42	19.1	80	36.4	400	182
2	0.9	12	5.5	24	10.9	44	20.0	85	38.6	450	205
3	1.4	13	5.9	26	11.8	46	20.9	90	40.9	500	227
4	1.8	14	6.4	28	12.7	48	21.8	95	43.2	600	273
5	2.3	15	6.8	30	13.6	50	22.7	100	45.5	700	318
6	2.7	16	7.3	32	14.5	55	25.0	150	68.2	800	364
7	3.2	17	7.7	34	15.5	60	27.3	200	90.9	900	409
8	3.6	18	8.2	36	16.4	65	29.5	250	114	1000	455
9	4.1	19	8.6	38	17.3	70	31.8	300	136	1500	682
10	4.5	20	9.1	40	18.2	75	34.1	350	159	2000	909

ANSWER KEY

CHAPTER 1: INTRODUCTION TO ANESTHESIA

1. d
2. a
3. c
4. b
5. b
6. d
7. b
8. b
9. a, b, d
10. a, d

CHAPTER 2: PATIENT PREPARATION

1. c
2. b
3. d
4. c
5. b
6. b
7. c
8. c
9. a
10. a
11. c
12. d
13. a
14. c
15. b
16. d
17. d
18. b
19. b
20. d

CHAPTER 3: ANESTHETIC AGENTS AND ADJUNCTS

1. b
2. c
3. a
4. False
5. True

6. b
7. a
8. True
9. d
10. b
11. c
12. d
13. a
14. c
15. True
16. a
17. c
18. a
19. c
20. d
21. a
22. a, b, c, d
23. c
24. a, b, c, d
25. a, c
26. a, b, c, d
27. a, b
28. b, d
29. a, c, d
30. b, d

CHAPTER 4: ANESTHETIC EQUIPMENT

1. d
2. a
3. b
4. b
5. a
6. c
7. d
8. c
9. b
10. a
11. b
12. d
13. b
14. a
15. d
16. c
17. b
18. b
19. c
20. a, b, c
21. b, c

22. a, b
23. d
24. b, d
25. a, b, d

CHAPTER 5: WORKPLACE SAFETY

1. d
2. a
3. c
4. a
5. b
6. False
7. a
8. True
9. d
10. False
11. a
12. b
13. c
14. d
15. b
16. c
17. a, b, c, d
18. a, d
19. a, b, c
20. a, b

CHAPTER 6: ANESTHETIC MONITORING

1. d
2. c
3. b
4. c
5. a
6. d
7. b
8. a
9. b
10. c
11. d
12. a
13. d
14. a
15. b
16. c
17. b

18. c
19. a, b, c
20. a, b, c, d
21. a, b, c
22. a, b, c, d
23. a, b, d
24. a, b, c
25. b, c

CHAPTER 7: SPECIAL TECHNIQUES

1. b
2. b
3. b
4. a
5. a
6. d
7. b
8. c
9. True
10. d
11. c
12. b
13. c
14. c
15. b
16. a
17. False
18. a
19. c
20. False
21. a, c, d
22. b, c, d
23. a, b, d
24. a, b, c, d
25. a, b, c

CHAPTER 8: ANALGESIA

1. b
2. c
3. c
4. c
5. b
6. b
7. d
8. d
9. c

10. False
11. d
12. c
13. c
14. d
15. True

CHAPTER 9: CANINE AND FELINE ANESTHESIA

1. c
2. a
3. d
4. d
5. b
6. c
7. b
8. d
9. c
10. b
11. d
12. d
13. a
14. c
15. a, b, c, d
16. b, c, d
17. a, c, d
18. a, b, c, d
19. a, b, d
20. a, c, d

CHAPTER 10: EQUINE ANESTHESIA

1. c
2. a
3. b
4. a
5. c
6. a
7. d
8. c
9. True
10. b

CHAPTER 11: ANESTHESIA OF RUMINANTS, CAMELIDS, AND SWINE

1. a
2. False
3. b
4. c
5. True
6. c
7. a
8. d

9. d
10. c
11. d
12. a

CHAPTER 12: RODENT AND RABBIT ANESTHESIA

1. b
2. a
3. b
4. d
5. b
6. c
7. b
8. b
9. c
10. a

CHAPTER 13: ANESTHETIC PROBLEMS AND EMERGENCIES

1. d
2. d

3. b
4. a
5. c
6. c
7. d
8. b
9. d
10. d
11. False
12. a, b, c, d
13. a, b
14. a, c
15. b, c, d
16. a, b, c, d
17. a, b, c, d
18. a, c
19. a, b, c
20. b, d
21. b
22. False
23. False
24. c

GLOSSARY

Academy of Veterinary Technicians in Anesthesia and Analgesia (AVTAA) A professional organization that exists to promote interest in the discipline of veterinary anesthesia. The AVTAA provides a process by which a veterinary technician may become certified as a Veterinary Technician Specialist (Anesthesia/Analgesia) through completion of an arduous set of requirements that demonstrates competency in the advanced practice of anesthesia and analgesia in animals.

Activated charcoal canister A type of passive scavenging system, consisting of a canister containing activated charcoal, designed to remove halogenated anesthetic agents from gases exiting from the adjustable pressure-limiting valve of a breathing circuit.

Acute pain Pain of immediate onset after tissue injury. Resolves when healing is complete.

Adaptive pain Pain that promotes survival by preventing injury and by promoting healing of the injured body part. Physiologic pain is an example of adaptive pain.

Adjunct A drug that is not a true anesthetic but that is used during anesthesia to produce other desired effects such as sedation, muscle relaxation, analgesia, reversal, neuromuscular blockade, or parasympathetic blockade. This term is also used to describe agents and modalities that can contribute to, or enhance, drugs that are primarily used to provide analgesia.

Adjustable pressure limiting (APL) valve Also known as *pressure relief valve, pop-off valve, exhaust valve,* or *overflow valve;* this valve is the point of exit of anesthetic gases from the breathing circuit.

Advanced Life Support (ALS) The phase of cardiopulmonary resuscitation that follows basic life support (BLS). This phase consists of ECG and end-tidal CO_2 monitoring, placement of an intravenous (IV) catheter, and administration of emergency drugs and fluids.

Agonal An abnormal breathing pattern seen during cardiopulmonary arrest, characterized by gasping and labored breathing.

Agonist A drug that binds to and stimulates tissue receptors.

Agonist-antagonist A drug that binds to more than one receptor type, simultaneously stimulating at least one and blocking at least one.

Algesia Sensitivity to pain.

Allodynia A phenomenon in which an uninjured area close to a site of tissue injury is painful if stimulated with a normally nonnoxious stimulus.

Alveolar dead space Space in alveoli that are inadequately perfused with pulmonary blood and in which, therefore no gas exchange occurs.

Alveolar ventilation The portion of the tidal volume that travels from the source of fresh gas to the alveoli and participates in gas exchange.

Ambu bag *See Manual resuscitator bag.*

American College of Veterinary Anesthesia and Analgesia (ACVAA) A professional organization with a mission to promote the highest standards of clinical practice of veterinary anesthesia and analgesia, and to define criteria used to designate veterinarians with advanced training as specialists in the clinical practice of veterinary anesthesiology.

Analeptic agent (a.k.a. analeptic) A drug that causes general central nervous system stimulation.

Analgesia Absence of pain.

Anatomic dead space Dead space in anatomic structures through which inhaled air travels on its way to the alveoli such as the nasal cavity, pharynx, larynx, trachea, and bronchi.

Anesthesia A loss of sensation.

Anesthetic agent Any drug used to induce a loss of sensation with or without unconsciousness.

Anesthetic chamber A clear, aquarium-like box used to induce general anesthesia in small patients that are feral, vicious, or intractable, or that cannot be handled without undue stress.

Anesthetic gas analyzer A machine that measures the concentration of inhalant anesthetic (isoflurane, sevoflurane, or desflurane) in the breathing circuit by sampling gas from a spacer placed between the endotracheal tube connector and the breathing circuit.

Anesthetic induction The process by which an animal loses consciousness and enters general anesthesia.

Anesthetic maintenance The process of keeping a patient in a state of general anesthesia. The period between induction and recovery.

Anesthetic mask A cone-shaped device, ideally made of transparent material, used to administer oxygen and anesthetic gases to nonintubated patients via the nose and mouth. Also used to administer pure oxygen to dyspneic, hypoxic, or other critically ill patients requiring supplemental oxygen.

Anesthetic protocol A list of the anesthetic agents and adjuncts prescribed for a particular patient including doses, routes, and order of administration.

Anesthetic recovery The period between the time the anesthetic is discontinued and the time the animal is able to stand and walk without assistance.

Anesthetic safety checklist A document designed to improve outcomes and decrease anesthetic complications by ensuring that critical elements of preparation, completion of a complex task, and communication are not overlooked.

Anesthetic vaporizer A component of the anesthetic machine system that vaporizes liquid inhalant anesthetic and mixes it with the carrier gases. Vaporizers are classified as precision or nonprecision and vaporizer-out-of-circuit (VOC) or vaporizer-in-circuit (VIC).

Anisocoria The presence of pupils of unequal sizes.

Antagonist A drug that binds to but does not stimulate receptors.

Anticholinergic An adjunct that lessens parasympathetic effects by blocking muscarinic receptors of the parasympathetic nervous system. Also known as a *parasympatholytic.*

Anxiolysis Drug-induced reduction of anxiety. Synonymous with light tranquilization.

APL occlusion valve A valve, often placed between the APL valve and scavenging hose or built into the APL valve that, when pressed, temporarily prevents air escaping from the APL valve. Used to increase the ease with which a patient is manually ventilated.

Apnea A temporary absence of spontaneous breathing.

Apneustic respiration A breathing pattern, most often seen during dissociative anesthesia, in which there is a pause for several seconds at the end of the inspiratory phase, followed by a short, quick expiratory phase.

Asphyxiation The act of cutting off the supply of oxygen; suffocation.

Assisted ventilation A type of ventilation in which the anesthetist ensures that an adequate volume of air is delivered to the patient, although the patient initiates each inspiration.

Ataxia Inability to coordinate movement.

Atelectasis Collapse of a portion, or all, of one or both lungs.

Attending veterinarian The veterinarian responsible for the management and welfare of a particular patient.

Auscultation The act of listening to sounds made by internal organs with a stethoscope, especially the heart and lungs.

Ayre's T-piece A nonrebreathing circuit with a fresh gas inlet entering at the patient end of the breathing tube at a 90-degree angle (like the base of the letter T) and without a reservoir bag at the opposite end of the breathing tube; Mapleson E circuit.

Bagging Inflating the patient's lungs by squeezing the reservoir bag. Manual, positive-pressure ventilation.

Bain block *See Universal control arm.*

Bain coaxial circuit (Bain circuit) A nonrebreathing circuit with a "tube within a tube" configuration that discharges fresh gas at the patient end of the breathing tube. Both the overflow valve and the reservoir bag are located away from the patient at the opposite end of the breathing tube; modified Mapleson D circuit.

Balanced anesthesia Administration of multiple drugs concurrently in smaller quantities than would be required if each were given alone to produce sedation, tranquilization, muscle relaxation, analgesia, or a variety of other effects needed for a particular patient.

Barotrauma   Damage to the lungs, such as ruptured alveoli, due to excess pressure in the airways. Often a result of misuse of equipment, such as inadvertently leaving the APL valve closed.

Basic life support   The first phase of cardiopulmonary resuscitation (CPR). This phase consists of recognition that the patient is in cardiopulmonary arrest, application of heart compressions, and manual ventilation. In the anesthetized patient, all anesthetic drug administration should cease during this phase of CPR.

Behavioral disinhibition   Expression of previously inhibited behavior (such as aggression) which may result from administration of select anesthetic agents and adjuncts.

Blood gas analysis   Measurement of the pH, bicarbonate level, and partial pressures of oxygen and carbon dioxide in the blood (most often arterial blood obtained via an intraarterial catheter).

Blood pressure (BP)   The force exerted by flowing blood on vessel walls.

Body condition score   A numeric assessment of the patient's body weight compared with the ideal body weight.

Bolus   A pharmaceutical in the form of a large solid tablet or mass for oral administration; a relatively large volume of a liquid pharmaceutical for intravenous administration all at once; or a large mass of food ready to be swallowed.

Borborygmus   Intestinal noises audible with or without a stethoscope, caused by gas moving through the intestinal tract.

Brachycephalic obstructive airway syndrome (BOAS)   A constellation of abnormalities involving the skull and upper airway that impede air exchange and that result in stertor and difficulty breathing. Seen in brachycephalic (short-nosed) animals.

Breathing circuit   The anesthetic machine system that conveys the carrier gases and inhalant anesthetic to the patient and removes exhaled carbon dioxide. Breathing circuits are classified as rebreathing circuits or nonrebreathing circuits.

Breathing tubes   Corrugated tubes that complete a rebreathing circuit by carrying the anesthetic gases to and from the patient. Each tube is connected to a unidirectional valve at one end and to the Y-piece at the other end.

Cachexia   Weight loss, loss of muscle mass, and general debilitation that may accompany chronic diseases.

Calculated oxygen content   The total volume of oxygen in the blood including both dissolved and bound forms (expressed in milliliters per deciliter). Cao_2 = Calculated oxygen content in arterial blood. Arterial oxygen content is calculated using the following formula: $Cao_2 = (Hb \times 1.39 \times Sao_2/100) + (Pao_2 \times 0.003)$, where Hb = hemoglobin in grams per deciliter, Sao_2 = oxygen saturation, and Pao_2 = partial pressure of oxygen.

Capnogram   The graphic representation of CO_2 levels generated by a capnograph.

Capnograph   Also known as an *end-tidal CO_2 monitor*. A monitoring device that measures the amount of CO_2 in the air that is breathed in and out by the patient by sampling air passing between the endotracheal tube connector and the breathing circuit.

Carbon dioxide absorber canister   The part of a rebreathing circuit that holds the carbon dioxide absorbent granules. These granules, primarily made of calcium hydroxide, remove expired CO_2.

Cardiac arrhythmia   Any pattern of cardiac electrical activity that differs from that of the healthy awake animal.

Cardiac output (CO)   Total blood flow from the heart per unit time.

Cardiac pump theory   In CPR when providing cardiac compressions, a theory which states that blood flow to the tissues is caused by direct compression of the ventricles between the left and right ribs (when patient is in lateral recumbency) or sternum and spine (when the patient is in dorsal recumbency).

Catabolic state   A metabolic state in which the rate of catabolism (the breakdown of body tissues and substances into simple molecules) exceeds the rate of anabolism (the synthesis of body tissues and substances from simple molecules).

Cataleptoid state   A state produced by dissociative agents in which a patient does not respond to external stimuli and has a variable degree of muscle rigidity.

Categorical numeric rating scale   A tool used to assess pain. Has a series of numeric rating scales with descriptions to rate each of several categories of behavior and/or physiologic changes separately, such as appearance, interaction, posture, and response to palpation of the wound. The points for each of the categories are totaled.

Cauda equina   A group of nerves located at the caudal termination of the spinal cord in the spinal canal, so called because they visually resemble a horse's tail.

Central nervous system hypersensitivity   A state, caused by constant nociceptive input from the periphery, in which neurons in the spinal cord become hyperexcitable and sensitive to low-intensity stimuli that would not normally elicit a pain response. Also referred to as secondary hyperalgesia or *windup*.

Central nervous system vital centers   Areas of the brain that control cardiovascular function, respiratory function, and thermoregulation.

Central venous pressure (CVP)   Blood pressure in a large central vein, usually the caudal vena cava. Used to assess blood return to the heart and heart function.

Circulation   Movement of blood through the body for the purpose of supplying all cells with oxygen.

Chronic pain   Pain that lasts weeks, months, or years and persists after the tissues have healed or when they will not heal (such as in cancer patients).

Colic   Severe abdominal pain of sudden onset caused by a variety of conditions including obstruction, twisting, or spasm of the intestinal tract.

Colloids   Large–molecular-weight plasma proteins that provide oncotic pressure.

Comatose   In a sleeplike state; unresponsive to all stimuli including pain.

Common gas outlet   The point where the oxygen, inhalant anesthetic, and other anesthetic gases exit the anesthetic machine on the way to the breathing circuit.

Comprehensive Oral Health Assessment and Treatment (COHAT)   A full assessment of oral health, including teeth, gums, throat, and tongue; followed by formulation of a treatment plan, which usually includes a complete dental cleaning, consisting of scaling above and below the gum line and polishing.

Compressed gas cylinder   A container that holds a large volume of highly pressurized gas. Oxygen, medical air, nitrous oxide, and carbon dioxide are examples of gases stored in compressed gas cylinders.

Compressed gas supply   The anesthetic machine system that supplies carrier gases (oxygen and in some cases medical air or nitrous oxide).

Consent form   A form signed by the client confirming that they have been told about and understand the nature of the procedure to be performed, including the risks involved. Commonly includes a statement releasing the attending veterinarian, the hospital, and other healthcare providers from responsibility for uncontrollable outcomes.

Constant rate infusion (CRI)   Slow, continuous administration of a drug at a rate sufficient to achieve the desired effect.

Controlled ventilation   A type of ventilation in which the anesthetist controls the respiratory rate, the tidal volume, and the peak inspiratory pressure. In this type of ventilation, the patient does not make spontaneous respiratory efforts.

Core rewarming   Use of various devices and practices to manage hypothermia by either warming a patient internally or preventing excessive heat loss from the respiratory tract.

Cortisol   A natural steroid hormone, secreted by the adrenal cortex, which plays a role in protein, carbohydrate, and fat metabolism.

Crystalloids   Fluids that contain water and small–molecular-weight solutes (such as NaCl) and that pass freely through vascular endothelium.

Cyanosis   Blue discoloration of the mucous membranes.

Dead space   Equipment, tubes, trachea, bronchi, and other spaces through which inhaled and exhaled gases travel but in which no gas exchange occurs. In these areas, airflow is bidirectional (it travels toward the alveoli during inspiration and away from the alveoli during expiration). Consists of the sum total of anatomic dead space, alveolar dead space, and mechanical dead space.

Debilitated   Lacking strength; weak.

Demand valve   A valve attached to the endotracheal tube during anesthetic recovery that is used to deliver oxygen at a high flow rate; used most commonly for equine patients.

Dependent   The lowermost part (in reference to an anatomical structure or region such as the lungs); the part nearest the table or floor.

Desiccated   Dried or dehydrated.

Diastolic blood pressure   Arterial blood pressure when the heart is in its resting phase between contractions. (Compare with *Systolic blood pressure*.)

Distress   An extreme form of stress that leads to anxiety and suffering.

Doppler blood flow detector   A monitoring device that uses ultrasound frequency to convert the motion of red blood cells in small arteries into an audible "whooshing" sound. Used to monitor pulse rate and, if used in conjunction with a sphygmomanometer, systolic blood pressure.

Drip rate   A measurement of the rate at which fluids are administered (in drops per unit time; e.g., gtt/min or gtt/s). Used to set the roller clamp on a fluid administration set.

Dysphoria   Anxiety, uneasiness, and restlessness most often produced by opioids; the opposite of euphoria.

Dyspnea   Difficult or labored breathing.

Ecchymoses   Large bruises. Discolorations of the skin or mucous membranes caused by leakage of blood into the tissues.

Emergence delirium   Disorientation that occurs during anesthetic recovery as consciousness returns. May be characterized by vocalization, aggression, thrashing, and locomotor activity.

Enantiomer   One of a pair of molecules that are mirror images of one another. The dextrorotatory enantiomer is a molecule that rotates the plane of polarized light to the right, and a levorotatory molecule rotates it to the left.

Endotracheal tube (ET tube)   A flexible tube placed inside the trachea of an anesthetized patient and used to transfer anesthetic gases directly from the breathing circuit into the patient's trachea, bypassing the oral and nasal cavities, pharynx, and larynx.

End-tidal CO_2 monitor   *See Capnograph.*

Epidural anesthesia   Regional anesthesia produced by injection of a local anesthetic or analgesic into the epidural space surrounding the spinal cord.

Epistaxis   Nosebleed.

Eructate   Eject gas from the stomach; burp. Used most commonly in reference to ruminants.

Esophageal stethoscope   A monitoring device used to detect and amplify heart sounds via a catheter placed in the esophagus.

Eutectic mixture   A mixture of two substances with a melting point that is lower than the individual melting points. In the case of lidocaine and prilocaine, which are both solids at room temperature, mixture of the two drugs results in an oil that has a melting point of 16°C.

External active rewarming   Use of external heat-producing devices (such as circulating warm water blankets or warm air blankets) to raise body temperature of a hypothermic patient.

External passive warming   Use of various methods (such as the use of towels, blankets, or bubble wrap) to conserve body heat of anesthetized patients.

Extralabel drug use   The use of an approved drug in a manner that is not in accordance with the approved label directions.

Fasciculation   Involuntary muscle twitching.

Field anesthesia   General anesthesia performed away from the veterinary hospital at a farm or stable; used most commonly for short procedures (20 to 45 minutes) in large animal patients.

Flaccid   Lacking any muscle tone.

Flowmeter   A glass cylinder of graduated diameter that indicates carrier gas flow expressed in liters of gas per minute (L/min). Reduces the pressure of the gas in the intermediate-pressure line from about 50 psi (about 345 kPa) to 15 psi (about 100 kPa).

Fluanisone   A sedative that is combined with the opioid fentanyl in the product Hypnorm. Used to provide chemical restraint and analgesia for minor procedures in laboratory animals.

Fresh gas inlet   The point at which the carrier and anesthetic gases enter the breathing circuit.

Full rebreathing system   A rebreathing system in which the flow of oxygen is very low, providing only the volume necessary to meet the patient's metabolic needs. When using this system, the APL valve may be open, partially open, or nearly or completely closed. Also known as a complete, closed, or total rebreathing system.

Functional residual volume   The amount of air left in the lungs after expiration.

Gas exchange   The diffusion of oxygen from the alveoli to the blood and carbon dioxide from the blood to the alveoli during ventilation.

Gastric dilatation-volvulus   A dangerous gastrointestinal condition, occurring primarily in deep-chested, large-breed dogs in which the stomach swells with air and twists on its long axis, leading to shock, loss of blood supply, and respiratory compromise.

General anesthesia   A reversible state of unconsciousness, immobility, muscle relaxation, and loss of sensation throughout the entire body produced by administration of one or more anesthetic agents.

High pressure alarm   A device that measures pressure in the breathing circuit and thus the patient airways. Warns the anesthetist of pressure above a safe maximum.

Homeostasis   A constant state within the body created and maintained by normal physiologic processes.

Hypercarbia   Elevated carbon dioxide levels in the blood.

Hypnosis   A sleeplike state from which the patient can be aroused with sufficient stimulation.

Hypostatic congestion   Pooling of blood in the dependent lung and tissues (those nearest the floor or table).

Hypotension   Low blood pressure; the opposite of hypertension.

Hypothermia   Low body temperature; the opposite of hyperthermia.

Hypoventilation   Slow and/or shallow ventilation, resulting in decreased respiratory minute volume; the opposite of hyperventilation.

Hypoxemia   Low blood oxygen level.

Hypoxia   Low tissue oxygen level.

Icterus   Yellow discoloration of the skin and mucous membranes.

Idiopathic pain   Pain of unknown or unidentifiable cause.

Ileus   Intestinal obstruction caused by inhibition of bowel motility; also referred to as *gastrointestinal stasis*.

Infiltration   Injection of local anesthetic into tissues, often in proximity to a nerve.

Inflammatory mediators   Chemical substances released from damaged cells or inflammatory cells that cause a response, such as increasing the sensitivity of peripheral pain receptors.

Inflammatory pain   Pain that occurs at the site of tissue injury due to the release of chemical mediators such as prostaglandin and histamine.

Infusion rate   The rate at which fluids should be administered expressed in milliliters per unit time, most often mL/h.

Inotropy   Force of heart muscle contraction.

Insufflation   Provision of oxygen by placement of an oxygen supply tube inside an endotracheal tube, nasopharyngeal tube, or nostril.

Intact   Possessing gonads; not spayed or castrated.

Intermittent mandatory ventilation   Positive pressure ventilation throughout the entire anesthetic period as the sole source of the patient's ventilatory needs.

Intraosseous   In the bone marrow cavity. A route of administration sometimes used as an alternative to intravenous injection. Especially useful for very small patients (e.g., small exotic mammals and neonatal patients) in which venipuncture is difficult.

Intraperitoneal   In the intraperitoneal space of the abdominal cavity. A route of administration used primarily in small laboratory mammals for some drugs and fluids.

Intraperitoneal splash block (Also known as intraperitoneal lavage)   A local anesthetic block performed by squirting the local anesthetic into the abdominal cavity through an open incision.

Jackson-Rees circuit   A nonrebreathing circuit with a fresh gas inlet at the patient end of the breathing tube and a reservoir bag at the opposite end. The fresh gas inlet enters the breathing tube at a 45- to 90-degree angle; Mapleson F circuit.

Lack circuit   A nonrebreathing circuit with the fresh gas inlet, the overflow valve, and the reservoir bag located away from the patient at the opposite end of the breathing tube. Modified Mapleson A circuit.

Laryngeal mask airway   *See Supraglottic airway device.*

Laryngoscope   A device consisting of a handle, a blade, and a light source; used to increase visibility of the larynx during placement of an endotracheal tube.

Laryngospasm   A reflexive closure of the glottis in response to contact with any object or substance.

Lethargic   Depressed but able to be aroused with minimal difficulty.

Level of consciousness The patient's responsiveness to stimuli. How easily the patient can be aroused. Often used to assess brain function.

Line block Injection of a continuous line of local anesthetic in the subcutaneous or subcuticular tissues immediately proximal to the target area.

Line pressure gauge A gauge that indicates the pressure in the intermediate-pressure gas lines of an anesthetic machine between the pressure-reducing valve and the flow meters.

Local anesthesia A loss of sensation in a small area of the body produced by administration of a local anesthetic agent in proximity to the area of interest.

Locomotor Relating to movement from place to place.

Macrodrip A fluid administration set that delivers fluids at a rate of 10 or 15 drops per milliliter. Generally used for infusion rates equal to or more than 100 mL/h.

Macroemulsion A type of emulsion (a fine dispersion of minute droplets of one liquid in another with which it does not mix) in which the particles of one liquid are large enough to scatter light, causing the liquid to look cloudy.

Magill circuit A nonrebreathing circuit with an overflow valve at the patient end of the breathing tube. Both the fresh gas inlet and the reservoir bag are located away from the patient at the opposite end of the breathing tube; Mapleson A circuit.

Maladaptive pain Pain that is due to malfunction of or damage to the nervous system and that serves no useful function but causes suffering and is often difficult to treat.

Manual resuscitator bag A self-inflating reservoir bag used to provide manual ventilation when an anesthetic machine is not available (e.g., Ambu bag).

Manual ventilation Forced delivery of oxygen and anesthetic gases by squeezing of the reservoir bag of the anesthetic machine; may be used to provide periodic or intermittent mandatory ventilation.

Mapleson classification system A system developed by W.W. Mapleson that is used to classify nonrebreathing circuits based on the position of the fresh gas inlet, the reservoir bag, and the pressure-limiting valve.

Mean arterial pressure (MAP) The average arterial blood pressure. It may be calculated using the following equation: MAP = diastolic pressure + $\frac{1}{3}$ (systolic pressure - diastolic pressure).

Mechanical dead space Dead space in equipment such as the Y-piece, ETT connector, portion of the ETT extending beyond the incisors, respiratory monitor adaptors, moisture and heat exchangers, right angle adaptors, and the patient connector of nonrebreathing circuits.

Mechanical ventilation Forced delivery of oxygen and anesthetic gases by use of a mechanical ventilator. Usually used to provide intermittent mandatory ventilation.

Microdrip A fluid administration set that delivers fluids at a rate of 60 drops per milliliter. Generally used for infusion rates less than 100 mL/h.

Microemulsion A type of emulsion (a fine dispersion of minute droplets of one liquid in another with which it does not mix) in which the particles of the dispersed liquid are so small that they do not scatter light, resulting in a liquid that appears clear.

Minimal rebreathing system A rebreathing system in which the flow of oxygen meets or exceeds the respiratory minute volume, resulting in a system that functions in a similar way to a nonrebreathing system. When using this system, the APL valve should be open.

Minimum patient database A compilation of pertinent information from the patient history, physical examination, and diagnostic tests. Used to diagnose and manage a case.

Miosis Constriction of the pupil of the eye; opposite of mydriasis.

Modulation The third step in nociception, in which sensory nerve impulses are amplified or suppressed by other neurons.

Monitor A process of tracking physiologic and reflex responses to anesthetics for the purpose of keeping a patient safe and ensuring appropriate anesthetic depth.

Morbidity The incidence of disease.

Moribund Near death.

Mortality The death rate.

Motor neuron A neuron that conveys impulses from the brain to muscle fibers and is responsible for initiating and controlling voluntary movements.

Multimodal therapy Treatment of pain with analgesics that target different receptors in two or more steps of the pain pathway.

Multiparameter monitor An anesthetic monitor capable of measuring and displaying multiple machine-generated parameters (such as HR; ECG tracing; SAP, DAP, and MAP; Spo_2; Fio_2; RR; $ETco_2$; and body temperature).

Mydriasis Dilatation of the pupil of the eye; opposite of miosis.

Myoclonus Spontaneous muscle twitching.

Myopathy Muscle disease. In the context of anesthesia, this term refers to muscle damage caused by excessive pressure on dependent muscle tissue or insufficient blood flow to muscle tissue during the intraoperative period in large animals, particularly horses. Manifests during recovery as muscle hardness, pain, and weakness. Also known by the lay term "tying up."

Narcosis A drug-induced sleep from which the patient is not easily aroused and that is most often associated with the administration of narcotics.

National Institute for Occupational Safety and Health (NIOSH) The US federal agency responsible for conducting research and making recommendations for the prevention of work-related injury and illness.

Nerve block Loss of sensation in a particular anatomic site, produced by injection of local anesthetic in proximity to a nerve.

Neuroleptanalgesia A state of profound sedation and analgesia induced by the simultaneous administration of an opioid and a tranquilizer.

Neuromuscular blocking agent An adjunct used to paralyze skeletal muscles, including the diaphragm, as a part of balanced anesthesia.

Neuropathic pain Pain resulting from injury of a nerve.

Neuropathy Disease or injury of a peripheral nerve.

Nociception Detection by the nervous system of the potential for or actual tissue injury.

Nonrebreathing system An anesthetic machine fitted with a nonrebreathing circuit. In this system, minimum or no exhaled gases are returned to the patient but are instead removed from the circuit by use of appropriately high flow rates of carrier gas and evacuated by a scavenger connected to an adjustable pressure-limiting valve or other exit port. Used most commonly for patients under 3 kg in body weight.

Norman elbow A nonrebreathing circuit with a fresh gas inlet at the patient end of the breathing tube and a reservoir bag at the opposite end. The fresh gas inlet enters the breathing tube at a 45- to 90-degree angle, travels inside the patient connector, and discharges fresh gas very near the endotracheal tube; Mapleson F circuit.

North American Veterinary Anesthesia Society (NAVAS) A nonprofit organization whose mission is to make evidence-based guidelines regarding the safe administration of anesthesia and analgesia available to all interested professionals and caregivers.

Noxious Painful or physically harmful.

Numeric rating scale A tool used to assess pain. The intensity of the pain is assigned to one of several levels that are identified by a number (e.g., no pain = 0; mild pain = 1; moderate pain = 2; severe pain = 3).

Nystagmus A rhythmic, involuntary oscillation of both eyes.

Obtunded Depressed and unable to be fully aroused.

Occupational Safety and Health Administration (OSHA) US federal agency responsible for ensuring a safe and healthful working environment for working people.

Oncotic pressure A form of osmotic pressure provided by large–molecular-weight colloids such as albumin. Sometimes referred to as colloid osmotic-pressure.

Opisthotonus A severe spasm in which the back arches and the feet and head flex dorsally. Has several causes, including drug reactions and brain lesions.

Oscillometer A monitoring device used to measure systolic, mean, and diastolic blood pressure by detecting and analyzing pulsations of blood in the arteries of an extremity.

Osmolarity A measurement of the number of dissolved solute particles per unit water in body fluids; usually expressed as osmoles or milliosmoles per liter (mOsm/L) of water.

Osmotic pressure The pressure required to prevent water flow through a semipermeable membrane from a region of lower solute concentration to a region of higher solute concentration.

Oxygen analyzer A machine that measures the percent oxygen in inspired gases (fraction of inspired oxygen or Fio_2) by sampling gas from a spacer that can be placed between the tubing of the inspiratory limb and the Y-piece of a rebreathing system.

Oxygen flush valve A button or lever that rapidly delivers a large volume of pure oxygen (at a flow rate of 35 to 75 L/min) directly to the common gas outlet or breathing circuit of a rebreathing system, bypassing the anesthetic vaporizer and oxygen flow meters.

Oxygenation The physiologic process of supplying the lungs and blood with oxygen.

Pain An aversive sensory and emotional experience that elicits protective motor actions, results in learned avoidance, and may modify species-specific behavior.

Pain scale Any assessment tool used to rate the intensity of pain.

Paralysis Inability to move a particular muscle group or body part such as a limb because of loss of nerve function. May also involve a loss of sensation in the affected part.

Parasympatholytic *See Anticholinergic.*

Paresis Weakness of a body part caused by loss of nerve function; partial paralysis.

Paresthesia An abnormal sensation of tingling, pain, or irritation that may be apparent during recovery from local anesthesia.

Partial agonist A drug that binds to and partially stimulates tissue receptors.

Partial intravenous anesthesia (PIVA) Use of inhalant and injectable agents in combination to maintain anesthesia.

Partial pressure of oxygen(Po_2) A measurement of the unbound O_2 molecules dissolved in the plasma expressed in millimeters of mercury (mmHg). $Pao_2 = Po_2$ in arterial blood; $Pvo_2 = Po_2$ in venous blood.

Partial rebreathing system A rebreathing system in which the flow of oxygen exceeds that which is necessary to meet the patient's metabolic needs, and the APL valve is open or partially open. Also known as a semiclosed rebreathing system.

Passive dosimeter A device used to detect waste anesthetic gases such as nitrous oxide, isoflurane, and sevoflurane in the breathing zone of hospital personnel. After a defined exposure time (often 2 to 8 hours), the badge is recapped and returned for analysis. Results are given as a time-weighted average in parts per million.

Pathologic pain Pain that is amplified and persistent. This type of pain is due to malfunction of or damage to the nervous system and is maladaptive because it serves no useful function and causes suffering.

Percent oxygen saturation So_2; A measurement of the percentage of the total hemoglobin binding sites occupied by oxygen molecules. $Sao_2 = So_2$ in arterial blood; $Svo_2 = So_2$ in venous blood; $Spo_2 = So_2$ as measured by a pulse oximeter; $Sto_2 = So_2$ in the tissues.

Perception The final step of nociception in which sensory impulses are transmitted to the brain, where they are processed and recognized.

Perioperative analgesia Pain control before, during, and/or after surgery.

Peripheral hypersensitivity Increased sensitivity to a painful stimulus that occurs when the threshold of the peripheral pain receptors is lowered as a result of injury to peripheral tissues; also known as primary hyperalgesia.

Petechiae Small or pinpoint purple discolorations of the skin or mucous membrane resulting from hemorrhage; smaller than purpura.

Pharmacodynamics The effect that a drug has on the body; drug action.

Pharmacokinetics The effect that the body has on a drug, including movement of a drug within the body.

Physical status classification A graded assessment of a patient's physical condition. Used to plan patient management prior to administering anesthetics and to gauge patient risk.

Physiologic anemia A relative decrease in red blood cell (RBC) mass caused by an increase in plasma volume without a corresponding increase in the number of RBCs; seen in pregnant patients.

Physiologic dead space Spaces within the body through which inhaled and exhaled gases travel but in which no gas exchange occurs. In these areas, airflow is bidirectional (it travels toward the alveoli during inspiration and away from the alveoli during expiration). The sum total of anatomic dead space and alveolar dead space.

Physiologic pain The protective sensation of pain that normally occurs when there is a possibility of or actual tissue injury. Physiologic pain is adaptive because it promotes survival by preventing injury and by promoting healing of the injured body part.

Pleural effusion Abnormal accumulation of fluid in the space between the lungs and the chest wall (pleural space).

Pneumomediastinum The presence of air in the space between the lungs that contains the heart, great vessels, and esophagus.

Pneumothorax The presence of air in the space between the lungs and the chest wall (pleural space) associated with collapse of one or both lungs.

Porcine stress syndrome Also known as *malignant hyperthermia.* A hereditary, metabolic condition of swine caused by a mutation in one of the genes that controls calcium metabolism in muscle fibers. Occurs in affected swine in response to some anesthetic agents, including inhalant agents. Signs include muscle rigidity, rapid rise in temperature, hypercapnia, hyperkalemia, and death.

Positive inotrope A drug that increases inotropy (the force of heart muscle contractions).

Positive pressure ventilation (PPV) Any procedure by which the anesthetist assists or controls the delivery of oxygen and anesthetic gas to the patient's lungs; includes both manual and mechanical ventilation.

Postarrest care In cardiopulmonary resuscitation, steps taken following return of spontaneous circulation to minimize permanent adverse effects of cardiopulmonary arrest and maximize the likelihood of recovery and discharge from the hospital.

Preanesthetic medication An anesthetic agent or adjunct administered during the preanesthetic period to provide one or more of a variety of desired effects, including analgesia, sedation, and muscle relaxation.

Preemptive analgesia Provision of analgesia before tissue injury, including surgery.

Pressure manometer A gauge that indicates the pressure of the gases within the breathing circuit and by extension the pressure in the animal's airways and lungs. Expressed in centimeters of water (cm H_2O), millimeters of mercury (mmHg), or kilopascals (kPa).

Pressure-reducing valve A valve that reduces the pressure of a compressed gas to a constant safe operating pressure of 40 to 58 psi (276 to 400 kPa) regardless of pressure changes within the tank.

Pressure transducer An instrument designed to measure blood pressure. Converts the pressure exerted on the walls of a blood vessel into an electrical signal that is usually displayed as a waveform.

Primary hyperalgesia *See Peripheral hypersensitivity.*

Pulmonary contusion Bruising of lung tissue caused by blunt trauma.

Pulmonary thromboembolism The presence of a blood clot in the lungs.

Pulse oximeter A monitoring device used to estimate (1) the percent oxygen saturation of hemoglobin (Spo_2) by measuring differences in light absorption, and (2) the pulse rate by detecting blood pulsations in the small arterioles.

Purpura Purple discolorations of the skin or mucous membrane caused by hemorrhage; larger than petechiae.

Rebreathing system (circle system) An anesthetic machine fitted with a rebreathing circuit. In this system, exhaled gases minus carbon dioxide are recirculated and rebreathed by the patient, along with variable amounts of fresh oxygen and inhalant anesthetic. Appropriate for most patients 3 kg in body weight or over.

Recommended exposure limit (REL) The maximum concentration of any volatile gas anesthetic (in parts per million) to which employees should be exposed as recommended by the National Institute for Occupational Safety and Health (NIOSH) or other agency.

RECOVER Initiative Reassessment Campaign on Veterinary Resuscitation. A comprehensive ongoing study designed to develop a draft set of evidence-based clinical guidelines for veterinary CPR based on consensus of specialists and scientific research.

Regional anesthesia A loss of sensation in a limited area of the body produced by administration of a local anesthetic or other agent in proximity to sensory nerves.

Regurgitation Flow of stomach contents into the esophagus and mouth unaccompanied by retching; as distinguished from vomiting, which is a forceful expulsion of stomach contents into the esophagus and mouth preceded by retching.

Regurgitus Regurgitated stomach or ruminal contents consisting of saliva and ingesta.

Reproductive status Whether or not the patient has been spayed or castrated. If intact, whether or not the patient is being used for breeding. In the case of female patients, whether pregnant or not.

Reservoir bag Also called a *breathing bag*. A rubber or plastic bag that serves as a flexible storage reservoir for expired and inspired gases. It also allows the anesthetist to observe respirations, confirm proper endotracheal tube placement, and manually ventilate for the patient.

Respiration The processes by which oxygen is supplied to and used by the tissues and carbon dioxide is eliminated from the tissues.

Respiratory minute volume (RMV) The amount of air that moves into and out of the lungs in 1 minute; the tidal volume multiplied by the respiratory rate.

Respirometer A monitoring device used to measure the tidal volume and respiratory minute volume.

Return of spontaneous circulation (ROSC) The return of effective tissue perfusion with oxygenated blood after cardiopulmonary arrest and subsequent successful cardiopulmonary resuscitation.

Reversal agent A drug used to lessen or abolish the effects of anesthetic agents or adjuncts, and which is therefore used to wake the patient after sedation or anesthesia.

Ring block A type of line block that completely encircles an anatomic part, such as a digit or teat.

Safety pressure relief valve A device designed to passively limit the maximum pressure in the breathing circuit and by extension, the patient's lungs with no action required on the part of the anesthetist.

Scavenging system The anesthetic machine system that disposes of excess and waste anesthetic gases outside of the building, so that inhalation by occupationally exposed individuals is minimized.

Scoliosis Lateral curvature of the spine; seen in cattle following paravertebral block with local anesthetic.

Secondary hyperalgesia *See Central nervous system hypersensitivity.*

Sedation A drug-induced central nervous system depression and drowsiness.

Sensory neuron A neuron that conveys sensations (i.e., pain, heat, cold, and pressure) from the skin, muscles, and other peripheral tissues to the brain.

Sequestration Loss of blood or plasma into tissues or spaces within the body, resulting in a decreased circulating blood volume (e.g., hemorrhage into the abdominal cavity).

Signalment The species, breed, age, sex, and reproductive status of a patient.

Simple descriptive scale A tool used to assess pain by rating its severity (e.g., absent, mild, moderate, or severe).

Sloughing Separation and loss of dead tissue from surrounding live tissue in a wound. Often used in reference to tissue death and loss secondary to drug-induced damage (e.g., due to perivascular injection of a vesicant).

Solute An atom or molecule dissolved in body water.

Somatic analgesia Absence of pain of the skin, muscle, bone, and connective tissue.

Somatic pain Pain originating from the musculoskeletal or integumentary system; subclassified as superficial (i.e., skin) and deep (i.e., joints, muscles, bones).

Sphygmomanometer A monitoring device consisting of a pressure gauge and cuff used to measure arterial blood pressure in conjunction with a Doppler blood flow detector.

Splash block Local anesthesia produced by direct application of local anesthetic to a wound or open surgical site. Most often applied as a spray or with a soaked gauze sponge.

Standing chemical restraint A type of chemical restraint used in horses in which the patient is heavily sedated but remains standing throughout the procedure.

Status epilepticus Continuous seizures or a series of seizures in rapid succession.

Stertor A heavy snoring sound during inspiration; often caused by partial upper airway obstruction. Seen in patients with laryngospasm, laryngeal edema, and in brachycephalic dogs.

Stridor Noisy breathing caused by turbulent air flow in the upper airways.

Stuporous In a sleeplike state; can be aroused only with a painful stimulus.

Supraglottic airway device (a.k.a. laryngeal mask airway) A device used to maintain an open airway in an anesthetized patient that encompasses the opening of the glottis, but unlike an endotracheal tube, does not invade the tracheal lumen.

Surgical anesthesia A specific stage of general anesthesia in which there is a sufficient degree of analgesia and muscle relaxation to allow surgery to be performed without patient pain or movement.

Sympathetic blockade Loss of function of sympathetic nerves supplying the heart and blood vessels resulting from diffusion of local anesthetic into the thoracic spinal cord. Signs include bradycardia, decreased cardiac output, and hypotension. Blockade of the caudal sympathetic nerves results in less severe hypotension and tachycardia.

Syncope Fainting episodes caused by brain hypoxia.

Synergistic (a.k.a. supra-additive) An interaction between two drugs in such a way that the total effect is greater than the sum of the individual effects.

Systolic blood pressure Arterial blood pressure during contraction of the ventricles. (Compare with *Diastolic blood pressure.*)

Tachyarrhythmia Any arrhythmia in which the heart rate is abnormally increased.

Tachycardia Rapid heart rate; the opposite of bradycardia.

Tachypnea Rapid respiratory rate.

Tank pressure gauge A device attached to the yoke of an anesthetic machine or the pressure regulator of an H tank. Indicates the pressure of gas remaining in a compressed gas cylinder measured in pounds per square inch (psi) or kilopascals (kPa).

Therapeutic index (TI) A ratio of the toxic to therapeutic dose of a drug, used to measure relative safety. A drug with a wide therapeutic index (much more of the drug is required to intoxicate a patient than is required to treat it) is relatively safer than a drug with a narrow therapeutic index (one for which the toxic and therapeutic doses are similar).

Thoracic pump theory In CPR, when providing cardiac compressions, a theory which states that blood flow to the tissues is caused indirectly by compression of the chest wall with subsequent compression of the aorta resulting from increased intrathoracic pressure.

Thoracocentesis Surgical puncture of the pleural space with a needle or tube for the purpose of removing fluid or air.

Thrombocytopenia Low platelet count.

Tidal volume (V_T) The volume of a normal breath; approximately 10 to 15 mL/kg body weight in a patient that is awake and may be decreased by as much as one-third in the anesthetized patient.

Tilt table A specialized table used to restrain cattle, and occasionally horses, undergoing anesthetic procedures by securing the patient to the table with ropes and straps and tilting the table to the desired angle.

Titration Administration of an anesthetic agent in small increments until the desired depth of anesthesia is reached, as opposed to administration of the entire calculated dose.

TKX A combination of Telazol, ketamine, and xylazine, widely used to produce heavy sedation and total injectable anesthesia in pigs.

Topical anesthesia A loss of sensation of a localized area produced by administration of a local anesthetic directly to a body surface or to a surgical or traumatic wound.

Total injectable anesthesia Induction and maintenance of anesthesia by intramuscular injection of an anesthetic agent or combination of agents with no concurrent use of inhalant agents; a technique commonly employed in swine and for neutering in cats.

Total intravenous anesthesia Induction and maintenance of anesthesia by intravenous injection of short-acting anesthetics with no concurrent use of inhalant agents. Accomplished using repeat bolus injections or a constant rate infusion.

Tranquilization A drug-induced state of calm in which the patient is reluctant to move and is aware of but unconcerned about its surroundings.

Transdermal patch A reservoir of analgesic or other drug enclosed in plastic that is applied to clipped skin. The drug is released slowly through the back of the patch and absorbed transcutaneously. Especially useful for drugs with a short half-life.

Transduction   The first step in nociception, in which noxious thermal, chemical, or mechanical stimuli are transformed into electrical signals called *action potentials*.

Transmission   The second step in nociception, in which sensory impulses are conducted to the spinal cord.

Ultrapotent opioids   Injectable drugs used for the restraint and capture of wildlife, particularly large ungulates. Exposure of personnel to even minute quantities of these drugs carries a very high risk of severe or even life-threatening toxicity, requiring that strict safety procedures are followed.

Unidirectional valve   The inspiratory valve or expiratory valve of a rebreathing circuit; controls the direction of gas flow through a rebreathing circuit as the patient breathes.

Universal control arm (a.k.a. Bain block)   A device that, when attached to a Bain coaxial circuit, provides a conventional APL valve and manometer, increasing the ease and accuracy with which manual ventilation can be provided.

Validate   A process of evaluating the effectiveness and reliability of something such as a scale used to assess pain in animals. A valid pain scale is one that has been shown to accurately measure the quality and intensity of pain.

Vaporizer-in-circuit (VIC)   A vaporizer that is located in the breathing circuit. Nonprecision vaporizers are often positioned this way.

Vaporizer-out-of-circuit (VOC)   A vaporizer in which carrier gas from the flow meters flows into the vaporizer before entering the breathing circuit. Precision vaporizers are positioned this way.

Vasodilation (also *vasodilatation*)   Dilation of the blood vessels; the opposite of vasoconstriction.

Ventilation   The movement of gases into and out of the alveoli.

Ventilation-perfusion mismatch   A lack of equality in the volume of oxygen that reaches the alveoli per minute and the volume of blood that perfuses the alveoli per minute. Results in alveoli that are oxygenated but are not perfused and/or alveoli that are perfused but are atelectatic and not oxygenated.

Vesicants   Drugs that damage tissues if injected perivascularly.

Visceral analgesia   Absence of pain in the internal organs.

Visceral pain   Pain originating from the internal organs.

Visual analog scale   A tool used to assess pain that consists of a "ruler," the left end of which equates to no pain, and the right end to the worst pain imaginable for the specific disease or surgical procedure. The assessor places a mark (usually an X) on the ruler corresponding to the level of pain that the assessor feels the animal is experiencing.

Waste anesthetic gas (WAG)   Any inhalation anesthetic (including isoflurane, other halogenated compounds, and nitrous oxide) that is breathed out by the patient or that escapes from the anesthetic machine.

Wasting   A decrease in body mass, energy, or vigor, often caused by disease.

Windup   *See Central nervous system hypersensitivity.*

Note: Page numbers followed by "b", "f" and "t" indicate boxes, figures, and tables respectively.